SPORTS
NUTRITION

Sports Nutrition: A Handbook for Professionals, Sixth Edition

ISBN 978-0-88091-975-3 (print)

ISBN 978-0-88091-976-0 (eBook)

Catalog Number 411417, 411417e

Unless otherwise noted, the nutrient and energy data in this book were derived from the US Department of Agriculture, Agricultural Research Service, 2016. USDA Food Composition Databases, USDA National Nutrient Database for Standard Reference, Release 28, ndb.nal.usda.gov/ndb

For more information on the Academy of Nutrition and Dietetics, visit www. eatright.org

Library of Congress Cataloging-in-Publication Data

Names: Karpinski, Christine, editor. | Rosenbloom, Christine, 1951- editor. | Academy of Nutrition and Dietetics.
Title: Sports Nutrition : A Handbook for Professionals / [edited by] Christine Karpinski, Christine A. Rosenbloom.
Other titles: Sports Nutrition (1986)
Description: Sixth edition. | Chicago : Academy of Nutrition and Dietetics, [2017] | Description based on print version record and CIP data provided by publisher; resource not viewed.
Identifiers: LCCN 2017017459 (print) | LCCN 2017018805 (ebook) | ISBN 9780880919760 (eBook) | ISBN 9780880919753 (print)
Subjects: | MESH: Nutritional Physiological Phenomena | Exercise--physiology | Sports
Classification: LCC TX361.A8 (ebook) | LCC TX361.A8 (print) | NLM QU 145 | DDC 613.2024/796--dc23
LC record available at https://lccn.loc.gov/2017017459

6TH EDITION

SPORTS NUTRITION

A Handbook for Professionals

**SPORTS, CARDIOVASCULAR, AND WELLNESS
NUTRITION DIETETICS PRACTICE GROUP**

Editor-in-Chief
Christine Karpinski, PhD, RDN, CSSD, LDN

Assistant Editor
Christine A. Rosenbloom, PhD, RDN, CSSD, FAND

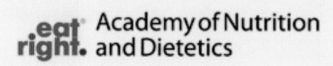
Academy of Nutrition and Dietetics

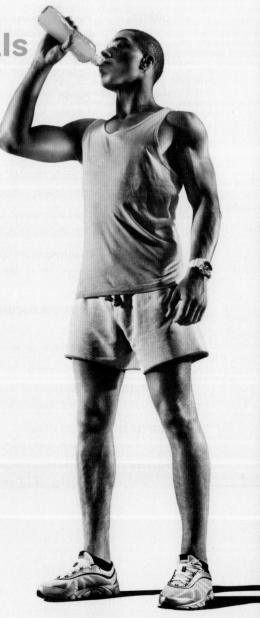

CONTENTS

SECTION I: SPORTS NUTRITION BASICS

SECTION 2: SPORTS NUTRITION ASSESSMENT AND ENERGY BALANCE

CONTRIBUTORS

Elizabeth Abbey, PhD, RDN
Assistant Professor, Health Sciences Department
Whitworth University
Spokane, WA

Roberta Anding, MS, RD, LD, CDE, CSSD, FAND
Director of Sports Nutrition
Texas Children's Hospital
Sports Dietitian, Houston Astros
Sports Dietitian, Rice University
Houston, TX

Katherine A. Beals, PhD, RDN, CSSD, FACSM
Associate Professor, University of Utah
Salt Lake City, UT

Nicholas A. Burd, PhD
Department of Kinesiology and Community Health
Division of Nutritional Sciences
University of Illinois at Urbana-Champaign
Urbana, IL

Louise M. Burke, OAM, PhD, APD, FACSM
Head of Sports Nutrition
Australian Institute of Sport
Canberra, Australia
And Chair of Sports Nutrition, Mary McKillop
Institute for Health Research
Australian Catholic University
Melbourne, Australia

Ellen J. Coleman, MA, MPH, RD, CSSD
Sports Dietitian
Riverside, CA

Abigail Duffine Gilman, MS, RD, LDN
Doctoral Student and Program Manager
Drexel University
Philadelphia, PA

Marie Dunford, PhD, RD
Sports Nutrition Educator
Alameda, CA

Rebecca Foright, MS
University of Colorado, Anschutz Medical Campus
Denver, CO

Carrie M. Hamady, MS, RD, LD
Director, Undergraduate Didactic Program in
Nutrition and Dietetics
Department of Public and Allied Health
Bowling Green State University
Bowling Green, Ohio

Sally Hara, MS, RDN, CSSD, CDE
Proactive Nutrition
Kirkland, WA

Christine A. Karpinski, PhD, RD, CSSD, LDN
Associate Professor and Chair Department of
Nutrition
West Chester University
West Chester, PA

Jennifer Ketterly, MS, RDN, CSSD
Director of Sports Nutrition
University of Georgia
Athens, GA

Laura J. Kruskall, PhD, RDN, CSSD, LD, FACSM, FAND, ACSM EP-C
Associate Professor and Director of UNLV
Nutrition Sciences
University of Nevada, Las Vegas
Las Vegas, NV

D. Enette Larson-Meyer, PhD, RDN, CSSD, FACSM
Associate Professor and Director of Nutrition and
Exercise Laboratory
University of Wyoming
Laramie, WY

Michele A. Macedonio, MS, RDN, CSSD
Nutrition Consultant, Sports Dietitian
Nutrition Strategies
Loveland, OH

Caroline Mandel, MS, RD, CSSD
Director of Performance Nutrition
University of Michigan
Ann Arbor, MI

Christopher Melby, DrPH
Professor, Department of Food Science and
Human Nutrition
Nutrition and Metabolic Fitness Laboratory
Colorado State University
Fort Collins, CO

Amy L. Morgan, PhD, FACSM
Professor, Exercise Science
Bowling Green State University
Bowling Green, OH

Kimberly Mueller, MS, RD, CSSD
Road Runners Club of America Certified
Running Coach
Owner, Fuel Factor Custom Nutrition &
Training Plans
Wilmington, NC

Bob Murray, PhD, FACSM
Sports Science Insights, LLC
Crystal Lake, IL

Kris Osterberg, PhD, RDN, CSSD
Team Sports Manager
Gatorade Sports Marketing
Blacksburg, VA

Hunter L. Paris, MS
Associate Instructor, Department of Kinesiology
Indiana University
Bloomington, IN

Eve Pearson, MBA, RDN, CSSD
Sports Dietitian
Nutriworks, Inc.
Dallas, TX

Stuart M. Phillips, PhD, FACN, FACSM
Professor and Canada Research Chair,
Department of Kinesiology
McMaster University
Hamilton, ON, Canada

Karen Reznik Dolins, EdD, RD, CSSD, CDN
Sports Dietitian
Adjunct Associate Professor, Nutrition and
Exercise Physiology
Teachers College, Columbia University
New York, NY

Christine A. Rosenbloom, PhD, RDN, CSSD, FAND
Professor Emerita, Division of Nutrition
Georgia State University
Atlanta, GA

David M. Schnell, PhD
Department of Pharmacology
and Nutritional Sciences
University of Kentucky
Lexington, KY

Christina Scribner, MS, RDN, CSSD, CEDRD
Instructor, College of Health Solutions, Arizona
State University
Nutrition Consultant, Encompass Nutrition LLC,
Littleton, CO

Greg Shaw, BHSc
Senior Sport Dietitian, Sport Nutrition
Australian Institute of Sport
Canberra, Australia

D. Travis Thomas, PhD, RDN, CSSD, LD, FAND
Associate Professor, College of Health Sciences
University of Kentucky
Lexington, KY

Stella Lucia Volpe, PhD, RD, LDN, FACSM
Professor and Chair, Department of
Nutrition Sciences
Drexel University
Philadelphia, PA

Janet Walberg Rankin, PhD, FACSM
Professor, Human Nutrition, Foods, and Exercise
Virginia Tech
Blacksburg, VA

Sheryl Akagi Allen, PhD
Nutrition Scientist
Santa Clara, CA

Jessica Bachman, PhD, RD
Assistant Professor, Department of Exercise Science and Sport
The University of Scranton
Scranton, PA

Hope Barkoukis, PhD, RDN
Interim Department Chair and Associate Professor
Case Western Reserve University, Nurition Department
Cleveland, OH

Charlotte Caperton-Kilburn, MS, RDN, CSSD
NFL Performance
Charleston, SC

Carolyn Cardona, MS, RD, CSSD
Dietitian III
Mental Health Institute
Pueblo, CO

Lynn Cialdella-Kam, PhD, MA, MBA, RDN, LD
Assistant Professor, Department of Nutrition
Case Western Reserve University School of Medicine
Cleveland, OH

Nancy Clark, MS, RD, CSSD
Sports Nutritionist
Sports Nutrition Services, LLC
Boston, MA

Kaitlyn L. Davis, MS, RDN, CSSD, LDN
Owner
RDKate Sports Nutrition
Fowler, MI

Stephanie R. De Leon, MS, RDN, CSSD, LD, CDE
Certified Diabetes Educator
InVentiv Health, Inc.
San Antonio, TX

Lisa Dorfman, MS, RD, CSSD, LMHC, FAND
CEO
Food Fitness International, Inc.
Miami, FL

Amanda Downing Tyler, MEd, RD, CSSD, LD, LAT
Owner
Sports Nutrition Consulting
Bulverde, TX

Cristen Harris, PhD, RDN, CSSD, CD, CEP, FAND
Associate Professor
Bastyr University
Kenmore, WA

Lisa Heaton, MS, RD, CSSD, LDN
Scientist and Sports Dietitian
Barrington, IL

Susan Kleiner, PhD, RD, FACN, CNS, FISSN
Author and Owner
High Performance Nutrition, LLC
Mercer Island, WA

Theresa Logan, MS, RD, CSSD
Sports Dietician
University of South Carolina
Columbia, SC

JJ Mayo, PhD, RD, CSCS
Associate Professor
Department of Nutrition
University of Central Arkansas
Conway, AR

Cindy Milner, MSEd, RDN, CSSD, CDN
Outpatient and Sports Dietitian
Sports Medicine and Athletic Performance of Cayuga Medical
Ithaca, NY

Stephanie Mull, MS, RD, CSSD
Nutrition and Exercise Consultant
Smull Nutrition
Round Hill, VA

Margaret O'Bryan Murphy, PhD, RD, LD
Postdoctoral Scholar, Department of Pharmacology and Nutrition Sciences
University of Kentucky
Lexington, KY

Kortney Parman, RDN, RN, MS, FNP-C
Nurse Practitioner and Dietitian
Academic Medical Center
San Francisco, CA

Karen Reznik Dolins, EdD, RD, CSSD
Nutrition and Exercise Physiology, Teacher's College, Columbia University
New York, NY

Megan T. Robinson, MS, RDN, CDE, LDN
Clinical Dietitian
The Children's Hospital of Philadelphia
Philadelphia, PA

Monique Ryan, MS, RDN, CSSD, LDN
Personal Nutrition Designs, LLC
Evanston, IL

Stacy Sims, PhD
CRO-Director of Research, Design and Innovation
OSMO Nutrition
Fairfax, CA

Sherri Stastny, PhD, RD, CSSD, LRD
Associate Professor
North Dakota State University
Fargo, ND

Marta D. Van Loan, PhD, FACSM
Research Physiologist
USDA–Western Human Nutrition Research Center
Davis, CA

Patrick B. Wilson, PhD, RD
Assistant Professor of Exercise Science
Old Dominion University
Norfolk, VA

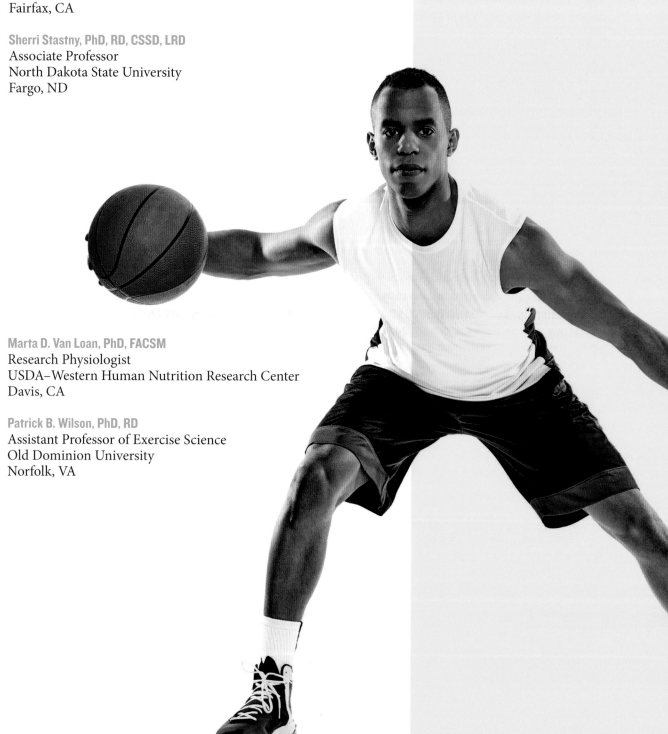

FOREWORD

The sixth edition of *Sports Nutrition: A Handbook for Professionals* is an evidence-based complete reference manual written by experienced sports dietitians and others with acclaimed expertise in their respective practice areas. The unique feature of this manual is the focus on key takeaways at the end of every chapter to guide the reader on how to apply the principles presented. Balancing the evidence-based information with practical application points will be valuable for all professionals interested in the health and performance of athletes, including sports medicine professionals, sports dietitians, athletic and fitness trainers, coaches, and educators.

This edition provides a comprehensive overview of the expected core topics, such as nutrition assessment, energy balance, macronutrient and micronutrient basics, and body composition, and it also includes emerging areas of interest. Some of these newly featured topics include detailed discussions on nine endurance events, emerging areas of opportunity for the sports registered dietitian nutritionist, the gut microbiome, and the most recent considerations in weight management.

Your understanding of sports nutrition practice will undoubtedly grow, and you will benefit from owning this sixth edition. I strongly recommend this as the best sports nutrition reference manual available and an absolute must for your professional library! This copy will replace the lovingly worn and repeatedly highlighted fifth edition in my own library. I can't wait to startreading this edition again in its published format!

Hope Barkoukis, PhD, RDN, LD
Interim Department Chair and Associate Professor
School of Medicine, Nutrition Department
Case Western Reserve University
Cleveland, OH

PREFACE

Effectively delivering evidence-based guidelines translated into practical information for athletes is critical for improving their health and performance. The sixth edition of *Sports Nutrition: A Handbook for Professionals* is a joint venture between the Academy of Nutrition and Dietetics and the Sports, Cardiovascular, and Wellness Nutrition (SCAN) dietetic practice group. All six editions of this manual have involved SCAN registered dietitian nutritionists, and this edition offers *even more* chapters written or reviewed by SCAN registered dietitian nutritionists. We are pleased with the changes to the sixth edition and hope that you will find this updated edition useful.

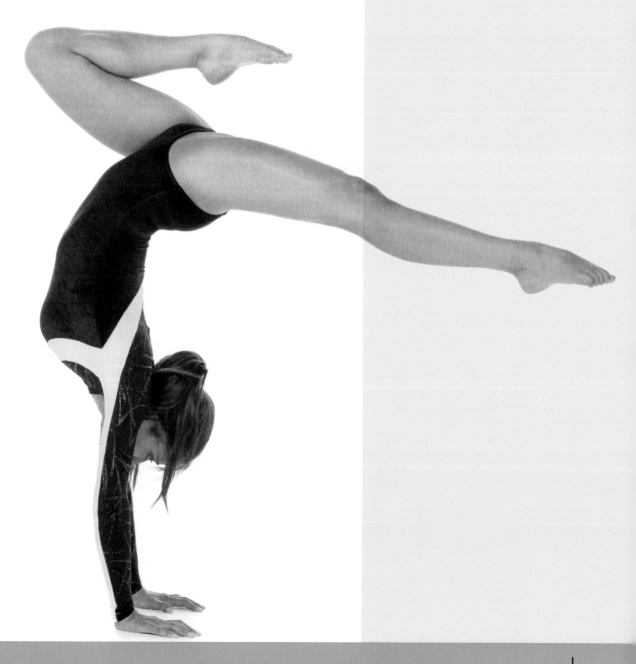

ACKNOWLEDGMENTS

The sixth edition of *Sports Nutrition: A Handbook for Professionals* builds on the previous five editions of a book that belongs on the shelf of any health and sports professional. This edition continues to provide evidence-based information, as well as practical applications, for a broad range of athletes of all ages. We would like to extend a special thanks to the following individuals:

- The SCAN executive committee, past and present chairwomen (Carol Lapin, Eve Pearson, and Karen Collins), for their support and recognition of the value of this project

- The SCAN office and our past Executive Director, Athan Barkoukis, for his persistence and attention to detail

- The returning authors and the 11 new authors who provided their time, talent, and expertise in writing such high-quality chapters

- The reviewers who played such a critical role in the process of creating the manual

- The Academy of Nutrition and Dietetics Publications, Resources, and Products Team

- The athletes, coaches, and families of all the athletes we have worked with over the years who motivate us to remain current and relevant

Note from Christine Karpinski:

I cannot thank Chris Rosenbloom, 5th edition editor-in-chief, enough for her invaluable advice, support, and context.

Christine A. Karpinski, PhD, RDN, CSSD, LDN, Editor-in-Chief
Christine A. Rosenbloom, PhD, RDN, CSSD, FAND, Assistant Editor

OVERVIEW OF THE SIXTH EDITION

The sixth edition of *Sports Nutrition: A Handbook for Professionals* is organized in four sections and designed to be a complete reference manual for practicing professionals that can also be used as resource for undergraduate and graduate sports nutrition classes. We think that we have made some excellent changes to this new edition:

- We have increased the number of authors who are SCAN registered dietitian nutritionists (RDNs), featuring 11 new lead authors. The manual is anchored by our esteemed returning authors who are a mix of SCAN RDNs, international sports RDNs, and our exercise physiologist colleagues.

- We have incorporated more practical information that you can implement into your daily practice. One way we accomplished this was to have authors provide several takeaway points at the end of the chapters.

- This edition includes updated references. If a related study was conducted since the last edition, you will most likely see it in the sixth edition.

- We completely revised seven chapters (Chapters 1, 5, 8, 9, 12, 17, and 19).

- A brand new chapter (Chapter 23) discusses emerging opportunities in sports nutrition.

- We include guidelines from the most current position and practice papers, including the 2016 Position Statement of the American College of Sports Medicine, Academy of Nutrition and Dietetics, and Dietitians of Canada: Nutrition and Athletic Performance.

Section 1 covers sports nutrition basics. It begins with a completely revised overview of exercise physiology (Chapter 1), including a description of training principles and an important discussion about scope of practice for sports RDNs. Chapters 2 through 4 cover the basics and sports applications of dietary carbohydrates, protein, and fat, with updated literature and practical advice. Chapter 4 also contains a significantly expanded discussion of high-fat diets and fat adaptation. A completely revamped vitamin and mineral chapter is featured in this edition (Chapter 5). Instead of an alphabetical review of the micronutrients, the chapter is organized into categories based on risk (due to training, risk factors, and dietary intake) and function. Chapter 7 completes this section of the manual, focusing on the regulation of sports supplements and featuring the Australian Institute of Sport classification system.

Section 2 focuses on nutrition assessment and energy balance. Chapter 8 has an increased focus on how sports RDNs can translate and incorporate the Nutrition Care Process and the Standards of Practice and Standards of Professional Performance into a sports nutrition practice. A sports RDN and an exercise scientist collaborated to provide a different approach to the assessment of body size and composition (Chapter 9). Three authors worked together to update Chapters 10, which includes a discussion of the emerging research on gut microbiome. Lastly, the seasoned authors of Chapter 11 provide new research in the area of weight management.

Section 3 has been renamed *Principles in Practice* to better reflect the approach of its chapters. Chapters 12 through 19 provide practical application of the sports nutrition basics discussed in Sections 1 and 2. To that end, we have kept the same population-specific topics as we had in the previous edition. It took the collaborative efforts of nine experienced sports RDNs to complete this section, which offers you a plethora of information that you can incorporate into your practice.

Section 4 digs deep into sport-specific recommendations. Chapters 20 and 21 feature updated research for sprint, power, and intermittent sports. Chapter 22 discusses the research behind fueling endurance athletes, and brand new to this edition is an in-depth discussion about considerations for specific endurance events, such as adventure racing, obstacle course racing, cross-country skiing, endurance cycling, endurance running, marathon rowing, triathlons, endurance mountain biking, and multiday events. This section concludes with a new chapter (Chapter 23), which explores emerging areas of opportunities for sports RDNs, such as CrossFit, obstacle course races, motorsports, performance artists (eg, dancers, marching band), first responders, and more.

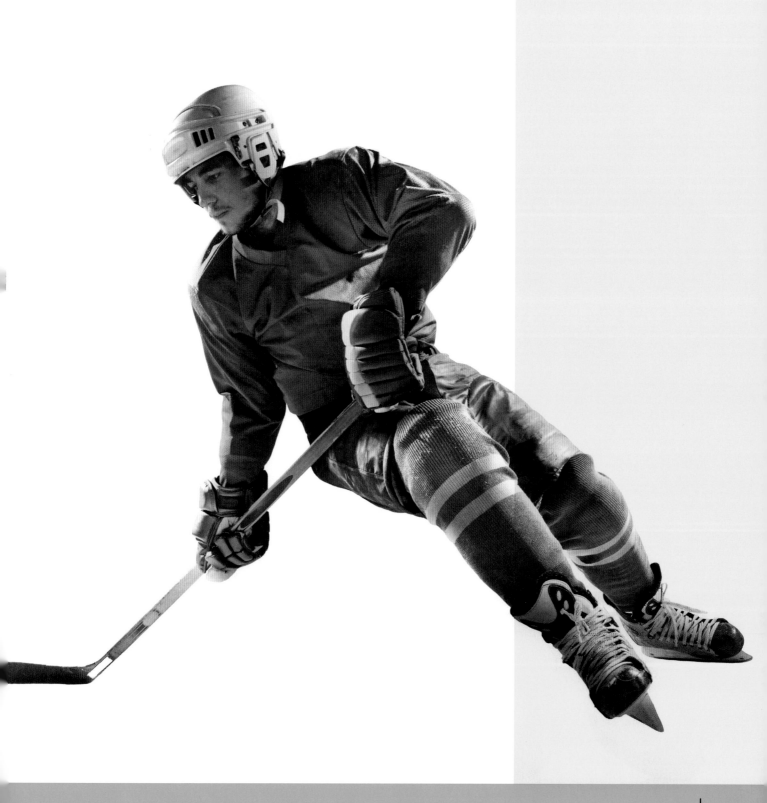

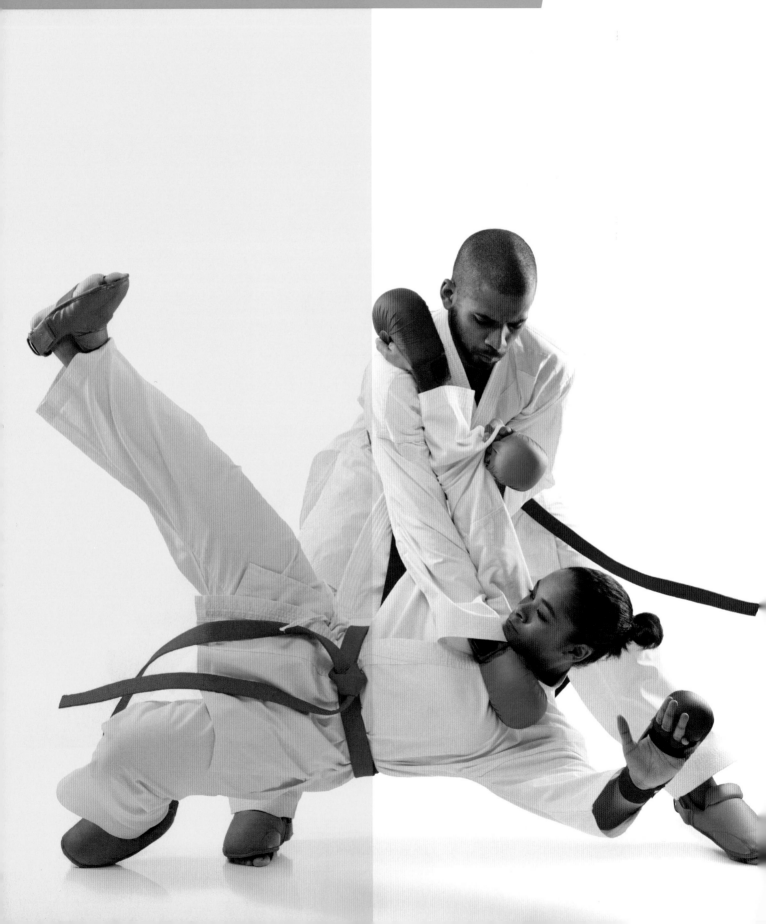

SPORTS NUTRITION BASICS

A thorough understanding of exercise physiology and the way nutrients support training and competition is essential for the registered dietitian nutritionist working with active people. Because of the importance of this topic, the first section of *Sports Nutrition* examines the critical role of macronutrients and micronutrients in exercise performance.

The physiology of exercise includes more than just energy production. Athletic success depends on proper nutrition for growth and development and for an effective immune system function (Chapter 1). Our knowledge of the interrelated roles of dietary carbohydrate, protein, and fat has increased tremendously in the past decade, and this new information is incorporated into Chapters 2, 3, and 4. Micronutrients are covered in detail in Chapter 5, which presents the most current research on how vitamins and minerals affect sports performance. The most essential nutrient for athletes, water, is explained in both scientific and practical terms in the chapter on hydration, electrolytes, and exercise (Chapter 6). Lastly, this section concludes with a comprehensive look at dietary supplements and ergogenic aids that athletes use in the hope of improving performance (Chapter 7). This chapter discusses how the sports dietitian can critically evaluate dietary supplements and provide sound advice to athletes about using these supplements.

CHAPTER 1

PHYSIOLOGY OF EXERCISE

Laura J. Kruskall, PhD, RDN, CSSD, LDN, FACSM, FAND, ACSM EP-C

INTRODUCTION

The human body is a dynamic organism composed of molecules, cells, tissues, whole organs, and systems working together to regulate the environment within itself—a process called homeostasis. Many factors can threaten the inner environment of the body; the body's response is always to attempt to maintain homeostasis. External extremes and challenges include changes in temperature and altitude. One deliberate challenge is participation in physical activity and exercise, when homeostasis in systems such as the cardiorespiratory and musculoskeletal are challenged, triggering a body response. With these challenges, the organ systems must coordinate and adjust to meet the increased energy and metabolic demands of the body.

Exercise physiology is the study of these alterations and the responses to exercise that result from acute bouts of activity, as well as the chronic adaptations that occur from repeated exercise and long-term training.[1] This chapter will provide a brief overview of the basics of the physiology of exercise and will include a discussion of the role of the registered dietitian nutritionist (RDN) or certified specialist in sports dietetics and appropriate application to practice.

ACUTE RESPONSE TO EXERCISE

Even at rest, the body is in a constant state of flux, metabolically active to maintain physiological function. This requires a continual supply of energy. During exercise, the energy demands of skeletal muscle greatly increase, and the respiratory and cardiovascular systems must work harder to allow for increased respiration and blood supply to the working muscles with a concomitant reduction of blood flow to the gastrointestinal tract. This can continue for minutes to hours depending on the intensity of exercise and the condition of the individual. In some sports or events, the increased energy demand is relatively constant for an extended time (eg, a marathon), while in others it is not constant and is often characterized by periods of high intensity followed by periods of active recovery or rest (eg, soccer, tennis). During both endurance and stop-and-go activities, the energy demand increase can be 2 to 20 times that at rest. Very high-intensity activities can exceed this range but can only be sustained for seconds to minutes. Ultimately, the body systems must work together to meet the increased energy demands.[1-5]

Skeletal Muscle and Exercise

Skeletal muscles are attached to the skeleton. These muscles allow movement of the body as they contract and relax. The human body has over 600 skeletal muscles that allow fine and gross movement. We often think of a muscle or muscle group (like the biceps or quadriceps) as a single unit. These units, however, are made of many complex components working together to complete a single contraction. Muscle fiber is the term to describe a muscle cell. A single nerve and the group of muscle fibers it innervates are referred to as a motor unit. Each muscle cell contains organelles, including mitochondria for aerobic energy production, and hundreds to thousands of myofibrils. Sarcomeres, the functional unit of a myofibril, are responsible for the contractile properties of the muscle. Sarcomeres are comprised of thin and thick filaments called actin and myosin, respectively. Activation of the motor unit causes these filaments to "slide" over one another, allowing the muscles to shorten or contract. This slide, referred to as the sliding filament theory, is an energy-requiring process. Not all available motor units are activated at once—only those needed to generate the appropriate force will be used. The force and speed of movement needed will determine the extent of the motor unit recruitment. The higher the force or speed of contraction required, the greater the number of individual muscle fibers that must be recruited for contraction. Muscle groups in opposition cannot contract at the same time—one contracts while the other relaxes or lengthens (eg, biceps and triceps). Nerve transmission is coordinated, so it is unlikely to stimulate the contraction of two antagonistic muscles at any time.[1,6-9]

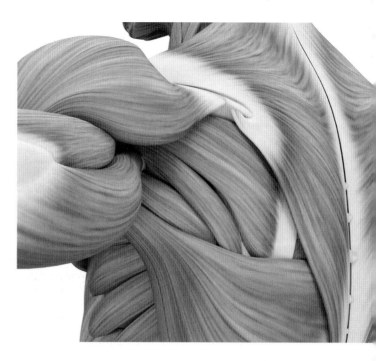

Different types of muscle fibers contract at different speeds, producing varying amounts of force. Type I fibers, sometimes referred to as slow-twitch fibers, have a high level of aerobic endurance; they can use a continuous supply of energy from the aerobic metabolism of carbohydrate and fat. These fibers allow prolonged muscular contraction for long periods. They are primarily used with activities of daily living, like walking, or during lower-intensity endurance events, like bike riding or jogging. Type II fibers, sometimes referred to as fast-twitch, have relatively poor endurance capacity and work better anaerobically. While these fiber types can be further classified as type IIa, type IIx, and type IIc, the differences between the types are not fully understood and are a subject of research.

Most skeletal muscles comprise approximately 50% type I fibers, 25% type IIa fibers, 22% to 24% type IIx, and only 1% to 3% type IIc. The precise percentages of fibers can vary greatly among individuals, even within the specific muscle, and we often see extreme variation in athletes from different sports. Type IIa fibers are recruited most frequently but are secondary to type I fibers, and type IIc are recruited least frequently. Type IIa fibers generate more force than type I but fatigue more easily. They tend to be recruited during higher-intensity events of short duration, such as a half-mile run or a strength-training workout. The significance of type IIx fibers is poorly understood. It appears they are used with explosive activities such as a 50-meter dash or weightlifting. Most muscle groups contain both types of fibers and recruit the type needed for the activity.[1,6-11]

It is plausible to suspect a difference in skeletal muscle fiber types between different types of athletes and untrained individuals. Most studies show little to no difference in the proportion of type I muscle fibers between athletes and controls (but, in contrast, some studies show large differences).[12-18] One study examining bodybuilders reported extremely high values of type IIx fibers,[18] yet other similar studies do not support this finding.[14,16,19] There does, however, appear to be proportional differences in type IIa and type IIx muscle fibers between strength and power athletes and untrained control subjects. Studies support the notion that strength and power athletes have a greater proportion of type IIa and a smaller proportion of type IIx fibers, while others do not.[12-18] The majority of studies show a shift from type IIx to type IIa fibers with long-term resistance training.[12-17,19]

Endurance athletes tend to possess a greater proportion of type I muscle fibers, but the difference does not appear to be caused by training for shifts between type II and type I. Furthermore, it seems that endurance athletes do not have significant changes in their type IIa fiber profile.[20-23] Lack of concrete evidence leads many to scientists ask: Is there a relationship between fiber type and endurance performance success? We would expect that more type I fibers would enhance long-endurance performance activities and more type II fibers would benefit high-intensity activities. Studies reporting on muscle fiber types in the gastrocnemius muscle in distance runners and sprinters support this concept: Endurance athletes have more type I fibers and sprinters have more type II fibers. It is important to keep in mind that fiber type is just one piece of the puzzle. Other factors, such as training, nutrition, and motivation, also affect performance.[1,6-9,24]

Cardiovascular and Respiratory Systems

The cardiovascular and respiratory systems work together seamlessly to deliver oxygen and nutrients to the working muscle and all tissues and to remove metabolic waste products and carbon dioxide from these tissues. These systems working together, often called the cardiorespiratory system, consist of the heart, blood vessels, airways, and lungs. Pulmonary ventilation is the term to describe breathing (air moving in and out of the lungs). Ventilation happens in two phases: inspiration and expiration. Inspiration is an active process

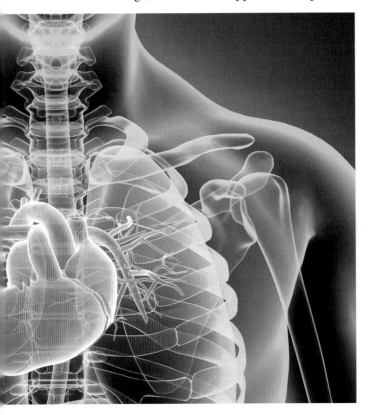

involving the activation of the diaphragm and external intercostal muscles, while expiration is usually a passive process as muscles relax and air is expelled from the lungs. Most of the oxygen in the blood is bound to hemoglobin and delivered to the working muscle. Once inside the muscle, oxygen is transported to the mitochondria by myoglobin and is then available for aerobic energy production in the muscle cell.[1,9]

The cardiorespiratory system has many functions and supports all other physiological systems. In addition to those already identified, key functions include transportating hormones and other compounds, assisting thermoregulation and fluid balance, and maintaining acid-base balance. The cardiac cycle occurs during each heartbeat and includes both electrical and mechanical events.[1,9]

Heart rate is the number of heartbeats per unit of time, usually measured and expressed as beats per minute (bpm). Heart rate is based on the number of contractions of the ventricles (the lower chambers of the heart). Normal range for heart rate is 60 to 100 bpm. A heart rate that is faster than normal is called tachycardia; a heart rate this is slower than normal is called bradycardia. Volume of blood pumped during one heartbeat is called stroke volume. Cardiac output is the total volume of blood pumped from one heartbeat, a product of the heart rate and the stroke volume. Resting cardiac output averages 5 L/min but can vary with body size. Cardiac output increases with exercise and can range from less than 20 L/min in an untrained, sedentary person to 40 L/min or more for those with elite endurance training.[1,25]

The volume of blood distributed throughout the body depends on the metabolic demands of the tissues, with the most active tissues receiving the greatest amount. At rest, many organs require more blood than skeletal muscles. At rest, the muscle receives approximately 15% of the cardiac output, but this can increase to as much as 80% during intense exercise to deliver oxygen and nutrients to the active muscle.[1,26]

Cardiovascular and Respiratory Responses to Acute Exercise

The initiation of exercise requires increased muscle oxygen and nutrient demand and the removal of more metabolic waste products. Almost immediately upon beginning exercise, ventilation increases to meet the oxygen demand of the muscle. During lower-intensity activities, this can be accomplished by simply moving more air in and out of the lungs. As exercise intensity increases, respiration rate increases. During most common forms of endurance exercise, pulmonary ventilation is usually not at its maximum capacity and therefore not the limiting factor in performance. The exception may occur during very high-intensity exercise. Usually the respiratory muscles can withstand fatigue during prolonged endurance exercise. There is a point where athletes cannot take in any higher volume of air and respiration rate cannot be any faster. At this point, they are at aerobic capacity, and the energy required for any activity in excess of this must come entirely from anaerobic metabolism. The term to describe this is maximal oxygen uptake (VO_2 max). VO_2 max, an important consideration for performance lasting more than a few minutes, can be measured in an exercise physiology laboratory. It is considered the best measurement of cardiovascular or aerobic fitness.[1,27-29] VO_2 max is usually expressed as $mL \times kg^{-1} \times min^{-1}$. A sedentary person may see a 10-fold increase in maximal oxygen transport with exercise, while an endurance athlete may see a 23-fold increase. A sedentary man has an average VO_2 max of $35\ mL \times kg^{-1} \times min^{-1}$, while a world-class endurance athlete can have one as high as $80\ mL \times kg^{-1} \times min^{-1}$.[30,31]

The lungs–gas exchange is not considered a limiting factor in exercise performance. Instead, with longer-term endurance exercise, glycogen availability, or its utilization by the working skeletal muscles, is the more important factor. The key element seems to be the maximum cardiac output (heart rate multiplied by stroke volume) that can be achieved, as this is closely related to both VO_2 max and endurance performance. Heart rate increases linearly as exercise intensity increases, but ultimately a maximum rate is achieved, and the heart rate plateaus. Maximum heart rate differs little between trained and untrained individuals, although the intensity level at which these individuals will reach maximum heart rate will vary. For example, both a trained and untrained person may have a maximum heart rate of 170 bpm, but the trained person can work at a higher oxygen uptake before reaching that maximum heart rate.

Stroke volume is also a determining factor for cardiovascular endurance capacity. In untrained persons, stroke volume increases proportionally as exercise intensity increases but usually does not further increase once a person is exercising at 40% to 60% of his or her VO_2 max. In trained individuals, stroke volume can increase even further as exercise intensity increases. Since heart rate and stroke volume increase with exercise, total increased cardiac output parallels the intensity of the exercise to meet the increased blood flow demands of the working muscle. Individuals do not usually exercise at maximum heart rate; instead, they perform submaximal exercise for an extended time. The point where the cardiovascular system is delivering the optimal amount of oxygen and nutrients to the muscle is called steady-state heart rate.[1,27,30-32]

FUEL FOR EXERCISE

The biologically usable form of energy in the human body is adenosine triphosphate (ATP). Each time skeletal muscles contract or relax, ATP is required. All movement, including intentional exercise, requires an increased energy demand on skeletal muscles. If energy cannot be supplied in a timely manner and in adequate amounts, movement will cease. As the intensity or duration of exercise increases, the body may have difficulty keeping up with this increased energy demand, and ultimately fatigue ensues. One of the limiting factors in ATP production is exogenous fuel from the energy nutrients once endogenous carbohydrate stores are exhausted.[1,5,33]

Energy Substrates

Plants rely on the process of photosynthesis to convert light from the sun into chemical energy. Humans obtain energy from consuming plants and animals, thereby taking in energy nutrients. Energy nutrients come in the form of carbohydrate, fat, or protein. All cells in the body have the ability to oxidize these nutrients, causing a breakdown and release of stored energy. The cells also have metabolic pathways to process these energy substrates, resulting in the generation of ATP. In muscle cells, ATP is hydrolyzed, releasing a phosphate group, adenosine diphosphate (ADP), and energy.[1,3,5,33]

In addition to gaining energy from the ingestion of nutrients from foods and beverages (exogenous sources), the human body has the ability to store and utilize substrates for later use (endogenous sources). Under normal circumstances, the primary nutrients for energy production come from carbohydrate and fat. Usually, protein contributes less than 5% to 10% to the body's energy needs because it has so many other important functions, such as acting as enzymes, hormones, and immune proteins and performing functions such as tissue maintenance, growth, and repair. The exception to this is during the later stages of prolonged endurance exercise where proteins can contribute up to 15% of the energy needs if exogenous carbohydrate is not consumed and glycogen stores become depleted. In this chapter, we will focus on carbohydrate and fat being the fuel sources for working muscle during exercise.

The storage form of carbohydrate in humans, glycogen, is found in both skeletal muscle and liver. Glycogen storage has a maximum capacity, and, on average, these organs can store approximately 1,600 to 2,500 kcal of energy. The liver can store up to 75 to 100 g (300 to 400 kcal) of glycogen, while skeletal muscle can hold up to 300 to 400 g (1,200 to 1,600 kcal). Plasma glucose is a small source of carbohydrate, containing approximately 5 to 25 g (20 to 100 kcal). Under normal circumstances, we cannot fully depend on any of these stores to fuel exercise because the brain and central nervous system require glucose and take priority. Fat (adipose tissue) is stored as triglycerides within adipose tissue and skeletal muscle. Unlike glycogen, adipose tissue triglyceride is limitless and can provide 70,000 kcal of energy or more.[3,34,35]

Energy Systems

ATP is stored in body cells in very limited quantities, so the body must constantly have the ability to generate ATP to meet the demands of cellular metabolism and especially muscle contraction during exercise. During rest, most of the cells and organs use a constant supply of ATP. With increased activity, skeletal muscle ATP demand can increase greatly, depending on the intensity and duration of exercise. As ATP is used—with each muscle contraction generating ADP and a single phosphate group—the ADP and phosphate group must be rephosphorylized to ATP. There are three basic metabolic pathways to accomplish this: those that generate ATP without the use of oxygen, called anaerobic; those that require oxygen involvement, called aerobic; and those that rely on the large amount of creatine found in muscle cells, called the phosphocreatine (PC) system. Approximately 95% of the body's creatine is found in skeletal muscle and can easily be replenished by the diet. Athletes who include meat in their diet obtain plenty of creatine, but creatine can also be synthesized from the amino acids methionine, arginine, and glycine, which are obtained from other dietary sources.[1,3,34,35]

ADENOSINE TRIPHOSPHATE–PHOSPHOCREATINE SYSTEM

The most rapid method that the body uses to produce ATP is the ATP-PC system. This anaerobic system is used during intensive, explosive movements, such as a tennis serve or a power lift. This system generates ATP rapidly; however, it is very limited and only supplies ATP for up to 10 seconds. A key component in the ATP-PC system is PC, which is stored in skeletal muscle. PC is simply a molecule of creatine attached to a single molecule of phosphate. A creatine kinase enzyme breaks the two molecules apart, and the free phosphate molecule then combines with ADP, forming new ATP. The ATP-PC system is limited because there is a very small pool of PC stored in the skeletal muscle. Once all PC molecules have donated their phosphate group to ADP, the system can no longer facilitate further ATP production until PC is replenished, which normally happens during recovery with rest and dietary intake.[1,3]

ANAEROBIC GLYCOLYSIS

This system oxidizes one glucose molecule (six carbons) to form two pyruvic acid molecules (three carbons). Glucose can come from dietary intake (circulating blood glucose) or from glycogen stored in the muscle or liver. In the process, potential energy is generated in two ways. First, ATP is directly generated from the breakdown process of glucose to pyruvate. Second, while glucose is being oxidized, hydrogen molecules are being removed. Nicotinamide adenine dinucleotide (NAD) is a coenzyme that carries electrons. NAD receives these molecules, accepts an electron (hydrogen molecule [H]), and forms NADH, transporting hydrogen to a mitochondrial location, called the electron transport chain (ETC), where the body can generate ATP aerobically. This pathway does not produce large amounts of ATP but does generate it fairly rapidly. This system and the ATP-PC system are the predominant energy systems for the first few minutes of intense, continuous activity.[1,3,36] Anaerobic glycolysis also provides energy during the first few moments of moderate, longer-duration activity as the aerobic system begins to generate ATP.[3,37,38]

Another limitation of this system is the production and accumulation of lactate during high-intensity situations, when skeletal muscle ATP demand is high. Production of pyruvic acid is not problematic when oxygen is present and metabolism continues. When oxygen is limited, such as during very high-intensity activity, the pyruvic acid gets converted to lactic acid. Lactic acid is relatively unstable at normal body pH: it loses a hydrogen ion or dissociates to lactate. As hydrogen molecules accumulate, the pH of the muscle

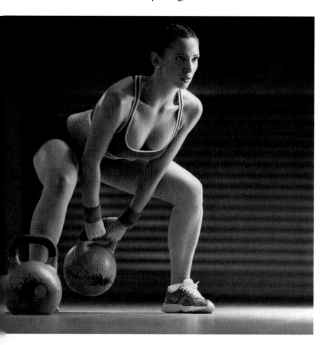

cell drops, glycolytic enzymatic activity is hampered, and skeletal muscle fatigue results. The body must slow down to recover before intense activity can continue. Lactate is constantly being produced, but, fortunately, it is easily cleared with time by a few mechanisms. First, lactate is taken up and oxidized by the mitochondria in the same muscle cell. This occurs primarily in type I muscle fibers. Second, much more lactate is produced in the type II muscle fibers, but that lactate is transported to the type I fibers or to other cells in the body for oxidation. Third, via the Cori cycle, lactate travels from the muscle to the liver, gets converted to glucose via gluconeogenesis, and then is sent back to the working muscle for fuel. Once lactate is cleared, activity can continue.[3,37,38]

AEROBIC METABOLISM

The system described in the preceding section is also known as oxidative phosphorylation. Oxidative phosphorylation can break down carbohydrate, fats, or proteins with the involvement of oxygen. It uses the Krebs cycle and the ETC. Unlike the other two energy systems, oxidative phosphorylation can supply ATP on a fairly limitless basis as long as macronutrients and oxygen are available. Acetyl coenzyme A (CoA), a metabolic intermediate from both glucose and fat oxidation, is ultimately oxidized via aerobic metabolism. This compound combines with oxaloacetate to begin the Krebs cycle. Many hydrogen molecules produced during the Krebs cycle are shuttled by NAD and flavin adenine dinucleotide (FAD) to the ETC. As the hydrogen molecules are passed along the chain, ATP is generated. Oxygen, the final hydrogen acceptor, combines to form water. The ETC is the most efficient way that our bodies produce ATP because there are no metabolic by-products that produce fatigue.[1,3,34]

CROSSOVER CONCEPT

All metabolic systems work concurrently. One system does not shut off as another turns on; rather, all the systems are working at any given time. The relative contribution of each system will depend on the physiological need for ATP. Fatty acid oxidation produces more ATP per gram than carbohydrate oxidation, but it is a much slower process and requires more oxygen to complete. Oxidation of a 6-carbon glucose molecule nets approximately 32 molecules of ATP, but a 16-carbon fatty acid can produce 106 ATP molecules. More ATP can be produced with increased carbon length of the fatty acid. ATP can only be generated from fat aerobically. A glucose molecule does not yield as much ATP, but it can be oxidized rapidly and without oxygen when necessary.[3,39]

During rest or low-intensity activity, ATP demand is low, and oxygen is plentiful. As a result, fat is the preferred fuel source at this time. As exercise intensity increases, skeletal muscle ATP demand increases and oxygen delivery becomes more limited. In this case, there is more reliance on carbohydrate for fuel because glucose is oxidized more rapidly and is more oxygen efficient (more ATP is generated per oxygen molecule used) than fat. Remember, both carbohydrate and fat are always being used, but the ATP demand and oxygen availability will determine which substrate and metabolic system is predominant in ATP generation.[34,36]

FATIGUE

Muscular fatigue refers to the impairment or inability to produce force at the level of the muscle. At rest and lower-intensity exercise, humans are capable of producing enough ATP to fuel activity without muscular fatigue, as long as there are sufficient energy substrates (primarily carbohydrate and fat) readily available in our bodies. At low exercise intensity, carbon-containing pyruvate is consistently oxidized to acetyl CoA. At the same time, hydrogen molecules are shuttled smoothly within cells to the ETC by the compounds NAD and FAD. At such low exercise intensities, ATP is readily produced in required amounts, and there are no metabolic by-products that contribute to fatigue.[1,40-42]

Short-Term Fatigue

Short-term fatigue occurs when exercise intensity rises to levels that disturb our body's ability to derive energy from our primary exercise fuel substrates: carbohydrate and fat. Possible causes include the accumulation of metabolic products such as inorganic phosphate and lactate, depletion of creatine phosphate, and changes in cellular calcium. The primary culprit in metabolic fatigue is the limited ability to inspire and transport oxygen to working muscles at a rate sufficient to keep up with increased ATP demand as exercise intensity rises. When oxygen levels at the working muscle are insufficient, hydrogen molecules that normally bind with oxygen to form water start to accumulate and eventually overwhelm the capacity for NAD and FAD to accept and transport the hydrogen molecules. Pyruvate's normal metabolism to acetyl CoA diminishes, and instead, pyruvate accepts these hydrogen molecules and forms lactic acid, which rapidly dissociates to lactate. Lactate is formed faster than it can be cleared, and the acidic environment in the cell disrupts glycolysis enzymatic activity. At this point, ATP production is hindered, and skeletal muscle contraction is impaired. The only way to restore homeostasis is to reduce exercise intensity to enhance oxygen uptake and clear metabolic by-products. Lactate is not just a waste product of metabolism; it is a fuel source for resting tissues and contracting cardiac and skeletal muscles, and endurance-trained individuals can better utilize lactate for energy. Once the lactate is cleared—and this is a rapid process—the fatigue dissipates and the skeletal muscle can once again contract.[1,40-42]

Long-Term Fatigue

Lactate accumulation is not significantly related to fatigue in prolonged endurance activities. Long-term fatigue or substrate fatigue, sometimes referred to as "hitting the wall" or "bonking," is thought to be a consequence of glycogen depletion. Because liver and muscle glycogen storage capacity is limited, depletion can occur fairly rapidly. Once glycogen stores are depleted, dietary carbohydrate absorption and gluconeogenesis cannot keep up with the skeletal muscle ATP demand, and movement must stop. The body cannot continue to perform until more carbohydrate (glucose) becomes available for ATP production. For endurance athletes, any strategy to maximize glycogen stores and provide a continuous supply of glucose during exercise will help delay the onset of substrate depletion.[1,40-42]

PRINCIPLES OF EXERCISE TRAINING

Exercise training refers to the body's response to physical activity repeated over time, resulting in positive physiological adaptations. Appropriate training, coupled with proper fueling and adequate rest and recovery, generally results in improved performance. Overtraining or undertraining will not result in a desired effect. The principles of exercise training apply to the novice beginning an exercise program to improve health as well as to the elite athlete wishing to compete.

Individuality

Both genetic and environmental factors contribute to body composition. While genetics creates starting points and boundaries that determine our fat patterning and muscularity, this does not mean that our ultimate body shape and size are completely outside our control. We have the ability to alter our physique, to an extent, with nutrition and training. It is, however, important to understand that we must be realistic about our genetic potential. People have different body shapes, separated into three categories: the ectomorph is generally tall and lean; the endomorph is rounder; and the mesomorph is somewhere in between. People from different categories can respond differently to the same training. For example, a very tall and lean person may never be able to participate in a resistance training regimen resulting in the physique of a professional bodybuilder. On the other hand, a stout, muscular person may never be light or fast enough to compete as an elite marathon runner. Furthermore, some people are considered higher responders to training and seem to achieve desired results more than lower responders. Being realistic in terms of body type and accomplishments for specific types is an important consideration.[43,44]

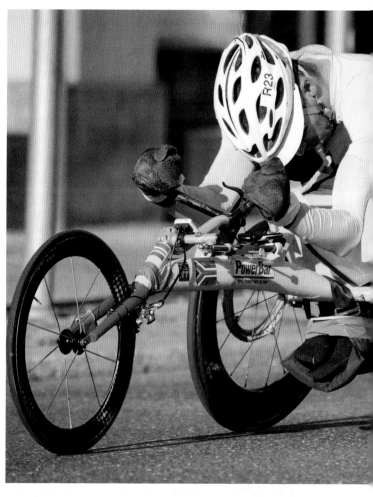

Specificity

This principle dictates that physiological adaptations and performance enhancements are specific to the mode, intensity, and duration of the exercise training. A training regimen must induce a physical stress specific to the system needed for performance gains. For example, a distance runner must perform endurance activities long enough in duration to promote cellular training adaptations, such as increases in mitochondrial density. Anaerobic sprints or weight lifting promote increased muscle strength and hypertrophy, which are detrimental to an endurance athlete. Similarly, cardiovascular training will not result in the increased muscular strength and hypertrophy desired for high-intensity activity and stop-and-go sport athletes. The training program must mimic the desired activity.[1,45]

Progressive Overload

To see improvements, athletes need to overload the system being trained (eg, cardiovascular, muscular), resulting in continuous demands on that system. For example, if a person wants to gain strength, he or she may initially bench press 100 lbs for 8 repetitions, and, over time, he or she will be able to do 12 to 15 repetitions before fatigue. As training continues, he or she needs to add weight until again reaching fatigue at 8 repetitions. In addition to the weight and number of repetitions performed, muscle can reach fatigue in other ways. For example, one can increase the number of sets of the exercise, decrease the rest period between sets, or emphasize the eccentric contraction by slowing the speed of the lowering motion. With endurance performance, one must increase the total training volume with intensity, duration, or both to see an improvement.[1,45]

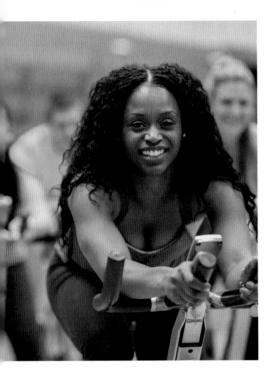

Variation/Periodization

The principle of periodization involves exercise training for a particular sport or event in smaller periods based on the desired outcome. Proper periodization allows for the intensity of training needed for the desired performance outcome while working in adequate rest and recovery to prevent overtraining. Traditional periodization usually consisted of a long time frame, such as 1 to 4 years. Within that time, there were various cycles of months (macrocycles), weeks (mesocycles), days (microcycles), and individual training sessions. This plan may work well for individuals training for a specific, single competition like a marathon. The focus here is on the cardiovascular system. This is not as effective for well-rounded athletes who wish to compete in multiple types of events across seasons. Well-rounded athletes require many systems and skills that make use of a combination of aerobic, anaerobic, and strength training.

A newer area of training uses training blocks (or block periodization) that can be individualized based on the desired sport or event. These blocks can focus on a minimum number of performance outcomes. Training consists of performing a small number of blocks at one time (eg, three or four), and the blocks may last a few weeks. The sequence can be customized for the sport or event. One example comes from top-performing canoe and kayak paddlers. The first block of their training focused on accumulating the skills needed for the sport with general conditioning for aerobic endurance and muscular strength and endurance. Block two focused on specialized movements and proper technique, combining anaerobic and aerobic conditioning along with continued muscular strength and endurance. Block three emphasized specific race modeling and obtaining optimal speed and recovery between sessions. This regimen resulted in outstanding performance outcomes.[1,46]

Detraining

As both resistance and aerobic training result in increased strength and cardiovascular endurance, stopping this training (detraining) results in the opposite. Continued training is necessary to prevent this detraining effect. Systematically increasing the physical demands on the body with training will be necessary for further improvements, while maintenance-level training regimens prevent physiological decline from the trained state. Detraining can be defined as partial or full reductions in training-induced physiological adaptations in response to a lower training load or inactivity. It appears there is a more significant loss of cardiorespiratory endurance gains than loss of muscular endurance, strength, and power. While these data are not concrete, some research shows that athletes can lose approximately 25% of cardiorespiratory gains in about 10 to 20 days of inactivity. Data vary regarding muscle strength, power, and endurance, but 2 weeks of inactivity often results in declines in muscular endurance and strength. Fortunately, three training session per week at approximately 70% VO_2 max can maintain cardiorespiratory fitness levels and provide adequate skeletal muscle stimulatory load to retain any gains made with strength training.[1,45]

PHYSIOLOGICAL ADAPTATIONS TO ENDURANCE TRAINING

Cardiorespiratory fitness is the term for the ability to perform prolonged endurance exercise using large muscle groups. VO_2 max is one of the best measures of cardiorespiratory endurance. As discussed previously, with acute responses to exercise, both the respiratory and cardiovascular systems play an important role in facilitating endurance activity. Training has minimal effect on lung structure and function, but maximal effort does increase pulmonary ventilation, pulmonary diffusion, distribution of arterial blood away from inactive tissue toward active skeletal muscle, and the ability of the muscle to take up delivered oxygen.[1,29]

The cardiovascular system has numerous adaptations to regular endurance training, summarized below. All changes result in greater delivery of oxygen and nutrients to the working skeletal muscle.[1,29]

- Increases in left ventricular internal space, wall thickness, and mass allow for a stronger contraction and ultimately greater stroke volume. Increased stroke volume in trained individuals is seen at rest and exercise.
- Resting heart rate decreases with endurance training; the rate and can be 40 bpm or lower (compared with the 60 to 80 bpm in the typical sedentary person).
- Exercise heart rate is also lower at a given training load (eg, 60% VO_2 max) with endurance training, but maximum heart rate does not drastically change.
- Cardiac output does not change much during rest and submaximal exercise but does increase considerably during maximal effort and is a significant contributor to the increased VO_2 max with training.
- Resting blood pressure is reduced.
- Increased capillarization, blood volume, plasma volume, and red blood cell volume, improve tissue perfusion and oxygen delivery.
- There are increases in percentage and cross-sectional area of type I muscle fibers (those primarily used in endurance activities).
- There are increases in mitochondria, oxidative enzymes, and myoglobin content (more machinery for ATP production).

PHYSIOLOGICAL ADAPTATIONS TO RESISTANCE TRAINING

Individuals undergo regular resistance training to improve muscular strength and power. Strength can be defined as the maximum force generated by the muscle, whereas power is a product of muscle force × velocity and, therefore, is an indicator of the rate at which the work is performed. Changes in strength and power require numerous adaptations in the neuromuscular system depending on the type of resistance training. The neuromuscular system is highly responsive to training, and improvements can be seen within months. Skeletal muscle is very dynamic. Training can improve size (hypertrophy) and strength, while disuse or immobility can result in decreased size (atrophy) and strength. Muscle size and strength are somewhat related: Training causes an increase in both and detraining causes a decrease in both. The primary neuromuscular adaptations to regular resistance training include:

- improved neural adaptations (increased motor unit recruitment, decreasing neurologic inhibition) with strength gains, with or without hypertrophy, especially in the early stages of training;
- strength gains related to muscle hypertrophy in later stages of training; and
- increased size of the individual skeletal muscle fibers and increased myofibrils and actin and myosin filaments from hypertrophy.

Muscles can be trained to improve strength and size, but there is a limit beyond which further adaptation is not possible. Genetic potential plays a large role in body type. For example, it may be impossible for a tall, slender person to look like a professional bodybuilder, and likewise it may be impossible for a large muscular person to become a lean, slim runner.[43,44]

OVERTRAINING

It is clear that proper training and adequate recovery result in increased performance, but many athletes develop the belief that more is better and that there is not a ceiling for performance enhancement. Excessive training usually results in a performance decrement, which the athlete often follows with even more effort to compensate. The American College of Sports Medicine (ACSM) and the European College of Sports Science issued a Joint Consensus Statement on this topic.[47] The two terms to describe this condition are overreaching and overtraining. Overreaching describes excessive training that results in short-term performance decrements that can be reversed in several days to several weeks with proper training and rest. In addition, adequate fluid to restore hydration, adequate carbohydrate to replenish glycogen stores, and adequate protein to optimize protein synthesis and healing are critical. The symptoms leading to performance decrements include overall fatigue, muscular fatigue, chronic muscle tenderness and soreness, lack of concentration, and disrupted eating habits or loss of interest in eating. This is characteristic during periods of competition training. Overtraining results in a series of symptoms referred to as the overtraining syndrome (OTS). OTS is more serious because long-term decrements in performance can take several weeks or months to recover from. OTS includes both physiological maladaptations and often psychological factors stemming from stress of competition, family and social relationships, and other life demands. There are no set diagnostic criteria for OTS because symptoms vary from person to person and are highly individualized. It is important for an athlete with suspected OTS to seek medical care to rule out other confounding diseases or conditions and to develop a sound recovery plan.[47,48] See Box 1.1 for a list of some symptoms.

Box 1.1 Signs and Symptoms of Overtraining Syndrome[47,48]

These are some of the common signs and symptoms of overtraining syndrome:

- Decline in performance despite continued training
- Fatigue, with loss of skeletal muscle strength, endurance capacity, and overall coordination
- Decrease in appetite
- Weight or fat loss
- Anxiousness, restlessness, and sleep disruption
- Inability to concentrate, loss of motivation, and even depression

---

SCOPE OF PRACTICE FOR REGISTERED DIETITIAN NUTRITIONISTS

Scope of practice is an important issue for all health professionals. States that license the various health professions have a very specific defined scope of practice for each profession. For RDNs interested in sports dietetics, there is a natural desire to discuss exercise with patients and clients, regardless of whether the RDN has the appropriate educational training or certification to do so. Current Didactic Programs in Nutrition and Dietetics do not require courses in exercise science, and student learning outcomes do not have a knowledge requirement for this area. As a result, many RDNs graduating from traditional dietetics programs are not qualified to discuss detailed issues regarding fitness assessment and exercise prescription.

It is critical for the practitioner to understand the laws of the state or states where they live and practice. The exercise profession relies largely on self-regulated certification. Many states regulate the profession of dietetics, yet most states (except Louisiana) do not regulate the practice of exercise professionals. If you live in a state that licenses any health profession, licensure supersedes any registration or certification.

Physical Activity Guidance

RDNs with an interest in sports dietetics should be comfortable discussing some aspects of exercise and physical activity with their patients and clients. They should, at a minimum, be familiar with the current federal Physical Activity Guidelines for Americans[45] and the overall health benefits of exercise. From a general standpoint, RDNs should assist medically cleared patients and clients with planning and implementing ways to increase their physical activity levels to match these guidelines. RDNs should use the patient or client's current level of physical activity and stage of readiness to change as a basis for physical activity plans and goals. When should an RDN refer a client to a qualified exercise professional? It is critical for the RDN to fully assess their current knowledge and scope of practice in the area of exercise science. Most RDNs who specialize in sports dietetics should be able to discuss the health benefits of exercise and the principles of exercise training discussed earlier in this chapter. Conducting a fitness assessment and prescribing exercise require specialized knowledge and skills and, ideally, an appropriate certification.

Fitness Assessment and Exercise Prescription

Fitness assessments and exercise prescriptions may be out of the scope of practice for RDNs, depending on whether or not they hold additional training and certification. A fitness assessment measures cardiorespiratory fitness, musculoskeletal strength and endurance, flexibility, balance, and body composition. This information is used to develop a detailed exercise plan, known as an exercise prescription, tailored to the individual's current fitness level and health goals. This should be created by qualified exercise professionals. There are two reputable places to find qualified exercise professionals: The ACSM ProFinder (http://certification.acsm.org/pro-finder) and the US Registry of Exercise Professionals (USREPS) website (www.usreps.org/Pages/default.aspx).[49,50] ACSM has certified over 32,000 health professionals in 44 countries. The USREPS is a nationally recognized registry of exercise professionals and an advocate for the exercise professionals who hold accredited exercise certifications from the National Commission of Certifying Agencies (NCCA).

Reputable Exercise and Fitness Certifications

Unlike nutrition and dietetics, no single accrediting body for programs in kinesiology or exercise science results in a nationally recognized credential. These academic programs may voluntarily become accredited through the Commission on Accreditation of Allied Health Education Programs (CAAHEP)[51] with the goal to have some consistency among all exercise science programs. Many CAAHEP-accredited programs provide a track for students to prepare for and earn an exercise-based certification.

It is important for the RDN who is not qualified to conduct fitness assessments and provide exercise prescriptions to have a network of qualified exercise professionals for patient/client referral, and this should be documented when using the Nutrition Care Process. There are numerous exercise-related certifications available, so it is important to research the qualifications for certification and the knowledge and skills assessed in the process. The NCCA governs many of the exercise certifications. A few reputable organizations and their certifications are listed in Table 1.1.

Table 1.1 Examples of Reputable Organizations that Certify Exercise Professionals[a]

Name of Organization	Name of Certification	Qualifications	Purpose
American College of Sports Medicine	Certified Personal Trainer	18 years old High school diploma or equivalent Adult CPR[b]/AED[c] certification	Plan and implement exercise programs for healthy individuals
American College of Sports Medicine	Certified Group Exercise Instructor	18 years old High school diploma CPR/AED	Supervise participants or lead instructional sessions for healthy individuals
American College of Sports Medicine	Certified Exercise Physiologist	Bachelor of science degree in exercise science, exercise physiology, or kinesiology CPR/AED	Fitness assessments, exercise plans, personal training for those with medically controlled diseases

Continued on next page

Name of Organization	Name of Certification	Qualifications	Purpose
American College of Sports Medicine	Certified Clinical Exercise Physiologist	Bachelor of science degree in exercise science, exercise physiology, or kinesiology 400–500 hours of supervised experience Basic Life Support certification	Fitness assessments, exercise plans, personal training for those with medically controlled diseases and those with cardiovascular, pulmonary, and metabolic diseases
American College of Sports Medicine	Registered Clinical Exercise Physiologist	Master of Science degree in exercise science, exercise physiology, or kinesiology 600 hours of supervised experience Basic Life Support certification	Fitness assessments, exercise plans, personal training for those with medically controlled diseases and those with cardiovascular, pulmonary, and metabolic diseases Rehabilitative strategies
American College of Sports Medicine	Specialty Certifications Exercise Is Medicine Credential Certified Cancer Exercise Trainer Certified Inclusive Fitness Trainer Certified Physical Activity in Public Health Specialist	Bachelor of Science degree in exercise science, exercise physiology, or kinesiology Another American College of Sports Medicine certification or National Commission of Certifying Agencies–accredited health and fitness certification CPR/AED	See American College of Sports Medicine website for specifics (www.acsm.org)
National Strength and Conditioning Association	Certified Personal Trainer	18 years old High school diploma CPR/AED	Work with healthy clients in one-on-one situations
National Strength and Conditioning Association	Certified Special Population Specialist	Current National Strength and Conditioning Association certification or RDN[d] credential CPR/AED Supervised practice experience	Use an individualized approach to assess, motivate, educate, and train special population clients
National Strength and Conditioning Association	Certified Strength and Conditioning Specialist	Bachelor of science from an accredited institution CPR/AED	Implement strength and conditioning programs for athletes in a team setting
American Council on Exercise	Personal Trainer Certification	18 years old High school diploma CPR/AED	One-on-one or small-group training for healthy individuals

Continued on next page

Table 1.1 Examples of Reputable Organizations that Certify Exercise Professionals[a] (Continued)

Name of Organization	Name of Certification	Qualifications	Purpose
American Council on Exercise	Group Fitness Instructor Certification	18 years old High school diploma CPR/AED	Lead fitness classes for healthy individuals
American Council on Exercise	Health Coach Certification	18 years old CPR/AED Current National Strength and Conditioning Association–accredited certification or license in nutrition (RDNs may qualify) or associates of science degree or higher in nutrition 2 years of work experience	Lead healthy clients to sustainable, healthy change by applying knowledge in behavior change, physical activity, and nutrition
American Council on Exercise	Specialty Certifications Mind Body Fitness Nutrition Weight Management	National Strength and Conditioning Association–accredited certification or equivalent professional credentials, including NDTR[e] and RDN	See American Council on Exercise website for specifics (www.nsca.org)

[a] This is not an all-inclusive list. Please see the organization websites for updated information.

[b] CPR = cardiopulmonary resuscitation

[c] AED = automated external defibrillator

[d] RDN = registered dietitian nutritionist.

[e] NDTR = nutrition dietetic technician, registered;

Physical Activity Guidance and the Nutrition Care Process

The first step in the Nutrition Care Process is assessment. During this step, the RDN should refer to the current Nutrition Terminology Reference Manual (eNCPT) website (http:\\ncpt.webaturhor.com).[52] The RDN may assess readiness to change, weight and body composition, and physical activity history and current level of physical activity. During the diagnosis step, the RDN can document any problems and create a diagnostic statement. Usually the diagnosis refers to level of physical activity or inactivity, readiness to change, or something in the behavioral domain. For the intervention step, the RDN can choose to provide education if it is within his or her scope, can refer to a qualified exercise professional, or can do a combination of both. For most RDNs, education can include the health benefits of exercise, how to start an exercise program, the key concepts presented in the Physical Activity Guidelines for Americans, and provision of additional resources (eg, handouts, names of community centers, list of professionals). Monitoring and evaluation should include follow-up on the physical activity–related goals set for the patient or client.

Federal Physical Activity Guidelines

RDNs with an interest in sports dietetics should be familiar with the federal Physical Activity Guidelines for Americans and be comfortable discussing these guidelines with their patients or clients.[45] The guidelines may be downloaded for free at the Health.gov website (http://health.gov/paguidelines). Some key concepts from this document are discussed in this section. Principles of training were discussed previously and are again presented in these guidelines. Box 1.2 provides definitions of the levels, components, and intensity of physical activity.

Another way of defining exercise intensity is the use of metabolic equivalents (METs). MET is the ratio of rate of energy expended during exercise to the rate of energy expended at rest. One MET is equivalent to a VO_2 of 3.5 mL $\times$ kg^{-1} $\times$ min^{-1}. Multiples of this value can be used to quantify energy expenditure and will be discussed in detail in Chapter 10. METs are a simple concept: 1 MET is the work at rest, while 5 METs would be work at 5 times rest. The Physical Activity Guidelines also use MET-minutes for guidance. MET-minutes take into account both physical activity intensity and duration. For example, a 4-MET activity for 30 minutes equals 120 MET-minutes, and an 8-MET activity for 15 minutes also equals 120 MET-minutes. For health benefits, one can exercise at a lower intensity for longer periods of time or at a higher intensity for shorter periods of time. Keep in mind, these physical activity guidelines are for health and are not exercise training guidelines for optimal performance. The goal for health is to achieve a minimum of 500 to 1,000 MET-min/week, with potential greater health benefits found at greater than 1,000 MET-min/week. The relationship between intensity and METs is summarized here:

- Light intensity = 1.1 to 2.9 METs
- Moderate intensity = 3.0 to 5.9 METs
  - For example, walking 3 mph requires 3.3 METs of energy expenditure
- Vigorous intensity ≥6.0 METs
  - For example, running a 10-minute mile (6 mph) is a 10 MET activity

Box 1.2 Definitions of Levels, Components, and Intensity of Physical Activity [45]

Levels of Physical Activity

Inactive	No activity beyond baseline (This is considered unhealthy.)
Low	Beyond baseline but fewer than 150 min/w (Better for health than inactive.)
Medium	150–300 min/wk (Additional and possible extensive health benefits.)
High	>300 min/wk (Additional and possible extensive health benefits.)

Components of Physical Activity

Intensity	How hard a person works
Frequency	How often an activity is performed
Duration	How long in one session or how many repetitions

Intensity of Physical Activity

Light	1.1–2.9 METs (1.1–2.9 times rest)
Moderate	3.0–5.9 METs
Vigorous	≥6.0 METs

KEY GUIDELINES FOR HEALTH

- Physical activity reduces the risk of many adverse health outcomes.
- Some physical activity is better than none.
- Additional benefits occur with increases in intensity, frequency, and duration.
- Both cardiorespiratory and resistance exercise are beneficial.
- Health benefits occur at all ages.
- Benefits far outweigh the possibility of adverse outcomes.
- Substantial health benefits are seen with 150 min/wk of moderate-intensity physical activity or 75 min/wk of vigorous physical activity or a combination.
- Additional health benefits are seen with 300 min/wk of moderate-intensity physical activity or 150 min/wk of vigorous physical activity or a combination.
- Resistance training—moderate or high in intensity—involving all major muscle groups is recommended 2 d/wk or more.
- For health, 2 minutes of moderate physical activity equals 1 minute of vigorous physical activity.

SUMMARY

Exercise physiology is the study of the alterations and responses to acute and chronic exercise. Exercise disrupts homeostasis resulting in increased energy needs to meet metabolic demands of active muscles. The respiratory and cardiovascular systems work in a coordinated fashion to supply oxygen and nutrients to working muscles in an attempt to meet demand. At low- or moderate-intensity exercise, the body can use carbohydrate and fat via aerobic metabolism, meeting the energy demands with ease. As exercise intensity increases, the body's reliance on carbohydrate for a fuel source with some ATP being generated through anaerobic glycolysis increases. Short-term or metabolic fatigue is a result of reliance on anaerobic metabolism, while long-term or substrate fatigue is a result of glycogen depletion. Exercise training results in positive physiological adaptations that improve performance. Several principles of exercise training are key for determining the performance outcome.

RDNs should be comfortable discussing exercise with their patients or clients while staying within their scope of practice. The extent of this discussion will depend on comfort level and any additional education and certification. All RDNs should be able to discuss the health benefits of exercise and the general principles in the federal Physical Activity Guidelines for Americans. Beyond this, if the RDN cannot complete a fitness assessment and exercise prescription, then the RDN should refer to a qualified exercise professional.

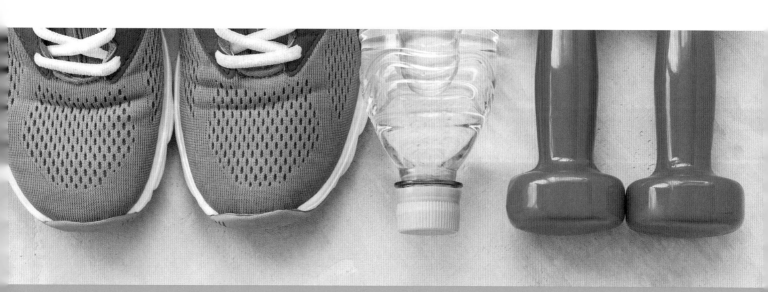

An understanding of exercise physiology basics is necessary for all RDNs interested in sports nutrition to understand the sports nutrition specific guidelines and their effects on performance.

Exercise results in increased skeletal muscle ATP demand, and the cardiovascular and respiratory systems work in a coordinated fashion to deliver oxygen and nutrients to the working skeletal muscle.

The key nutrients providing energy during exercise are carbohydrate and fat. Carbohydrate can provide ATP via both anaerobic and aerobic metabolism, but fat can only be fully oxidized aerobically.

At all times, the body is using a mixture of carbohydrate and fat. As exercise intensity increases, there is an increased reliance on carbohydrate for fuel (crossover concept). Carbohydrate is a more oxygen-efficient fuel and can produce ATP quickly.

Short-term or metabolic fatigue is a result of reliance on anaerobic metabolism under high exercise intensities. Long-term or substrate fatigue is a result of glycogen depletion.

Sound training results in physiological adaptations that improve performance. There are several principles of training that should be considered.

RDNs should include physical activity in their use of the Nutrition Care Process.

All RDNs interested in sports nutrition should be comfortable discussing the health benefits of exercise and the key principles presented in the federal Physical Activity Guidelines for Americans.

An RDN may or may not have the education and training to conduct fitness assessments and develop exercise prescriptions. If not, the RDN must refer to a qualified exercise professional.

REFERENCES

1. Kenny WL, Wilmore JH, Costill DL. *Physiology of Sport and Exercise.* 6th ed. Champaign, IL: Human Kinetics; 2015.

2. Achten J, Gleeson M, Jeukendrup AE. Determination of the exercise intensity that elicits maximal fat oxidation. *Med Sci Sports Exerc.* 2002;34(1):92-97.

3. Brooks GA. Bioenergetics of exercising humans. *Compr Physiol.* 2012;2(1):537-562.

4. Gollnick PD. Metabolism of substrates: energy substrate metabolism during exercise and as modified by training. *Fed Proc.* 1985;44(2):353-357.

5. Newsholme EA. The control of fuel utilization by muscle during exercise and starvation. *Diabetes.* 1979;28(suppl 1):1-7.

6. Fry AC, Allemeier CA, Staron RS. Correlation between percentage fiber type area and myosin heavy chain content in human skeletal muscle. *Eur J Appl Physiol Occup Physiol.* 1994;68(3):246-251.

7. Herzog W, Powers K, Johnston K, Duvall M. A new paradigm for muscle contraction. *Front Physiol.* 2015;6:1-11.

8. Staron RS, Karapondo DL, Kraemer WJ, et al. Skeletal muscle adaptations during early phase of heavy-resistance training in men and women. *J Appl Physiol (1985).* 1994;76(3):1247-1255.

9. Systrom DM, Lewis GD. Up to Date: Exercise Physiology. UpToDate website. www.uptodate.com/contents/exercise-physiology. Updated July 25, 2016. Accessed July 25, 2016.

10. Barnard RJ, Edgerton VR, Furukawa T, Peter JB. Histochemical, biochemical, and contractile properties of red, white, and intermediate fibers. *Am J Physiol.* 1971;220(2):410-414.

11. Brooke MH, Kaiser KK. Muscle fiber types: how many and what kind? *Arch Neurol.* 1970;23(4):369-379.

12. Fry AC, Schilling BK, Staron RS, Hagerman FC, Hikida RS, Thrush JT. Muscle fiber characteristics and performance correlates of male Olympic-style weightlifters. *J Strength Cond Res.* 2003;17(4):746-754.

13. Fry AC, Webber JM, Weiss LW, Harber MP, Vaczi M, Pattison NA. Muscle fiber characteristics of competitive power lifters. *J Strength Cond Res.* 2003;17(2):402-410.

14. Jurimae J, Abernethy PJ, Quigley BM, Blake K, McEniery MT. Differences in muscle contractile characteristics among bodybuilders, endurance trainers and control subjects. *Eur J Appl Physiol Occup Physiol.* 1997;75(4):357-362.

15. Kesidis N, Metaxas TI, Vrabas IS, et al. Myosin heavy chain isoform distribution in single fibres of bodybuilders. *Eur J Appl Physiol.* 2008;103(5):579-583.

16. Klitgaard H, Zhou M, Richter EA. Myosin heavy chain composition of single fibres from m. biceps brachii of male body builders. *Acta Physiol Scand.* 1990;140(2):175-180.

17. Shoepe TC, Stelzer JE, Garner DP, Widrick JJ. Functional adaptability of muscle fibers to long-term resistance exercise. *Med Sci Sports Exerc.* 2003;35(6):944-951.

18. D'Antona G, Lanfranconi F, Pellegrino MA, et al. Skeletal muscle hypertrophy and structure and function of skeletal muscle fibres in male body builders. *J Physiol.* 2006;570(pt 3):611-627.

19. MacDougall JD, Sale DG, Alway SE, Sutton JR. Muscle fiber number in biceps brachii in bodybuilders and control subjects. *J Appl Physiol Respir Environ Exerc Physiol.* 1984;57(5):1399-1403.

20. Costill DL, Coyle EF, Fink WF, Lesmes GR, Witzmann FA. Adaptations in skeletal muscle following strength training. *J Appl Physiol Respir Environ Exerc Physiol.* 1979;46(1):96-99.

21. Gollnick PD, Armstrong RB, Saubert CW, Piehl K, Saltin B. Enzyme activity and fiber composition in skeletal muscle of untrained and trained men. *J Appl Physiol.* 1972;33(3):312-319.

22. Harber MP, Gallagher PM, Creer AR, Minchev KM, Trappe SW. Single muscle fiber contractile properties during a competitive season in male runners. *Am J Physiol Regul Integr Comp Physiol.* 2004;287(5):R1124-R1131.

23. Trappe S, Harber M, Creer A, et al. Single muscle fiber adaptations with marathon training. *J Appl Physiol (1985).* 2006;101(3):721-727.

24. Saltin B, Gollnick PD. Skeletal muscle adaptability: significance for metabolism and performance. In: Peachey L, ed. *Handbook of Physiology.* Baltimore, MD: American Physiological Society; 1983:555-631.

25. Concu A, Marcello C. Stroke volume response to progressive exercise in athletes engaged in different types of training. *Eur J Appl Physiol Occup Physiol.* 1993;66(1):11-17.

26. Casey DP, Joyner MJ. Local control of skeletal muscle blood flow during exercise: influence of available oxygen. *J Appl Physiol (1985).* 2011;111(6):1527-1538.

27. Bassett DR Jr, Howley ET. Limiting factors for maximum oxygen uptake and determinants of endurance performance. *Med Sci Sports Exerc.* 2000;32(1):70-84.

28. Howley ET, Bassett DR Jr, Welch HG. Criteria for maximal oxygen uptake: review and commentary. *Med Sci Sports Exerc.* 1995;27(9):1292-1301.

29. Taylor HL, Buskirk E, Henschel A. Maximal oxygen intake as an objective measure of cardio-respiratory performance. *J Appl Physiol.* 1955;8(1):73-80.

30. Foster C, Kuffel E, Bradley N, et al. VO2max during successive maximal efforts. *European J Appl Physiol.* 2007;102(1):67-72.

31. Stromme SB, Ingjer F, Meen HD. Assessment of maximal aerobic power in specifically trained athletes. *J Appl Physiol Respir Environ Exerc Physiol.* 1977;42(6):833-837.

32. Wilmore JH, Stanforth PR, Gagnon J, et al. Cardiac output and stroke volume changes with endurance training: the HERITAGE Family Study. *Med Sci Sports Exerc.* 2001;33(1):99-106.

33. Gollnick PD, Riedy M, Quintinskie JJ, Bertocci LA. Differences in metabolic potential of skeletal muscle fibres and their significance for metabolic control. *J Exp Biol.* 1985;115:191-199.

34. Baar K. Nutrition and the adaptation to endurance training. *Sports Med.* 2014;44(suppl 1):5S-12S.

35. Bergstrom J, Hermanssen L, Saltin B. Diet, muscle glycogen, and physical performance. *Acta Physiol Scand.* 1967;71(2):140-150.

36. Jeukendrup AE. Performance and endurance in sport: can it all be explained by metabolism and its manipulation? *Dialog Cardiovasc Med.* 2012;17(1):40-45.

37. Brooks GA. Lactate production under fully aerobic conditions: the lactate shuttle during rest and exercise. *Fed Proc.* 1986;45(13):2924-2929.

38. Stainsby WN, Brooks GA. Control of lactic acid metabolism in contracting muscles and during exercise. *Exerc Sport Sci Rev.* 1990;18:29-63.

39. Brooks GA, Mercier J. Balance of carbohydrate and lipid utilization during exercise: the "crossover" concept. *J Appl Physiol (1985).* 1994;76(6):2253-2261.

40. Allen DG, Lamb GD, Westerblad H. Skeletal muscle fatigue: cellular mechanisms. *Physiol Rev.* 2008;88(1):287-332.

41. Enoka RM, Stuart DG. Neurobiology of muscle fatigue. *J Appl Physiol (1985).* 1992;72(5):1631-1648.

42. Fitts RH. Cellular mechanisms of muscle fatigue. *Physiol Rev.* 1994;74(1):49-94.

43. Manore MM. Weight management in the performance athlete. *Nestle Nutr Inst Workshop Ser.* 2013;75:123-133.

44. Manore MM. Weight management for athletes and active individuals: a brief review. *Sports Med.* 2015;45(suppl 1):83-92.

45. Office of Disease Prevention and Health Promotion, US Department of Health and Human Services. 2008 Physical Activity Guidelines for Americans. http://health.gov/paguidelines. Published 2008. Accessed May 30, 2016.

46. Issurin VB. New horizons for the methodology and physiology of training periodization. *Sports Med.* 2010;40(3):189-206.

47. Meeusen R, Duclos M, Foster C, et al. Prevention, diagnosis, and treatment of the overtraining syndrome: joint consensus statement of the European College of Sports Medicine and the American College of Sports Medicine. *Med Sci Sports Exerc.* 2013;45(1):186-205.

48. Kreher JB, Schwartz JB. Overtraining syndrome: a practical guide. *Sports Health.* 2012;(2):128-138.

49. American College of Sports Medicine. ACSM ProFinder. ACSM Certification website. http://certification.acsm.org/pro-finder. Accessed February 2, 2016.

50. US Registry of Exercise Professionals. USREPS website. www.usreps.org/Pages/Default.aspx. Accessed February 2, 2016.

51. Commission on Accreditation of Allied Health Education Programs. www.caahep.org. Accessed July 25, 2016.

52. Academy of Nutrition and Dietetics. Nutrition Terminology Reference Manual (eNCPT): Dietetics Language for Nutrition Care. 2014; http://ncpt.webauthor.com. Accessed July 24, 2016.

CHAPTER 2

CARBOHYDRATE AND EXERCISE

Ellen J. Coleman, MA, MPH, RD, CSSD

INTRODUCTION

Adequate carbohydrate stores (muscle and liver glycogen and blood glucose) are critical for optimum performance during both intermittent high-intensity work and prolonged endurance exercise. Nutritional strategies to enhance the availability of carbohydrate before, during, and after exercise are recommended.

Consuming carbohydrate before exercise can help performance by topping off existing muscle and liver glycogen stores. Consuming carbohydrate during exercise can improve performance by maintaining blood glucose levels and carbohydrate oxidation, sparing muscle glycogen, or activating reward centers in the central nervous system. Ingesting carbohydrate after glycogen-depleting exercise facilitates rapid glycogen restoration, especially among athletes engaged in daily hard training or tournament activity.

CARBOHYDRATE AVAILABILITY DURING EXERCISE

Muscle glycogen represents the major source of carbohydrate in the body (300 to 400 g or 1,200 to 1,600 kcal), followed by liver glycogen (75 to 100 g or 300 to 400 kcal), and, lastly, blood glucose (5 g or 20 kcal). These amounts vary substantially among individuals, depending on factor per kilogram of wet muscle weight. Carbohydrate loading increases muscle glycogen stores to 210 to 230 mmol/kg of wet muscle weight.[1]

The energy demands of exercise dictate that carbohydrate is the predominant fuel for exercise.[2] Muscle glycogen and blood glucose provide about half of the energy for moderate-intensity exercise (65% of maximal oxygen uptake [VO_2 max]) and two-thirds of the energy for high-intensity exercise (85% of VO_2 max). It is impossible to meet the adenosine triphosphate (ATP) requirements for high-intensity, high-power output exercise when these carbohydrate fuels are depleted.[2] Utilization of muscle glycogen is most rapid during early stages of exercise, exponentially related to exercise intensity.[1,3]

Liver glycogen stores maintain blood glucose levels both at rest and during exercise. At rest, the brain and central nervous system utilize most of the blood glucose, and muscle accounts for less than 20% of blood glucose utilization. During exercise, however, muscle glucose uptake can increase 30-fold, depending on exercise intensity and duration. Initially, the majority of hepatic glucose output comes from glycogenolysis; however, as exercise duration increases and liver glycogen decreases, the contribution of glucose from gluconeogenesis increases.[1,3]

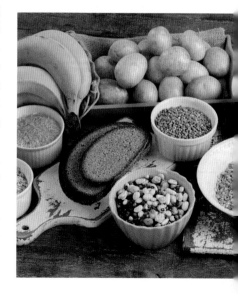

At the beginning of exercise, hepatic glucose output matches the increased muscle glucose uptake, so blood glucose levels remain near resting levels.[3] Although muscle glycogen is the primary source of carbohydrate during exercise intensities between 65% and 75% of VO_2 max, blood glucose becomes an increasingly important source of carbohydrate as muscle glycogen stores decrease.[2] Hypoglycemia occurs when the hepatic glucose output can no longer keep up with muscle glucose uptake during prolonged exercise.[3]

Liver glycogen stores can be depleted by a 15-hour fast, decreasing from a typical level of 490 mmol on a mixed diet to 60 mmol on a low-carbohydrate diet. A high-carbohydrate diet can increase liver glycogen content to approximately 900 mmol.[1]

DAILY CARBOHYDRATE RECOMMENDATIONS

Consuming adequate carbohydrate daily is necessary to replenish muscle and liver glycogen between training sessions and competitive events and to help meet the energy requirements of an athlete's training program.[4-9]

An athlete's carbohydrate status is determined by his or her total daily intake and the timing of carbohydrate intake relative to exercise. A diet with high carbohydrate availability maintains an adequate supply of carbohydrate substrate for the muscle and central nervous system for exercise. Conversely, carbohydrate fuel sources are depleted or limited for exercise in a diet with low carbohydrate availability.[4]

Carbohydrate availability is increased by (1) consuming carbohydrate in the hours or days before exercise; (2) ingesting carbohydrate during exercise; and (3) consuming carbohydrate after exercise. High carbohydrate availability is recommended for competition and key training sessions to promote optimal performance.[4] Targets for daily carbohydrate intake should be based on the athlete's body weight (to account for the size of the athlete's muscle mass) and the athlete's training load.[4,5]

Carbohydrate recommendations for athletes range from 3 to 12 g of carbohydrate per kilogram of body weight per day.[4,5] Athletes with very light training programs (low-intensity exercise or skill-based exercise) should consume 3 to 5 g/kg/d.[4,5] These targets may also be suitable for athletes with a large body mass or athletes who need to reduce energy intake to lose weight.[4] Athletes engaged in moderate-intensity training programs for 60 min/d should consume 5 to 7 g/kg/d. During moderate- to high-intensity endurance exercise lasting for 1 to 3 hours, athletes should consume 6 to 10 g/kg/d.[4,5] Athletes participating in moderate- to high-intensity endurance exercise for 4 to 5 h/d or more (eg, the Tour de France) should consume 8 to 12 g/kg/d.[4,5,10] These are general recommendations and should be adjusted with consideration for the athlete's total energy needs, specific training needs, and feedback from their training performance.[4,5]

Carbohydrate intake can be strategically adjusted around important exercise sessions to enhance performance and promote recovery. An athlete's carbohydrate requirement may also change based on alterations in daily, weekly, or seasonal exercise goals.[4]

Recommended daily carbohydrate intake is summarized in Box 2.1.

Box 2.1 Recommended Daily Carbohydrate Intake for Trained Athletes[4,5]

Recommended daily carbohydrate intake ranges from 3 to 12 g/kg. Adjust with consideration for the athlete's total energy needs, specific training needs (see chart), and feedback from training performance. Carbohydrate intake should be spread over the day to promote fuel availability for key training sessions—before, during, or after exercise.

Type of Activity	Recommended Carbohydrate Intake, g/kg
Very-light training program (low-intensity or skill-based exercise)	3–5
Moderate-intensity training programs, 60 min/d	5–7
Moderate- to high-intensity endurance exercise, 1–3 h/d	6–10
Moderate- to high-intensity exercise, 4–5 h/d	8–12

Athletes should consume sufficient energy as well as carbohydrate.[10] Consumption of a reduced-energy diet impairs endurance performance due to muscle and liver glycogen depletion.[4,5,11] Adequate carbohydrate intake is also important for athletes in high-power activities (eg, wrestling, gymnastics, and dance) who have lost weight due to negative energy balances.[12] Weight loss and consumption of low-energy diets are prevalent among athletes in high-power activities. A negative energy balance can harm high-power performance due to impaired acid-base balance, reduced glycolytic enzyme levels, selective atrophy of type II muscle fibers, and abnormal sarcoplasmic reticulum function. In practical terms, the athlete cannot sustain high-intensity exercise. However, adequate dietary carbohydrate may ameliorate some of the damaging effects of energy restriction on the muscle.[12]

Foods that provide approximately 25 g of carbohydrate per serving are shown in Box 2.2. These are typical serving sizes, making it easy for the sports dietitian or athlete to understand how much carbohydrate is in a typical serving when planning meals and snacks.

Box 2.2 Carbohydrate-Rich Foods: 25-g Portions

Grains
- 2 slices whole-wheat bread
- ½ deli-style bagel
- 2-oz English muffin
- 1 cup oatmeal
- 1 cup ready-to-eat breakfast cereal
- 1 package snack-type cheese crackers (6 to a package)
- 2 fig cookie bars
- ½ cup rice
- ½ cup cooked pasta
- 5 cups popcorn
- ½ large soft pretzel
- 17 mini pretzels
- 1 flour tortilla (12-in diameter)
- 1 oz tortilla chips and ¼ cup salsa

Dairy Products and Other Beverages
- 2 cups milk (low-fat or nonfat)
- 1 cup low-fat chocolate milk
- 4.5-oz container fruit-flavored yogurt
- 6 oz plain yogurt
- 1 cup vanilla-flavored soy milk
- 1 package instant hot chocolate (made with water)

Beans and Starchy Vegetables
- ½ cup black beans
- ½ cup baked beans
- ¾ cup kidney beans
- ½ cup lima beans
- 1 cup green peas
- ½ cup corn
- ¾ cup mashed potatoes
- ½ medium baked potato with skin

Sports Drinks, Bars, and Gels
- 2 cups sports drink (6%–8% carbohydrate-containing sports drink)
- 1 energy bar[a]
- 1 carbohydrate gel
- ½ can nutrition shake
- ½ can meal replacement shake

Mixed Dishes
- 1 slice thin-crust pizza with meat or veggie toppings
- ½ slice thick-crust pizza with meat or veggie toppings
- 1 small bean and rice burrito
- ½ cup black beans and rice
- 1½ cups canned chicken noodle soup
- ¾ cup tomato soup
- 1 cup cooked ramen noodles
- ½ 6-in submarine sandwich
- ½ cup macaroni and cheese

Fruit and Juice
- 2 cups fresh strawberries
- 1 large orange
- ¾ cup orange juice
- ½ cup cranberry-apple juice
- 1 medium apple

a = 25 g is an average, taken from many energy bars; individual brands may vary in exact carbohydrate portion size

COMMUNICATING CARBOHYDRATE RECOMMENDATIONS

Population dietary guidelines generally express goals for macronutrient intake as a percentage of total energy. However, the *absolute quantity* of carbohydrate, rather than the percentage of energy from carbohydrate, is important for exercise performance. Carbohydrate guidelines based on grams per kilogram of body weight are also user-friendly and practical. It is relatively easy to determine the carbohydrate content of meals and snacks to daily carbohydrate goals.[4,5]

Another problem with using percentages is that an athlete's energy and carbohydrate requirements are not always matched. Athletes with large muscle mass and heavy training regimens generally have very high energy requirements and can meet their carbohydrate needs with a lower percentage of energy from carbohydrate. When an athlete consumes 4,000 to 5,000 kcal/d, even a diet providing 50% of energy from carbohydrate will supply 500 to 600 g/d. This translates into 7 to 8 g/kg for a 70-kg athlete, which should be adequate to maintain muscle glycogen stores from day to day.[5]

Conversely, when a 60-kg athlete consumes fewer than 2,000 kcal/d, even a diet providing 60% of energy from carbohydrate (4 to 5 g/kg/d) may not provide sufficient carbohydrate to maintain optimal carbohydrate stores for daily training. This situation is particularly common in female athletes who restrict energy intake to achieve or maintain a low body weight or percentage of body fat.[5]

GLYCEMIC INDEX AND GLYCEMIC LOAD

The glycemic index (GI) provides a way to rank carbohydrate-rich foods according to the blood glucose response after these foods are consumed. GI is calculated by measuring the incremental area under the blood glucose curve after ingestion of a test food providing 50 g carbohydrate compared with a reference food (glucose or white bread). Foods with a low GI cause a slower, sustained release of glucose to the blood, whereas foods with a high GI cause a rapid, short-lived increase in blood glucose.[13]

Foods are usually divided into those that have a high GI (glucose, bread, potatoes, breakfast cereal, and sports drinks), a moderate GI (sucrose, soft drinks, oats, and tropical fruits, such as bananas and mangos), or a low GI (fructose, milk, yogurt, lentils, pasta, nuts, and fruits, such as apples and oranges). Tables of GI values for a large number of foods have been published and are available at the Glycemic Index Foun-

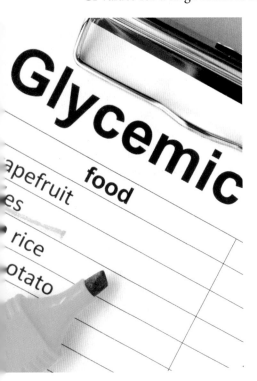

dation website (www.gifoundation.com); another useful resource is the GI site from the University of Sydney (www.glycemicindex.com).[14]

Some practitioners recommend manipulating the GI of food choices before, during, and after exercise to improve athletic performance. For example, low GI foods and low-carbohydrate foods are recommended before exercise to promote sustained carbohydrate availability. Moderate-to high-GI carbohydrate foods are recommended periexercise to promote carbohydrate oxidation and postexercise to promote glycogen repletion. However, the research data are mixed, and there is substantial debate about the benefit of manipulating GI to improve athletic performance.[5,13]

The glycemic load (GL) considers both GI and the amount of carbohydrate consumed.[14] The formula is: GL = GI × dietary carbohydrate content (GI is expressed as a decimal and dietary carbohydate content is expressed in grams). The GL of a food is almost always less than its corresponding GI and provides an overview of the daily diet.

The GI may be useful in sports as it may help athletes fine-tune food choices, but it should not be used exclusively to provide guidelines for intake before, during, and after exercise. Athletes should choose foods to match the practical demands of the event and individual preferences and experiences.[4,13]

Glycemic Effects of Modified Starches

Technological advances have allowed starches to be modified by various means (eg, hydrothermally or chemically). The type of modification produces either a fast-digesting starch (high GI) or a slow-digesting starch (low GI) with different effects on blood glucose and insulin responses.[15]

Stephens and colleagues evaluated the effect of postexercise consumption of a high molecular weight, fast-digesting (high GI) modified starch (Vitargo) on metabolic responses and subsequent time-trial performance. Consuming 100 g of the modified starch after glycogen-depleting exercise significantly increased serum glucose and insulin levels during a 2-hour recovery period and improved time-trial performance by 10%, compared with consuming 100 g of a low molecular-weight maltodextrin recovery drink. The authors speculated that the improved time-trial performance observed with modified starch group was due to greater resynthesis of muscle glycogen during recovery.[16]

Roberts and associates evaluated the effect of preexercise consumption of a high-molecular-weight, slow-digesting (low GI) modified starch (UCAN) on metabolic responses during submaximal exercise and time-trial performance. Consuming 1 g/kg of the modified starch 30 minutes before prolonged exercise (150 minutes at 70% VO_2 peak) significantly blunted the initial spike in serum glucose and insulin levels and increased fat breakdown compared with consuming 1 g/kg of a maltodextrin drink. However, there was no significant difference in time-trial performance between the modified starch group and the maltodextrin drink group.[17]

Modifying starches appears to enhance carbohydrate availability in multiple ways. A high-GI modified starch could enhance muscle glycogen storage postexercise, and a low-GI modified starch could sustain blood glucose levels during prolonged endurance exercise.[16,17] Further research is warranted due to the limited data on modified starches and athletic performance.[15]

MUSCLE GLYCOGEN SUPERCOMPENSATION

Muscle glycogen depletion is a well-recognized limitation to endurance performance.[3-5] Carbohydrate loading (glycogen supercompensation) can increase muscle glycogen stores from resting levels of 130 to 135 mmol/kg to approximately 210 to 230 mmol/kg and improve performance in endurance events exceeding 90 minutes.[13,18-20]

For endurance athletes, carbohydrate loading is an extended period of fueling up to prepare for competition.[13] The regimen can postpone fatigue and extend the duration of steady-state exercise by about 20% and improve endurance performance by about 2% to 3% in which a set distance is covered as quickly as possible.[18] Carbohydrate loading enables the athlete to maintain high-intensity exercise longer but will not affect pace for the first hour.[19]

The classical regimen of carbohydrate loading involved a 3-day depletion phase of hard training and a low carbohydrate intake. The athlete finished with a 3-day loading phase of tapered training and a high-carbohydrate intake before the event.[4] Subsequent research found that high glycogen concentrations can be achieved without a depletion phase by tapering training for 3 days and consuming a high carbohydrate diet of 10 g/kg/d.[21]

More recent studies suggest that endurance athletes can carbohydrate load in as little as 24 to 36 hours, provided that the athlete does not train and consumes adequate carbohydrate.[22,23] A high-carbohydrate diet of 10 g/kg/d significantly increased muscle glycogen from preloading levels of approximately 90 mmol/kg to approximately 180 mmol/kg after 1 day.[22] A high-carbohydrate intake of 10.3 g/kg after a 3-minute bout of high-intensity exercise enabled athletes to increase muscle glycogen levels from preloading levels of approximately 109 mmol/kg to 198 mmol/kg in 24 hours.[23]

The new carbohydrate loading guidelines recommend that athletes rest for 36 to 48 hours and consume 10 to 12 g/kg/d.[4,5] These updated guidelines are summarized in Table 2.1.

Table 2.1 Carbohydrate-Loading Guidelines

Day	Training	Carbohydrate
1	Rest	10–12 g/kg/d
2	Rest	10–12 g/kg/d
3	Competition	Follow carbohydrate guidelines for intake before competition, during competition, and after competition

It may not be possible to carbohydrate load repeatedly within a short time. Cyclists could not achieve high muscle glycogen levels following glycogen-depleting exercise when a second carbohydrate loading session was undertaken within 48 hours of the first session. However, the cyclists maintained their performance on the successive exercise test when a high-carbohydrate diet (12 g/kg/d) was consumed between trials.[24]

Most athletes need to eat frequently throughout the day to consume adequate carbohydrate and energy for glycogen supercompensation. To avoid gut distress, the athlete may benefit from consuming low-fiber foods such as pasta, white rice, pancakes, cereal and fruit bars, sports nutrition bars and gels, yogurt, baked goods, and low-fat or nonfat sweets (eg, hard candy). Carbohydrate-rich fluids, such as sports drinks, low-fat chocolate milk, liquid meals, liquid high-carbohydrate supplements, yogurt drinks, and fruit smoothies, augment carbohydrate and energy intake.[5,13]

Although some bodybuilders use carbohydrate loading to increase muscle size and enhance appearance, there was no increase in the girths of seven muscle groups after a carbohydrate-loading regimen in resistance-trained bodybuilders.[25] Carbohydrate loading will also not enhance performance in events lasting less than 90 minutes and may harm performance due to the associated stiffness and weight gain.[13]

Endurance training promotes glycogen supercompensation by increasing the activity of glycogen synthase, but the athlete must be trained or the regimen will not be effective. Because glycogen stores are specific to the muscle groups used, the exercise used to deplete the stores must be the same as the athlete's competitive event. Some athletes note a feeling of stiffness and heaviness associated with the increased glycogen storage (since additional water is stored with glycogen), but these sensations dissipate with exercise.[13]

As with other nutrition strategies, athletes should test their carbohydrate-loading regimen during a prolonged workout or a low priority race.[13]

CARBOHYDRATE SUPPLEMENTS

Athletes who train heavily and have difficulty eating enough food to consume adequate carbohydrate and energy can utilize a high-carbohydrate liquid supplement.[26] Most products contain glucose polymers (maltodextrins) or modified starches to reduce the solution's osmolality and potential for gastrointestinal distress.

High-carbohydrate supplements do not replace regular food, but they do help supplement energy, carbohydrate, and liquid during heavy training or carbohydrate loading. If the athlete has no difficulty eating enough conventional food, these products offer only the advantage of convenience.

Liquid high-carbohydrate supplements should be consumed before or after exercise, either with meals or between meals. Although ultraendurance athletes may also use them during exercise to obtain energy and carbohydrate, these products are too concentrated in carbohydrate to double as a fluid-replacement beverage.

Consuming carbohydrate-rich foods and fluids in the 4 hours before exercise helps to (1) restore liver glycogen, especially for morning exercise when liver glycogen is depleted from an overnight fast; (2) increase muscle glycogen stores if they are not fully restored from the previous exercise session; (3) prevent hunger, which may in itself impair performance; and (4) provide glucose for the central nervous system. Including some low-GI foods *may* be beneficial in promoting a sustained release of glucose into the bloodstream when carbohydrate cannot be consumed during exercise.[13]

Consuming carbohydrate on the morning of an endurance event may help to maintain blood glucose levels during prolonged exercise. Compared with an overnight fast, ingesting a meal containing 200 to 300 g of carbohydrate 2 to 4 hours before exercise improves endurance performance.[27-29]

The preexercise meal should contain 1 to 4 g carbohydrate per kilogram body weight and be consumed 1 to 4 hours before exercise.[4,28,30] To avoid potential gastrointestinal distress when blood is diverted from the gut to the exercising muscles, the carbohydrate and energy content of the meal should be reduced the closer to exercise that it is consumed. For example, a carbohydrate feeding of 1 g/kg is appropriate 1 hour before exercise, whereas 4 g/kg can be consumed 4 hours before exercise. Athletes may also need to avoid foods high in fat, protein, and fiber to reduce the risk of gastrointestinal issues during exercise.[4] Recommendations for carbohydrate intake before exercise are summarized in Box 2.3.

If the athlete is unable to eat breakfast before early morning exercise, consuming approximately 30 g of an easily digested carbohydrate-rich food or fluid, such as a banana, carbohydrate gel, or sports drink, 5 minutes before exercise may improve endurance performance.[31]

The performance benefits of a preexercise meal may be additive to consuming carbohydrate during prolonged exercise. Although the combined feedings provided the greatest benefit, the preexercise feeding was less effective than carbohydrate consumed during exercise. Thus, to obtain a continuous supply of glucose, the endurance athlete should consume carbohydrate during exercise.[29]

A number of commercially formulated liquid meals satisfy the requirements for preexercise food: they are high in carbohydrate and provide both energy and fluid. Some were designed for hospital patients (eg, Ensure and Sustacal), whereas others have been specifically created for and marketed to athletes (eg, Myoplex Original and Muscle Milk).

Liquid meals can be consumed closer to competition than regular meals due to a shorter gastric emptying time. This may help avoid precompetition nausea for athletes who are tense or anxious and have an associated delay in gastric emptying.[5]

Box 2.3 Recommended Carbohydrate Intake Before Exercise

- Consider both the amount and timing of carbohydrate intake. See the chart for general recommendations.
- If you are unable to eat breakfast before early morning exercise, consuming approximately 30 g of easily digested carbohydrate 5 minutes before exercise may improve performance.
- Low glycemic index foods may be beneficial when carbohydrate cannot be consumed during exercise.

Timing Before Exercise	Carbohyrate
1 hour	1 g/kg
2 hours	2 g/kg
3 hours	3 g/kg
4 hours	4 g/kg

Liquid meals produce a low stool residue, thereby minimizing immediate weight gain. This is especially advantageous for athletes who need to "make weight." Liquid meals are convenient for athletes competing in day-long tournaments, meets, and ultraendurance events (eg, Ironman Triathlon). Liquid meals can also be used for nutritional supplementation during heavy training when energy requirements are extremely elevated.

Carbohydrate in the Hour Before Exercise

Based primarily on the results of only one early study, athletes have been cautioned to avoid eating carbohydrate in the hour before exercise. In the late 1970s, researchers found that consuming 75 g of glucose 30 minutes before cycling at 80% of VO_2 max caused initial rapid decrease in blood glucose and reduced exercise time by 19%. High blood insulin levels induced by preexercise carbohydrate feeding were blamed for this chain of events.[32] However, subsequent studies have contradicted these findings. Preexercise carbohydrate feedings either improve performance or have no detrimental effect. In most cases, the decrease in blood glucose observed during the first 20 minutes of exercise is self-correcting and has no apparent effects on the athlete.[13,30,33]

A small number of athletes react negatively to carbohydrate feedings in the hour before exercise and experience symptoms of hypoglycemia and fatigue. The reason for this unusual reaction is not known. Preventive strategies include the following[34]:

1. Choose low-GI carbohydrate sources before exercise because they produce more stable glucose and insulin responses.

2. Consume carbohydrate a few minutes before exercise.

3. Wait until exercising to consume carbohydrate.

The metabolic and performance effects of ingesting carbohydrate shortly before exercise are similar to consuming carbohydrate during exercise. The exercise-induced increase in the hormones epinephrine, norepinephrine, and growth hormone inhibit the release of insulin and thus counter insulin's effect in reducing blood glucose.[34]

Preexercise Carbohydrate and the Glycemic Index

A 1991 study sparked interest in the use of the GI in sports.[35] Consumption of 1 g carbohydrate per kilogram from lentils (low GI) 1 hour before cycling at 67% of VO_2 max promoted more stable blood glucose levels during exercise and increased endurance performance compared with an equal amount of carbohydrate from potatoes (high GI). Few studies have reported enhanced endurance from consuming low GI meals before exercise, although most studies have failed to show improvements in exercise performance.[4,13,36]

The overall importance of the preexercise meal for maintaining carbohydrate availability is questionable because endurance athletes also consume carbohydrate-rich foods and fluids during prolonged exercise.[4] When carbohydrate is ingested *during* exercise, according to sports nutrition guidelines, there is no difference in performance or carbohydrate oxidation between low- and high-GI preexercise meals. Thus, consuming carbohydrate during exercise negates the glycemic effects of the preexercise meal on performance and metabolism.[13,36-38]

A low-GI preexercise meal may be beneficial when it is difficult to consume carbohydrate during prolonged exercise or when the athlete reacts negatively to carbohydrate feedings. However, there is no evidence that athletes will universally benefit from low-GI preexercise meals, especially when athletes can refuel during exercise. The type, timing, and amount of carbohydrate in the preexercise meal should be individualized based on the athlete's specific event, gut comfort, and individual preferences.[4,13]

Consuming a high-GI carbohydrate (eg, glucose) immediately before anaerobic exercise, such as sprinting or weight lifting, will not provide athletes with a quick burst of energy, allowing them to exercise harder. There is adequate ATP, creatine phosphate, and muscle glycogen already stored for these anaerobic tasks.

It is well established that consuming carbohydrate during exercise can increase exercise capacity and improve performance. For exercise lasting longer than 2 hours, the effects are primarily metabolic: carbohydrate ingestion prevents hypoglycemia, maintains high rates of carbohydrate oxidation, and improves endurance.[39-43]

During prolonged exercise, blood glucose becomes an increasingly important fuel source as muscle glycogen stores decrease. Carbohydrate feedings maintain blood glucose levels at a time when muscle glycogen stores are diminished. Thus, carbohydrate oxidation (and, therefore, ATP production) can continue at a high rate, and performance is enhanced.[39,40,43]

Carbohydrate feedings may also improve performance during high-intensity (more than 75% VO_2 max), relatively short-duration exercise (approximately 1 hour). Since this type of activity is not limited by the availability of muscle glycogen or blood glucose, the underlying mechanism for performance benefit is not metabolic, though it may be tied to the central nervous system.[4,43]

When individuals rinse their mouths with a carbohydrate solution, the improvements in performance are very similar to those seen with carbohydrate ingestion. Experts speculate that carbohydrate receptors in the oral cavity signal the central nervous system to positively modify motor output, thereby improving performance. The precise receptors in the oral cavity have not yet been identified, and the exact role of various brain areas is not clearly understood. Further research is warranted.[43,44]

Current evidence suggests that using a carbohydrate mouth rinse or consuming very small amounts of carbohydrate during high-power exercise lasting 30 to 75 minutes may improve performance by 2% to 3%. The benefits are more pronounced after an overnight fast but are evident even after a preexercise meal.[45]

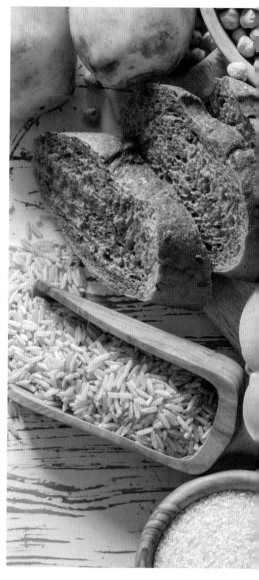

Although it makes sense that athletes should consume high-GI carbohydrates to promote carbohydrate oxidation, glycemic response to carbohydrate feedings during exercise has not been systematically studied. However, most athletes choose carbohydrate-rich foods (sports nutrition bars and gels) and fluids (sports drinks) that would be classified as having a moderate to high GI.[36]

Carbohydrate During Intermittent, High-Intensity Sports

Most team sports, such as basketball, soccer, hockey, and football, have bursts of very high-intensity exercise followed by relatively low-intensity recovery periods. A large number of studies have demonstrated that consuming carbohydrate during intermittent, high-intensity running delays fatigue and increases time to exhaustion.[43,46-50]

Consuming carbohydrate improved performance during a shuttle-running test designed to replicate the activity pattern of intermittent, high-intensity sports.[47] Carbohydrate ingestion also enhanced endurance capacity during intermittent high-intensity running, possibly by maintaining blood glucose levels toward the end of exercise.[48,49] During the fourth quarter of a sodium-dependent glucose transporter, intermittent, high-intensity shuttle run designed to replicate basketball, carbohydrate feedings resulted in longer run time to fatigue and faster sprint time.[50] These studies establish that the benefits of carbohydrate feedings are not limited to prolonged endurance exercise.

Carbohydrate feedings may improve performance in intermittent, high-intensity sports by decreasing muscle glycogen utilization, increasing muscle glycogen resynthesis during rest or low-intensity periods, or increasing blood glucose. The beneficial effects of carbohydrate ingestion may also be mediated by the central nervous system. Further research is warranted to determine the mechanisms by which carbohydrate feedings influence intermittent, high-intensity performance.[46]

Multiple Transportable Carbohydrates for Endurance and Ultraendurance Performance

Since exogenous carbohydrate oxidation is limited by intestinal absorption of carbohydrates, a high rate of carbohydrate absorption is necessary to increase exogenous carbohydrate oxidation. The maximum amount of glucose that can be absorbed during exercise is about 1 g/min (60 g/h) because the sodium-dependent glucose transporter 1 (SGLT1) responsible for glucose absorption becomes saturated. However,

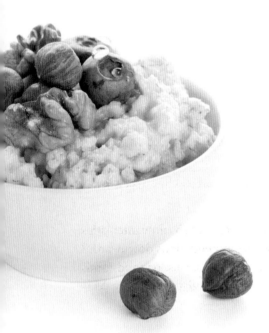

when glucose is consumed with fructose (absorbed by a transport mechanism called GLUT5), the maximum rate of carbohydrate oxidation exceeds 1 g/min.[51]

A series of studies determined the maximal rate of exogenous carbohydrate oxidation. The rate of carbohydrate ingestion varied, as did the types and combinations of carbohydrates. These studies confirmed that consuming multiple transportable carbohydrates resulted in up to 75% higher oxidation rates compared with carbohydrates that only use SGLT1.[43,52]

Currell and Jeukendrop showed that increased exogenous oxidation rates observed with multiple transportable carbohydrates delays fatigue and enhances endurance performance. Ingestion of glucose and fructose (1.8 g/min) during 2 hours of cycling at 55% of VO$_2$ max improved subsequent time-trial performance by 8% compared with an isocaloric amount of glucose.[53] This was the first study to show that increased exogenous carbohydrate oxidation improves endurance performance.

The performance benefits of multiple transportable carbohydrates are observed during endurance exercise lasting 2.5 hours or longer, becoming apparent during the third hour of exercise. Multiple transportable carbohydrates provide the same performance benefits as other carbohydrate sources during shorter duration exercise.[43,52]

Guidelines for Intake During Exercise

There is no relationship between body weight and exogenous carbohydrate use. Thus, guidelines for intake during exercise can be absolute (g/h) and not based on body weight.[4,5,43]

Recommendations for carbohydrate intake during exercise depend upon exercise duration, absolute exercise intensity, individual gut tolerance to intake, as well as the sport and its rules and regulations. In general, carbohydrate intake should increase as the duration of exercise increases. Duration of exercise also influences the type of carbohydrate consumed (single or multiple transportable carbohydrates) and determines advice for nutritional training.[4,5,43]

Consuming carbohydrate is not necessary during exercise lasting less than 30 minutes. During sustained high-intensity exercise lasting 30 to 75 minutes, consuming small amounts of single or multiple transportable carbohydrates or a carbohydrate mouth rinse may enhance performance.[43]

Athletes should consume 30 g of single or multiple transportable carbohydrates per hour during endurance and intermittent, high-intensity exercise lasting 1 to 2 hours. During endurance exercise lasting 2 to 3 hours, athletes should consume up to 60 g of single or multiple transportable carbohydrates per hour.[43]

As the duration of exercise increases, so does the amount of carbohydrate required to fuel performance.[4,5,43] There is evidence of a dose-response relationship between carbohydrate intake and performance in endurance events lasting 2.5 hours or longer.[54,55] The ingestion of carbohydrate significantly improves performance in a dose-dependent manner, and the greatest benefit is observed with between 60 and 90 g of carbohydrate per hour.[43,54,55] Thus, during endurance and ultraendurance exercise lasting 2.5 hours or more, athletes should consider consuming up to 90 g of multiple transportable carbohydrates per hour. Products providing multiple transportable carbohydrates help achieve high rates of carbohydrate oxidation during prolonged exercise.[4,5,43] Recommendations for carbohydrate intake during exercise are listed in Table 2.2.

Table 2.2 Recommended Carbohydrate Intake During Exercise

Type of Activity	Recommended Carbohydrate Intake
Exercise lasting less than 30 minutes	Not necessary or practical
High-intensity exercise lasting 30–75 minutes	Small amounts of carbohydrate orcarbohydrate mouth rinse—single or multiple transportable carbohydrates
Endurance and intermittent, high-intensity exercise lasting 1–2 hours	30 g/h—single or multiple transportable carbohydrates
Endurance exercise lasting 2–3 hours	60 g/h—single or multiple transportable carbohydrates
Endurance and ultraendurance exercise lasting 2.5 hours or more	Up to 90 g/h—multiple transportable carbohydrates, which help achieve high rates of carbohydrate oxidation

These recommendations are for well-trained athletes. Athletes who perform at lower absolute intensities will have lower carbohydrate oxidation rates and may need to adjust these recommendations downward.[43]

Athletes can achieve the recommended carbohydrate intake by consuming drinks, gels, or solid foods low in fat, protein, and fiber. Fuel selection should be guided by personal preference and gut tolerance. Various combinations of foods and fluids can be used to achieve carbohydrate intake goals.[4,5,43,56,57]

Carbohydrate intake must be balanced with hydration. Solid foods and highly concentrated carbohydrate solutions reduce the absorption of fluid. Using products with multiple transportable carbohydrates optimizes gastric emptying and intestinal absorption. Athletes should test their nutrition strategy in training to reduce the risk of gastrointestinal distress.[43]

The carbohydrate content of selected foods is listed in Table 2.3 (see page 32).

CARBOHYDRATE AFTER EXERCISE

The restoration of muscle and liver glycogen is essential for recovery between training sessions or competitive events, particularly when the athlete works out multiple times a day and has limited time to recover before the next exercise session. Utilizing effective refueling strategies after strenuous exercise promotes optimal glycogen resynthesis.[4,58-60]

When strenuous workouts or competitions occur less than 8 hours apart, athletes should consume carbohydrate *as soon as possible* after the first exercise session to maximize effective recovery time between sessions. For speedy refueling after glycogen-depleting exercise, athletes should consume 1 to 1.2 g of carbohydrate per kilogram per hour for the first 4 hours.[4] Consuming carbohydrate at frequent intervals (every 15 to 30 minutes for up to 4 hours postexercise also enhances muscle glycogen synthesis.[4,58] During longer recovery periods (24 hours or more), the timing, pattern, and type of carbohydrate intake can be chosen according to what is practical and enjoyable, provided the athlete consumes adequate carbohydrate and energy.[4,58]

Table 2.3 Examples of Carbohydrate Content of Selected Foods

Food	Portion	Carbohydrate
Sports drink	1 qt (~1 L)	60 g
Protein bar	1 bar	47 g
Energy gel pack	2 gels	50 g
Caffeinated jelly beans	28 pieces	50 g
Energy chews	6 chews	50 g
Graham crackers	3 large	66 g
Fig bars	4 bars	42 g
Banana	1 whole	30 g

Carbohydrate-rich foods with a moderate to high GI supply, a readily available source of carbohydrate for muscle glycogen synthesis, may help to maximize glycogen storage for athletes who have limited recovery time between workouts.[4,36,61] Adequate energy intake is necessary to optimize glycogen storage. Restrained eating practices interfere with meeting carbohydrate intake goals and glycogen restoration.[11]

The foods consumed during recovery meals and snacks should contribute to an athlete's overall nutrient intake. Nutrient-dense carbohydrates, lean meat, and reduced-fat dairy products also contain vitamins and minerals essential for performance and health.[13]

There is no difference in glycogen synthesis when liquid or solid forms of carbohydrate are consumed.[62] However, liquid forms of carbohydrate may be appealing when athletes have decreased appetite due to fatigue or dehydration.[26]

There are several reasons that glycogen repletion occurs faster after exercise: the blood flow to the muscles is much greater immediately after exercise; the muscle cells are more likely to take up glucose; and the muscle cells are more sensitive to the effects of insulin, which enhances the action of glycogen synthase.

Recommendations for carbohydrate intake postexercise are summarized in Box 2.4.

Box 2.4 Recommended Carbohydrate Intake After Glycogen-Depleting Exercise

- When exercise sessions are less than 8 hours apart, start consuming carbohydrate immediately after exercise to maximize recovery time.
- Consume 1 to 1.2 g of carbohydrate per kilogram per hour for the first 4 hours after glycogen-depleting exercise.
- Early refueling may be enhanced by consuming small amounts of carbohydrate more frequently (every 15 to 30 minutes) for up to 4 hours postexercise.
- Medium- to high-glycemic index foods *may* help to maximize glycogen storage for athletes who have limited time to recover between workouts.
- Add a small amount of protein (20 g) to the first feeding to stimulate muscle protein synthesis and repair.

Protein in Postexercise Feedings

The addition of protein in recovery feeding does not further enhance muscle glycogen synthesis when carbohydrate intake is at the recommended level (≥ 1.2 g/kg/h) for glycogen repletion.[4,58,63-66] However, when carbohydrate intake is suboptimal for refueling (< 1.2 g/kg/h), adding a small amount of protein (≥ 0.3 g/kg/h or about 20 g) will enhance glycogen storage.[4,58,67,68]

It is not always possible to consume large amounts of carbohydrate after exercise. Consuming a small amount of protein (~0.3 g/kg/h) with a lesser amount of carbohydrate (~0.8 g/kg/h) may represent a more practical approach to optimize glycogen repletion. This strategy promotes rates of muscle glycogen synthesis similar to those achieved with high intakes ($\geq$ 1.2 g/kg/h) of carbohydrate.[58]

Consuming protein after exercise also helps stimulate mixed muscle protein synthesis, inhibit protein breakdown, and enhance net muscle protein accretion.[58] In addition to carbohydrate, athletes' initial recovery snack or meal should include 0.25 to 0.3 g/kg (~15 to 25 g) of a high-quality protein containing all of the essential amino acids.[5,58] This amount can be provided by 24 oz of nonfat milk (20 g), three large eggs (21 g), or 3 oz of lean red meat (21 g).

CONTROVERSY: TRAINING WITH LOW CARBOHYDRATE AVAILABILITY

Endurance training causes a number of adaptations in skeletal muscle that improve exercise capacity. The most important of these adaptations is the increase in mitochondrial mass (mitochondrial biogenesis) that enables individuals to exercise longer at higher absolute intensities. Training-induced increases in mitochondrial biogenesis are thought to be due to the accumulative responses of transient changes in gene expression that follow each exercise bout.[69]

A growing body of evidence indicates that training with low carbohydrate availability ("training low") promotes greater training adaptation (eg, mitochondrial biogenesis) than when subjects undertake a similar training regimen with normal or elevated glycogen levels.[69] Training with reduced carbohydrate availability during short-term endurance training for 3 to 10 weeks enhances the activation of cell signaling pathways for mitochondrial biogenesis, upregulates oxidative enzymes, and increases whole–body and intramuscular lipid oxidation.[70-76] These findings support utilizing training low during specific exercise sessions to maximize the physiological adaptations to endurance training.[69]

There are many ways to reduce carbohydrate availability for exercise: training after an overnight fast, training twice per day so that the second session is performed with reduced glycogen stores, restricting carbohydrate intake during exercise, or restricting carbohydrate intake after exercise. Athletes can also "sleep low" by training in the evening to deplete carbohydrate stores, going to sleep without refueling, and then training in the fasted state the next morning.[69,77-79]

Although commencing some training sessions with reduced carbohydrate availability enhances skeletal muscle adaptations, the effect on exercise performance is less apparent.[69,77,78] Only one study in trained endurance athletes has found that 3 weeks of sleeping low promoted significant improvements in submaximal cycling economy, supramaximal cycling capacity, and 10-km running time.[79] Another study in active adults has shown that manipulating carbohydrate availability between twice-daily sessions of high-intensity interval training over 2 weeks improved cycling time-trial performance.[80] However, previous studies have found that improvements in cycling and running performance are independent of carbohydrate availability.[73-76]

Over time, training with reduced carbohydrate availability may limit the athlete's ability to maintain a desirable training intensity and lower the overall training stimulus.[73,75] Performing long-duration or high-intensity training sessions in a carbohydrate-restricted state may also compromise immune function and increase the risk of illness.[81] Exercising with reduced muscle glycogen levels increases muscle protein breakdown and long-term training on a low-carbohydrate diet may cause loss of skeletal muscle mass.[69,82] Lastly, withholding carbohydrate feedings during exercise impairs the athlete's ability to oxidize exogenous carbohydrate (an important fuel source for prolonged exercise) and may harm endurance performance.[83]

Training low is best regarded as an example of nutritional periodization where carbohydrate is deliberately withheld before, during, or after carefully selected training sessions to enhance training adaptations. Bartlett and colleagues suggest the following recommendations to incorporate training low into the training regimen[69]:

1. Athletes may benefit from including elements of training low when exercise intensity and duration lend them to the approach so that training loads are not compromised.

2. To minimize exercise-induced immunosuppression, training low should be undertaken during sessions that are not dedicated to heavy training loads.

3. Athletes can consume caffeine before exercise or use a carbohydrate mouth rinse during exercise to partially offset the reduced exercise intensity that accompanies training with low carbohydrate availability.

4. To attenuate muscle protein breakdown and promote protein synthesis, athletes should consume 20 to 25 g of protein before, during, or immediately after exercise.

5. Training low should be combined with sessions of training high (glycogen-loaded, preexercise meal or carbohydrate feedings during exercise) to simulate the competition fueling schedule.[84] These sessions are best undertaken when the intensity and duration of training replicate the physiological demands of competition.

There are many unanswered questions about training low that limit the ability to effectively apply the regimen. There is no definitive research regarding the optimal way to periodize elements of training low into an athlete's training program. The optimal practical strategies to train low are not currently known. Most importantly, it is not clear whether training low enhances real-world measures of exercise performance.[69]

The ability to generate high power outputs and work rates is a critical component of a periodized training program. Furthermore, the strategic moves that occur during competition depend on the athlete's ability to work at high intensities fueled by carbohydrate. Thus, a diet with high carbohydrate availability is recommended during periods of heavy training and when an athlete is preparing to peak for competition.[69,77,78]

SUMMARY

Carbohydrate is the predominant fuel for moderate- to high-intensity endurance exercise and repeated bouts of moderate- to high-intensity exercise. The strategic moves that occur during both endurance and stop-and-go sports depend on the athlete's ability to work at high intensities, which are, in turn, fueled by carbohydrate. Because the depletion of endogenous carbohydrate stores (muscle and liver glycogen and blood glucose) can impair athletic performance, fueling strategies should optimize carbohydrate availability before, during, and after exercise.

KEY TAKEAWAYS

Athletes with very light training programs (low-intensity exercise or skill-based exercise) should consume 3 to 5 g of carbohydrate per kilogram per day. Athletes engaged in moderate-intensity training programs for 60 min/d should consume 5 to 7 g/kg/d. During moderate- to high-intensity endurance exercise for 1 to 3 hours, athletes should consume 6 to 10 g/kg/d. Athletes participating in moderate- to high-intensity endurance exercise for 4 to 5 h/d or more (eg, Tour de France) should consume 8 to 12 g/kg/d.

One to 4 hours prior to endurance and intermittent, high-intensity exercise, athletes should consume 1 to 4 g of carbohydrate per kilogram to top off muscle and liver glycogen stores.

Consuming carbohydrate is not necessary during exercise lasting less than 30 minutes. During sustained high-intensity exercise lasting 30 to 75 minutes, consuming small amounts of single or multiple transportable carbohydrates or a carbohydrate mouth rinse may enhance performance. Athletes should consume 30 g of single or multiple transportable carbohydrates per hour during endurance and intermittent, high-intensity exercise lasting 1 to 2 hours. During endurance exercise lasting 2 to 3 hours, athletes should consume 60 g of single or multiple transportable carbohydrates per hour. During endurance and ultraendurance exercise lasting 2.5 hours and longer, athletes should consider consuming up to 90 g of multiple transportable carbohydrates per hour. Products providing multiple transportable carbohydrates help achieve high rates of carbohydrate oxidation during prolonged exercise.

When strenuous workouts or competitions are less than 8 hours apart, the athlete should consume carbohydrate as soon as possible after the first exercise session to maximize the effective recovery time between sessions. For speedy refueling after glycogen-depleting exercise, the athlete should consume 1 to 1.2 g of carbohydrate per kilogram per hour for the first 4 hours. Consuming carbohydrate at frequent intervals (every 15 to 30 minutes) for up to 4 hours postexercise also enhances muscle glycogen synthesis. During longer recovery periods (24 hours or more), it does not matter how carbohydrate intake is spaced throughout the day as long as the athlete consumes adequate carbohydrate and energy.

In addition to carbohydrate, the athlete's initial recovery snack or meal should include 0.25 to 0.3 g/kg (~15 to 25 g) of a high-quality protein containing all the essential amino acids to stimulate mixed muscle protein synthesis, inhibit protein breakdown, and enhance net muscle protein accretion.

These are general recommendations. They should be adjusted with consideration of the athlete's total energy needs, specific training needs, gut tolerance, and feedback from training and competition.

REFERENCES

1. Jacobs KA, Sherman WM. The efficacy of carbohydrate supplementation and chronic high carbohydrate diets for improving endurance performance. *Int J Sport Nutr.* 1999;9(1):92-115.

2. Coyle EF. Substrate utilization during exercise in active people. *Am J Clin Nutr.* 1995;61(suppl 4):968S-979S.

3. Hargreaves M. Exercise physiology and metabolism. In: Burke L, Deakin V, eds. *Clinical Sports Nutrition.* 4th ed. Sydney, Australia: McGraw-Hill; 2010;1-15.

4. Burke LM, Hawley JA, Wong S, Jeukendrup AE. Carbohydrates for training and competition. *J Sports Sci.* 2011;29(suppl 1):17S-27S.

5. Thomas DT, Erdman KA, Burke LM. Position of the Academy of Nutrition and Dietetics, Dietitians of Canada, and the American College of Sports Medicine: nutrition and athletic performance. *J Acad Nutr Diet.* 2016;116(3):501-528.

6. Costill DL, Sherman WM, Fink WJ, Maresh C, Whitten M, Miller JM. The role of dietary carbohydrate in muscle glycogen resynthesis after strenuous running. *Am J Clin Nutr.* 1981;34(9):1831-1836.

7. Fallowfield JL, Williams C. Carbohydrate intake and recovery from prolonged exercise. *Int J Sports Nutr.* 1993;3(2):150-164.

8. Achten J, Halson SH, Moseley L, Casey A, Jeukendrup AE. Higher dietary carbohydrate content during intensified running training results in better maintenance of performance and mood state. *J Appl Physiol.* 2004;96(4):1331-1340.

9. Simonsen JC, Sherman WM, Lamb DR, Dernbach AR, Doyle JA, Strauss R. Dietary carbohydrate, muscle glycogen, and power output during rowing training. *J Appl Physiol.* 1991;70(4):1500-1505.

10. Saris WHM, van Erp-Baart MA, Brouns F, Westerterp KR, ten Hoor F. Study of food intake and energy expenditure during extreme sustained exercise: the Tour de France. *Int J Sport Med.* 1989;10(suppl):26S-31S.

11. Costill DL, Flynn MJ, Kirwan JP, et al. Effect of repeated days of intensified training on muscle glycogen and swimming performance. *Med Sci Sports Exerc.* 1988;20(3):249-254.

12. Walberg-Rankin J. Dietary carbohydrate as an ergogenic aid for prolonged and brief competitions in sport. *Int J Sport Nutr.* 1995;5(suppl1):13S-28S.

13. Burke LM. Preparation for competition. In: Burke L, Deakin V, eds. *Clinical Sports Nutrition.* 4th ed. Sydney, Australia: McGraw-Hill; 2010:304-326.

14. Atkinson FS, Foster-Powell K, Brand-Miller JC. International tables of glycemic index and glycemic load values: 2008. *Diabetes Care.* 2008;31(12):2281-2283.

15. Ormsbee MJ, Bach CW, Baur DA. Pre-exercise nutrition: the role of macronutrients, modified starches and supplements on metabolism and endurance performance. *Nutrients.* 2014;6(5):1782-1808.

16. Stephens FB, Roig M, Armstrong G, Greenhaff PL. Post-exercise ingestion of a unique, high molecular weight glucose polymer solution improves performance during a subsequent bout of cycling exercise. *J Sports Sci.* 2008;26(2):149-154.

17. Roberts MD, Lockwood C, Dalbo VJ, Volek J, Kerksick CM. Ingestion of a high-molecular-weight hydrothermally modified waxy maize starch alters metabolic responses to prolonged exercise in trained cyclists. *Nutrition.* 2011;27(6):659-665.

18. Hawley JA, Schabort EJ, Noakes TD, Dennis SC. Carbohydrate-loading and exercise performance. An update. *Sports Med.* 1997;24(2):73-81.

19. Karlsson J, Saltin B. Diet, muscle glycogen, and endurance performance. *J Appl Physiol.* 1971;31(2):203-206.

20. Bergstrom J, Hermansen L, Saltin B. Diet, muscle glycogen, and physical performance. *Acta Physiol Scand.* 1967;71(2):140-150.

21. Sherman WM, Costill DL, Fink WJ, Miller JM. The effect of exercise and diet manipulation on muscle glycogen and its subsequent use during performance. *Int J Sport Med.* 1981;2(2):114-118.

22. Bussau VA., Fairchild TJ, Rao A. Steele P, Fournier PA. Carbohydrate loading in human muscle: an improved 1 day protocol. *Eur J Appl Physiol.* 2002;87(3):290-295.

23. Fairchild TJ, Fletcher S, Steele P, Goodman C, Dawson B, Fournier PA. Rapid carbohydrate loading after a short bout of near maximal-intensity exercise. *Med Sci Sport Exerc.* 2002;34(6):980-986.

24. McInerney P, Lessard SJ, Burke LM, et al. Failure to repeatedly supercompensate muscle glycogen stores in highly trained men. *Med Sci Sport Exerc.* 2005;37(3):404-411.

25. Balon TW, Horowitz JF, Fitzsimmons KM. Effects of carbohydrate loading and weight-lifting on muscle girth. *Int J Sport Nutr.* 1992;2(4):328-334.

26. Brouns F, Saris WH, Stroecken J, et al. Eating, drinking, and cycling: a controlled Tour de France simulation study, part II. Effect of diet manipulation. *Int J Sport Med.* 1989;10(suppl 1):41S-48S.

27. Nuefer PD, Costill DL, Flynn MG, Kirwan JP, Mitchell JB, Houmard J. Improvements in exercise performance: effects of carbohydrate feedings and diet. *J Appl Physiol.* 1987;62(3):983-988.

28. Sherman WM, Brodowicz G, Wright DA, Allen WK, Simonsen J, Dernbach A. Effects of 4 hour pre-exercise carbohydrate feedings on cycling performance. *Med Sci Sports Exerc.* 1989;21(5):598-604.

29. Wright DA, Sherman WM, Dernbach AR. Carbohydrate feedings before, during, or in combination improves cycling performance. *J Appl Physiol.* 1991;71(3):1082-1088.

30. Sherman WM, Peden MC, Wright DA. Carbohydrate feedings 1 hour before exercise improves cycling performance. *Am J Clin Nutr.* 1991;54(5):866-870.

31. Anantaraman R, Carimines AA, Gaesser GA, Weltman A. Effects of carbohydrate supplementation on performance during 1 hour of high-intensity exercise. *Int J Sport Med.* 1995;16(7):461-465.

32. Foster C, Costill DL, Fink WJ. Effects of pre-exercise feedings on endurance performance. *Med Sci Sport Exerc.* 1979;11(1):1-5.

33. Hargreaves M, Costill DL, Fink WJ, King DS, Fielding RA. Effects of pre-exercise carbohydrate feedings on endurance cycling performance. *Med Sci Sports Exerc.* 1987;19(1):33-36.

34. Jeukendrup AE, Killer S. The myths surrounding pre-exercise carbohydrate feeding. *Ann Nutr Metab.* 2011;57(suppl 2):18S-25S.

35. Thomas DE, Brotherhood JR, Brand JC. Carbohydrate feeding before exercise: effect of glycemic index. *Int J Sport Med.* 1991;12(2):180-186.

36. Donaldson CM, Perry TL, Rose MC. Glycemic index and endurance performance. *Int J Sport Nutr Exerc Metab.* 2010;20(2):154-165.

37. Burke LM, Claassen A, Hawley JA, Noakes TD. Carbohydrate intake during exercise minimizes effect of glycemic index of pre-exercise meal. *J Appl Physiol.* 1998;85(6):2220-2226.

38. Wong SH, Chan OW, Chen YJ, Hu HL, Lam CW, Chung PK. Effect of preexercise glycemic-index meal on running when CHO-electrolyte solution is consumed during exercise. *Int J Sport Nutr Exerc Metab.* 2009;19:(3)222-242.

39. Coyle EF, Hagberg JM, Hurley BF, Martin WH, Ehsani AA, Holloszy JO. Carbohydrate feeding during prolonged strenuous exercise can delay fatigue. *J Appl Physiol.* 1983;55(1 Pt 1):230-235.

40. Coyle EF, Coggan AR, Hemmert WK, Ivy JL. Muscle glycogen utilization during prolonged strenuous exercise when fed carbohydrate. *J Appl Physiol.* 1986;61(1):165-172.

41. Wilber RL, Moffat RJ. Influence of carbohydrate ingestion on blood glucose and performance in runners. *Int J Sport Nutr.* 1992;2(4):317-327.

42. Millard-Stafford ML, Sparling PB, Rosskopf LB, Hinson BT, Dicarlo LJ. Carbohydrate-electrolyte replacement improves distance running performance in the heat. *Med Sci Sports Exerc.* 1992;24(8):934-940.

43. Jeukendrup AE. A step towards personalized sports nutrition: carbohydrate intake during exercise. *Sports Med.* 2014;44(suppl 1):25S-33S.

44. Jeukendrup AE, Chambers ES. Oral carbohydrate sensing and exercise performance. *Curr Opin Clin Nutr Metab Care.* 2010;13(4):447-451.

45. Jeukendrup AE. Oral carbohydrate rinse: placebo or beneficial? *Curr Sports Med Rep.* 2013;12(4):222-227.

46. Baker LB, Rollo I, Stein KW, Jeukendrup AE. Acute effects of carbohydrate supplementation on intermittent sports performance. *Nutrients.* 2015;7(7):5733-5763.

47. Nicholas CW, Williams C, Lakomy HK, Phillips G, Nowitz A. Influence of ingesting a carbohydrate-electrolyte solution on endurance capacity during intermittent, high-intensity shuttle running. *J Sport Sci.* 1995;13(4):283-290.

48. Foskett A, Williams C, Boobis L, Tsintzas K. Carbohydrate availability and muscle energy metabolism during intermittent running. *Med Sci Sports Exerc.* 2008;40(1):96-103.

49. Patterson SD, Gray SC. Carbohydrate-gel supplementation and endurance performance during intermittent high-intensity shuttle running. *Int J Sport Nutr Exerc Metab.* 2007;17(5):445-455.

50. Welsh RS, Davis JM, Burke JR, Williams HG. Carbohydrates and physical/mental performance during intermittent exercise to fatigue. *Med Sci Sports Exerc.* 2002;34(4):723-731.

51. Jentjens RL, Moseley L, Waring RH, Harding LK, Jeukendrup AE. Oxidation of combined ingestion of glucose and fructose during exercise. *J Appl Physiol.* 2004;96(4):1277-1284.

52. Jeukendrup AE. Carbohydrate and exercise performance: the role of multiple transportable carbohydrates. *Curr Opin Clin NutrMetab Care.* 2010;13(4):452-457.

53. Currell K, Jeukendrup AE. Superior endurance performance with ingestion of multiple transportable carbohydrates. *Med Sci Sports Exerc.* 2008;40(2):275-281.

54. Smith JW, Zachwieja JJ, Peronnet F, et al. Fuel selection and cycling endurance performance with ingestion of [13C] glucose: evidence for a carbohydrate dose response. *J Appl Physiol.* 2010;108(6):1520-1529.

55. Smith JW, Pascoe DD, Passe DH, et al. Curvilinear dose-response relationship of carbohydrate (0-120 g·h(-1)) and performance. *Med Sci Sports Exerc.* 2013;45(2):336-341.

56. Pfeiffer B, Stellingwerff T, Zaltas E, Jeukendrup AE. CHO oxidation from a CHO gel compared with a drink during exercise. *Med Sci Sports Exerc.* 2010;42(11):2038-2045.

57. Pfeiffer B, Stellingwerff T, Zaltas E, Jeukendrup AE. Oxidation of solid versus liquid CHO sources during exercise. *Med Sci Sports Exerc.* 2010;42(11):2030-2037.

58. Beelen M, Burke LM, Gibala MJ, van Loon L JC. Nutritional strategies to promote postexercise recovery. *Int J Sport Nutr Exerc Metab.* 2010;20(6):515-532.

59. Ivy JL, Katz AL, Cutler CL, Sherman WM, Coyle EF. Muscle glycogen synthesis after exercise: effect of time of carbohydrate ingestion. *J Appl Physiol.* 1988;6(4):1480-1485.

60. Ivy JL, Lee MC, Broznick JT, Reed MJ. Muscle glycogen storage after different amounts of carbohydrate ingestion. *J Appl Physiol.* 1988;65(5):2018-2023.

61. Burke LM, Collier GR, Hargreaves M. Muscle glycogen storage after prolonged exercise: effect of glycemic index. *J Appl Physiol.* 1993;75(2):1019-1023.

62. Reed MJ, Broznick JT, Lee MC, Ivy JL. Muscle glycogen storage postexercise: effect of mode of carbohydrate administration. *J Appl Physiol.* 1989;66(2):720-726.

63. van Loon LJ, Saris WH, Kruijshoop M, Wagenmakers A. Maximizing postexercise muscle glycogen synthesis: carbohydrate supplementation and the application of amino acid or protein hydrolysate mixtures. *Am J Clin Nutr.* 2000;72(1):106-111.

64. van Hall G, Shirreffs S, Calbet J. Muscle glycogen resynthesis during recovery from cycle exercise: no effect of additional protein ingestion. *J Appl Physiol.* 2000;88(5):1631-1636.

65. Jentjens RL, van Loon LJ, Mann CH, Wagenmakers AJ, Jeukendrup AE. Additional protein and amino acids to carbohydrates does not enhance postexercise muscle glycogen synthesis. *J Appl Physiol.* 2001;91(2):839-846.

66. Carrithers JA, Williamson DL, Gallagher P,M Godard MP, Schulze KE, Trappe SW. Effects of postexercise carbohydrate-protein feedings on muscle glycogen restoration. *J Appl Physiol.* 2000;88(6):1976-1982.

67. Howarth KR, Moreau NA, Phillips SM, Gibala MJ. Coingestion of protein with carbohydrate during recovery from endurance exercise stimulates skeletal muscle protein synthesis in humans. *J Appl Physiol.* 2009;106(4):1394-1402.

68. Betts JA, Williams C. Short-term recovery from prolonged exercise: exploring the potential for protein ingestion to accentuate the benefits of carbohydrate supplements. *Sports Med.* 2010;40(11):941-959.

69. Bartlett JD, Hawley JA, Morton JP. Carbohydrate availability and exercise training adaptation: too much of a good thing? *Eur J Sport Sci.* 2015;15(1):3-12.

70. Bartlett JD, Louhelainen J, Iqbal Z, et al. Reduced carbohydrate availability enhances exercise-induced p53 signaling in human skeletal muscle: implications for mitochondrial biogenesis. *Am J Physiol Regul Integr Comp Physiol.* 2013;304(6):R450-R458.

71. Yeo WK, McGee SL, Carey AL, et al. Acute signaling responses to intense endurance training commenced with low or normal muscle glycogen. *Exp Physiol.* 2010;95(2):351-358.

72. Hansen AK, Fischer CP, Plomgaard P, Andersen JL, Saltin B, Pedersen BK. Skeletal muscle adaptation: training twice every second day vs. training once daily. *J Appl Physiol.* 2005;98(1):93-99.

73. Yeo WK, Paton CD, Garnham AP, Burke LM, Carey AL, Hawley JA. Skeletal muscle adaptation and performance responses to once a day versus twice every second day endurance training regimens. *J Appl Physiol.* 2008;105(5):1462-1470.

74. Morton JP, Croft L, Bartlett JD, et al. Reduced carbohydrate availability does not modulate training-induced heat shock protein adaptations but does upregulate oxidative enzyme activity in human skeletal muscle. *J Appl Physiol.* 2009;106(5):1513-1521.

75. Hulston CJ, Venables MC, Mann CH, et al. Training with low muscle glycogen enhances fat metabolism in well-trained cyclists. *Med Sci Sports Exerc.* 2010;42(11):2046-2055.

76. Van Proeyen K, Szlufcik K, Nielens H, Ramaekers M, Hespel P. Beneficial metabolic adaptations due to endurance exercise training in the fasted state. *J Appl Physiol.* 2011;110(1):236-245.

77. Hawley JA, Burke LM. Carbohydrate availability and training adaptation: effects on cell metabolism. *Exerc Sport Sci Rev.* 2010;38(4):152-160.

78. Burke LM. Fueling strategies to optimize performance: training high or training low? *Scand J Med Sci Sports.* 2010;20(suppl 2):48S-58S.

79. Marquet LA, Brisswalter J, Louis J, et al. Enhanced endurance performance by periodization of CHO intake: "sleep low" strategy [published online ahead of print January 7, 2016]. *Med Sci Sports Exerc.* 2016;48(4):663-672. doi: 10.1249/MSS.0000000000000823.

80. Cochran AJ, Myslik F, MacInnis MJ, et al. Manipulating carbohydrate availability between twice-daily sessions of high-intensity interval training over two weeks improves time-trial performance. *Int J Sport Nutr Exerc Metab.* 2015;25(5):463-470.

81. Gleeson M, Nieman DC, Pedersen BK. Exercise, nutrition and immune function. *J Sports Sci.* 2004;22(1):115-125.

82. Howarth KR, Phillips SM, MacDonald MJ, Richards D, Moreau NA, Gibala MJ. Effect of glycogen availability on human skeletal muscle protein turnover during exercise and recovery. *J Appl Physiol.* 2010;109(2):431-438.

83. Cox GR, Clark SA, Cox AJ, et al. Daily training with high carbohydrate availability increases exogenous carbohydrate oxidation during endurance cycling. *J Appl Physiol.* 2010;109(1):126-134.

84. Stellingwerff T. Case study: nutrition and training periodization of three elite marathon runners. *Int J Sport Nutr Exerc Metab.* 2012;22(5):392-400.

CHAPTER 3

PROTEIN AND EXERCISE

Nicholas A. Burd, PhD, and Stuart M. Phillips, PhD, FACN, FACSM

INTRODUCTION

The energy for muscle contraction was originally hypothesized to be derived from the "explosive breakdown of protein molecules."[1] Indeed, the evaluation of daily dietary protein intake among certain cohorts of athletes (eg, bodybuilders, power and strength athletes) suggests that many athletes are still firm believers in the afore-mentioned thesis, reflected by their excessively high protein intakes.[2] However, scientists and sports dietitians generally regard protein intake to be inconsequential with respect to providing energy for muscle contraction. For instance, amino acids provide only a minor portion of energy contribution (~2% to 4%) during prolonged dynamic exercise.[3,4] This is despite the capacity of human skeletal muscle to oxidize at least seven amino acids during exercise, including the branched-chain amino acids—leucine, valine, and isoleucine—the amino acids oxidized to the greatest extent.[5] Despite the relatively low use of amino acids as fuel during exercise, exercise does have a profound influence on muscle protein synthesis (MPS) and muscle protein breakdown (MPB) (or, collectively, skeletal muscle protein turnover). For example, distinct phenotypic adaptations occur in response to divergent exercise training stimuli. Resistance exercise leads to hypertrophy, and endurance exercise leads to an enhanced oxidative capacity. However, to maximize skeletal muscle adaptation induced by a training stimulus, regardless of the mode of exercise, intake of dietary protein is fundamental to facilitate the repair, remodeling, or accretion of muscle protein and to maintain muscle throughout the life span.

This chapter is a practical reference tool that discusses protein and exercise for scientists, athletes, and general fitness enthusiasts. A general overview of muscle protein turnover with regards to both resistance and endurance exercise is provided. Further details on such topics as protein quality, quantity, and timing of ingestion in relation to both resistance and endurance exercise are provided where relevant. Human studies are emphasized; however, other animal models are examined when human research is inadequate.

MUSCLE PROTEIN TURNOVER

Muscle protein turnover (MPS and MPB) is a synchronous and continuous process in human muscle. During the course of the day, fasted-state losses of muscle protein are counterbalanced by fed-state gains of muscle protein so that over time the muscle net protein balance (NPB) equation (NPB = MPS – MPB) is zero and skeletal muscle mass remains essentially unchanged (Figure 3.1).[6]

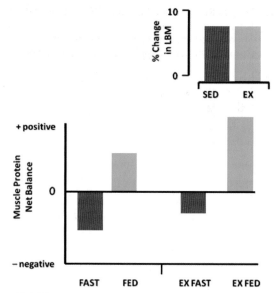

FIGURE 3.1 Muscle Net Protein Balance at Rest and After Feeding and Resistance Exercise Resistance exercise is fundamentally anabolic, such that muscle net protein balance becomes less negative in the fasted state. The inset illustrates the training-induced changes in lean body mass that manifest from the synergistic effect of feeding dietary amino acids and exercise. However, in the absence of an anabolic stimulus, lean body mass remains essentially unchanged, such as in sedentary individuals.

LBM = lean body mass
SED = sedentary
EX = exercise
FAST = fasting for 12 hours
FED = feeding dietary amino acids
EX FAST = exercise in fasting state
EX FED = exercise and feeding.

A detailed description of the regulation of muscle protein turnover is beyond the scope of this chapter; however, a general understanding of the protein pools controlling protein turnover will solidify the concepts presented throughout the chapter. Briefly, consumption of dietary protein is followed by an increase in the concentration of amino acids in the blood, which are subsequently transported into the muscle and ultimately double the rate of MPS.[7] Scientists generally assume that the muscle intracellular free amino acid pool functions as a link between the environment and muscle proteins. The amino acid inputs to the muscle intracellular free amino acid pool can come from the blood amino acids during feeding or from the breaking down of muscle proteins during the fasting state. Of course, not all amino acids are used for building muscle proteins. For example, de novo synthesis can occur for certain nonessential amino acids, and amino acids can be used in intermediary metabolism or oxidized. It is noteworthy that aminoacyl-transfer RNA in the muscle is the true free amino acid pool leading to MPS.[8]

Resistance Exercise

Resistance exercise is fundamentally anabolic. For instance, after an isolated bout of resistance exercise, NPB becomes more positive, lasting as long as 2 days after the stimulus in untrained subjects.[9] Chronic application of resistance exercise (ie, training) results in myofibrillar protein (the predominant protein in skeletal muscle) accretion, an increase in skeletal muscle fiber size, and, ultimately, increased lean body mass.[9,10,11] Recent research has illustrated that resistance training can have profound effects on muscle protein turnover. Resting MPS is chronically elevated in resistance trained subjects, whereas MPB is attenuated compared with untrained subjects.[12-15] Furthermore, resistance training seems to shorten duration and amplitude of elevation of MPS after acute resistance exercise.[16] Smaller amplitude and duration of the MPS with training suggests a need for increased attention to training-based variables such as load, intensity, and exercise order to maintain a relatively unique exercise stimulus. In addition, the importance of timing with regards to feeding dietary protein, such as essential amino acids (EAAs), close to the completion of exercise also becomes important in maximizing protein accretion and the subsequent gains in muscle mass. The EAAs are the primary stimulators of muscle protein synthesis rates.[17] As highlighted in Figure 3.2, postexercise feeding is important in supporting a positive NPB and ultimately eliciting an adaptation that could include muscle hypertrophy, changes in strength, or increases in oxidation capacity. However, certain feeding patterns may be superior to others in inducing positive effects on skeletal muscle, discussed later in the chapter.

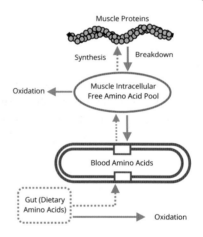

FIGURE 3.2 General Overview of the Fate of Dietary Amino Acids and Protein Pools in the Body *Muscle proteins* is a collective term referring to myofibrillar, sarcoplasmic, and mitochondrial proteins. These specific protein subfractions make up approximately 60%, 30%, and 10% of skeletal muscle, respectively. Solid arrows represent anabolic destinations. Dashed arrows represent catabolic destinations.

Endurance Exercise

Carbohydrate- and fat-based fuels provide the majority of the energy required for muscle contraction during sustained endurance exercise events. However, the oxidation of some classes of amino acids, such as branched-chain amino acids, can contribute up to 10% of total energy during endurance exercise.[18] Amino acid oxidation rates during exercise are influenced by several factors including: intensity and duration of aerobic exercise, sex, muscle glycogen availability, energy availability, and training status.[3,19-23] Of note is that amino acid oxidation rates are reduced during aerobic exercise in trained athletes because there is a greater reliance on fat-based fuels to provide the energy for muscle contraction.[23] However, regardless of training status, the increased amino acid oxidation rates during aerobic exercise are thought to partly contribute to the elevated protein requirements of endurance athletes.[18,24] Daily dietary protein requirements of an endurance athlete are further discussed later in this chapter.

Studies examining muscle protein turnover using stable isotope methodology after acute aerobic exercise suggest that aerobic exercise can induce increases in MPS, although the response is smaller in both amplitude and duration compared with resistance exercise.[9,13-15,25-28] This remodeling of muscle proteins during recovery from aerobic exercise is essential to replace damaged proteins and synthesize myofibrillar- and mitochondrial-related proteins and enzymes, as well as angiogenic proteins, thereby leading to increased oxidative capacity of skeletal muscle with prolonged aerobic training.

Recent work has shown that aerobic exercise intensity influences the duration of the postexercise MPS response, where high-intensity exercise elicits a more sustained MPS response than low-intensity aerobic exercise.[29] This work supports a hypothesis that there is a relationship between the force placed on the muscle and the subsequent stimulation of MPS during postexercise recovery. Thus, greater forces or intensities elicit greater and apparently longer-lasting increases in MPS compared with lower-intensity aerobic exercise.

PROTEIN TIMING: THE CLOCK IS TICKING

Resistance Exercise

Research on maximizing hypertrophy emphasizes the timing of postexercise protein intake. Some findings include extreme recommendations, such as periworkout nutrition, which describe the concept of feeding protein both preexercise and postexercise. Historically, dietary protein recommendations for athletes focused on total daily protein intake, deemphasizing timing of protein intake. Recently, considerable research has explored optimal timing of protein intake to maximize acute posttraining anabolic response and hypertrophy.

PREEXERCISE FEEDING

Numerous studies have examined protein ingestion pre- and postresistance exercise in an attempt to determine the best time to deliver dietary amino acids to exercised muscle to optimize anabolism.[6] Early work demonstrated that administering 6 g of EAAs (equivalent to ~15 g of high-quality protein, such as eggs) and 35 g of sucrose before resistance exercise induced a 160% greater increase in muscle anabolism compared with a similar drink consumed after exercise. This effect was attributed to the preexercise supplement promoting an exercise-induced hyperemia and subsequently an almost four fold increase in the delivery and uptake of amino acids to the muscle.[30] In a subsequent study, Tipton and colleagues examined the influence of intact proteins fed immediately before or after resistance exercise. Both feeding patterns induced similar anabolic responses because there was no stimulation of hyperemia with exercise. However, there were large individual differences in the anabolic responses to feeding pre- and postresistance exercise, which led the researchers to speculate that certain individuals may be more responsive to preexercise feeding to induce muscle anabolism.[31]

DURING EXERCISE FEEDING

Just as feeding pre- vs postresistance exercise is controversial, so too is the physiological relevance of feeding during acute resistance exercise. Indeed, in the fasting state, research demonstrates that the energy-consuming process of MPS is not elevated during resistance exercise, and this down regulation of MPS may be attributed to activation of adenosine monophosphate protein kinase, the energy sensor in muscle cells.[28,32,33] However, coingestion of carbohydrate (50% glucose and 50% maltodextrin) and casein protein hydrolysate during a combined endurance and whole-body resistance exercise session stimulated sustained postworkout MPS when the participants had a preexercise meal. Some researchers speculate, however, that this result may actually have been attributed to an enhanced MPS during the rest periods between exercise sets. It is noteworthy that this accelerated MPS during exercise did not further augment net muscle protein accretion during the subsequent overnight recovery.[34] In conclusion, there seems to be little benefit to feeding during resistance exercise to induce muscle hypertrophy.

POSTEXERCISE FEEDING

Early work by Esmarck and colleagues demonstrated the importance of consuming protein near the time of exercise. Elderly patients in a 12-week study who consumed a supplement immediately after training sessions had significant increases in thigh muscle mass, whereas delaying protein supplementation by as little as 2 hours after training resulted in no change in muscle mass.[35] Indeed, these data are difficult to reconcile because increases in muscle mass and strength are hallmark adaptations to resistance exercise, regardless of whether a specific nutrition intervention is used in the young or elderly patients.[36-41] Furthermore, in elderly men who habitually consume adequate dietary protein (1.1 ± 0.1 g/kg/d), 10 g of additional protein supplementation both before and after training had no additional effect on muscle mass or strength gains compared with the nonsupplemented group.[42]

Research has shown the importance of a positive energy balance during a resistance training regimen. One study suggested that an increase of approximately 15% in total energy intake may be necessary to maintain body weight and support muscle protein accretion during a training period.[43] A 2006 study

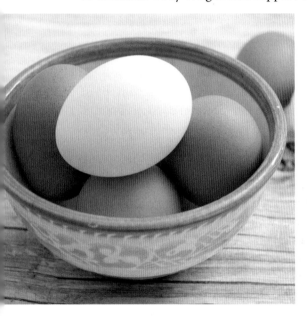

demonstrated that women between 49 and 74 years of age undergoing resistance training for 21 weeks benefited from appropriate nutritional intake, guided by nutrition counseling.[44] Women who were counseled displayed greater increases in thigh muscle mass (~9.5%) compared with the group without counseling (~6.8%). The authors suggested that these results were due to increases in energy from protein and the ratio of polyunsaturated to saturated fatty acids. However, research has demonstrated that a positive energy balance is not obligatory for lean mass accretion during exercise training.[45]

Men who had previously undergone resistance training participated in a 12-week training program where they were randomly assigned to groups consuming a protein supplement that included whey protein, glucose, and creatine, either before breakfast and late evening before bed or pre- and postworkout. The periworkout nutrition induced superior gains in lean body mass and strength.[46] However, in a study using a similar design, researchers found no difference between the groups consuming the protein supplement—a proprietary blend of whey and casein—in mornings and evenings or following a periworkout nutrition protocol after a 10-week resistance training program. The authors noted, however, that low energy intakes (~29 kcal/kg/d) were less than the recommended values for active individuals, regardless of training group.[47] Another study attempted to delineate the importance of protein timing in relation to resistance training used a randomized within-subject crossover design. Young men in one group consumed a protein supplement (~40 g casein) twice daily in the morning and evening (timing of protein intake was not immediately pre- or postworkout). A second group consumed the same supplement immediately before a training session. The first group (the group spacing out supplement intake) experienced greater increases in fat-free mass than the group following the other supplement protocol after 8 weeks of resistance training.[48]

SUMMARY OF FINDINGS

Marked differences in study designs, training length, and type of protein consumed during the training periods in these studies make it difficult for practitioners to make accurate recommendations about the timing of protein ingestion.[46-48] A meta-analysis found that there is no evidence that protein ingestion before or immediately after resistance exercise (≤ 1 hour) augments skeletal muscle hypertrophy or strength with prolonged resistance training.[49] These results are not surprising because the nutrient timing window for protein supplementation to further enhance postexercise MPS is not limited to this immediate and narrow (< 1 hour) timing window.[50] Cermak and colleagues showed that protein supplementation during a program of resistance exercise training positively affects increases for both skeletal muscle mass and strength.[51] Thus, total daily protein intake distributed throughout the day is important to optimize training adaptations, and less emphasis should be placed on a narrow pre- or postworkout protein supplementation window (< 1 hour).[52] Study results generally demonstrate that protein intake close to exercise, in particular up to 3 hours after exercise, seems to offer some benefit in lean mass and strength gain and facilitates adequate daily intake of protein by the athlete.

Other evidence, in which timing of protein ingestion was not the major manipulated variable, supports the conclusion that ingesting protein close to exercise matters in determining lean mass gains. Hartman and colleagues reported lean mass gains in a large cohort of young men (N = 56) after 13 weeks of intense resistance training.[10] To test whether milk was superior to soy or protein-free carbohydrates at inducing gains in lean mass, subjects were randomly assigned to consume 500 mL of fat-free milk (18 g protein); an isonitrogenous, isoenergetic fat-free soy drink; or a carbohydrate control (0 g protein) immediately after resistance exercise and again 1 hour after exercise. In this study, milk induced superior increases in type II fiber size and fat- and bone-free mass compared with soy. These data illustrate that the intake of a high-quality protein within 2 hours of training is fundamental in maximizing the hypertrophic adaptations, but these results also highlight a previously unrecognized benefit of milk proteins vs soy protein. Furthermore, studies show that resistance exercise and feeding are synergistic and that MPS is elevated to the greatest extent within the initial hours after exercise, so it would seem that eating protein early offers substantial benefits.[6,53] That is not to say, however, that feeding protein later does not offer benefits, as illustrated in Figure 3.3. It seems that the synergistic effect of exercise and feeding occurs even on the day after resistance exercise. Burd and colleagues studied a group of young people who consumed 15 g of whey protein after an acute bout of resistance exercise. The results demonstrated that the muscle remains more "anabolically sensitive" for up to 24 hours.[50] The exact underlying mechanisms behind this synergism of exercise and feeding are unknown but may be due to anabolic signaling molecules that "turn on" muscle protein synthesis and are more sensitive to feeding. Moreover, research demonstrated that resistance exercise and protein ingestion are both capable of up regulating skeletal muscle amino acid transporters, which may assist in the transport of amino acids into the free amino acid pool.[54,55] Therefore, the resistance exercise–mediated increase in amino acid transport proteins in skeletal muscle tissue during late exercise recovery may ultimately sensitize the muscle to dietary protein–derived amino acids in the subsequent meal.[56] However, it is important to recognize that the role of increased skeletal muscle amino acid transporter expression in modulating the postexercise or postprandial MPS response is not completely understood.

Interestingly, Beelen and colleagues examined the impact of resistance exercise performed in the evening and the effectiveness of protein ingestion during and immediately after exercise on MPS during overnight recovery.[34] Results showed that the MPS response was reduced in the evening compared with the MPS response commonly observed in the morning during the later stages of exercise recovery, up to 24 or 48 hours later.[9] This work provided the basis to assess the capacity of protein ingestion before sleep to optimize MPS during overnight recovery. Res and colleagues demonstrated that protein consumed before sleep is efficiently digested and absorbed into circulation and augments the subsequent postexercise MPS response during overnight recovery.[58] This result was observed despite

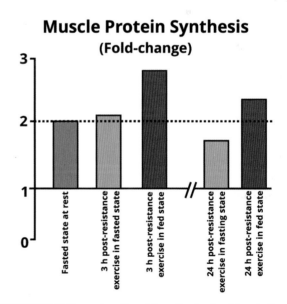

FIGURE 3.3 Fold-Change from Fasted-State Resting Conditions in Muscle Protein Synthesis After Feeding and Resistance The anabolic sensitizing effect of resistance exercise is greatest during the immediate acute recovery period; however, this sensitizing effect is still conferred more than 1 day after exercise. The dashed line illustrates the summation of the fed response following exercise.

participants receiving a full day of standardized nutritional intake, including adequate protein intake and immediate postexercise nutrition (20 g protein, 60 g carbohydrate).[57] Therefore, protein supplementation before sleep may be an effective nutrient timing strategy to further modulate the skeletal muscle adaptive response to exercise training.[58]

Endurance Exercise

As with resistance exercise, the importance of protein consumption soon after endurance exercise is most likely equally as important. Hallmark adaptations that occur with aerobic training are increases in capillarization, mitochondrial biogenesis, and increased abundance of glucose and fat transporters.[59-61] These adaptations require turning over proteins and net addition of new proteins; in other words, a positive NPB to support optimum adaptation. Providing support for this notion, recent data demonstrated that after 2 hours of cycling, participants who consumed 36 g/h of protein (an excessively high dose) during the cycling with carbohydrates during postexercise recovery had enhanced rates of MPS, greater than rates seen after consumption of carbohydrates alone.[62] Unfortunately, only mixed MPS was determined, and, as such, researchers cannot determine whether the additional protein enhanced the synthesis of myofibrillar or mitochondrial proteins. Of note, the additional protein did not enhance glycogen replenishment during the 4-hour postexercise recovery period, but it did facilitate the net synthesis of proteins.[62]

Aerobic exercise seems to affect nutrient-sensitizing in skeletal muscle. A 2007 study by Fujita and colleagues demonstrated that normal muscle protein synthetic response to hyperinsulinemia in older individuals was restored the day after a 45-minute bout of low-intensity aerobic exercise. Results suggested that exercise has a nutrient-sensitizing effect on skeletal muscle. However, the researchers only examined mixed MPS, and, therefore, which protein fractions (myofibrillar, sarcoplasmic, or mitochondrial) were being affected could not be determined.[63] Recent studies suggest that this response may have been confined to the mitochondrial or sarcoplasmic protein pools. Data reveal that aerobic exercise preferentially stimulates the synthesis of mitochondrial proteins.[13] Elderly test subjects (71 years old) performing 12 weeks of training on a cycle ergometer and reaching 60% to 80% of their heart-rate reserve for 20 minutes had ~12% increase in thigh muscle volume but had a significant decline in myofibrillar concentration. These data indicate that other proteins (such as mitochondrial) were accrued or possibly that aerobic exercise enhanced sensitivity to feeding after each exercise, which resulted in protein accretion.[64] Effects of aerobic exercise on enhancing amino acid sensitivity of muscle protein synthesis during postexercise recovery has not been established in healthy young adults. Collectively, these data suggest that, similar to resistance exercise, aerobic exercise can improve the receptiveness of the protein synthetic machinery to feeding for at least a day after exercise.[63,64] However, the intensity or duration of the endurance exercise may determine if the amino acid sensitivity of skeletal muscle tissue is sustained in the subsequent day of recovery.[29]

DURING EXERCISE

Some research suggests that feeding protein during endurance exercise may offer some additional performance benefits compared with feeding carbohydrate alone. For example, a 2003 study by Ivy and colleagues demonstrated that consumption of protein (3.8 g) with carbohydrate (16 g) in small doses during 3 hours of intense cycling increased time to exhaustion vs placebo and carbohydrate-only trials in trained male cyclists.[65] Other studies confirm the presumed beneficial effects of protein supplementation during exercise on performance.[66,67] In contrast, a well-designed, double-blind, repeated-measures, placebo-controlled, crossover study showed that there was no additional benefit from protein ingested with carbohydrate compared with carbohydrate alone.[68] Another study established that in moderately well-trained cyclists, ingestion of protein with carbohydrate, compared with carbohydrate alone, during 90 minutes of cycling did not influence the magnitude of glycogen or phosphocreatine utilization or a performance in 20-km time trial measured approximately 24 hours after the first exercise bout.[69] These findings are replicated in other studies where data illustrate no beneficial effect on performance.[70,71] Conflicting evidence from a variety of studies suggests that ingesting protein with carbohydrate during endurance exercise is not beneficial to performance gains when adequate amounts of carbohydrate are consumed. However, as explained in the following section, protein is fundamental in replacing exercise-induced amino acid oxidative loss and supporting a positive NPB and the subsequent adaptation to aerobic exercise.

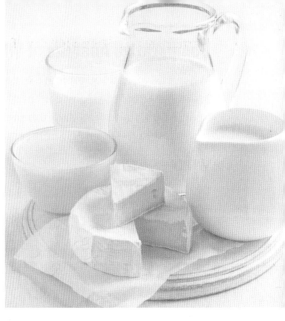

DURING ULTRAENDURANCE EXERCISE ACTIVITY

In a recent study, researchers sought to determine the response of whole-body protein turnover in triathletes, ultramarathon runners, cyclists, and others who exercise for greater than 5 hours per day during competition or training. Participants were given carbohydrates or carbohydrates and protein before, during, and after exercise. Prolonged exercise neither increased protein breakdown nor protein synthesis compared with resting in these highly trained endurance athletes. However, protein and carbohydrate coingestion affected whole-body NPB by increasing whole-body MPS and decreasing whole-body MPB, resulting in a net positive whole-body NPB during exercise recovery. These results illustrate the potential of feeding even a small amount of protein during endurance exercise to augment the remodeling of whole-body protein pools, despite not having a performance benefit.[72]

SUMMARY OF FINDINGS

From a practical perspective, the caloric demands of aerobic exercise are generally greater than those of high-intensity or resistance exercise that lasts 30 to 60 minutes because a single session of aerobic exercise can be sustained for much longer than resistance exercise. Therefore, it is paramount that energy needs are met after aerobic exercise to ensure that the dietary protein is being used for protein synthesis and not being unnecessarily oxidized to meet energy needs.[73] Lastly, an individual's diet should be assessed before making recommendations on supplemental protein. Timing of protein intake immediately after exercise greatly affects protein synthesis. However, the postexercise "window of anabolic opportunity" is greater than what is commonly believed. The synergistic effect of exercise and feeding on MPS rates is less effective than feeding up to 24 hours after exercise.[50] Take time after exercise to prepare a well-balanced meal that includes high-quality dietary proteins, rather than focusing on supplemental powders or drinks.

PROTEIN TYPE AND QUALITY

Leucine as an Anabolic Trigger

The consumption of dietary protein results in a dose-dependent hyperaminoacidemia compared with fasting levels. Different types of proteins have different digestion kinetics; thus, the rate of appearance of amino acids in the blood differs substantially based on the type of dietary protein consumed.[74-77] The essential nature and signaling role of leucine in the stimulation of MPS is intriguing. Indeed, the exact explanation behind leucine as an anabolic signal remains somewhat elusive. Leucine is insulinogenic, but insulin is not particularly anabolic above levels already present while fasting (5 mcU/mL). Additionally, its influence on MPB fully manifests at insulin levels of approximately 30 mcU/mL, a concentration commonly obtained after a mixed meal.[78] Leucine may also serve as an anabolic mediator through its ability to increase the transport of other amino acids into muscle, where they can accumulate in the muscle-free amino acid pool and be used for protein synthesis.[79] Moreover, research shows that the amino acid transporter responsible for bringing leucine into the muscle cell, LAT1, may serve as an amino acid sensor to communicate to the protein synthetic machinery.[80] Thus, foods that have a lot of leucine are generally considered anabolic toward muscle.

Comparative Analysis of Whey, Casein, and Soy

Whey, casein, and soy protein isolates are the most commonly studied proteins on MPS after recovery from resistance exercise.[76] Milk contains approximately 20% whey and 80% casein proteins. Based on their rate of digestion, these proteins are commonly referred to as fast and slow proteins, respectively.[81] Soy is considered a fast digested protein source.

WHEY PROTEIN

In recent years, whey protein, the soluble fraction extracted from milk as a result of cheese manufacturing, has become exceedingly popular among athletes as a dietary supplement. Whey proteins are available as concentrates (generally >70% protein), isolates (generally >90% protein), and hydrolysates (varies in protein content but typically >80% protein) in powder form; however, the protein content of these preparations can vary. For this chapter, the term *whey protein* will be used to describe all three types. Whey protein is considered high quality due to its protein digestibility corrected amino acid score. This means that its amino acid composition is close to or, in most cases, exceeds the digestibility of human body proteins and is rapidly and easily digested. Whey protein contains very high concentrations of EAAs, and its total amino acid composition has a surprisingly disproportionate amount of leucine (14%) compared with other high-quality protein sources. For example, milk and beef contain 10% and 9% leucine, respectively, by total amino acid content.[82] In one study, consumption of whey protein induced a superior increase in MPS compared with soy or casein after a single bout of resistance exercise.[76] Similarly, a rapid increase in the EAAs (leucine, in particular) was shown after whey protein consumption compared with soy or casein alone. Studies have shown that consumption of only the EAAs is necessary to stimulate MPS, which highlights the importance of consuming a high-quality protein.[17] The significance of leucine as a modulator of MPS has made it a popular supplement among strength-training individuals.[83] This practice is a case of false reasoning. For example, if one assumes that de novo synthesis of nonessential amino acids could keep pace with the stimulatory effect of leucine in its free form on muscle protein synthesis, it would be inevitable that the muscle intracellular free amino acid pool would become depleted of the other EAAs, and muscle protein synthesis would actually be impaired. A superior method of supplementing a diet is to simply consume high-quality proteins that contain all the amino acids to build muscle protein and are rich in leucine, such as chicken, beef, egg, and milk proteins.

It is interesting to consider that a certain threshold of EAAs or, more likely, simply leucine in the blood must be reached to maximally initiate protein synthesis; this leucine trigger hypothesis is illustrated in Figure 3.4. A recent report illustrated a graded response relationship between protein dose and rates of MPS.[84] Research suggests that there is a direct relationship between the concentration of extracellular amino acids, particularly leucine, and rates of muscle protein synthesis.[85] Carbohydrate ingestion with protein does not modulate the postexercise MPS response, despite slowing dietary protein digestion and amino acid absorption rates and thus lowering the rate at which leucine enters circulation.[86] Thus, carbohydrate ingestion with protein did not affect the leucine trigger hypothesis.

CASEIN

Casein, the acid-insoluble fraction of protein, is produced from the solid fraction of milk after exposure to an acidic environment; it is less commonly used in sports drinks or bars because of solubility issues and production cost.[87] Casein is

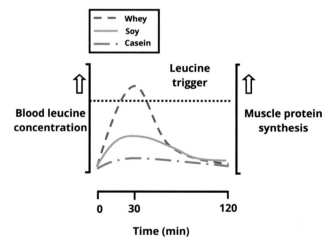

FIGURE 3.4 The Leucine Trigger Hypothesis After consumption of whey protein (which is higher in leucine content than soy or casein), there is a rapid increase in plasma leucine concentration, and this increase corresponds to the extent to which muscle protein synthesis is stimulated. The amount of leucine needed to achieve the trigger is about 2 to 3 g in a meal.

commonly recommended for consumption in the late evening because it takes a long time to digest.[77,81] The slow and prolonged release of amino acids into systemic circulation is hypothesized to promote a positive NPB during the overnight fast/recovery period and thus a greater accretion of muscle proteins; however, this supposition has very little scientific support.

SOY

Soy, a vegetable protein, contains a single protein fraction, and the rate of digestion more closely resembles that of whey than casein.[88] However, the total amino acid content of soy protein contains a lower proportion of leucine compared with milk-derived proteins and thus is thought to have a lower potential anabolic effect on skeletal muscle tissue.[89]

The superiority of higher-quality, animal-based proteins in inducing maximal responses after resistance exercise is not a novel phenomenon. Wilkinson and colleagues demonstrated that young men who consumed 500 mL of nonfat milk exhibited a greater anabolic response after strength training than when they consumed an isonitrogenous, isoenergetic, and macronutrient-matched soy beverage.[90] A training study confirmed these acute findings in men and women.[10,91] Similar to these findings, another study found that young men who consumed 500 mL milk (~17.5 g protein, ~25.7 g carbohydrate, ~0.4 g fat) within 2 hours after full-body resistance training showed the greatest gains in lean body mass and significantly more loss of fat mass compared with training groups that consumed a soy- or carbohydrate-only product.[10] These data suggest that examining the acute muscle protein synthetic response can qualitatively predict long-term training adaptations, at least to prolonged resistance exercise training.[10,90] The effectiveness of milk in inducing superior training adaptations is not sex-specific; it has been established that young women who consumed 500 mL nonfat milk immediately after exercise and an hour later had greater increases in bench press strength, greater loss of fat mass, and greater accretion of muscle protein compared with a group that consumed a carbohydrate (isoenergetic maltodextrin) drink at similar times after whole-body resistance strength training. The women who drank the milk did not gain any weight with strength training, and those in the carbohydrate group had a slight increase in weight. The truly interesting portion of the data is the comparison of the lean mass gains and fat mass losses in both groups, which were far greater in the milk group that the carbohydrate group. Collectively, these data illustrate that women can clearly benefit by consuming a diet high in healthy low-fat dairy protein, especially when coupled with an anabolic stimulus such as resistance training. This is at odds with the belief of some young women that dairy foods are fattening.[91-93]

One typical question related to the beneficial effect of supplementing with milk vs whey after a training period is: Would consuming approximately 20 g whey induce superior training adaptations vs consuming, for example, 500 mL of milk? Although, this comparison (whey vs milk) has never been investigated, the examination of the current literature would suggest that gains in lean body mass and loss of fat mass would be relatively similar.[10,46,91,94-96] Of note, however, is that low-fat dairy seems to be exceptionally potent in decreasing fat mass, especially in young women who consume relatively low amounts of dairy.[91] This effect may be related to the interplay between calcium and vitamin D and how it affects adipocyte metabolism and inhibition of lipid accretion.[97,98] Thus, the consumption of protein/nutrient-dense whole foods (milk, beef, chicken, seafood, etc) may offer additional benefits beyond simply stimulating the postprandial MPS response compared with the consumption of isolated protein sources that have lost many nutritional factors during processing. Although there has been an interest in the use of protein blends (partly to reduce industrial manufacturing cost of single higher-quality protein sources) to augment the skeletal muscle adaptive response, these protein blends will likely not offer any benefit beyond that of simply ingesting protein-dense foods.[99] However, protein blends, such as those with added whey, are likely valuable to increase the anabolic potential of casein and/or isolated plant-based proteins.[89,99] It is important to note, however, the need to confirm the purity of a protein supplement product. Products that are NSF Certified for Sport or are certified by Informed-Choice are logical choices.

Finally, it would seem that plant-based proteins (eg, soy) are relatively inferior at eliciting training adaptations compared with animal proteins.[10,100] This supposition leaves a vegetarian athlete at odds with the exact type of protein that should be consumed for optimal recovery from exercise; however, lean mass gains with soy protein consumption are superior over those obtained by simply consuming carbohydrate after exercise, suggesting that supplementing with soy protein is not entirely without benefit.[10,100] Of particular interest to a vegetarian athlete may be a plant-based protein, quinoa, which has a leucine, lysine, and methionine content superior to that of soy and similar to that of milk.[89,101] Assuming, as with isolated soy protein, that the antinutritional components of the quinoa plant can be removed, mainly fiber, then isolated quinoa may be a very beneficial protein source. To date, however, this protein (and many other plant-derived proteins) has yet to be produced in supplemental form and has yet to be systematically tested against animal proteins for the anabolic response after exercise. Overall, more work is required to assess how ingesting a wider variety of plant-derived proteins affects the skeletal muscle adaptive response to training. In addition, fortification of plant-based proteins with free amino acids or genetic manipulation or cross-breeding of plants, such as high-quality maize protein, to improve the amino acid composition—leucine in particular—may serve as useful strategies to enhance the postprandial MPS response to ingesting plant-derived proteins during exercise recovery.

PROTEIN QUANTITY

How Much Protein Should an Athlete Consume After Resistance Training?

The optimal dose of protein to maximize the acute anabolic response after exercise is a classic debate within groups ranging from sport scientists to fitness enthusiasts. Resistance-trained athletes often believe the more protein they eat, the more lean mass they will gain because the amino acids in protein are the building blocks for muscle. Recent data would suggest quite the contrary.[84] Research shows that experienced weight-trained men, weighing on average 85 kg, who consumed varying doses of high-quality isolated egg protein experienced the greatest degree of stimulation of MPS at 20 g. No further benefit was gained from consuming 40 g of protein vs 20 g after acute resistance exercise (Figure 3.5). Of interest, however, is that consuming excess amounts of protein actually increased leucine oxidation, which means excess amino acids are being utilized for energy production or are being wasted. This finding of a graded response relationship with the dose of protein consumed and the extent of stimulation of MPS agrees with other data that illustrated that MPS is twice as great when 6 g of EAA is consumed compared with approximately 3 g of EAA, which is equivalent to approximately 15 g and 7.5 g of a high-quality protein, respectively.[102]

A common and relevant question when attempting to advise athletes about the quantity of protein to consume is, "How does body mass, or, more appropriately, lean body mass factor into this recommendation?" That is to say, do individuals with a greater degree of lean body mass ($\geq$ 90 kg) require more protein than their smaller counterparts ($\leq$ 50 kg)? This is an intriguing question that remains to be systematically investigated. However, considering that larger individuals have a greater absolute volume of blood—based on the notion that the blood amino acid concentrations after dietary protein consumption (specifically the leucine trigger hypothesis [Figure 3.4]) are a primary

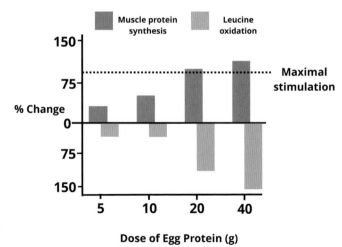

FIGURE 3.5 The Relationship Between Protein Dose and Muscle Protein Synthesis
Twenty grams of egg protein maximizes the anabolic response to resistance exercise. There is no additional benefit from consuming 40 g of egg protein. Protein consumed in excess is either used for energy or wasted (excreted).

factor in determining the increase in MPS after acute exercise—it is reasonable that larger individuals require more protein than their smaller counterparts (Figure 3.6).[103] The maximal dose of protein, as noted in Figure 3.6, is most likely not too far off (± 5 g) from the maximal dose of 20 g that has been previously demonstrated.[84] Importantly, Moore and colleagues have recently provided insight into meal-based protein requirements to optimize the postprandial MPS response relative to body weight.[104] Their research demonstrated that about 0.24 g protein per kilogram in a meal (range: 0.18 to 0.30 g protein per kilogram) is sufficient to maximize postprandial MPS in young adults. Indeed, these results were not obtained in the postexercise state but likely provide reasonable estimates of the protein requirements of skeletal muscle tissue during recovery from resistance exercise as well.[104]

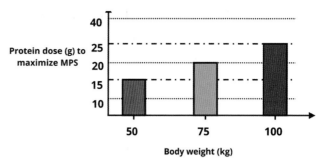

FIGURE 3.6 Theoretical model illustrating the dose of protein needed to maximally stimulate muscle protein synthesis (MPS) after an acute bout of resistance or endurance exercise (~0.25 g protein/kg per meal) Note that this thesis has never been systematically tested and as such is purely speculative.

Recommendations for individuals who have been training for a period of ≥ 8 weeks may require special consideration. If a sports dietitian were to base recommendations on the fact that resistance exercise increases protein synthesis, then it would be possible that higher protein intakes are required to support this elevated response.[6,105] However, recent data suggest that this hypothesis is fallacious. Hartman and colleagues demonstrated that 12 weeks of resistance training decreases both whole-body protein synthesis and breakdown, resulting in a greater NPB measured over the course of 24 hours compared with the untrained state.[106] These findings imply a greater retention of dietary nitrogen (protein) after resistance training than before a person begins a training program, which is consistent with the anabolic nature of resistance exercise in stimulating muscle to hang on to more of its protein mass. Researchers have established that turnover of whole-body leucine decreases in both the fasting and fed states after 12 weeks of resistance training, with a concomitant increase in fiber size.[107] This suggests greater use of amino acids for protein accretion or simply a greater net retention, which further suggests that protein requirements are not elevated in strength-trained individuals.[108,109] The underlying mechanisms for the decreased protein requirements with training may be two-fold: (1) resistance exercise in the fasted state increases NPB, suggesting a more efficient use of intracellular amino acids, and (2) aerobic exercise and resistance training preferentially stimulate specific muscle proteins.[9,13,14] This indicates that skeletal muscle has the ability to direct signals to turn on specific proteins in response to a specific exercise stimulus. Thus, it would not be completely unlikely that repeated bouts of an anabolic stimulus on skeletal muscle may predispose muscle tissue to become a greater site of disposition of amino acids than in the untrained state.

Finally, from a practical standpoint, combining differing research findings can illustrate how much and how often an individual could consume protein within a given day. Specifically, it is reasonable to hypothesize that an individual could consume 20 g of protein no more than five or six times a day to maximize MPS without excess loss to oxidation for an 80-kg athlete.[84] See Box 3.1 for examples of high-quality protein.

Box 3.1 Sources of High-Quality Protein

The following foods provide 20 g of high-quality protein when consumed in the portions indicated:

- 500 mL (about 2 cups) nonfat milk
- 3 oz beef
- 2.5 oz chicken or turkey
- ¾ cup cottage cheese

Is Protein Consumption Necessary After Endurance Exercise?

Carbohydrates and fats are the primary fuels used during endurance exercise, and protein consumption is often not of primary concern as a fuel source for endurance athletes.[4,23,110] However, it is worth considering that if dietary protein is not consumed in adequate quantities, then MPB is the only alternative to supply the amino acids to the intracellular free amino acid pool to ultimately support protein synthesis. Recommendations for nutrition practices in endurance athletes point to studies in nitrogen balance that report that these athletes require as much as 60% to 100% more protein than the Recommended Dietary Allowance (0.8 g/kg/d) to sustain nitrogen balance.[111] Furthermore, research has established that mitochondrial protein synthesis is stimulated after endurance exercise, and this protein fraction is responsive to protein feeding.[13,112] Therefore, consumption of dietary protein after endurance exercise is recommended to ensure an optimal adaptation and exploitation of the protein synthetic stimulus of the exercise itself. The quantity of protein to recommend to endurance athletes largely depends on the athlete's training status, training intensity, and workout duration. As highlighted by Tarnopolsky in a recent review, a recreational athlete training at a very moderate intensity (~40% VO_2 max) for approximately 1 hour per day, 4 days per week, would expend approximately 2,000 kcal per week, whereas an elite athlete training at intensities of 60% to 80% VO_2 max for 8 to 40 hours per week would expend approximately an additional 6,000 to 40,000 kcal per week more than resting energy requirements.[18] The body size of the athlete should be considered because bigger athletes burn more energy than smaller athletes.[113] For these reasons, it is clear that any recommendation should be made on an individual basis and confirmed by monitoring body weight to ensure that the athlete is obtaining adequate energy. Finally, if athletes who are expending large quantities of energy are matching this expenditure with intake, it is unlikely, even at low percentage of total dietary energy derived from protein, that they are consuming insufficient protein. For example, a 70-kg athlete consuming 4,500 kcal/d and 15% energy from protein still would be consuming 170 g protein (2.4 g/kg) daily.

Current recommendations for endurance athletes' protein requirements are largely based on nitrogen balance studies because studies using direct measures of muscle protein synthesis are lacking.[18,114,115] If the dietary protein consumed contains amino acids and every amino acid contains nitrogen, then it seems quite reasonable that nitrogen balance would be a valid method to assess need. A positive nitrogen balance indicates that consumption of dietary protein was adequate or more than needed, and negative nitrogen balance indicates an inadequate protein intake. However, assessing dietary protein needs utilizing nitrogen balance methodology does have its shortcomings, and this topic has been reviewed elsewhere.[2,18,116,117]

A study using stable isotope methodology demonstrated that active young men who performed two 90-minute cycling bouts daily (one in the morning and one in the afternoon) and consumed 1.0 g protein per kilogram per day achieved nitrogen balance during a 24-hour period.[114] Another study compared subjects who were habitually fed a high-protein (1.8 g/kg/d) or low-protein (0.7 g/kg/d) diet for 7 days and then walked on a treadmill for 2 hours at a moderate intensity. In this study, leucine oxidation increased after the high-protein diet, which indicates that the excess protein was utilized for energy during the exercise bout.[118] Although not directly determined, the low-protein diet was likely inadequate to meet the protein requirements to optimize performance in these participants. Bolster and colleagues recruited endurance athletes (running ≥ 56 km/wk) and had them consume a low-protein (0.8 g/kg/d), moderate-protein (1.8 g/kg/d), or high-protein (3.6 g/kg/d) diet for 4 weeks.[119] Subsequently, the researchers had the athletes perform a 75-minute treadmill run at 70% VO_2 peak. In this study, the fasted-state, mixed-muscle, fractional synthetic rate (a direct measure of muscle protein synthesis) was attenuated during the recovery period following the high-protein dietary intervention vs the low or moderate protein intakes.[119] This result was in contrast to the authors' hypothesis, which was that habitually consuming a high-protein diet would ultimately expand the free amino acid pool and therefore support greater rates of muscle protein synthesis.[119] Researchers noted in a review of a small subset of these participants (n = 4) that fractional breakdown rate (a direct measure of muscle protein breakdown) was attenuated after high protein intakes, such that NPB was improved to a greater extent compared with moderate or low protein intakes.[73] These preliminary findings are not entirely surprising because MPS and breakdown have been shown to be tightly coordinated.[9] Lastly, studies of highly trained cyclists who engaged in an exercise protocol similar to the Tour de France (ie, long, exhausting cycling) demonstrated that daily protein requirements of 1.5 to 1.8 g/kg are needed to maintain nitrogen balance under such vigorous exercise conditions.[120,121]

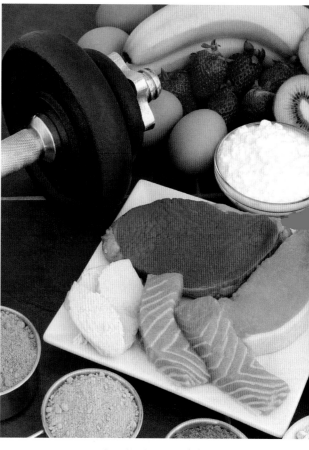

It seems that diet manipulation can influence the anabolic response to endurance exercise, but moderate endurance exercise does not increase dietary protein requirements above those of the general population. Athletes engaged in vigorous training may need slightly more dietary protein; however, provided that the athletes are consuming adequate daily energy and that 10% to 15% is coming from dietary protein, these individuals will be meeting their daily protein requirements.

Overall, dietary protein requirements for an endurance athlete have not been clearly defined. In particular, there are no data that describe the ingested protein dose-response curves on the postprandial MPS response during recovery from endurance exercise. Additional work is required to assess the effects of intensity or duration of the endurance exercise bout on dietary protein requirements for a specific athlete, which may vary based on their specific phase of training. In particular, higher-intensity or longer-duration endurance exercise training increases oxidation of amino acids to be used for hepatic gluconeogenesis (or deamination) or as a fuel source for skeletal muscle mitochondria. As such, exercise intensity or duration may modulate dietary protein requirements for an endurance athlete. Moreover, Rowlands and Wadsworth demonstrated that the daily protein requirements of female endurance athletes may be slightly higher than those of male athletes.[122] However, it seems likely that approximately 0.25 g protein per kilogram per meal provides a reasonable recommendation to optimize repair, remodeling, or muscle protein accretion during recovery from endurance exercise until additional work that is specific to an endurance athlete is completed in this area.

INDIVIDUAL AMINO ACID SUPPLEMENTATION: FACT OR FICTION?

Glutamine and arginine are amino acids purported to have ergogenic effects if consumed in supplemental form, especially during recovery from injury. Glutamine, a highly abundant amino acid in the body, is largely synthesized in skeletal muscle and released in plasma during exercise.[123,124] Muscle glutamine concentrations have been related to rates of MPS in skeletal muscle of rats, some of which were protein deficient, endotoxemic, or starved, which begs the question of whether the findings can be extended to humans.[125] Glutamine supplementation combined with 6 weeks of resistance training in young adults had no added effect on muscle strength and fat-free mass accretion compared with a placebo group.[126] Furthermore, data demonstrated that glutamine ingestion in healthy adult men and women was associated with an approximately four-fold increase (compared with control participants) in plasma growth hormone.[127] It was suggested that an increase in plasma growth hormone concentrations following glutamine supplementation may be significant for strength athletes to maximize training adaptations.[87] However, it is not entirely clear whether elevated concentrations of growth hormone within normal physiological concentrations would benefit strength-training athletes. Specifically, West and colleagues have established that exercise-induced anabolic hormones (ie, growth hormone, testosterone, insulin-like growth factor), within the physiological limits seen with protein or exercise-induced increments, have no influence on MPS, strength gains, or muscle hypertrophy.[11,128] Furthermore, recombinant growth hormone has no effect on myofibrillar protein synthesis after resistance exercise in young men.[129] Therefore, dietary supplementation with glutamine to maximize muscle hypertrophy or strength gains after resistance training is not recommended.

L-arginine, considered a conditionally essential amino acid, is in high demand after periods of rapid growth or physical or pathologic insult such that de novo synthesis cannot be met by normal dietary intake.[130-132] However, in healthy adults, arginine can be synthesized in sufficient quantity to meet needs.[132-134] Similar to glutamine, a purported benefit of administering arginine intravenously is its ability to stimulate growth hormone release.[135] One study demonstrated that oral arginine could stimulate growth hormone; these results, however, could not be repeated in another study.[136,137] Furthermore, oral arginine administration in doses ≥ 10 g resulted in unwanted side effects (ie, abdominal cramps and diarrhea).[137] Regardless of the method of administration, the relevance of stimulating growth hormone release in healthy non-deficient adults within physiological limits, insofar as muscle hypertrophy and strength are concerned, is questionable.[11,128] Research has established that arginine is not required or stimulatory for muscle protein synthesis.[138] Therefore, any ergogenic effect of L-arginine supplementation must be indirect and may be related to the stimulation of nitric oxide production.[132] For example, L-arginine is the primary substrate for nitric oxide synthase, the enzyme responsible for nitric oxide production. This leads to the release of nitric oxide from the vascular endothelium, leading to vasodilation and subsequent increase in local blood flow. However, in a randomized and double-blind study, Tang and colleagues found that after resistance exercise in young men, consumption of 10 g EAAs in combination with 10 g L-arginine or an isonitrogenous amount of glycine as a control had no influence on femoral artery blood flow despite an approximate five-fold increase in blood L-arginine after L-arginine consumption.[139] Furthermore, there was no effect on any markers of nitric oxide (nitrate, nitrite, endothelin-1) and no stimulatory effect on MPS at rest or after exercise.[139] Therefore, L-arginine supplementation, provided that sufficient EAAs are consumed, has no influence on the anabolic response after resistance exercise. As with glutamine supplementation, supplementation with free-form L-arginine cannot be recommended.

SUMMARY

Recommendations for dietary protein intake should be individualized, but general recommendations are presented in Table 3.1.

Table 3.1 Daily Protein Recommendations for Endurance-Training and Resistance-Training Athletes[a,27,28,33,45,46,80,85]

Type of Training	Protein Recommendation, g/kg/d	Example of Total Daily Protein Intake
Endurance	1.2–1.4	84–98 g for 70-kg (154-1b) endurance athlete
Resistance	1.6–1.7	146–155 g for 91-kg (200-lb) strength athlete

[a] Emphasis should be placed on timing and distribution of dietary protein ingestion over the course of the day (eg, approximately 0.25 g protein per kilogram per meal × 4 to 5 meals per day) to optimize the skeletal muscle adaptive response in an athlete.

Resistance and endurance exercise both have the ability to stimulate MPS, but the type of proteins that are accrued is related to the nature and stress of the stimulus as noted by diverse adaptations that occur after different modes of exercise. Specifically, resistance exercise preferentially stimulates myofibrillar proteins to aid in force production, and endurance training stimulates the accretion of mitochondria proteins to assist in sustained energy production during exercise. Ingesting dietary protein after exercise, however, is paramount in supporting a high rate of MPS, which would elicit an optimal adaptation to the exercise stimulus. For example, many researchers have established that consuming protein soon after performing resistance exercise results in a greater hypertrophic response than when no protein is consumed or when protein is not consumed close to the exercise stimulus.[10,140,141] High-quality proteins such as milk, whey, casein, and soy can positively influence the MPS response, but differences in digestion rates and the subsequent rate at which amino acids appear in the blood may also influence the MPS response such that milk and its isolated forms, such as whey, may confer a further advantage to muscle anabolism. The leucine content of the protein meal may also be an important component to consider in regards to muscle anabolism. Approximately 2 to 3 g leucine per meal should allow for the leucine threshold to be met without excessive leucine oxidation rates; this is an amount that is contained in most protein-dense foods when 20 to 30 g protein is ingested. The quantity of protein to consume after exercise is less than what is commonly believed. However, consuming dietary protein within 1 to 2 hours after exercise may be of primary concern to elicit optimal training adaptations, provided the athlete is consuming adequate energy throughout the course of the day. Finally, supplementing dietary needs with individual amino acids, specifically glutamine and arginine, has no ergogenic effect in healthy adults.

KEY TAKEAWAYS

Athletes should ingest sufficient protein as part of each meal (~0.25 g protein per kilogram body mass) with 4 to 5 meals daily to optimize the skeletal muscle adaptive response.

The optimal timing window to consume protein during recovery from exercise is not known. The anabolic effect of exercise diminishes with increasing time during recovery, and, therefore, ingestion of protein is recommended within 4 hours of recovery.

There is no evidence to suggest that ingestiong isolated protein powders or supplements is necessary to enhance the skeletal muscle adaptive response to prolonged exercise training. Instead, the regular consumption of protein as part of nutrient-dense foods that contain all essential amino acids and are high in leucine is recommended.

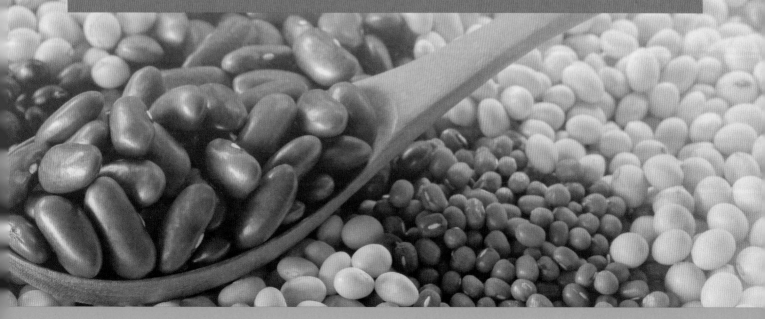

1. Von Liebig J. *Animal Chemistry or Organic Chemistry in its Application to Physiology.* London: Taylor and Walton; 1842.

2. Phillips SM. Protein requirements and supplementation in strength sports. *Nutrition.* 2004;20(7-8):689-695.

3. Phillips SM, Atkinson SA, Tarnopolsky MA, MacDougall JD. Gender differences in leucine kinetics and nitrogen balance in endurance athletes. *J Appl Physiol (1985).* 1993;75(5):2134-2141.

4. Tarnopolsky MA, Atkinson SA, Phillips SM, MacDougall JD. Carbohydrate loading and metabolism during exercise in men and women. *J Appl Physiol (1985).* 1995;78(4):1360-1368.

5. Goldberg AL, Chang TW. Regulation and significance of amino acid metabolism in skeletal muscle. *Fed Proc.* 1978;37(9):2301-2307.

6. Burd NA, Tang JE, Moore DR, Phillips SM. Exercise training and protein metabolism: influences of contraction, protein intake, and sex-based differences. *J Appl Physiol (1985).* 2009;106(5):1692-1701.

7. Rennie MJ, Edwards RH, Halliday D, Matthews DE, Wolman SL, Millward DJ. Muscle protein synthesis measured by stable isotope techniques in man: the effects of feeding and fasting. *Clin Sci (Lond).* 1982;63(6):519-523.

8. Martini WZ, Chinkes DL, Wolfe RR. The intracellular free amino acid pool represents tracer precursor enrichment for calculation of protein synthesis in cultured fibroblasts and myocytes. *J Nutr.* 2004;134(6):1546-1550.

9. Phillips SM, Tipton KD, Aarsland A, Wolf SE, Wolfe RR. Mixed muscle protein synthesis and breakdown after resistance exercise in humans. *Am J Physiol.* 1997;273(1 pt 1):e99-a107.

10. Hartman JW, Tang JE, Wilkinson SB, et al. Consumption of fat-free fluid milk after resistance exercise promotes greater lean mass accretion than does consumption of soy or carbohydrate in young, novice, male weightlifters. *Am J Clin Nutr.* 2007;86(2):373-381.

11. West DW, Burd NA, Tang JE, et al. Elevations in ostensibly anabolic hormones with resistance exercise enhance neither training-induced muscle hypertrophy nor strength of the elbow flexors. *J Appl Physiol (1985).* 2010;108(1):60-67.

12. Kim PL, Staron RS, Phillips SM. Fasted-state skeletal muscle protein synthesis after resistance exercise is altered with training. *J Physiol.* 2005;568(pt 1):283-290.

13. Wilkinson SB, Phillips SM, Atherton PJ, et al. Differential effects of resistance and endurance exercise in the fed state on signalling molecule phosphorylation and protein synthesis in human muscle. *J Physiol.* 2008;586(pt 15):3701-3717.

14. Phillips SM, Parise G, Roy BD, Tipton KD, Wolfe RR, Tamopolsky MA. Resistance-training-induced adaptations in skeletal muscle protein turnover in the fed state. *Can J Physiol Pharmacol.* 2002;80(11):1045-1053.

15. Phillips SM, Tipton KD, Ferrando AA, Wolfe RR. Resistance training reduces the acute exercise-induced increase in muscle protein turnover. *Am J Physiol.* 1999;276(1 pt 1):e118-124.

16. Tang JE, Perco JG, Moore DR, Wilkinson SB, Phillips SM. Resistance training alters the response of fed state mixed muscle protein synthesis in young men. *Am J Physiol Regul Integr Comp Physiol.* 2008;294(1):R172-R178.

17. Tipton KD, Gurkin BE, Matin S, Wolfe RR. Nonessential amino acids are not necessary to stimulate net muscle protein synthesis in healthy volunteers. *J Nutr Biochem.* 1999;10(2):89-95.

18. Tarnopolsky M. Protein requirements for endurance athletes. *Nutrition.* 2004;20(7-8):662-668.

19. Lamont LS, McCullough AJ, Kalhan SC. Relationship between leucine oxidation and oxygen consumption during steady-state exercise. *Med Sci Sports Exerc.* 2001;33(2):237-241.

20. Haralambie G, Berg A. Serum urea and amino nitrogen changes with exercise duration. *Eur J Appl Physiol Occup Physiol.* 1976;36(1):39-48.

21. Howarth KR, Phillips SM, MacDonald MJ, Richards D, Moreau NA, Gibala MJ. Effect of glycogen availability on human skeletal muscle protein turnover during exercise and recovery. *J Appl Physiol (1985).* 2010;109(2):431-438.

22. Moore DR. Nutrition to support recovery from endurance exercise: optimal carbohydrate and protein replacement. *Curr Sports Med Rep.* 2015; 14(4):294-300.

23. McKenzie S, Phillips SM, Carter SL, Lowther S, Gibala MJ, Tarnopolsky MA. Endurance exercise training attenuates leucine oxidation and BCOAD activation during exercise in humans. *Am J Physiol Endocrinol Metab.* 2000;278(4):e580-e587.

24. Moore DR, Camera DM, Areta JL, Hawley JA. Beyond muscle hypertrophy: why dietary protein is important for endurance athletes. *Appl Physiol Nutr Metab.* 2014;39(9):987-997.

25. Carraro F, Stuart CA, Hartl WH, Rosenblatt J, Wolfe RR. Effect of exercise and recovery on muscle protein synthesis in human subjects. *Am J Physiol.* 1990;259(4 pt 1):e470-e476.

26. Harber MP, Konopka AR, Jemiolo B, Trappe SW, Trappe TA, Reidy PT. Muscle protein synthesis and gene expression during recovery from aerobic exercise in the fasted and fed states. *Am J Physiol Regul Integr Comp Physiol.* 2010;299(5):R1254-R1262.

27. Miller BF, Olesen JL, Hansen M, et al. Coordinated collagen and muscle protein synthesis in human patella tendon and quadriceps muscle after exercise. *J Physiol.* 2005;567(pt 3):1021-1033.

28. Dreyer HC, Fujita S, Cadenas JG, Chinkes DL, Volpi E, Rasmussen BB. Resistance exercise increases AMPK activity and reduces 4E-BP1 phosphorylation and protein synthesis in human skeletal muscle. *J Physiol.* 2006;576(pt 2):613-624.

29. Di Donato DM, West DW, Churchward-Venne TA, Breen L, Baker SK, Phillips SM. Influence of aerobic exercise intensity on myofibrillar and mitochondrial protein synthesis in young men during early and late postexercise recovery. *Am J Physiol Endocrinol Metab.* 2014;306(9):e1025-e1032.

30. Tipton KD, Rasmussen BB, Miller SL, et al. Timing of amino acid-carbohydrate ingestion alters anabolic response of muscle to resistance exercise. *Am J Physiol Endocrinol Metab.* 2001;281(2):e197-e206.

31. Tipton KD, Elliott TA, Cree MG, Aarsland AA, Sanford AP, Wolfe RR. Stimulation of net muscle protein synthesis by whey protein ingestion before and after exercise. *Am J Physiol Endocrinol Metab.* 2007;292(1):e71-e76.

32. Durham WJ, Casperson SL, Dillon EL, et al. Age-related anabolic resistance after endurance-type exercise in healthy humans. *FASEB J.* 2010;24(10):4117-4127.

33. Rasmussen BB, Tipton KD, Miller SL, Wolf SE, Wolfe RR. An oral essential amino acid-carbohydrate supplement enhances muscle protein anabolism after resistance exercise. *J Appl Physiol (1985).* 2000;88(2):386-392.

34. Beelen M, Tieland M, Gijsen AP, et al. Coingestion of carbohydrate and protein hydrolysate stimulates muscle protein synthesis during exercise in young men, with no further increase during subsequent overnight recovery. *J Nutr.* 2008;138(11):2198-2204.

35. Esmarck B, Andersen JL, Olsen S, Richter EA, Mizuno M, Kjaer M. Timing of postexercise protein intake is important for muscle hypertrophy with resistance training in elderly humans. *J Physiol.* 2001;535(pt 1):301-311.

36. Frontera WR, Meredith CN, O'Reilly KP, Knuttgen HG, Evans WJ. Strength conditioning in older men: skeletal muscle hypertrophy and improved function. *J Appl Physiol (1985).* 1988;64(3):1038-1044.

37. Trappe S, Williamson D, Godard M. Maintenance of whole muscle strength and size following resistance training in older men. *J Gerontol A Biol Sci Med Sci.* 2002;57(4):B138-B143.

38. Kosek DJ, Kim JS, Petrella JK, Cross JM, Bamman MM. Efficacy of 3 days/wk resistance training on myofiber hypertrophy and myogenic mechanisms in young vs. older adults. *J Applied Physiol.* 2006;101(2):531-544.

39. Fiatarone MA, Marks EC, Ryan ND, Meredith CN, Lipsitz LA, Evans WJ. High-intensity strength training in nonagenarians. Effects on skeletal muscle. *JAMA.* 1990;263(22):3029-3034.

40. Kalapotharakos VI, Michalopoulou M, Godolias G, Tokmakidis SP, Malliou PV, Gourgoulis V. The effects of high- and moderate-resistance training on muscle function in the elderly. *J Aging Phys Act.* 2004;12(2):131-143.

41. Slivka D, Raue U, Hollon C, Minchev K, Trappe S. Single muscle fiber adaptations to resistance training in old (>80 yr) men: evidence for limited skeletal muscle plasticity. *Am J Physiol Regul Integr Comp Physiol.* 2008;295(1):R273-R280.

42. Verdijk LB, Jonkers RA, Gleeson BG, et al. Protein supplementation before and after exercise does not further augment skeletal muscle hypertrophy after resistance training in elderly men. *Am J Clin Nutr.* 2009;89(2):608-616.

43. Campbell WW, Crim MC, Young VR, Evans WJ. Increased energy requirements and changes in body composition with resistance training in older adults. *Am J Clin Nutr.* 1994;60(2):167-175.

44. Sallinen J, Pakarinen A, Fogelholm M, et al. Serum basal hormone concentrations and muscle mass in aging women: effects of strength training and diet. *Int J Sport Nutr Exerc Metab.* 2006;16(3):316-331.

45. Josse AR, Atkinson SA, Tarnopolsky MA, Phillips SM. Increased consumption of dairy foods and protein during diet- and exercise-induced weight loss promotes fat mass loss and lean mass gain in overweight and obese premenopausal women. *J Nutr.* 2011;141(9):1626-1634.

46. Cribb PJ, Hayes A. Effects of supplement timing and resistance exercise on skeletal muscle hypertrophy. *Med Sci Sports Exerc.* 2006;38(11):1918-1925.

47. Hoffman JR, Ratamess NA, Tranchina CP, Rashti SL, Kang J, Faigenbaum AD. Effect of protein-supplement timing on strength, power, and body-composition changes in resistance-trained men. *Int J Sport Nutr Exerc Metab.* 2009;19(2):172-185.

48. Burk A, Timpmann S, Medijainen L, Vahi M, Oopik V. Time-divided ingestion pattern of casein-based protein supplement stimulates an increase in fat-free body mass during resistance training in young untrained men. *Nutr Res.* 2009;29(6):405-413.

49. Schoenfeld BJ, Aragon AA, Krieger JW. The effect of protein timing on muscle strength and hypertrophy: a meta-analysis. *J Int Soc Sports Nutr.* 2013;10(1):53.

50. Burd NA, West DW, Moore DR, et al. Enhanced amino acid sensitivity of myofibrillar protein synthesis persists for up to 24 h after resistance exercise in young men. *J Nutr.* 2011;141(4):568-573.

51. Cermak NM, Res PT, de Groot LC, Saris WH, van Loon LJ. Protein supplementation augments the adaptive response of skeletal muscle to resistance-type exercise training: a meta-analysis. *Am J Clin Nutr.* 2012;96(6):1454-1464.

52. Areta JL, Burke LM, Ross ML, et al. Timing and distribution of protein ingestion during prolonged recovery from resistance exercise alters myofibrillar protein synthesis. *J Physiol.* 2013;591(pt 9):2319-2331.

53. Kumar V, Selby A, Rankin D, et al. Age-related differences in the dose-response relationship of muscle protein synthesis to resistance exercise in young and old men. *J Physiol.* 2009;587(pt 1):211-217.

54. Drummond MJ, Fry CS, Glynn EL, et al. Skeletal muscle amino acid transporter expression is increased in young and older adults following resistance exercise. *J Appl Physiol (1985).* 2011;111(1):135-142.

55. Drummond MJ, Glynn EL, Fry CS, Timmerman KL, Volpi E, Rasmussen BB. An increase in essential amino acid availability upregulates amino acid transporter expression in human skeletal muscle. *Am J Physiol Endocr Metab.* 2010;298(5):e1011-e1018.

56. Dickinson JM, Gundermann DM, Walker DK, et al. Leucine-enriched amino acid ingestion after resistance exercise prolongs myofibrillar protein synthesis and amino acid transporter expression in older men. *J Nutr.* 2014;144(11):1694-1702.

57. Res PT, Groen B, Pennings B, et al. Protein ingestion before sleep improves postexercise overnight recovery. *Med Sci Sports Exerc.* 2012;44(8):1560-1569.

58. Snijders T, Res PT, Smeets JS, et al. Protein ingestion before sleep increases muscle mass and strength gains during prolonged resistance-type exercise training in healthy young men. *J Nutr.* 2015;145(6):1178-1184.

59. Holloszy JO, Coyle EF. Adaptations of skeletal muscle to endurance exercise and their metabolic consequences. *J Appl Physiol Respir Environ Exerc Physiol.* 1984;56(4):831-838.

60. Hood DA. Invited review: contractile activity-induced mitochondrial biogenesis in skeletal muscle. *J Appl Physiol (1985).* 2001;90(3):1137-1157.

61. Hood DA, Takahashi M, Connor MK, Freyssenet D. Assembly of the cellular powerhouse: current issues in muscle mitochondrial biogenesis. *Exerc Sport Sci Rev.* 2000;28(2):68-73.

62. Howarth KR, Moreau NA, Phillips SM, Gibala MJ. Coingestion of protein with carbohydrate during recovery from endurance exercise stimulates skeletal muscle protein synthesis in humans. *J Appl Physiol (1985).* 2009;106(4):1394-1402.

63. Fujita S, Rasmussen BB, Cadenas JG, et al. Aerobic exercise overcomes the age-related insulin resistance of muscle protein metabolism by improving endothelial function and Akt/mammalian target of rapamycin signaling. *Diabetes.* 2007;56(6):1615-1622.

64. Harber MP, Konopka AR, Douglass MD, et al. Aerobic exercise training improves whole muscle and single myofiber size and function in older women. *Am J Physiol Regul Integr Comp Physiol.* 2009;297(5):R1452-R1459.

65. Ivy JL, Res PT, Sprague RC, Widzer MO. Effect of a carbohydrate-protein supplement on endurance performance during exercise of varying intensity. *Int J Sport Nutr Exerc Metab.* 2003;13(3):382-395.

66. Saunders MJ, Kane MD, Todd MK. Effects of a carbohydrate-protein beverage on cycling endurance and muscle damage. *Med Sci Sports Exerc.* 2004;36(7):1233-1238.

67. Saunders MJ, Luden ND, Herrick JE. Consumption of an oral carbohydrate-protein gel improves cycling endurance and prevents postexercise muscle damage. *J Strength Cond Res.* 2007;21(3):678-684.

68. van Essen M, Gibala MJ. Failure of protein to improve time trial performance when added to a sports drink. *Med Sci Sports Exerc.* 2006;38(8):1476-1483.

69. Cermak NM, Solheim AS, Gardner MS, Tarnopolsky MA, Gibala MJ. Muscle metabolism during exercise with carbohydrate or protein-carbohydrate ingestion. *Med Sci Sports Exerc.* 2009;41(12):2158-2164.

70. Breen L, Tipton KD, Jeukendrup AE. No effect of carbohydrate-protein on cycling performance and indices of recovery. *Med Sci Sports Exerc.* 2010;42(6):1140-1148.

71. Jeukendrup AE, Tipton KD, Gibala MJ. Protein plus carbohydrate does not enhance 60-km time-trial performance. *Int J Sport Nutr Exerc Metab.* 2009;19(4):335-337; author reply 337-339.

72. Koopman R, Pannemans DL, Jeukendrup AE, et al. Combined ingestion of protein and carbohydrate improves protein balance during ultra-endurance exercise. *Am J Physiol Endocrinol Metab.* 2004;287(4):e712-e720.

73. Rodriguez NR, Vislocky LM, Gaine PC. Dietary protein, endurance exercise, and human skeletal-muscle protein turnover. *Curr Opin Clin Nutr Metab Care.* 2007;10(1):40-45.

74. Dangin M, Boirie Y, Garcia-Rodenas C, et al. The digestion rate of protein is an independent regulating factor of postprandial protein retention. *Am J Physiol Endocrinol Metab.* 2001;280(2):e340-e348.

75. Dangin M, Boirie Y, Guillet C, Beaufrere B. Influence of the protein digestion rate on protein turnover in young and elderly subjects. *J Nutr.* 2002;132(10):3228S-3233S.

76. Tang JE, Moore DR, Kujbida GW, Tarnopolsky MA, Phillips SM. Ingestion of whey hydrolysate, casein, or soy protein isolate: effects on mixed muscle protein synthesis at rest and following resistance exercise in young men. *J Appl Physiol (1985).* 2009;107(3):987-992.

77. Pennings B, Boirie Y, Senden JM, Gijsen AP, Kuipers H, van Loon LJ. Whey protein stimulates postprandial muscle protein accretion more effectively than do casein and casein hydrolysate in older men. *Am J Clin Nutr.* 2011;93(5):997-1005.

78. Greenhaff PL, Karagounis LG, Peirce N, et al. Disassociation between the effects of amino acids and insulin on signaling, ubiquitin ligases, and protein turnover in human muscle. *Am J Physiol Endocrinol Metab.* 2008;295(3):e595-e604.

79. Hagenfeldt L, Eriksson S, Wahren J. Influence of leucine on arterial concentrations and regional exchange of amino acids in healthy subjects. *Clin Sci.* 1980;59(3):173-181.

80. Hundal HS, Taylor PM. Amino acid transceptors: gate keepers of nutrient exchange and regulators of nutrient signaling. *Am J Physiol Endocrinol Metab.* 2009;296(4):e603-e613.

81. Boirie Y, Dangin M, Gachon P, Vasson MP, Maubois JL, Beaufrere B. Slow and fast dietary proteins differently modulate postprandial protein accretion. *Proc Natl Acad Sci U S A* 1997;94(26):14930-14935.

82. Burd NA, Gorissen SH, van Vliet S, Snijders T, van Loon LJ. Differences in postprandial protein handling after beef compared with milk ingestion during postexercise recovery: a randomized controlled trial. *Am J Clin Nutr.* 2015;102(4):828-836.

83. Smith K, Barua JM, Watt PW, Scrimgeour CM, Rennie MJ. Flooding with L-[1-13C]leucine stimulates human muscle protein incorporation of continuously infused L-[1-13C]valine. *Am J Physiol.* 1992;262(3 pt 1):e372-e376.

84. Moore DR, Robinson MJ, Fry JL, et al. Ingested protein dose response of muscle and albumin protein synthesis after resistance exercise in young men. *Am J Clin Nutr.* 2009;89(1):161-168.

85. Bohe J, Low A, Wolfe RR, Rennie MJ. Human muscle protein synthesis is modulated by extracellular, not intramuscular amino acid availability: a dose-response study. *J Physiol.* 2003;552(pt 1):315-324.

86. Staples AW, Burd NA, West DW, et al. Carbohydrate does not augment exercise-induced protein accretion versus protein alone. *Med Sci Sports Exerc.* 2011;43(7):1154-1161.

87. Paul GL. The rationale for consuming protein blends in sports nutrition. *J Am Coll Nutr.* 2009;28(4):464S-472S.

88. Bos C, Metges CC, Gaudichon C, et al. Postprandial kinetics of dietary amino acids are the main determinant of their metabolism after soy or milk protein ingestion in humans. *J Nutr.* 2003;133(5):1308-1315.

89. van Vliet S, Burd NA, van Loon LJ. The skeletal muscle anabolic response to plant-versus animal-based protein consumption. *J Nutr.* 2015;145(9):1981-1991.

90. Wilkinson SB, Tarnopolsky MA, Macdonald MJ, Macdonald JR, Armstrong D, Phillips SM. Consumption of fluid skim milk promotes greater muscle protein accretion after resistance exercise than does consumption of an isonitrogenous and isoenergetic soy-protein beverage. *Am J Clin Nutr.* 2007;85(4):1031-1040.

91. Josse AR, Tang JE, Tarnopolsky MA, Phillips SM. Body composition and strength changes in women with milk and resistance exercise. *Med Sci Sports Exerc.* 2010;42(6):1122-1130.

92. Gulliver P, Horwath C. Women's readiness to follow milk product consumption recommendations: design and evaluation of a "stage of change" algorithm. *J Hum Nutr Diet.* 2001;14(4):277-286.

93. Gulliver P, Horwath CC. Assessing women's perceived benefits, barriers, and stage of change for meeting milk product consumption recommendations. *J Am Diet Assoc.* 2001;101(11):1354-1357.

94. Rankin JW, Goldman LP, Puglisi MJ, Nickols-Richardson SM, Earthman CP, Gwazdauskas FC. Effect of post-exercise supplement consumption on adaptations to resistance training. *J Am Coll Nutr.* 2004;23(4):322-330.

95. Cribb PJ, Williams AD, Carey MF, Hayes A. The effect of whey isolate and resistance training on strength, body composition, and plasma glutamine. *Int J Sport Nutr Exerc Metab.* 2006;16(5):494-509.

96. Cribb PJ, Williams AD, Stathis CG, Carey MF, Hayes A. Effects of whey isolate, creatine, and resistance training on muscle hypertrophy. *Med Sci Sports Exerc.* 2007;39(2):298-307.

97. Teegarden D. The influence of dairy product consumption on body composition. *J Nutr.* 2005;135(12):2749-2752.

98. Zemel MB. Role of calcium and dairy products in energy partitioning and weight management. *Am J Clin Nutr.* 2004;79(5):907S-912S.

99. Reidy PT, Walker DK, Dickinson JM, et al. Soy-dairy protein blend and whey protein ingestion after resistance exercise increases amino acid transport and transporter expression in human skeletal muscle. *J Appl Physiol (1985).* 2014;116(11):1353-1364.

100. Candow DG, Burke NC, Smith-Palmer T, Burke DG. Effect of whey and soy protein supplementation combined with resistance training in young adults. *Int J Sport Nutr Exerc Metab.* 2006;16(3):233-244.

101. Ruales J, Nair BM. Nutritional quality of the protein in quinoa (*Chenopodium quinoa*, Willd) seeds. *Plant Foods Hum Nutr.* 1992;42(1):1-11.

102. Borsheim E, Tipton KD, Wolf SE, Wolfe RR. Essential amino acids and muscle protein recovery from resistance exercise. *Am J Physiol Endocrinol Metab.* 2002;283(4):E648-E657.

103. Mier CM, Domenick MA, Turner NS, Wilmore JH. Changes in stroke volume and maximal aerobic capacity with increased blood volume in men and women. *J Appl Physiol (1985).*1996;80(4):1180-1186.

104. Moore DR, Churchward-Venne TA, Witard O, et al. Protein ingestion to stimulate myofibrillar protein synthesis requires greater relative protein intakes in healthy older versus younger men. *J Gerontol A Biol Sci Med Sci.* 2015;70(1):57-62.

105. Lemon PW, Tarnopolsky MA, MacDougall JD, Atkinson SA. Protein requirements and muscle mass/strength changes during intensive training in novice bodybuilders. *J Appl Physiol (1985).*1992;73(2): 767-775.

106. Hartman JW, Moore DR, Phillips SM. Resistance training reduces whole-body protein turnover and improves net protein retention in untrained young males. *Appl Physiol Nutr Metab.* 2006;31(5):557-564.

107. Moore DR, Del Bel NC, Nizi KI, et al. Resistance training reduces fasted and fed state leucine turnover and increases dietary nitrogen retention in previously untrained young men. *J Nutr.* 2007;137(4):985-991.

108. Campbell WW, Crim MC, Young VR, Joseph LJ, Evans WJ. Effects of resistance training and dietary protein intake on protein metabolism in older adults. *Am J Physiol.* 1995;268(6 pt 1):e1143-e1153.

109. Campbell WW, Trappe TA, Jozsi AC, Kruskall LJ, Wolfe RR, Evans WJ. Dietary protein adequacy and lower body versus whole body resistive training in older humans. *J Physiol.* 2002;542(pt 2):631-642.

110. Tarnopolsky LJ, MacDougall JD, Atkinson SA, Tarnopolsky MA, Sutton JR. Gender differences in substrate for endurance exercise. *J Appl Physiol (1985).* 1990;68(1):302-308.

111. Rodriguez NR, Di Marco NM, Langley S. American College of Sports Medicine position stand. Nutrition and athletic performance. *Med Sci Sports Exerc.* 2009;41(3):709-731.

112. Burd NA, Tardif N, Rooyackers O, van Loon LJ. Optimizing the measurement of mitochondrial protein synthesis in human skeletal muscle. *Appl Physiol Nutr Metab.* 2015;40(1):1-9.

113. Loftin M, Sothern M, Koss C, et al. Energy expenditure and influence of physiologic factors during marathon running. *J Strength Cond Res.* 2007;21(4):1188-1191.

114. el-Khoury AE, Forslund A, Olsson R, et al. Moderate exercise at energy balance does not affect 24-h leucine oxidation or nitrogen retention in healthy men. *Am J Physiol.* 1997;273(2 pt 1):e394-e407.

115. Forslund AH, El-Khoury AE, Olsson RM, Sjodin AM, Hambraeus L, Young VR. Effect of protein intake and physical activity on 24-h pattern and rate of macronutrient utilization. *Am J Physiol.* 1999;276(5 pt 1):e964-e976.

116. Phillips SM, Moore DR, Tang JE. A critical examination of dietary protein requirements, benefits, and excesses in athletes. *Int J Sport Nutr Exerc Metab.* 2007;17(suppl):58S-76S.

117. Elango R, Humayun MA, Ball RO, Pencharz PB. Evidence that protein requirements have been significantly underestimated. *Curr Opin Clin Nutr Metab Care.* 2010;13(1):52-57.

118. Bowtell JL, Leese GP, Smith K, et al. Effect of oral glucose on leucine turnover in human subjects at rest and during exercise at two levels of dietary protein. *J Physiol.* 2000;525(pt 1):271-281.

119. Bolster DR, Pikosky MA, Gaine PC, et al. Dietary protein intake impacts human skeletal muscle protein fractional synthetic rates after endurance exercise. *Am J Physiol Endocrinol Metab.* 2005;289(4):e678-e683.

120. Brouns F, Saris WH, Stroecken J, et al. Eating, drinking, and cycling. A controlled Tour de France simulation study, Part II. Effect of diet manipulation. *Int J Sports Med.* 1989;10(suppl 1):41S-48S.

121. Brouns F, Saris WH, Stroecken J, et al. Eating, drinking, and cycling. A controlled Tour de France simulation study, Part I. *Int J Sports Med.* 1989;10(suppl 1):32S-40S.

122. Rowlands DS, Wadsworth DP. Effect of high-protein feeding on performance and nitrogen balance in female cyclists. *Med Sci Sports Exerc.* 2011;43(1):44-53.

123. Bergstrom J, Furst P, Hultman E. Free amino acids in muscle tissue and plasma during exercise in man. *Clin Physiol.* 1985;5(2):155-160.

124. Henriksson J. Effect of exercise on amino acid concentrations in skeletal muscle and plasma. *J Exp Biol.* 1991;160:149-165.

125. Jepson MM, Bates PC, Broadbent P, Pell JM, Millward DJ. Relationship between glutamine concentration and protein synthesis in rat skeletal muscle. *Am J Physiol.* 1988;255(2 pt 1):e166-e172.

126. Candow DG, Chilibeck PD, Burke DG, Davison KS, Smith-Palmer T. Effect of glutamine supplementation combined with resistance training in young adults. *Eur J Appl Physiol.* 2001;86(2):142-149.

127. Welbourne TC. Increased plasma bicarbonate and growth hormone after an oral glutamine load. *Am J Clin Nutr.* 1995;61(5):1058-1061.

128. West DW, Kujbida GW, Moore DR, et al. Resistance exercise-induced increases in putative anabolic hormones do not enhance muscle protein synthesis or intracellular signalling in young men. *J Physiol.* 2009;587(pt 21):5239-5247.

129. Doessing S, Heinemeier KM, Holm L, et al. Growth hormone stimulates the collagen synthesis in human tendon and skeletal muscle without affecting myofibrillar protein synthesis. *J Physiol.* 2010;588(pt 2):341-351.

130. Saito H, Trocki O, Wang SL, Gonce SJ, Joffe SN, Alexander JW. Metabolic and immune effects of dietary arginine supplementation after burn. *Arch Surg.* 1987;122(7):784-789.

131. Witte MB, Barbul A. Arginine physiology and its implication for wound healing. *Wound Repair Regen.* 2003;11(6):419-423.

132. Paddon-Jones D, Borsheim E, Wolfe RR. Potential ergogenic effects of arginine and creatine supplementation. *J Nutr.* 2004;134(suppl 10):2888S-2894S; discussion 2895S.

133. Castillo L, Ajami A, Branch S, et al. Plasma arginine kinetics in adult man: response to an arginine-free diet. *Metab.* 1994;43(1):114-122.

134. Castillo L, deRojas TC, Chapman TE, et al. Splanchnic metabolism of dietary arginine in relation to nitric oxide synthesis in normal adult man. *Proc Natl Acad Sci U S A.* 1993;90(1):193-197.

135. Kanaley JA. Growth hormone, arginine and exercise. *Curr Opin Clin Nutr Metab Care.* 2008;11(1):50-54.

136. Isidori A, Lo Monaco A, Cappa M. A study of growth hormone release in man after oral administration of amino acids. *Curr Med Res Opin.* 1981;7(7):475-481.

137. Gater DR, Gater DA, Uribe JM, Bunt JC. Effects of arginine/lysine supplementation and resistance training on glucose tolerance. *J Appl Physiol (1985).* 1992;72(4):1279-1284.

138. Volpi E, Kobayashi H, Sheffield-Moore M, Mittendorfer B, Wolfe RR. Essential amino acids are primarily responsible for the amino acid stimulation of muscle protein anabolism in healthy elderly adults. *Am J Clin Nutr.* 2003;78(2):250-258.

139. Tang JE, Lysecki PJ, Manolakos JJ, MacDonald MJ, Tarnopolsky MA, Phillips SM. Bolus arginine supplementation affects neither muscle blood flow nor muscle protein synthesis in young men at rest or after resistance exercise. *J Nutr.* 2011;141(2):195-200.

140. Holm L, Esmarck B, Suetta C, et al. Postexercise nutrient intake enhances leg protein balance in early postmenopausal women. *J Gerontol A Biol Sci Med Sci.* 2005;60(9):1212-1218.

141. Cribb PJ, Williams AD, Hayes A. A creatine-protein-carbohydrate supplement enhances responses to resistance training. *Med Sci Sports Exerc.* 2007;39(11):1960-1968.

CHAPTER 4

DIETARY FAT AND EXERCISE

D. Travis Thomas, PhD, RDN, CSSD, LD, FAND, and David M. Schnell, PhD

INTRODUCTION

Fat, also known as lipid, is a major fuel source for athletes. It constitutes a broad range of molecules that play vital roles in multiple physiological functions. Indeed, the intricacies surrounding fat intake recommendations seem to be overshadowed by interest in carbohydrate and protein needs to support, sustain, and improve athletic performance. However, given the critical role of dietary fat in both energy metabolism and many other physiological functions, athletes should view fat as a necessary component of the diet—an essential dietary macronutrient that can affect overall wellness and performance during exercise and sport. Dietary fat, dietary carbohydrate, and endogenous fat stores all have the capacity to influence fat metabolism. They work separately and in concert to regulate substrate utilization and availability during exercise and at rest. Many details of how fatty acids serve as energy sources and how exercise intensity affects fatty acid metabolism during exercise and in postexercise recovery are well established in the scientific literature. There is emerging interest in researching the metabolic adaptations that may occur in response to a high-fat diet and the ways these changes may translate into improved training capacity and athletic performance.[1] This chapter provides a brief overview of lipids and reviews current evidence to help practitioners understand dietary strategies involving fat manipulation that may influence athletic performance and health.

PHYSICAL STRUCTURE OF DIETARY FAT AND FOOD SOURCES

Among the multiple varieties of lipids in our food supply, triglycerides, also known as triacylglycerols, make up over 90% of lipid consumed in the human diet.[2] Phospholipids and sterols are also classes of lipid found in food that exhibit essential functions in metabolism. Non–energy-producing metabolic functions of phospholipids include imparting structure to cell membranes, emulsification, molecular signaling, and participating in biochemical reactions and pathways, such as hormone synthesis. Phospholipids are found in a wide range of foods and are characterized by a polar, hydrophilic head group with hydrophobic tails composed of two longer-chain fatty acids. Cholesterol is only found in foods of animal origin and is highest in animal-based diets, while phytosterols are found in plant materials and are therefore more abundant in plant-based diets. Generally, all cholesterol needs are met through endogenous synthesis; the body uses cholesterol as an essential component of cell membrane structure and many physiological pathways, including the biosynthesis of steroid hormones. Given their plant-based origin, dietary intake of phytosterols depends on diet composition and may impart some health benefits by reducing low-density lipoprotein cholesterol.[3] Athletes generally consume enough fat in their diets to receive adequate amounts of both phospholipids and sterols or can synthesize these compounds. Because of the disproportionate amount of triglycerides and various fatty acids that make up dietary triglycerides, the focus of this chapter will be these lipids.

Triglycerides are composed of three fatty acid groups attached by ester bonds to a glycerol backbone (Figure 4.1). These lipids serve as a substantial source of energy and contribute to the essential fatty acids that we must consume to avoid a dietary deficiency. Many foods found in an athlete's diet are sources of

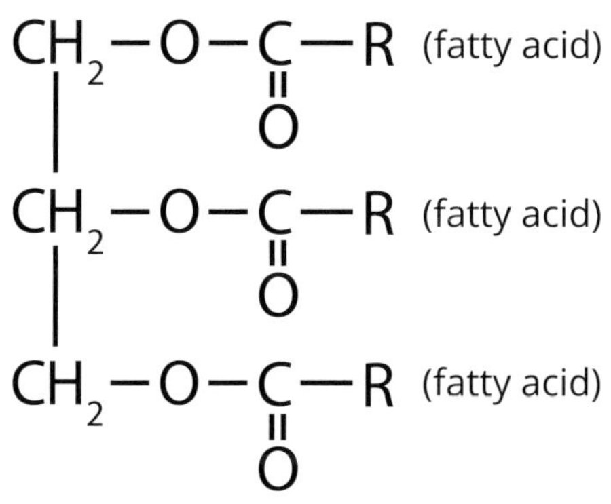

FIGURE 4.1 General Structure of a Triglyceride

dietary lipids, so it is important to carefully evaluate food labels and ingredient lists to understand and accurately assess lipid composition of an athlete's diet.

All fatty acid molecules are described by their physical structure and characterized by the presence of a hydrocarbon chain linked to a carboxylic acid group. Fatty acids can be classified based on the length of the hydrocarbon chain or based on their degree of saturation with hydrogen atoms. Fatty acids with one to three carbons are referred to as volatile fatty acids, while short-chain fatty acids have four to six carbons. Fatty acids can also be composed of 6 to 12 carbons (medium-chain fatty acids), 14 to 22 carbons (long-chain fatty acids), and more than 22 carbons (very-long-chain fatty acids). Small amounts of short- and medium-chain fatty acids are obtained as naturally occurring components of foods, such as dairy products and coconut oil. The majority of dietary fatty acids are 16 to 18 carbons in length (see Figures 4.2a-d).

A fatty acid that is saturated contains the maximal amount of hydrogen atoms possible and is thus "saturated" with hydrogens, whereas unsaturated fatty acids have one or more double bonds that displace hydrogen atoms. Unsaturated fatty acids are broadly characterized by the number of double bonds (unsaturated carbons) each molecule contains. Fatty acids with one double bond are monounsaturated fatty acids (MUFAs), and those with multiple double bonds are polyunsaturated fatty acids (PUFAs). Unsaturated fatty acids are further classified by the position of the first double bond within the hydrocarbon chain in relation to the omega carbon, as well as the *cis* or *trans* configurations of the double bonds (Table 4.1). For example, α-linolenic acid can be referred to as all-*cis* 18:3 or n-3. We will use n-3 in this book, but in some literature, n-3 takes the form Ω-3 (omega-3), used to represent the same information, where the number 3 refers to the position of the first double bond in relation to the terminal carbon, also known as the omega carbon. Most dietary sources of unsaturated fatty acids are found in *cis* conformation. However, partial hydrogenation of vegetable oils during the production of shortening and margarine produces unsaturated fatty acids containing *trans* bonds. The resulting fatty acids with one or more double

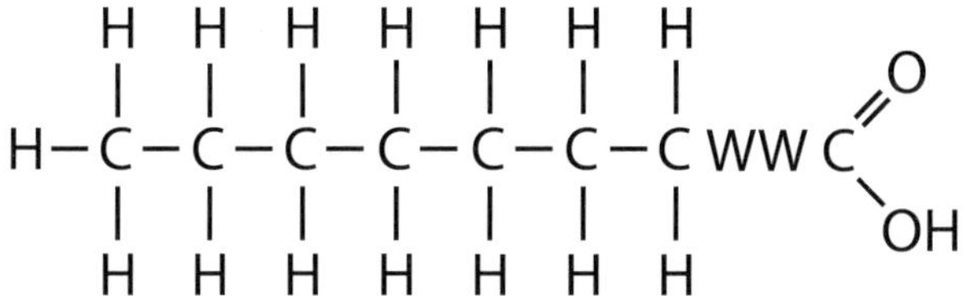

FIGURE 4.2a Structure of a Saturated Fatty Acid

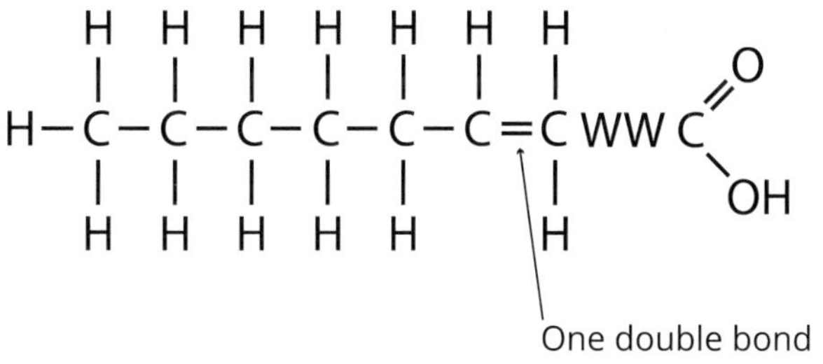

One double bond

FIGURE 4.2b Structure of a Monounsaturated Fatty Acid

Omega carbon   n-3 double bond   n-6 double bond

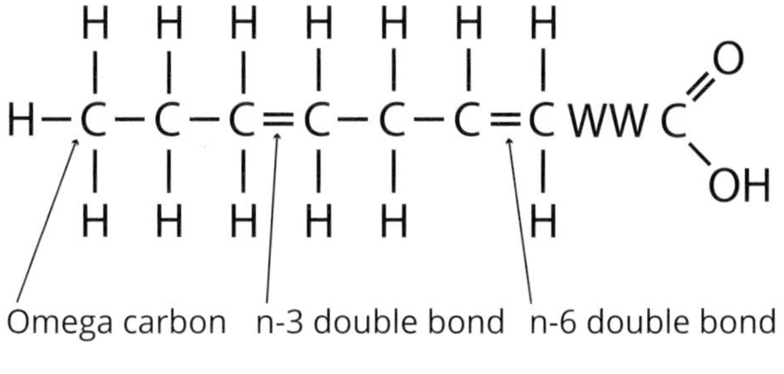

FIGURE 4.2c Structure of a Polyunaturated Fatty Acid

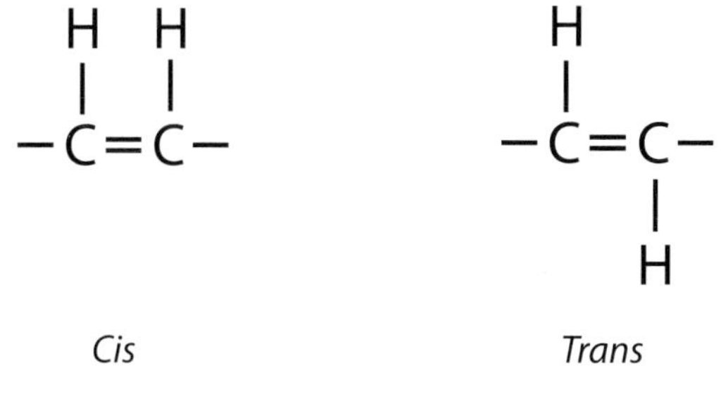

Cis   Trans

FIGURE 4.2d *Cis* vs *Trans* Double Bonds

bonds in the *trans* configuration are known as *trans* fatty acids. Although, these *trans* fats are primarily found in our food supply as artificial *trans* fats in processed foods from hydrogenation, a very small amount of naturally occurring *trans* fats exist in milk, butter, and beef fat. These *trans* bonds change the chemical and metabolic nature of the fats and are highly associated with increased risk of cardiovascular disease, and, as of 2015, are no longer recognized as safe by the US Food and Drug Administration.[4] The *2015-2020 Dietary Guidelines for Americans* suggest keeping *trans* fat intake as low as possible by limiting foods that contain synthetic sources of *trans* fats, such as partially hydrogenated oils in margarine, and by limiting other solid fats.[5] This is a prudent recommendation for athletes as well. Foods that are rich sources of various types of fatty acids are presented in Table 4.1.

Various foods contain different types of fatty acids, which should be balanced by consuming a complete, well-chosen diet. Foods that are rich sources of saturated fatty acids include many animal foods, cocoa butter, and tropical plant oils (eg, coconut oil, palm oil, and palm kernel oil). Plant foods such as canola oil, olives and olive oil, and avocados are good sources of MUFAs, whereas most other plant foods (eg, soy, corn, nuts, and seeds) and fish tend to be rich in PUFAs. Dietary sources of n-3 PUFAs include certain fatty fish, such as salmon and lake trout, as well as walnuts, canola oil, and flaxseed, whereas n-6 fatty acids are found in relatively high levels in most, but not all, other plant foods.

Examples of PUFAs include the essential fatty acids linoleic acid and α-linolenic acid. Although these are the only fatty acids required in the diet, a healthy diet includes a variety of longer, more unsaturated fatty acids. For example, eicosapentaenoic acid (EPA) and docosahexaenoic acid (DHA), both of which are abundant in fatty fish, can help meet n-3 fatty acid requirements. This serves as one example of why the types of fatty acids that make up the triglycerides within a particular food or diet are often as important as the total fat content.

The simple variations in fatty acid structure described previously can produce profoundly different metabolic effects that may directly influence chronic health and disease risk while indirectly influencing athletic performance. Long-term health implications are associated with both the amount and composition of the lipids consumed in the diet. Significant interest in performance and health outcomes associated with dietary fat continue to spark new research questions and debate. Some of the controversy is due to inconsistencies associated with public health messages surrounding fat intake guidelines and the latest fad diets that catch the eye of the public. Any confusion experienced by athletes and practitioners is likely exacerbated by the emergence of literature investigating the effects of a high-fat diet on athletic performance. This often leads to scenarios where wellness and athletic performance messages regarding proper fat intake are not aligned, contributing to mixed messages and misleading advice.

DIETARY FAT INTAKE PATTERNS AND CURRENT PUBLIC HEALTH RECOMMENDATIONS

Fat Intake Patterns

Data describing the macronutrient composition of the athlete's diet continue to emerge for various groups of athletes. In many cases, the quantity of fat athletes report consuming consistently falls within the range of 20% to 35% of total energy but is highly variable within this range. This range is consistent with the acceptable macronutrient distribution range (AMDR) established by the Institute of Medicine.[6] Fifteen studies since the previous edition of this textbook have documented fat intake in a diverse group of athletes ranging from 23% in Ethiopian distance runners to 33% in European rugby players.[7,8] In some cases, the variability of fat intake has extended above and below the AMDR. Total fat consumption has been reported as high as 36% in Spanish volleyball players and above 50% in ultraendurance athletes in Antartica.[9,10] Conversely, some athletes have reported fat intakes well below the AMDR.[11-13] At various phases of the training cycle, some athletes may choose to restrict their fat intake in an effort to lose body weight or improve

Table 4.1 Examples of Dietary Sources of Various Fatty Acids

Type of Fat	Food Sources	
Polyunsaturated (n-6) fatty acids	Corn oil	Sesame seeds
	Cottonseed oil	Soybean oil
	Pumpkin seeds	Walnuts
	Safflower oil	
Polyunsaturated (n-3) fatty acids	Anchovies	Mackerel
	Catfish	Salmon
	Flaxseed/flax oil	Sardines
	Herring	Shrimp
	High–n-3 eggs	Tuna
	Lake trout	
Monounsaturated (n-9) fatty acids	Almonds	Peanut oil
	Avocados	Peanuts
	Canola oil	Olive oil
	Cashews	Olives
	Peanut butter	
Saturated fatty acids	Bacon	Half-and-half
	Butter	Highly marbled steak
	Cheese	Ice cream
	Cheesecake	Palm kernel oil
	Cream	Poultry skin
	Cream cheese	Ribs
	Coconut	Sausage
	Coconut oil	
Trans unsaturated fatty acids	Commercial baked goods (cookies, cakes, pies)[a]	Snack crackers and chips
	Frozen breaded foods (chicken nuggets, fish sticks)	Stick and tub margarines containing partially hydrogenated fat
	Frozen french fries	
	Shortening	

[a] Many commercial baked goods no longer contain *trans* fats. The Food and Drug Administration has mandated that processed foods cannot contain added partially hydrogenated fats after June 18, 2018.

physique characteristics (ie, body size, shape, growth, and composition). This restriction is often well below the AMDR minimum of 20% total energy intake from fat.

Although there is limited evidence to support or refute the claim that acute consumption of 20% or less of energy intake from fat affects athletic performance, research widely supports the notion that chronic and extreme restriction of dietary fat contributes to a decrease in diet quality and can put the food intake range and quantity necessary to meet overall health and performance goals out of reach. For example, a study of endurance athletes found that fat intake was the major distinguishing factor between healthy female runners and those with menstrual dysfunction.[14] As a result of this study, researhers

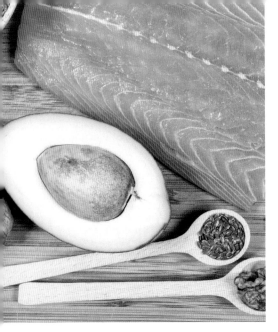

recommended that endurance athletes consume no less than 1 g/kg/d of fat. This is a practical and prudent recommendation, but other evidence to support this guideline is lacking. Most importantly, athletes should be discouraged from avoiding fat and implementating chronic extreme fat restriction. When acute fat restriction is practiced—common for athletes trying to make weight—it should be limited to very short-term scenarios. Fat restriction is widely considered acceptable in making-weight sports for the two to three days leading up to competition weigh-ins. Acute fat restriction may also be beneficial just before a sporting event or training session or during carbohydrate-loading, where considerations of preferred macronutrients or gastrointestinal comfort have priority. It is important to note that the requirements associated with extreme fat restriction will likely reduce the intake of a variety of nutrients and food components. Chronic fat restriction may also specifically limit the intake of key fat-related nutrients, such as fat-soluble vitamins, essential fatty acids (especially n-3 fatty acids), and fat-soluble phytonutrients. These nutrients are of value to the overall health of an athlete, and lack of these nutrients may lead to acute or chronic decrements in athletic performance.

Some athletes may be interested in following extremely high-fat diets based on claims that this practice can promote beneficial metabolic adaptations to support or improve athletic performance. Several human studies have investigated this over the last five years and have broadened our understanding of the concept.[15-19] Although it is clear that metabolic adaptations do occur in response to high-fat feeding, claims that extremely high-fat, carbohydrate-restricted diets provide a benefit to the performance of competitive athletes have not been proven. Current literature describing metabolic adaptations that occur in athletes on high-fat diets are outlined later in the chapter. However, given the variability in fat intake among athletes, different athlete types and training demands, and differences in fast- and slow-twitch muscle fat utilization, it is not easy to recommend a universal level for fat consumption that will optimize athletic performance. Furthermore, the way fat intake influences chronic health and disease and emerging evidence describing genetic differences in fat utilization add to the complexity.[20]

Public Health Recommendations: Total Fat Intake

The AMDR provides a good starting point for evaluating and recommending dietary fat intake for athletes. Total fat intake recommendations are often fine-tuned after other macronutrient demands are determined based on training macrocycles and microcycles and day-to-day training periodization. Consuming 20% to 35% of total energy from fat as part of a well-chosen diet will allow athletes to meet their needs for essential fatty acids without increasing their risk for coronary heart disease. The AMDR for total fat intake is in line with the 2014 American College of Cardiology (ACC) and American Heart Association (AHA) recommendations for total fat intake. These guidelines suggest that overall dietary pattern is more important than individual foods and call for a diet that emphasizes incorporating unsaturated, plant-based fats low in saturated fat and *trans* fat.[21] ACC/AHA guidelines allow for Mediterranean diet patterns that may provide up to 35% or more of total calories from fat, primarily from fatty fish, avocados, nuts, and olive and canola oils. These guidelines support the claim of some researchers that the type of dietary fat is much more important than the quantity in relation to heart health.[22] Given the elevated energy needs of most athletes, a well-chosen diet that includes dietary fat from many heart-healthy food sources aligned with the AMDR is likely to meet essential fatty acid needs without added risk for heart disease. When making recommendations for athletes, consider total fat intake demands for the training and competition stages of the training cycle, the importance of promoting gastrointestinal tolerance, whether added fat intake is displacing other essential macronutrients, and whether recommendations align with public health guidelines.

Public Health Recommendations: Lipid Composition of the Diet

Recommendations for athletes regarding fat composition can and should be centered on supporting both long-term cardiovascular health and athletic performance. Science in these areas continues to evolve, providing the basis for the types of dietary lipids athletes should strive to consume regularly during training and competition. The 2013 report from the ACC/AHA task force provides guidelines for lipid intake based on a large expert panel's comprehensive review of the literature.[21] Although the report centers on reducing risk factors for individuals at the highest risk for having a cardiovascular event, it also suggests that there is moderate to strong evidence that everyone would benefit from an energy intake relatively lower in saturated fatty acids than other dietary fatty acids. To be clear, this message is not to completely avoid saturated fat but to limit intake to align with the current AHA guidelines, which recommend less than 10% of total daily calories from saturated fat. Despite these guidelines, not all recommendations from the scientific literature or those expressed by the media are consistent with ACC/AHA guidelines. For example, the Dietary Guidelines Advisory Committee (DGAC) recently issued a report that addressed many questions consumers and professionals commonly have regarding dietary fat intake.[23] The report recommended a universal de-emphasis on saturated fat being classified as a nutrient of concern because the effect of saturated fat intake on disease end points is unclear.

What is lost in the saturated fat controversy is the consistent message for recommended dietary fat intake patterns. All organizations appear to agree that there should be a greater emphasis on consuming a larger proportion of MUFAs and PUFAs relative to total fat intake. This may be particularly helpful in supporting cardiovascular health when these fatty acids replace a portion of energy intake from refined carbohydrates and sugar. Most dietary fats should come from monounsaturated or polyunsaturated food sources as part of a diet emphasizing vegetables, fruits, whole grains, low-fat dairy, and seafood, with lower consumption of red meat and processed meat. Other prudent recommendations for both the general public and athletes are to limit *trans* fats to less than 1% of total calories and increase dietary intake of essential fatty acids to approximately 5% to 10% and 0.6% to 1.2% of energy for n-6 and n-3, respectively.[6]

These current lipid intake recommendations, on which most organizations seem to agree, not only promote cardiovascular health in athletes but also support athletic performance. Indeed, carbohydrate needs to support training demands and high-intensity efforts should be addressed first and not centered on high lipid consumption. Although the DGAC suggested that the most effective recommendation for the reducing cardiovascular disease would be to reduce carbohydrate intake and replace it with PUFAs, many athletes may experience performance decrements from following this strategy. Some athletes could instead benefit from reducing their intake of sugar-sweetened beverages (eg, soda) and confections in favor of carbohydrate-containing foods that are nutrient dense and higher in naturally occurring fiber. Widespread recommendation to reduce carbohydrate in favor of lipid intake should be cautioned against. Independent of carbohydrate considerations, there are many opportunities for sports dietitians to impact and influence the fat composition of an athlete's diet. By increasing the proportion of MUFAs and n-3 PUFAs consumed, athletes may benefit from the metabolic advantages of reduced inflammation and the maintenance of proper vascular function, which may indirectly support athletic performance.

The federal *2015-2020 Dietary Guidelines for Americans* provides additional guidance to further refine our practical recommendations regarding health messages associated with dietary fat intake. In general, the new guidelines focus on the recommendation of limiting saturated and *trans* fats while concomitantly modifying the diet to include more nutrient-dense versions of foods within each food group. The newest version of the Dietary Guidelines has not changed much from the last publication with regard to saturated fat intake. The guidelines state that the intake of saturated fats should be limited to less than 10% of calories per day and that these calories should be replaced with unsaturated fats, while keeping total dietary fats within the age-appropriate AMDR. Although the guidelines now state that "oils should replace solid fats rather than being added to the diet," the mention of solid fat consumption is no longer in the key recommendations and has been replaced with specific recommendations for saturated and *trans* fat intake reduction.[5]

Sports dietitians should consider the athlete's sport, goals for physique, and risk factors for chronic disease before recommending total and specific dietary fat intake. Professionals should also stay abreast of emerging science investigating the role of fat adaptation in athletic performance with special attention to protocol details such as scientific design, subject characteristics, and diet and exercise interventions. Such attention to details is imperative to promote critical evaluation of evidence and to clarify the applicability of the research findings to the athlete or athletic groups to whom sports dietitians are assigned.

INFLUENCE OF EXERCISE AND TRAINING ON LIPID METABOLISM

Fat has a variety of important roles in the body, but the key function for the athlete is energy production. Fat, in the form of plasma free fatty acids (FFAs), muscle lipid, and stored lipid in adipose tissue, provides a fuel substrate that is both relatively plentiful and readily available to the muscle as a result of endurance training. Triglyceride stored within muscle cells, called intramyocellular lipid (IMCL), represents a small fraction of body's triglyceride stores that increase with aerobic training. IMCLs can provide critical energy to the muscle cells in which they are stored, particularly during long endurance events. Muscle triglyceride is not only stored inside of muscle cells in lipid droplets but also within muscle tissues as an accumulation of adipocytes that appear as fatty streaks between muscle fibers, called intramyocellular triglyceride or extramyocellular lipid (EMCL). EMCL stores are typically low in young, healthy athletes, but they increase with aging, sedentary behavior, or muscular injury and are inversely associated with muscle functional performance.[24]

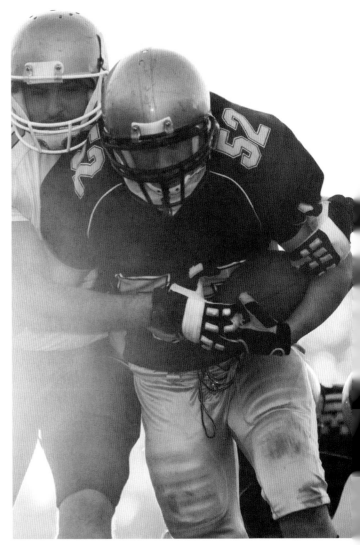

Adipose tissue triglycerides are exported into the circulation as protein-bound fatty acids by the action of hormone-sensitive lipase (HSL). HSL activity is stimulated by rising concentrations of epinephrine, norepinephrine, glucagon, adrenocorticotropic hormone, thyroxine, and growth hormones during exercise. These fatty acids can be taken up by muscle cells, where they are subsequently catabolized, which allows them to contribute to energy demands by providing adenosine triphosphate (ATP) for muscle movement. Fatty acids that enter muscle cells are linked to coenzyme A (CoA) by fatty acyl-CoA synthetase. These fatty acids must first be translocated to the mitochondrion via carnitine and the enzymes carnitine-acylcarnitine translocase, carnitine palmitoyltransferase I, and carnitine palmitoyltransferase II. These molecules work in concert to transfer the fatty acids across mitochondrial membranes and to reesterify them to CoA. Within the mitochondria, β oxidation results in one molecule of acyl-CoA, one reduced flavin adenine dinucleotide, and one reduced nicotinamide adenine dinucleotide for every two carbons cleaved from the fatty acid. These molecules can then undergo further mitochondrial oxidation via oxidative phosphorylation to regenerate ATP from adenosine diphosphate.

Factors Affecting Fat Metabolism in Exercise

The relative proportion of macromolecule energy sources (eg, carbohydrate, fat) oxidized during exercise is influenced by many variables. With regard to lipid, most of the relative contribution to energy turnover varies based on exercise intensity and duration. The contribution of different body stores of fat to energy turnover is influenced by many of the same factors influencing the proportion of substrate oxidation. Training, a function of exercise frequency, also influences fat metabolism principally by promoting metabolic adaptations that facilitate lipid delivery and lipid oxidation in working muscle. Although the effects of exercise intensity, duration, and training are the primary factors in determining the proportion and source of lipid utilized and total exercise energy expenditure, the contribution of the various lipid sources in the body to fat oxidation also depends on sex and dietary intake before and during exercise.

Lipid Sources and Integration with Macronutrient Metabolism

Fatty acids represent a major fuel for muscle contractions and the major type of lipids used for energy during exercise. These fatty acids come principally from adipose tissue, muscle lipid depots EMCL and IMCL, and lipoproteins. While albumin-bound fatty acids contribute more to fatty acid oxidation, very-low-density lipoprotein triglycerides can contribute up to 10% of total energy expenditure during prolonged exercise of moderate intensity.[25] With regard to muscle lipid depots at lower exercise intensity, IMCL generally contributes only a minor portion of energy expended compared with fatty acids obtained from the plasma. IMCLs, found in lipid droplets, are generally located next to the mitochondria. The overall amount of IMCL within muscle tissue varies by individual differences in fiber type content, diet, and training. In addition, females typically have more IMCL than males relative to aerobic capacity, fitness level, and training history. Each of these factors is known to dictate the relative contribution of IMCL to energy turnover. Furthermore, females tend to have higher fatty acid oxidation rates during moderate-intensity prolonged endurance events, likely due to more type I fibers and capillary density.[26] Type I muscle fibers, which are more oxidative than type II fibers, also contain more IMCL. IMCL fatty acids are liberated from their triglyceride bond via the sequential lipase hydrolyzation involving adipose tissue triglyceride lipase, HSL, and monoglyceride lipase. Endurance training increases IMCL concentration in athletes, and adipose triglyceride lipase protein content to increases with training, suggesting improved lipolysis efficiency in response to training. The relative energy contribution of IMCL increases as exercise intensity increases.[27,28] IMCL contribution to energy turnover decreases, however, with extended endurance events, such as those which occur at consistent intensities. During these events plasma FFA concentrations increase.[29]

The contribution of different stored fat sources to energy turnover is influenced by both the duration and intensity of the exercise bout, with plasma FFA contributing a higher percentage of fat utilization and a decrease in the relative utilization of muscle lipid as the duration progresses.[28] During prolonged endurance exercise in trained individuals, the carbohydrate to fat oxidation ratio is relatively stable, with carbohydrate contributing to a higher oxidation rate, particularly in exercise events lasting between 60 and 90 minutes. Generally, with regards to exercise duration, fatty acid oxidation is only significantly higher than carbohydrate in endurance events lasting more than 90 minutes. However, it should be noted that dietary intake both before and during exercise can have a significant effect on these observations, as can intensity of exercise and fitness of the individual.

During light to moderate exercise intensities and long-duration exercise, fatty acids are a major fuel for muscle contraction. This occurs as oxygen becomes more available to the working muscle, allowing the body to use more of the aerobic (oxidative) pathways and less of the anaerobic (phosphagen and glycolytic) pathways. The crossover shift toward greater carbohydrate oxidation at increasing intensity is a limitation in fatty acid utilization in high-intensity sporting activities. The limitation is partially explained by the inverse relationship between lipolysis and lactate concentrations. Lipolysis is also limited by inadequate blood perfusion of adipose tissue and the sympathetic response to high-intensity exercise.[30] Apart from limitations with lipolysis, other explanations include the inability of the mitochondria to completely oxidize fat with limited oxygen availability marked at exercise intensities over 85% of VO_2 peak. Despite limited changes in plasma free fatty acid availability, a decrease in total fatty acid oxidation during high-intensity exercise (72% of VO_2 peak) compared with moderate intensities of 44% to 55% of VO_2 peak suggests that reduced fatty acid oxidation cannot be fully explained by a decreased delivery of fatty acid to an exercising muscle.[31] As exercise intensity increases, there is a progressive increase in the respiratory exchange ratio (RER), indicating a shift to greater carbohydrate oxidation. However, even with greater carbohydrate oxidation, there is a benefit of elevated fatty acid oxidation lasting several hours after exercise. The maximum lipid contribution as an energy source is reached at approximately 60% to 65% of VO_2 with carbohydrate oxidation contribution maintained at about 50% of the energy expenditure of exercise. Fatty acid transport across the sarcolemma of the muscle does not appear to be a limiting factor for fatty acid oxidation at high intensity; instead, research continues to point toward traditionally defined mitochondrial regulatory steps. [28,31,32]

METABOLIC ADAPTATIONS TO A HIGH-FAT DIET

Exercise-induced adaptations do not appear to maximize oxidation rates since they can be further enhanced by dietary strategies, such as fasting, acute preexercise intake of fat, and chronic exposure to high-fat and low-carbohydrate diets.[33] Significant interest in the effects of high-fat feeding in promoting metabolic adaptation that may result in supporting or improving athletic performance has emerged over the past few decades, partially explained by limited endogenous stores of carbohydrate that can limit endurance performance. Most endurance events (>90 minutes) and ultraendurance events (>4 to 5 hours) are completed between 65% and 85% VO_2 max, at which approximately 50% of energy is acquired from muscle glycogen. Because a well-trained human can only store approximately 350 to 500 g (1,400 to 2,000 kcal) of glycogen in liver and muscle tissue, glycogen availability is often a limiting factor in performance duration and intensity. However, even a very lean athlete (eg, a 70-kg man with 6% body fat) holds over 4 kg of body fat, equivalent to over 35,000 kcal. In an effort to extend performance, athletes and sports nutrition professionals have attempted to implement dietary strategies to shift substrate utilization during exercise to favor fat utilization and carbohydrate sparing. Because fatty acids are digested slowly, acute dietary interventions to increase FFA availability and oxidation are not practical. Therefore, if availability and oxidation of FFA is to be increased during exercise, a multiday strategy to significantly increase fat intake is usually implemented.

The science investigating fat adaptation began in the early 1980s as an attempt to reduce athletes' reliance on exogenous carbohydrate during endurance events. An early study examining a ketogenic diet for weight loss in overweight and obese men and women recognized a drop in respiratory quotient (RQ) at VO_2 max from 0.76 at baseline to 0.66 after 5 weeks of a ketogenic diet (<10 g/d carbohydrate).[34] This was accompanied by a decrease in resting muscle glycogen from 1.53 mg/100 g to 1.04 mg/100 g wet weight and complete sparing of muscle glycogen during an uphill treadmill walk to exhaustion. A second study by the same group built upon this and identified a 30% decrease in glucose oxidation at rest during consumption of a ketogenic diet.[35] However, participants noted a 30% increase in mean serum cholesterol, despite a 28 mg/dL drop in mean serum triglyceride. Further examination of a ketogenic diet in endurance-trained humans showed a drop in the RER from 0.83 to 0.72 after 5 weeks of ketogenic adaptation. Further, ketosis-adapted athletes were shown to exhibit fat oxidation rates almost 50% higher (90 g/h vs 60 g/hr) during exercise than those eating a traditional diet.[36] These early studies showed potential metabolic advantages for athletes consuming a ketogenic diet and spurred several decades of research examining the metabolic and athletic adaptations to a high-fat diet. Recent strategies have diverged from this extreme carbohydrate restriction in hopes of better maintaining glycogen stores, as well as high-intensity capability.

Interest is raised periodically in the use of protocols for short-term or long-term adherence to low-carbohydrate, high-fat diets that increase the ability of fat to support the fuel needs of exercise.[16] Fat adaptation interventions have sparked the interest of endurance athletes and are generally described as a high-fat, low-carbohydrate diet for at least 5 to 14 days while maintaining normal training. Protocols may be implemented with or without carbohydrate restoration, coupled with a training taper leading up to competition.[17] While early efforts to identify a fat-adaptive diet strategy focused on ketogenic diets, more recent efforts have attempted less-restrictive approaches that maintain muscle glycogen for high-intensity training and competition. Historical dietary models that combined a period of fat-adaptation before restoring endogenous and exogenous carbohydrate availability for a simulated endurance task not only failed to find benefits to overall endurance performance despite robust increases in fat utilization during exercise but also resulted in impaired performance of higher-intensity pieces within the protocol.[37,38] This was later explained further by evidence of a down regulation of carbohydrate metabolism even when glycogen is available.[39] A recent review of the effects of low-carbohydrate, high-fat diets on performance noted that despite widespread anecdotal support and a surge in popularity on social media and non–peer reviewed sources, research failed to show an improvement in performance from low-carbohydrate, high-fat diets.[16]

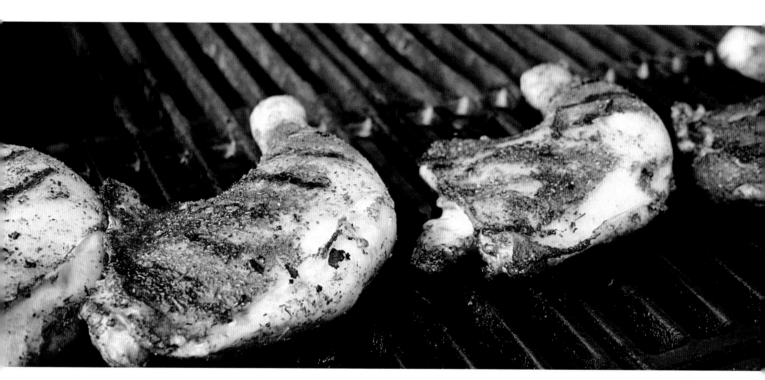

Ketogenic Diets

A high-fat, very-low-carbohydrate diet has the potential to induce ketosis. A diet containing less than 10 g/d of carbohydrate can increase β-hydroxybutyrate blood concentrations from 0.06 mm to approximately 2.5 mm and total ketone body concentration are typically more than 30 times higher after only 1 week.[34] Such a diet has the theoretical potential to negate the need for exogenous nutrients during extreme endurance events.[19] However, the only study that has evaluated the effect of a ketogenic, low-carbohydrate diet on well-trained athletes concluded that chronic adaptation to a diet providing more than 80% of energy from fat was able at best to maintain endurance capacity at only a moderate working intensity and sacrificed the ability and desire to exercise at higher workloads.[36]

One study reported weight loss and an increase in VO_2 max and lactic threshold (VO_2 LT) after 4 weeks of a ketogenic diet consisting of 70% fat and 15% carbohydrate in well-trained, off-road cyclists.[40] However, ketone bodies only exhibited a moderate increase (0.04 mM to 0.15 mM β-hydroxybutyrate) compared with other studies, and maximal power output was decreased following the ketogenic protocol, despite maintenance of absolute VO_2.[34,36] An additional study examining gymnasts on a very-low-carbohydrate diet (22 g/d carbohydrate, 54% fat calories) found no change in performance markers such as pull-ups, push-ups, and triceps dips.[41] The authors observed a significant body weight reduction from both fat and lean mass during consumption of a ketogenic diet. Similar results were found in trained men and women by Sawyer and colleagues, who observed a decrease in weight but no change in handgrip dynamometry, vertical jump, one-repetition maximum bench press and back squat, maximum-repetition bench press, or 30-second Wingate anaerobic cycling test after 7 days of a diet with 53% of calories from fat.[42] To date, very little peer-reviewed research has been published describing performance outcomes in power athletes. However, decreased high-intensity performance in endurance athletes suggests that no ergogenic effect would be seen in power athletes. More research must be conducted before sports nutrition professionals can make informed recommendations encouraging high-fat diets to these athletes. The limited data described previously suggest that performance in power athletes is either reduced or maintained as a result of following a ketogenic diet.

Training with Low-Carbohydrate Availability

The implementation of a high-fat diet is as much of a low-carbohydrate challenge as it is a high-fat challenge. Although training low does not explicitly refer to the practice of a high-fat diet, many times these practices overlap, particularly if the athlete is in energy balance. The restriction of exogenous carbohydrate availability while exercising in a fasted state promotes an extended signaling response, albeit less robustly than the case for exercise with low endogenous carbohydrate stores.[43] These strategies enhance the cellular outcomes of endurance training, such as increased maximal mitochondrial enzyme activities or mitochondrial content and increased rates of lipid oxidation, with the augmentation of responses likely to be explained by enhanced activation of key cell-signaling kinases (eg, AMPK, p38MAPK), transcription factors (eg, p53, PPARδ), and transcriptional coactivators (eg, PGC-1α).[43] Deliberate integration of such training low exercise and dietary strategies within a periodized training program is becoming a recognized part of sports nutrition practice, despite its potential for misuse.[43,44]

Exercising in a postabsorptive phase attempts to simulate a metabolic effect similar to that of a high-fat diet while allowing for moderate carbohydrate intake. Shimada and colleagues found that well-trained endurance athletes exhibited a metabolic shift away from glycogen oxidation when exercising before breakfast.[45] During a before breakfast 60-minute cycle ergometer training session at 50% VO_2 max, athletes exhibited a lower RQ (0.89 vs 0.94), increased 24-hour fat oxidation, and decreased 24-hour glycogen oxidation compared with the same workout performed in the afternoon. However, their study did not examine changes in performance. There is evidence that long-duration, low-intensity training in a fasted state increases mitochondrial biogenesis, and some researchers suggest that this pattern of training may improve performance.[46] A modified version of this strategy used a high-fat pretraining meal (as opposed to a high-carbohydrate meal) and found similar results.[47] The data showed that a high-fat meal consumed 90 minutes before a 185-minute cycling workout reaching 82% peak power produced a lower RER than a high-carbohydrate meal given at the same time. However, despite substantial effects on plasma hormone concentrations and fuel utilization, there were no observed effects on performance.

A variation to the training low strategy is to complete two training sessions in 1 day with a high-fat, low-carbohydrate diet and the inclusion of a carbohydrate restoration meal after the second training session. This strategy attempts to deplete muscle glycogen in the morning, creating an environment in which athletes rely more heavily on fat oxidation for the second workout. One study divided well-trained cyclists into two groups completing the same workouts on a different schedule, one training twice every other day (aerobic in the morning, high intensity in the afternoon) with a high-fat meal between the workouts, and the other completing an aerobic training session one day and a high-intensity session the next day with a regular diet. Cyclists who completed two training sessions every other day burned more fat and improved β-hydroxyacyl-CoA-dehydrogenase protein content compared with athletes who completed the same training regimen on separate days. While both groups showed performance improvements over the 3-week study, there was no difference in performance improvements between the two groups.[48]

Dietary Periodization and Carbohydrate Restoration

The metabolic perturbations favoring the oxidation of fat persist even in the face of restored endogenous carbohydrate stores and increased exogenous carbohydrate availability.[17] Thus, to maximize possible fat-adaptation benefits from a high-fat diet without sacrificing endogenous carbohydrate stores, some researchers have proposed a method of diet periodization in which a high-fat diet (approximately 70% energy from fat, 15% energy from carbohydrate) is consumed for 5 to 14 days, then replaced with a traditional carbohydrate-loading diet directly before an event. This model replenishes glycogen stores at the time of competition in combination with increased rates of fat oxidation, albeit lower rates than are observed without carbohydrate replenishment. One of the original studies investigating diet periodization showed successful increase of fat oxidation, a decrease in glucose oxidation, and a decrease in RER after 5 days of a high-fat diet with 1 day of carbohydrate restoration in well-trained cyclists. However, performance improvements in an approximately 30-minute cycling time trial after 120 minutes of riding at 70% VO_2 max were not significant.[49]

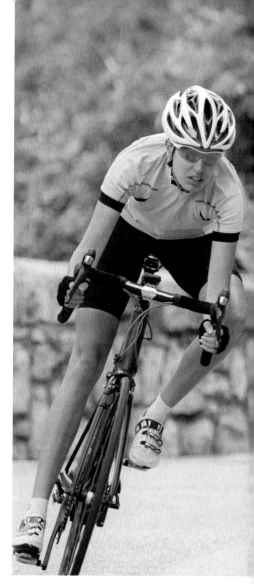

A variety of studies have produced similar results using this dietary strategy. A 5-day, high-fat diet followed by 1 day of rest and high-carbohydrate diet resulted in lowered RER and carbohydrate oxidation during both a 2-hour steady-state workout and the following time trial but did not have significant effects on time-trial performance.[50] Havemann and colleagues showed that a 7-day high-fat diet followed by 1 day of carbohydrate restoration increased fat oxidation and maintained endurance during a 100-km cycling time trial but compromised performance during intermediary sprints.[38] The authors also noted the possibility of increased sympathetic activation or altered contractile function. The same study showed that metabolic adaptation to a high-fat diet can be observed in the form of decreased RER at rest and during exercise in as little as 3 days.

While most studies have shown no significant increases in performance with high-fat diets, several have demonstrated moderate improvements. One of the strongest studies supporting dietary periodization for endurance athletes showed that an 11.5-day high-fat diet followed by a 2.5-day carbohydrate-loading regimen reported a nonsignificant 3% to 4% improvement during a 100-km time trial.[51] However, the high-fat–diet attenuated power decline observed during the high-carbohydrate condition and power output during the last 5 km of this time trial was 1.3-fold greater after the high-fat diet compared with the high-carbohydrate diet. Another study showed a 4% improvement in a 20-km time trial preceded by a 150-minute preload at 70% VO_2 max following a 10-day nonketogenic, high-fat diet with 3 days of carbohydrate loading.[52]

Potential Mechanisms of Fat Adaptation with Carbohydrate Restoration

Yeo and colleagues investigated mechanisms of fat adaptation with carbohydrate restoration. The authors studied a 5-day fat adaptation followed by 1 day of carbohydrate restoration with a 1-hour cycling workout at 70% VO_2 peak for 1 hour. Results revealed higher AMPK-α1 and AMPK-α2 activity, lower RER and glycogen utilization, increased resting muscle triglyceride stores, and fat oxidation but did not examine performance.[53] Bigrigg and colleagues observed a reduction in pyruvate dehydrogenase activity following 6 days of a high-fat protocol. These findings may partially explain decreased performance due to a reduction in glucose utilization observed in other trials. However, these effects were rapidly reversed after the reintroduction of carbohydrates.[54] More work is needed to determine the significance of changes in pyruvate dehydrogenase and pyruvate dehydrogenase kinases in athletes with varying metabolic demands, including those needing to train or compete at high intensity with a greater reliance on anaerobic metabolism. Multiple studies have shown increases in fat oxidation and decreases in RER in response to both chronic and acute high-fat feeding compared with high-carbohydrate diets. This is possibly in response to increased mitochondrial biogenesis activated through PGC-1α signaling.[46,55]

Another mechanism through which high-fat diets may improve performance is through increased muscle triglyceride stores. Increased storage of lipids in immediate proximity to mitochondria in muscle increases their availability during exercise and may decrease muscles' demand on glycogen for energy production. High-fat diet in combination with endurance training has been shown to increase intramyocellular triglyceride by 50% in type I fibers and 75% in type IIa muscle fibers over 6 weeks.[56] Other research has shown a 75% preexercise increase in total muscle triacylglycerol after 5 days of fat adaptation and 1 day of carbohydrate loading.

Summary of High-Fat Diet Literature and Need for Future Research

There seems to be very little contention that high-fat diets increase the amount of fat burned during exercise, but it remains unclear how this strategy directly affects athletic performance. This form of dietary periodization increases the rate of whole-body and muscle fat oxidation while attenuating the rate of muscle glycogenolysis during submaximal exercise. It is important to note that dietary periodization strategies similar to this represent a low-carbohydrate challenge as well as a high-fat challenge because muscle glycogen is reduced during the adaptation phase. Furthermore, simply increasing fat oxidation does not increase performance and cannot be assumed to improve long-term metabolic health, as has been suggested in some studies. These concerns may be even more pronounced in recreational athletes who may misunderstand their carbohydrate needs and associated claims about the potential benefits of fat adaptation. Much of the controversy surrounding whether or not this is a potentially helpful strategy for athletes is due to a long list of inconsistencies between study designs and outcomes. For example, research questions surrounding this topic have been studied in recreationally active subjects, well-trained cyclists, and ultraendurance athletes. Protocols have ranged from 1 day to several days, and the high-fat experimental groups have all experienced various degrees of carbohydrate restriction ranging from mild to ketogenic. Furthermore, some of the metabolic changes that have been reported use different methods for assigning high-fat treatment, many times using percent calories instead of dosing fat by body weight (g/kg). The discrepancies in research designs and lack of chronic studies make it difficult to translate the results into long-term effects on athletic performance and health.

Before recommending a fat adaptation diet to athletes, sports dietitians should consider several factors. Most importantly, there is no consensus on the performance benefits of a high-fat adaptation diet. There has been speculation that some athletes respond better than others to fat adaption diets in terms of tolerance, mood profile, and performance. However, these diets are associated with higher rated perceived exertion, especially at higher-intensity workouts, and athletes using these diets often need more encouragement to train.[57] Despite renewed attention and popular interest in this practice, recent reviews have concluded that there is no evidence to support widespread performance benefits.[19] This lack of evidence extends to the preparation of competitive athletes even in the face of metabolic adaptations to increase the mobilization, transport, and oxidation of fat as an exercise substrate.[37] Although there has been historical[35] and revived interest in chronic adaptation to high-fat, low-carbohydrate diets, present evidence suggests that enhanced rates of fat oxidation can only match exercise capacity/performance achieved by diets or strategies promoting high-carbohydrate availability at moderate intensities.[19,36] However, performance of exercise at the higher intensities representative of or important for competitive outcomes in most sporting activities seems to be impaired.[36,38]

Further research is warranted, both in view of the current discussions and the failure of recent studies to include an adequate reference diet that includes contemporary periodized dietary approaches.[19,37] Although specific scenarios may exist where high-fat diets offer some benefits or at least are not disadvantageous to performance, in general they appear to reduce rather than enhance metabolic flexibility by reducing carbohydrate availability and capacity to use it effectively as an exercise substrate. Therefore, competitive athletes would be unwise to sacrifice their ability to undertake high-quality training or high-intensity efforts during competition that could determine the competitive outcome.[37] Even when working at the highest intensities that can be supported by oxidative phosphorylation, carbohydrate offers advantages over fat as a substrate because it provides a greater yield of ATP per volume of oxygen that can be delivered to the mitochondria,[33] thus improving gross exercise efficiency.[58]

CHOOSING FAT IN SPORT

Dietary fat is essential for promoting both the health and performance of athletes. While no athlete's diet should be devoid of fat, there are certainly scenarios and acute time frames where recommending fat restriction as a temporary strategy is necessary. When acute fat restriction is practiced to make weight, it should be limited to very-short-term scenarios for the 2 to 3 days leading up to competition weigh-ins. Other examples where acute fat restriction may be beneficial are when considerations of preferred macronutrients or gastrointestinal comfort have priority, such as immediately before a sporting event or training session or during carbohydrate loading. Athletes who choose to excessively restrict their fat intake in an effort to lose body weight or improve physique should be cautioned about not meeting energy needs. Fat is a key energy provider, and restriction may lead to low energy availability, resulting in unwanted loss of muscle mass; menstrual dysfunction and hormonal disturbances; suboptimal bone density; increased risk of fatigue, injury, and illness; impaired adaptation; and a prolonged recovery process. Adequate energy availability is needed to optimize protein metabolism. When energy availability is reduced (eg, to reduce body weight or fat), performance can suffer.[59]

In most athletes, fat intakes associated with eating styles that accommodate public health recommendations typically range from 20% to 35% of total energy intake. Consuming less than 20% of energy intake from fat does not benefit performance, and extreme restriction of fat intake may limit the food range needed to meet overall health and performance goals. Claims that extremely high-fat (more than 35%), carbohydrate-restricted diets provide a benefit to the performance of competitive athletes are also not supported by current literature.

The choice of what fats to include in the diet should be based on taste preference while incorporating a wide range of foods consistent with the *2015-2020 Dietary Guidelines for Americans*. Many athletes would benefit from consuming more plant-based fatty acids and fewer foods containing significant sources of animal fat. Dietary sources of n-3 PUFAs include fish, walnuts, canola oil, and flaxseed, whereas n-6 fatty acids are found in relatively high levels in most, but not all, other plant foods.

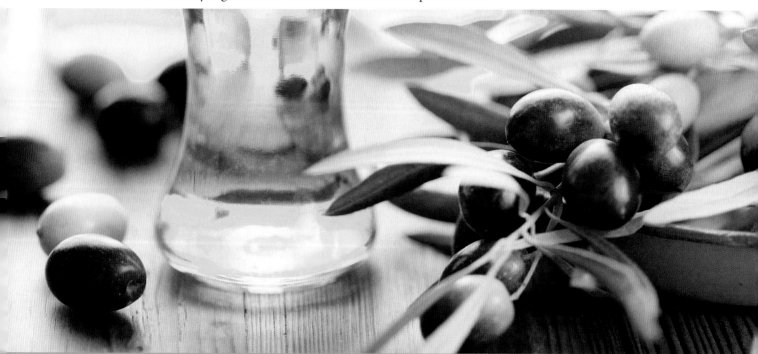

The daily fat intake for an athlete should help meet the energy demands of a periodized nutrition program to support proper training and competition. The percent energy consumed daily from fat will clearly fluctuate based on changing energy needs, with specific target amounts generally determined after carbohydrate and protein goals are established. Once a general gram per day amount is determined, athlctcs should modify their diet planning to incorporate more MUFA and PUFA food sources and devise a plan for consuming a dietary source of n-3 fatty acids several days per week. Sports dietitians might want to discuss the ratio of n-6 to n-3 when counseling athletes about diet planning because this may have a greater impact on fatty acid nutrition than a relatively small dose of an n-3 fatty acid supplement. With the possible exception of n-3 fatty acids, lipid-based dietary supplements have shown limited efficacy as ergogenic aids and should only be used with caution. If athletes remain interested in these types of dietary supplements, they should be assisted to undertake a cost-benefit analysis of the use of such products and to recognize that if they offer value, the greatest value will only be observed when added to a well-chosen eating plan. Research summaries on some popular lipid-based supplements are provided in Table 4.3.

Before exercise or competition, fat intake should be limited for one or two hours to prevent gastrointestinal distress. Athletes often benefit from liquid meal supplements, especially if they suffer from preevent anxiety or an uncertain preevent timetable, thus preferring a more quickly digested option. The amount of fat recommended in a meal or snack 3 to 4 hours before the event is variable and depends on individual tolerance. A prudent goal for meals 3 to 4 hours prior to training or competition would be to consume less than 30% calories from fat to promote gastric emptying at a rate unlikely to impede performance. Above all, athletes should choose a strategy that suits their situation and their past experiences and can be fine-tuned with further experimentation.[60,61] Generally, foods that are low-fat, low-fiber, and low to moderate in protein are preferred for a pre-event menu because they are less prone to cause gastrointestinal problems, including flatulence, bloating, nausea, vomiting, intestinal cramps, and diarrhea.[62]

n-3 and Other Lipid-Based Dietary Supplements

Athletes who chronically restrict their fat intake to below the acceptable macronutrient distribution range minimum of 20% energy from fat or who do not regularly consume sources of α-linolenic acid and EPA/DHA may benefit from taking n-3 fatty acid supplements. Depending on the extent of dietary limitations, n-3 fatty acid intake for vegetarians may be of concern. Supplementation with n-3 fatty acids may be useful in the prevention or treatment of nutrient deficiency under the supervision of an appropriate medical or nutritional expert. When choosing a supplement, it is important to note that 18:3 (n-3) (plant sources) of n-3 have limited conversion to EPA/DHA due to their entry point in the fatty acid conversion pathway that requires competition with n-6 fatty acids for the Δ^6 desaturase enzyme.[63,64] While EPA and DHA can be derived from algae, preparations usually have a low concentration compared with EPA/DHA derived from fish.[65] EPA and DHA are responsible for many bioactive end products, such as antiinflammatory resolvins and the antiarrhythmic, vasodilation, and platelet inhibitor effects of the PGH_3 family of molecules. Another potential concern is that n-3 supplements may be taken unnecessarily without appropriate supervision or monitoring.

Athletes who take supplemental n-3 fatty acids should be counseled that the antiinflammatory properties of these lipids have not been shown to enhance performance and that fish oil supplementation should not be viewed as ergogenic.[66-68] Due to inconclusive data, specific performance-based recommendations on the amount and duration of n-3 supplementation regimens are not available.[69] Moreover, some studies have indicated that large doses of n-3 supplements have increased oxidative stress markers after exercise, and some athletes who take high doses chronically may be at greater risk for immunosuppression and prolonged bleed times.[69-71] A prudent recommendation is that athletes who frequently restrict their energy intake may receive marginal benefits from increasing omega-3 intake via diet or supplementation. Up to 3 g of EPA/DHA from diet or supplements is considered safe and may help facilitate training and diet-induced performance improvements.

Table 4.3 Function, Efficacy, and Concerns of Common Lipid-Based Dietary Supplement

Supplement	Claims	Efficacy and Concerns	Evidence
Conjugated linoleic acid	May alter blood lipids and support immune function Helps to reduce body fat, change body composition, and improve athletic performance	Has not been shown to enhance aerobic exercise performance Body composition, immunity, and effects on lipid profile are equivocal May cause negative gastrointestinal (GI) side effects Evidence of effectiveness as a weight-loss aid is mixed in human studies	Jenkins ND, Buckner SL, Baker RB, et al. Effects of 6 weeks of aerobic exercise combined with conjugated linoleic acid on the physical working capacity at fatigue threshold. *J Strength Cond Res.* 2014;28(8):2127-2135. Onakpoya IJ, Posadzki PP, Watson LK, Davies LA, Ernst E.The efficacy of long-term conjugated linoleic acid (CLA) supplementation on body composition in overweight and obese individuals: a systematic review and meta-analysis of randomized clinical trials. *Eur J Nutr.* 2012;51(2):127-134. Song HJ, Grant I, Rotondo D, et al. Effect of CLA supplementation on immune function in young healthy volunteers. *Eur J Clin Nutr.* 2005;59(4):508-517. Petridou A, Mougios V, Sagredos A. Supplementation with CLA: isomer incorporation into serum lipids and effect on body fat of women. *Lipids.* 2003;38(8):805-811.
L-carnitine	Decreases heart rate Improves exercise performance Promotes recovery after exercise Increases fat metabolism and loss of body fat	Does not affect whole bodyfat utilization during short-duration exercise Safe at recommended doses of 2–4 g/d but is not effective for improving performance	Orer GE, Guzel NA. The effects of acute L-carnitine supplementation on endurance performance of athletes. *J Strength Cond Res.* 2014;28(2):514-519. Kraemer WJ, Volek JS, Dunn-Lewis C. L-carnitine supplementation: influence upon physiological function. *Curr Sports Med Rep.* 2008;7(4):218-223. Broad EM, Maughan RJ, Galloway S DR. Effects of exercise intensity and altered substrate availability on cardiovascular and metabolic responses to exercise after oral carnitine supplementation in athletes. *Int J Sport Nutr Exerc Metab.* 2011;21(5):385-397. Colombani P, Wenk C, Kunz I, et al. Effects of L-carnitine supplementation on physical performance and energy metabolism of endurance-trained athletes: a double-blind crossover field study. *J Appl Physiol Occup Physiol.* 1996;73(5):434-439.
Medium-chain triglyceride (MCT) oil	Can prolong performance and spare glycogen stores	MCT oils are ineffective in improving exercise performance in humans May cause GI distress in doses associated with performance enhancement Limited application to most sports Food sources may support healthy changes in body composition over other dietary lipids during a weight-loss program	Calbet JA, Mooren FC, Burke LM, Stear SJ, Castell LM. A-Z of nutritional supplements: dietary supplements, sports nutrition foods and ergogenic aids for health and performance: part 24. *Br J Sports Med.* 2011;45(12):1005-1007. Clegg ME. Medium-chain triglycerides are advantageous in promoting weight loss although not beneficial to exercise performance. *Int J Food Sci Nutr.* 2010;61(7):653-679. Dunford M, Coleman EJ. Ergogenic aids, dietary supplements, and exercise. In: Rosenbloom C, Coleman EJ, eds. *Sports Nutrition.* 5th ed. Chicago, IL: Academy of Nutrition and Dietetics; 2012:128-161. St-Onge MP, Bosarge A. Weight-loss diet that includes consumption of medium-chain triacylglycerol oil leads to a greater rate of weight and fat mass loss than does olive oil. *Am J Clin Nutr.* 2008;87(3):621-626.

Different lipids can produce profoundly different metabolic effects; therefore, it is very important for nutrition professionals to understand the differences between sources of dietary fat and make clear, evidence-based recommendations for both athletic performance and general wellness.

A well-chosen diet with balanced fatty acid intake includes a larger proportion of **MUFAs** and **PUFAs** relative to saturated fat intake as part of a mixed diet that emphasizes vegetables, fruits, whole grains, low-fat dairy, and seafood, with lower consumption of red and processed meat.

As exercise duration increases and intensity decreases, endogenous fat stores contribute a greater percentage of total energy relative to carbohydrate and amino acids.

Fat intake patterns may fluctuate daily to help the athlete meet the energy demands of a periodized nutrition program and support proper training and competition.

In very short-term scenarios (up to 72 hours), fat restriction may be effective for acutely reducing weight for weigh-ins or when preferred macronutrients or gastrointestinal comfort have priority.

Adequate fat consumption is crucial to health, and chronic fat restriction may contribute to low energy availability that can result in both decreased performance and serious, long-term health concerns.

While it is clear that metabolic adaptations do occur in response to high fat feeding, claims that high-fat, carbohydrate-restricted diets improve performance in competitive athletes have not been proven.

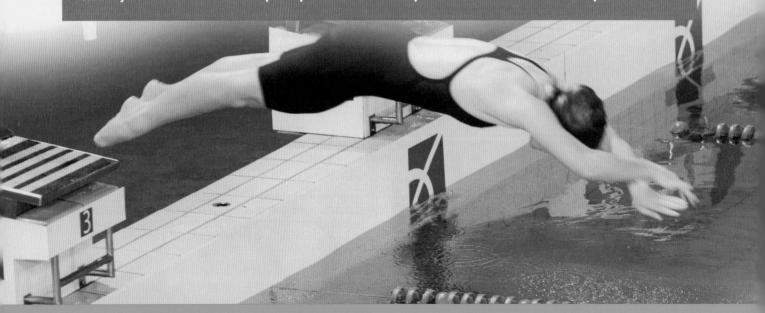

1. Nutrition and athletic performance. Joint position statement by the Academy of Nutrition and Dietetics, Dietitians of Canada, and American College of Sports Medicine. *Med Sci Sports Exerc.* 2016;48(3):543-568.

2. Jones PJ, Kubow S. Lipids, sterols and their metabolites. In: Shils M, Shike M, Ross AC, Caballero B, Cousins RJ, eds. *Modern Nutrition in Health and Disease.* 10th ed. Philadelphia, PA: Lippincott Williams & Wilkins; 2006:92-122.

3. Bard JM, Paillard F, Lecerf JM. Effect of phytosterols/stanols on LDL concentration and other surrogate markers of cardiovascular risk. *Diabetes Metab.* 2015;41(1):69-75.

4. Final determination regarding partially hydrogenated oils (removing trans fat). US Food and Drug Administration website. www.fda.gov/food/ingredientspackaginglabeling/foodadditivesingredients/ucm449162.htm. Revised June 16, 2015. Accessed June 7, 2016.

5. US Department of Health and Human Services and US Department of Agriculture. *2015-2020 Dietary Guidelines for Americans.* 8th ed. http://health.gov/dietaryguidelines/2015/guidelines/. Published December 2015. Accessed June 7, 2016.

6. Trumbo P, Schlicker S, Yates AA, Poos M, Food and Nutrition Board of the Institute of Medicine, The National Academy. Dietary reference intakes for energy, carbohydrate, fiber, fat, fatty acids, cholesterol, protein and amino acids. *J Am Diet Assoc.* 2002;102(11):1621-1630.

7. Beis LY, Willkomm L, Ross R, et al. Food and macronutrient intake of elite Ethiopian distance runners. *J Int Soc Sports Nutr.* 2011;8(1):1-7.

8. Bradley WJ, Cavanagh B, Douglas W, et al. Energy intake and expenditure assessed "in-season" in an elite European rugby union squad. *Eur J Sport Sci.* 2015;15(6):469-479.

9. Mielgo-Ayuso J, Zourdos MC, Calleja-Gonzalez J, Urdampilleta A, Ostojic SM. Dietary intake habits and controlled training on body composition and strength in elite female volleyball players during the season. *Appl Physiol Nutr Metab.* 2015;40(8):827-834.

10. Paulin S, Roberts J, Roberts M, Davis I. A case study evaluation of competitors undertaking an antarctic ultra-endurance event: nutrition, hydration and body composition variables. *Extrem Physiol Med.* 2015;4:3.

11. Kopp-Woodroffe SA, Manore MM, Dueck CA, Skinner JS, Matt KS. Energy and nutrient status of amenorrheic athletes participating in a diet and exercise training intervention program. *Int J Sport Nutr.* Mar 1999;9(1):70-88.

12. Wright HH, Garthe I. Weight-category sports. In: Maughan RJ, ed. *The Encyclopaedia of Sports Medicine: An IOC Medical Commission Publication, Volume 19.* Chichester, UK: John Wiley & Sons LTD; 2013:639-650.

13. Waly MI, Kilani HA, Al-Busafi MS. Nutritional practices of athletes in Oman: a descriptive study. *Oman Med J.* 2013;28(5):360-364.

14. Tomten SE, Høstmark AT. Energy balance in weight stable athletes with and without menstrual disorders. *Scand J Med Sci Sports.* 2006;16(2):127-133.

15. Burke LM. Fueling strategies to optimize performance: training high or training low? *Scand J Med Sci Sports.* 2010;20(suppl 2):48-58.

16. Burke LM. Re-examining high-fat diets for sports performance: did we call the 'nail in the coffin' too soon? *Sports Med.* 2015;45(suppl 1):33S-49S.

17. Yeo WK, Carey AL, Burke L, Spriet LL, Hawley JA. Fat adaptation in well-trained athletes: effects on cell metabolism. *Appl Physiol Nutr Metab.* 2011;36(1):12-22.

18. Noakes T, Volek JS, Phinney SD. Low-carbohydrate diets for athletes: what evidence? *Br J Sports Med.* 2014;48(14):1077-1078.

19. Volek JS, Noakes T, Phinney SD. Rethinking fat as a fuel for endurance exercise. *Eur J Sport Sci.* 2015;15(1):13-20.

20. Fumagalli M, Moltke I, Grarup N, et al. Greenlandic Inuit show genetic signatures of diet and climate adaptation. *Science.* 2015;349(6254):1343-1347.

21. Eckel RH, Jakicic JM, Ard JD, et al. 2013 AHA/ACC guideline on lifestyle management to reduce cardiovascular risk: a report of the American College of Cardiology/American Heart Association Task Force on Practice Guidelines. *J Am Coll Cardiol.* 2014;63(25 pt B):2960-2984.

22. Hu FB, Manson JE, Willett WC. Types of dietary fat and risk of coronary heart disease: a critical review. *J Am Coll Nutr.* 2001;20(1):5-19.

23. Dietary Guidelines Advisory Committe, 2010. Report of the Dietary Guidelines Advisory Committee on the Dietary Guidelines for Americans 2010, to the Secretary of Agriculture and the Secretary of Health and Human Services. www.cnpp.usda.gov/sites/default/files/dietary_guidelines_for_americans/2010DGACReport-camera-ready-Jan11-11.pdf. Published 2010. Accessed June 8, 2016.

24. Manini TM, Clark BC, Nalls MA, Goodpaster BH, Ploutz-Snyder LL, Harris TB. Reduced physical activity increases intermuscular adipose tissue in healthy young adults. *Am J Clin Nutr.* 2007;85(2):377-384.

25. Enevoldsen LH, Simonsen L, Bulow J. Postprandial triacylglycerol uptake in the legs is increased during exercise and post-exercise recovery. *J Physiol.* 2005;568(pt 3):941-950.

26. Roepstorff C, Thiele M, Hillig T, et al. Higher skeletal muscle alpha2AMPK activation and lower energy charge and fat oxidation in men than in women during submaximal exercise. *J Physiol.*2006;574(pt 1):125-138.

27. Alsted TJ, Nybo L, Schweiger M, et al. Adipose triglyceride lipase in human skeletal muscle is upregulated by exercise training. *Am J Physiol Endocrinol Metab.* 2009;296(3):445E-453E.

28. Romijn JA, Coyle EF, Sidossis LS, et al. Regulation of endogenous fat and carbohydrate metabolism in relation to exercise intensity and duration. *Am J Physiol.* 1993;265(3 pt 1):380E-391E.

29. Watt MJ, Heigenhauser GJ, Spriet LL. Effects of dynamic exercise intensity on the activation of hormone-sensitive lipase in human skeletal muscle. *J Physiol.* 2003;547(pt 1):301-308.

30. Frayn KN. Fat as a fuel: emerging understanding of the adipose tissue-skeletal muscle axis. *Acta Physiol (Oxf).* 2010;199(4):509-518.

31. van Loon LJ, Greenhaff PL, Constantin-Teodosiu D, Saris WH, Wagenmakers AJ. The effects of increasing exercise intensity on muscle fuel utilisation in humans. *J Physiol.* 2001;536(pt 1):295-304.

32. Kiens B, Jeppesen J. Fat metabolism during and after exercise. In: Maughan RJ, ed. *The Encyclopaedia of Sports Medicine: An IOC Medical Commission Publication, Volume 19.* Chichester, UK: John Wiley & Sons LTD; 2013:156-165.

33. Spriet LL. New insights into the interaction of carbohydrate and fat metabolism during exercise. *Sports Med.* 2014;44(suppl 1):87S-96S.

34. Phinney SD, Horton ES, Sims EA, Hanson JS, Danforth E Jr, LaGrange BM. Capacity for moderate exercise in obese subjects after adaptation to a hypocaloric, ketogenic diet. *J Clin Invest.* 1980;66(5):1152-1161.

35. Phinney SD, Bistrian BR, Wolfe RR, Blackburn GL. The human metabolic response to chronic ketosis without caloric restriction: physical and biochemical adaptation. *Metabolism.*1983;32(8):757-768.

36. Phinney SD, Bistrian BR, Evans WJ, Gervino E, Blackburn GL. The human metabolic response to chronic ketosis without caloric restriction: preservation of submaximal exercise capability with reduced carbohydrate oxidation. *Metabolism.* 1983;32(8):769-776.

37. Burke LM, Kiens B. "Fat adaptation" for athletic performance: the nail in the coffin? *J Appl Physiol* (1985). 2006;100(1):7-8.

38. Havemann L, West SJ, Goedecke JH, et al. Fat adaptation followed by carbohydrate loading compromises high-intensity sprint performance. *J Appl Physiol* (1985). 2006;100(1):194-202.

39. Stellingwerff T, Spriet LL, Watt MJ, et al. Decreased PDH activation and glycogenolysis during exercise following fat adaptation with carbohydrate restoration. *Am J Physiol Endocrinol Metab.* 2006;290(2):380E-388E.

40. Zajac A, Poprzecki S, Maszczyk A, Czuba M, Michalczyk M, Zydek G. The effects of a ketogenic diet on exercise metabolism and physical performance in off-road cyclists. *Nutrients.* 2014;6(7):2493-2508.

41. Paoli A, Grimaldi K, D'Agostino D, et al. Ketogenic diet does not affect strength performance in elite artistic gymnasts. *J Int Soc Sports Nutr.* 2012;9(1):34.

42. Sawyer JC, Wood RJ, Davidson PW, et al. Effects of a short-term carbohydrate-restricted diet on strength and power performance. *J Strength Cond Res.* 2013;27(8):2255-2262.

43. Bartlett JD, Hawley JA, Morton JP. Carbohydrate availability and exercise training adaptation: too much of a good thing? *Eur J Sport Sci.* 2015;15(1):3-12.

44. Stellingwerff T. Contemporary nutrition approaches to optimize elite marathon performance. *Int J Sports Physiol Perform.* 2013;8(5):573-578.

45. Shimada K, Yamamoto Y, Iwayama K, et al. Effects of post-absorptive and postprandial exercise on 24 h fat oxidation. *Metabolism.* 2013;62(6):793-800.

46. Baar K. Nutrition and the adaptation to endurance training. *Sports Med.* 2014;44(suppl 1):5S-12S.

47. Rowlands DS, Hopkins WG. Effect of high-fat, high-carbohydrate, and high-protein meals on metabolism and performance during endurance cycling. *Int J Sport Nutr Exerc Metab.* 2002;12(3):318-335.

48. Hulston CJ, Venables MC, Mann CH, et al. Training with low muscle glycogen enhances fat metabolism in well-trained cyclists. *Med Sci Sports Exerc.* 2010;42(11):2046-2055.

49. Burke LM, Angus DJ, Cox GR, et al. Effect of fat adaptation and carbohydrate restoration on metabolism and performance during prolonged cycling. *J Appl Physiol* (1985). 2000;89(6):2413-2421.

50. Burke LM, Hawley JA, Angus DJ, et al. Adaptations to short-term high-fat diet persist during exercise despite high carbohydrate availability. *Med Sci Sports Exerc.* 2002;34(1):83-91.

51. Rowlands DS, Hopkins WG. Effects of high-fat and high-carbohydrate diets on metabolism and performance in cycling. *Metabolism*. 2002;51(6):678-690.

52. Lambert EV, Goedecke JH, Zyle C, et al. High-fat diet versus habitual diet prior to carbohydrate loading: effects of exercise metabolism and cycling performance. *Int J Sport Nutr Exerc Metab*. 2001;11(2):209-225.

53. Yeo WK, Lessard SJ, Chen ZP, et al. Fat adaptation followed by carbohydrate restoration increases AMPK activity in skeletal muscle from trained humans. *J Appl Physiol* (1985). 2008;105(5):1519-1526.

54. Bigrigg JK, Heigenhauser GJ, Inglis JG, LeBlanc PJ, Peters SJ. Carbohydrate refeeding after a high-fat diet rapidly reverses the adaptive increase in human skeletal muscle PDH kinase activity. *Am J Physiol Regul Integr Comp Physiol*. 2009;297(3):885R-891R.

55. Margolis LM, Pasiakos SM. Optimizing intramuscular adaptations to aerobic exercise: effects of carbohydrate restriction and protein supplementation on mitochondrial biogenesis. *Adv Nutr*. 2013;4(6):657-664.

56. Van Proeyen K, Szlufcik K, Nielens H, et al. High-fat diet overrules the effects of training on fiber-specific intramyocellular lipid utilization during exercise. *J Appl Physiol* (1985). 2011;111(1):108-116.

57. Hawley JA. Fat adaptation science: low-carbohydrate, high-fat diets to alter fuel utilization and promote training adaptation. *Nestle Nutr Inst Workshop Ser*. 2011;69:59-71; discussion 71-77.

58. Cole M, Coleman D, Hopker J, Wiles J. Improved gross efficiency during long duration submaximal cycling following a short-term high carbohydrate diet. *Int J Sports Med*. 2014;35(3):265-269.

59. Nindl BC, Friedl KE, Frykman PN, Marchitelli LJ, Shippee RL, Patton JF. Physical performance and metabolic recovery among lean, healthy men following a prolonged energy deficit. *Int J Sports Med*. 1997;18(5):317-324.

60. Burke LM, Kiens B, Ivy JL. Carbohydrates and fat for training and recovery. *J Sports Sci*. 2004;22(1):15-30.

61. Ormsbee MJ, Bach CW, Baur DA. Pre-exercise nutrition: the role of macronutrients, modified starches and supplements on metabolism and endurance performance. *Nutrients*. 2014;6(5):1782-1808.

62. Rehrer NJ, van Kemenade M, Meester W, Brouns F, Saris WH. Gastrointestinal complaints in relation to dietary intake in triathletes. *Int J Sport Nutr*. 1992;2(1):48-59.

63. Goyens PL, Spilker ME, Zock PL, Katan MB, Mensink RP. Conversion of alpha-linolenic acid in humans is influenced by the absolute amounts of alpha-linolenic acid and linoleic acid in the diet and not by their ratio. *Am J Clin Nutr*. 2006;84(1):44-53.

64. Nakamura MT, Nara TY. Structure, function, and dietary regulation of delta6, delta5, and delta9 desaturases. *Annu Rev Nutr*. 2004;24:345-376.

65. Jump DB, Depner CM, Tripathy S. Omega-3 fatty acid supplementation and cardiovascular disease. *J Lipid Res*. 2012;53(12):2525-2545.

66. Nieman DC, Henson DA, McAnulty SR, Jin F, Maxwell KR. n-3 polyunsaturated fatty acids do not alter immune and inflammation measures in endurance athletes. *Int J Sport Nutr Exerc Metab*. 2009;19(5):536-546.

67. Bloomer RJ, Larson DE, Fisher-Wellman KH, Galpin AJ, Schilling BK. Effect of eicosapentaenoic and docosahexaenoic acid on resting and exercise-induced inflammatory and oxidative stress biomarkers: a randomized, placebo controlled, cross-over study. *Lipids Health Dis*. 2009;8:36.

68. Buckley JD, Burgess S, Murphy KJ, Howe PR. DHA-rich fish oil lowers heart rate during submaximal exercise in elite Australian Rules footballers. *J Sci Med Sport*. 2009;12(4):503-507.

69. Mickleborough TD. Omega-3 polyunsaturated fatty acids in physical performance optimization. *Int J Sport Nutr Exerc Metab*. 2013;23(1):83-96.

70. McAnulty SR, Nieman DC, Fox-Rabinovich M, et al. Effect of n-3 fatty acids and antioxidants on oxidative stress after exercise. *Med Sci Sports Exerc*. 2010;42(9):1704-1711.

71. Filaire E, Massart A, Portier H, et al. Effect of 6 weeks of n-3 fatty-acid supplementation on oxidative stress in judo athletes. *Int J Sport Nutr Exerc Metab*. 2010;20(6):496-506.

CHAPTER 5

VITAMINS, MINERALS, AND EXERCISE

Abigail Duffine Gilman, MS, RD, LDN, and Stella Lucia Volpe, PhD, RD, LDN, FACSM

INTRODUCTION

Micronutrients (vitamins and minerals) differ from macronutrients in that they are required in much smaller quantities. The use of macronutrients for all physiological processes is enabled by micronutrients.[1] Therefore, vitamins and minerals are necessary for numerous metabolic processes in the body as well as to support growth and development. Vitamins and minerals are also key regulators in many chemical reactions during exercise and physical activity, including energy metabolism, oxygen transfer and delivery, and tissue repair.[2]

The vitamin and mineral needs of people who are physically active is a subject of debate. Some researchers have reported that those who exercise require more vitamins and minerals than their sedentary counterparts; however, others have not reported greater micronutrient requirements. The intensity, duration, and frequency of activity, as well as overall energy and nutrient intake, affect micronutrient requirements.[2-4] This chapter will review vitamin and mineral needs of adults who are physically active.

DIETARY REFERENCE INTAKES

Recommendations for intake of all known vitamins and some essential minerals for healthy, moderately active people were updated beginning in 1997.[5-8] Updated references were established for calcium and vitamin D in 2010.[5]

In the United States, these recommendations are known as the Dietary Reference Intakes (DRIs). Adequate Intakes (AIs), Recommended Dietary Allowances (RDAs), Estimated Average Requirements (EARs), and Tolerable Upper Intake Levels (ULs) all fall under the umbrella of the DRIs. The RDA is the dietary intake level that is adequate for approximately 98% of healthy people. AI is an estimated value used when an RDA cannot be determined. EAR is used to approximate the nutrient needs of half of the healthy people in a group, from which an RDA is then established.[5] UL is the highest amount of a nutrient that most people can consume without adverse effects.[6] The National Academy of Medicine publishes DRI tables online (www.nationalacademies.org/hmd/Activities/Nutrition/SummaryDRIs/DRI-Tables.aspx).

In general, if energy intakes are adequate, vitamin and mineral needs of physically active people are similar to those of healthy, moderately active people; thus, DRI should be appropriate for micronutrient needs. Some athletes may have increased requirements because of excessive losses of nutrients in sweat and urine, and supplementation may be needed. Because many physically

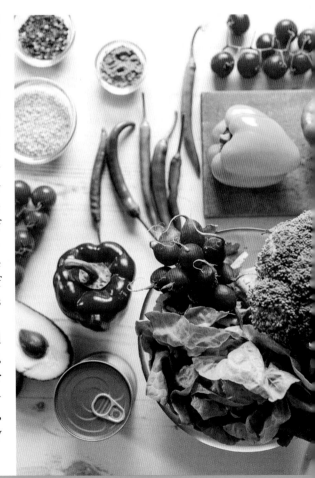

active people choose to supplement with vitamins and minerals, practitioners may use the ULs to give guidelines to those who take supplements to prevent adverse reactions from excess consumption.

The research on micronutrients for athletes has limitations. Many studies were conducted prior to 2000, which calls into question their relevance. Contradictory findings make it difficult for practitioners to give definitive advice to athletes. Research limitations include small sample sizes, mostly male subjects, differences in type of exercise performed or level of training and fitness, lack of strong longitudinal data, differences in assessment methodology or study design, and various types and amounts of supplements researched. In an effort to keep this chapter relevant, we did not include studies published prior to 2000 unless they were considered to be seminal. This eliminated more than 60 studies that were covered in previous editions of this book.

VITAMINS AND MINERALS OF CONCERN DURING TRAINING

Exercise can affect vitamin and mineral requirements because of increased physiological demands and the stress of exercise. In addition, there may be increased losses of certain micronutrients (eg, sodium through sweat) and decreased absorption due to diminished gastrointestinal tract function during exercise. The level of alteration depends on the volume of training and competition; athletes training or competing more than 20 hours per week are affected the most.

Energy Metabolism

Energy metabolism is the process of generating energy, in the form of adenosine triphosphate from nutrients. Energy metabolism is vital to life and is especially necessary during exercise. Interconnected pathways continuously produce energy with or without the presence of oxygen. While macronutrients are metabolized to produce energy, micronutrients play a crucial supporting role in the metabolic processes. This section will focus on the primary vitamins and minerals involved in energy metabolism as coenzymes and cofactors.

THIAMIN

Thiamin, also known as vitamin B-1, is a water-soluble vitamin that participates in several energy-producing reactions as part of thiamine diphosphate (also known as thiamine pyrophosphate), including the Krebs cycle (also known as the citric acid cycle), branched-chain amino acid (BCAA) catabolism, and the pentose phosphate pathway.[9] For example, thiamin is required to convert pyruvate to acetyl coenzyme A (CoA) during carbohydrate metabolism. It also aids in the conversion of α-ketoglutarate to succinyl-CoA in the Krebs cycle and in the decarboxylation of BCAAs, which increases with physical activity.[10] These conversions are all essential for the aerobic metabolism of glucose, BCAAs, and fatty acids as well as, in turn, exercise performance. Health and performance may be impaired if these conversions do not occur.[2] Researchers have not determined whether thiamin excretion increases due to exercise. Kim and colleagues showed that regular, moderate exercise training in rats elicited an increased urinary excretion of thiamin. However, this excretion was not significantly different ($P < .05$) from that of non–exercise-trained rats.[11]

Although research about the effects of exercise on thiamin is limited, especially in human trials, Sato and colleagues, conducted a cross-sectional study to evaluate the effect of high-intensity swim training on blood thiamin concentrations in 6 men and 13 women swimmers. The swimmers were assessed during a preparation period and an intensive-training period. Although anthropometric variables and dietary intake did not change during the training period, energy expenditure increased significantly. In addition, blood thiamin concentrations decreased significantly during the intensive-training period compared with the preparation period (41 ± 6 ng/mL vs 36 ± 3 ng/mL for males, $P = .048$; and 38 ± 10 ng/mL vs 31 ± 5 ng/mL for females, $P = .004$).[12] Although these results suggest that high-intensity training decreases blood thiamin concentrations, more research is required to determine if thiamin requirements are greater in people who exercise. Thiamin requirements may parallel the intensity, duration, and frequency of exercise, but because so little research has been conducted on thiamin and exercise, practitioners should not recommend thiamin intakes more than the DRI for physically active people unless a thiamin deficiency has been determined. Dietary sources of thiamin are listed in Table 5.1.

RIBOFLAVIN

Riboflavin, also known as vitamin B-2, is a water-soluble vitamin involved in several key metabolic reactions that are important during exercise: glycolysis, the Krebs cycle, and the electron transport chain. Riboflavin is the precursor in the synthesis of the flavin coenzymes, flavin mononucleotide, and flavin-adenine dinucleotide, which assist in oxidation-reduction reactions by acting as one- and two-electron transfers.[9]

Research has shown that initiating an exercise program may alter riboflavin status in humans; however, it is unclear if the effect is transient or long term.[9] Sato and colleagues reported no significant change in blood riboflavin concentrations in male and female participants during the off-season period compared with the intensive training period.[12] This could indicate that, unlike thiamin, riboflavin is less susceptible to changes in exercise habits or that riboflavin status is unaltered entirely by exercise. This research indicates that people who are physically active and consume adequate amounts of dietary riboflavin may not be at risk for depletion and may not require levels more than the RDA.[9] Riboflavin deficiency is uncommon in Western countries because it is found in a wide variety of foods; however, athletes who restrict their food intake for weight loss may be at greater risk for riboflavin deficiency. Dietary sources of riboflavin are listed in Table 5.1.

VITAMIN B-6

The three major forms of vitamin B-6 are pyridoxine, pyridoxal, and pyridoxamine. The active coenzyme forms of vitamin B-6 are pyridoxal 5′-phosphate and pyridoxamine 5′-phosphate. Vitamin B-6 is involved in approximately 100 metabolic reactions, including those involving gluconeogenesis, niacin synthesis, and lipid metabolism.[9] Pyridoxal 5′-phosphate is a required coenzyme of glycogen phosphorylase, the enzyme needed for glycogen metabolism.

The effects of maximal effort exercise on vitamin B-6 concentrations are unknown. Researchers have indicated that vitamin B-6 supplementation, in conjunction with a maltodextrin supplement in elite cyclists during maximal effort exercise, significantly increased available blood glucose concentrations compared with results for the control group. Nonetheless, there was no significant difference in performance between the maltodextrin-supplemented group compared with the maltodextrin plus vitamin B-6–supplemented group, suggesting that the maltodextrin provided the increased blood glucose concentrations.[13] Although supplementation with vitamin B-6 has not been found to enhance glucose availability, it has been shown that poor vitamin B-6 status can impair exercise performance.[14] Manore reported that vitamin B-6 plays a key role in producing energy during exercise, and therefore, people with an inadequate intake of vitamin B-6 have a decreased ability to perform physical activity optimally. Considering the limited amount of research that has been conducted, it seems that people who exercise do not have increased needs for vitamin B-6. However, Manore has reported that work capacity improves as vitamin B-6 status improves, while deficiencies of vitamin B-6 negatively affect aerobic capacity.[15] Therefore, if deficiencies exist, it may be necessary to supplement with vitamin B-6 at the level of the DRI. Dietary sources of vitamin B-6 are shown in Table 5.1.

NIACIN

Niacin, also known as vitamin B-3, is a family of molecules that include nicotinic acid and nicotinamide. The coenzyme forms of niacin are nicotinamide adenine dinucleotide and nicotinamide adenine dinucleotide phosphate. Both are involved in glycolysis, the pentose phosphate pathway, the Krebs cycle, lipid synthesis, and the electron transport chain. Pharmacologic doses of nicotinic acid may also augment the use of carbohydrate as a substrate during exercise by decreasing the availability of free fatty acids. Despite this strong connection to exercise metabolism, no solid data presently support increased niacin supplementation for people who exercise. Furthermore, pharmacologic doses of niacin can result in a "niacin flush," in which blood vessel dilation results in reddening of the face and extreme itching.[14] Athletes may

Vitamin	Effect of Exercise on Requirements	Recommended Intake for Athletes	Food Sources	Comments
Vitamin B-6	Exercise does not cause transient changes in vitamin B-6 status	Recommended Dietary Allowances (RDA); Supplementation may be necessary if deficiencies previously exist	Liver, chicken, bananas, potatoes, spinach	
Vitamin B-12	Exercise does not seem to increase needs for vitamin B-12	RDA	Fish, milk and milk products, eggs, meat, poultry, fortified breakfast cereals	Vegan athletes will likely need to supplement to ensure adequate intake
Folate	Exercise does not seem to increase folate needs	RDA	Leafy greens (eg, spinach, turnip greens), dry beans, peas, fortified cereals, grain products, strawberries	
Thiamin	Exercise does not seem to increase thiamin needs	RDA; Supplementation may be necessary if deficiencies previously exist	Wheat germ, brewer's yeast, oysters, beef liver, peanuts, green peas, raisins, collard greens	Ergogenic effects are equivocal
Riboflavin	Exercise does not seem to increase riboflavin needs	RDA	Organ meats, milk, cheese, oily fish, eggs, dark leafy green vegetables	
Niacin	Exercise does not seem to increase niacin needs	RDA	Beef, pork, chicken, wheat flour, eggs, milk	Does not seem to have ergogenic effects
Pantothenic acid	Not enough information	Adequate Intakes (AI)	Eggs, sunflower seeds, mushrooms, peanuts, brewer's yeast, yogurt, broccoli, whole grain cereals, meat	
Biotin	Not enough information	AI	Peanut butter, boiled eggs, toasted wheat germ, egg noodles, Swiss cheese, cauliflower	
Vitamin C	Increased vitamin C intakes may prevent upper respiratory tract infections	At least the Dietary Reference Intakes (DRIs); Ultraendurance athletes need more than the DRI, but below the Tolerable Upper Intake Levels	Brussels sprouts, broccoli, chili and bell peppers, kiwi, oranges, papaya, guava	Strong antioxidant properties reported for endurance and ultraendurance athletes
Choline	Exercise does not seem to increase needs.	AI	Liver, egg yolks, peanuts, cauliflower, soybeans, grape juice, and cabbage	Does not seem to have ergogenic effects

take high doses of niacin thinking "more is better." However, taking too much niacin, as with taking too much of any vitamin or mineral, can be detrimental to health and exercise performance.

More research is needed to determine how niacin affects the depletion of glycogen stores and, therefore, its potential to indirectly affect performance.[1] It is important for people who exercise to obtain the DRI for niacin to ensure adequate intake and prevent alterations in fuel utilization, but they should not exceed the UL. Dietary sources of niacin are listed in Table 5.1.

PANTOTHENIC ACID

Pantothenic acid, a water-soluble vitamin whose biologically active forms are CoA and acyl carrier protein, is involved in acyl group transfers, such as the acylation of amino acids.[9,16] Pantothenic acid coenzymes are also involved in lipid synthesis and metabolism and oxidation of pyruvate and α-ketoglutarate. Acetyl CoA is an important intermediate in fat, carbohydrate, and protein metabolism.[14] In a more recent human study, researchers confirmed that supplementation of D-pantothenic acid and L-cysteine did not affect fuel selection in the muscle or work output.[16] Although this research indicates that there may be an increased need for pantothenic acid with exercise, definite conclusions cannot be made for the human model. It would be prudent to suggest that athletes consume the AI for pantothenic acid. Dietary sources for pantothenic acid are listed in Table 5.1.

BETAINE

Betaine, a metabolic derivative of choline widely found in many plant food, acts similarly to choline (donating a methyl group in the same metabolic pathways), thus reducing the amount of choline required.[17] Betaine supplementation may work as an ergogenic (performance-enhancing) aid in improving power output.[18,19] Lee and colleagues conducted a randomized, double-blind, crossover study to determine if betaine supplementation increased strength and power performance. Significant increases ($P < .05$) in force and power production were observed in the upper but not the lower body.[20] While Lee and colleagues found significant changes in force and power production in the upper body, Hoffman and colleagues reported that the effects of betaine supplementation were more evident in the vertical jump vs the bench press throw.[21] Although the research designs and measures varied, these studies provide a foundation for future research on betaine supplementation in athletes.

Antioxidants and Oxidative Damage

Antioxidants are compounds that help counteract the damaging effects of free radicals in the body. Free radicals, reactive oxygen species, and reactive nitrogen species are compounds that contain one or more unpaired electrons that can lead to tissue damage and contribute to chronic disease.[22] Free radicals are endogenously produced in the body through oxidation reactions, such as energy metabolism; however, they are also created through exogenous sources, such as excess micronutrient intake (eg, vitamins C and A)[22,23] and exercise.[24,25] Exercise type, mode, duration, and intensity all affect the amount of free radicals produced.[25,26] When free-radical production overwhelms antioxidant availability, the resultant oxidation may decrease physical performance and health.[27] It is important to note, however, that regular exercise and conditioning may lead to responses that adapt to the increased oxidative stress and prevent associated damage.[28] It is also important to note that many in vivo experiments use fruit and vegetable extracts to elucidate the effect of individual antioxidants. This can be misleading because the combination of various micronutrients and phytochemicals may contribute to the desired outcomes. A number of researchers combine supplementation of vitamins and minerals in their research; therefore, caution must be used in attributing individual outcomes to one antioxidant or micronutrient.[17]

VITAMIN C

Vitamin C, also referred to as ascorbic acid, ascorbate, or ascorbate monoanion,[9] is a water-soluble vitamin involved in maintaining collagen synthesis, oxidizing fatty acids, and forming neurotransmitters. It is also an antioxidant.[9,14] Vitamin C protects against oxidative stress in endurance and ultraendurance athletes, especially in preventing upper respiratory tract infections.[29,30] Although aerobic exercise increases oxidative stress, it also increases enzymatic and nonenzymatic antioxidants as an adaptation to training.[28] Vitamin C concentrations in the blood can be increased up to 24 hours after exercise but may decrease to below preexercise concentrations in the days following prolonged exercise. Thus, caution must be used when blood measurements of vitamin C are used as assessment parameters in research studies because they may not be truly reflective of status.[29] This phenomenon is fairly common for all antioxidants; therefore, researchers must be cognizant of their measurement techniques and timing.

Robson and colleagues reported significantly greater neutrophil oxidative activity following exercise after 7 days of supplementing athletes with an antioxidant combination of 900 mg of vitamin C, 18 mg of β carotene, and 90 mg of vitamin E.[31] Because the researchers supplemented with β carotene and vitamin E, a definitive effect of vitamin C cannot be determined.

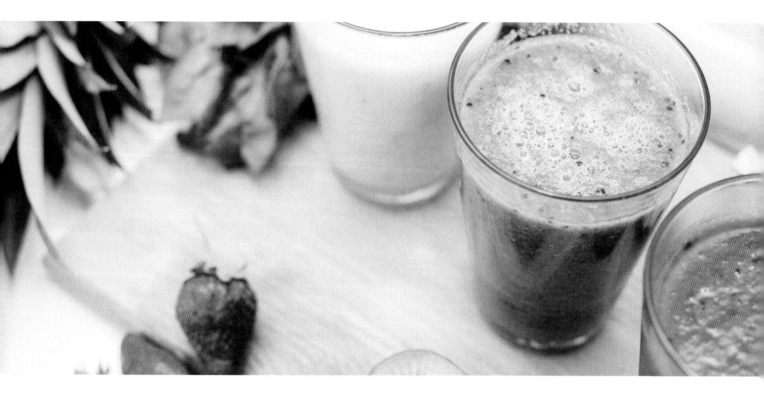

Conversely, Gomez-Cabrera and colleagues reported that vitamin C supplementation delayed the positive changes associated with exercise. The researchers studied the effects of vitamin C supplementation on training-induced increases in maximal oxygen consumption (VO$_2$ max) and skeletal muscle mitochondrial biogenesis in healthy sedentary men. They found that the maximal rate of oxygen consumption (VO$_2$ max) increased significantly ($P = .019$) after 8 weeks of training in both vitamin C–supplemented (1,000 mg/d) and nonsupplemented men. The researchers hoped to ascertain information regarding mitochondrial changes in skeletal muscle within both the supplemented and nonsupplemented participants, but due to ethical concerns, the researchers followed the training protocol on rats for this phase of the study. None of the expected changes associated with exercise, such as increased production of endogenous antioxidant enzymes, increased skeletal muscle protein concentrations, and increased protein concentration, indicative of mitochondrial adaptations, were seen in the supplemented rats. This study presents conflicting evidence regarding the use of vitamin C in athletes.[32]

Because of the conflicting evidence regarding vitamin C supplementation for athletic performance, athletes are not advised to consume vitamin C beyond the DRI. Vitamin C also plays a role in the immune system and will be discussed later in this chapter. Dietary sources of vitamin C are listed in Table 5.1 (page 83).

VITAMIN E

Vitamin E refers to a family of eight related fat-soluble compounds known as the tocopherols and the tocotrienols. Like vitamin C, vitamin E is well known for its antioxidant function in preventing free radical damage to cell membranes. Vitamin E also plays a role in immune function.[9] Dietary vitamin E intakes in athletes are generally low compared with the intake of other antioxidants. Researchers have reported that vitamin E intakes were lower than intake of other antioxidants in female figure skaters and heptathletes as well as male and female rowers.[33,34]

Although athletes have reported low dietary intakes of vitamin E, supplementation may be beneficial by reducing exercise-induced oxidative stress.[14] Garelnabi and colleagues sought to determine how vitamin E supplementation affects VO$_2$ max, oxidative stress, and lipid profile during short-duration, moderate-intensity activity. In the study, 455 healthy participants were randomized into two groups—placebo or vitamin E supplemented with 800 IU—and engaged in moderate aerobic exercise for at least 30 minutes per day, three times a week for 8 weeks. The researchers determined that myeloperoxidase (MPO), a protein released after oxidation of low-density lipoprotein cholesterol, increased in both the supplemented and placebo groups following the exercise regimen. MPO levels generally drop to clinically normal levels over time after oxidative stress; however, the vitamin E–supplemented participants had MPO concentrations that remained high after the 8-week intervention. The researchers had hoped to ascertain information regarding mitochondrial changes in skeletal muscle in the supplemented and nonsupplemented participants.[35]

Antioxidant combination therapies are frequently tested to assess the additive effects. Bryant and colleagues examined different levels and combinations of antioxidant supplements in seven trained male cyclists (approximately 22 years old) who participated in four separate supplementation phases. They ingested two capsules per day containing the following treatments: placebo (placebo plus placebo), vitamin C (1 g/day of vitamin C plus placebo), vitamins C and E (1 g/day of vitamin C plus 200 IU/kg of body weight of vitamin E), and vitamin E (400 IU/kg of vitamin E plus placebo). Researchers found that the vitamin E treatment was more effective than vitamin C alone or vitamin C and vitamin E together. Plasma malondialdehyde concentrations, a general measure of oxidative damage, were lowest with the vitamin E supplementation.[36]

The effects of vitamin E supplementation on resistance training performance are still unknown. Avery and colleagues assessed the effects of 1,200 IU/day of vitamin E vs a placebo on the recovery responses to repeated bouts of resistance training. No significant differences were found between the group taking the vitamin E supplement and the placebo group in muscle soreness, exercise performance, or plasma malondialdehyde concentrations.[37] The role of vitamin E in preventing oxidative damage due to exercise may be significant. Long-term research is needed to assess vitamin E supplementation on oxidative stress from exercise. Dietary sources of vitamin E are listed in Table 5.2.

VITAMIN A

Vitamin A, considered a subset of retinoids, is a fat-soluble vitamin best known for the role it plays in the visual cycle.[17] Other important functions of vitamin A include its roles in cellular differentiation, reproduction, gestation, fetal development, and bone formation; it also serves as an antioxidant.[17,38] Plants can synthesize carotenoids, which can serve as precursors of vitamin A; however, humans and other animals convert carotenoids to retinol or acquire preformed vitamin A from animal foods or supplements.[17] Assessment of vitamin A intake in people who are physically active has shown varied results, likely because the source of vitamin A (plant vs animal) was not specified.[14]

Vitamin A antioxidant status may alleviate the oxidative load associated with endurance training. Braakhuis and colleagues analyzed how antioxidant intake, including that of vitamin A, and training status affect total antioxidant capacity (TAC) in competitive rowers. TAC measures how well a food product or biological sample can reduce an oxidant and is measured by the moles of radicals neutralized per gram of tested sample. The researchers found that blood TAC was correlated with total dietary antioxidant intake

Table 5.2 Fat-Soluble Vitamin Needs for Athletes and Respective Food Sources

Vitamin	Effect of Exercise on Requirements	Recommended Intake for Athletes	Food Sources	Comments
Vitamin A	Exercise may increase vitamin A needs; results equivocal; β carotene may be better, but not definitive	Recommended Dietary Allowances (RDAs)	Carrots, broccoli, tomatoes	Although vitamin A can be an antioxidant, intakes more than the Dietary Reference Intakes may result in adverse effects in athletes
Vitamin D	Exercise does not seem to increase vitamin D needs	RDA; Higher levels may be needed in the winter if living in northern states (to prevent bone loss)	Oily fish, liver, eggs, fortified foods such as margarine, breakfast cereals, bread, milk, and powdered milk	
Vitamin E	Exercise may increase vitamin E needs	RDA	Plant oils (eg, soybean, corn, olive oils), nuts, seeds, wheat germ	Strong antioxidant effects in endurance athletes and older athletes
Vitamin K	Exercise does not seem to increase vitamin K needs	Adequate Intake	Leafy green vegetables (eg, spinach, turnip greens), cabbage, green tea, alfalfa, oats, cauliflower	Increased intakes may be needed for bone formation

(correlation factor, $r = 0.29$; 90% ± 0.27% confidence limit). A negative association was discovered between degree of training and TAC; this association was also reported between vitamin A intake and TAC but to a much lesser extent. These results indicate that, although dietary intake of vitamin A is correlated to the TAC of an individual, exercise training has a stronger influence on increasing the TAC.[34]

β carotene, a vitamin A precursor, is a weak antioxidant and may actually be a prooxidant if excessive amounts are consumed.[38] Aguiló and colleagues reported decreased blood concentrations of β carotene in well-trained professional cyclists after a 170-km endurance cycling bout, but this effect was not found in amateur cyclists.[39] Perhaps this is a preventive response for trained endurance athletes. Nonetheless, daily vitamin A supplementation (50,000 IU) for 60 days (in combination with 1,000 mg vitamin C and 200 mg vitamin E supplementation) was shown to be effective in decreasing the oxidative response after a 45-minute bout of cycling at 70% of VO_2 max in untrained, healthy people.[40] As with other studies where researchers combined antioxidants, it is difficult to determine if any one vitamin had a greater effect than another. In general, athletes are encouraged to consume fruits and vegetables containing β carotene; however, supplementation is not recommended. Because vitamin A is a fat-soluble vitamin that is stored in the body, athletes should not exceed the UL. Furthermore, of all the fat-soluble vitamins, vitamin A is the most toxic, and athletes need to be aware of this. Table 5.2 lists some dietary sources of vitamin A. Vitamin A will be further discussed later in the chapter.

SELENIUM

Selenium is a trace mineral well known for its role as an antioxidant in the body (metalloenzyme: glutathione peroxidase). Selenium also functions to maintain normal thyroid hormone metabolism.[2] Limited data are available about whether people who exercise require more selenium than those who are sedentary.

Researchers have reported that 150 mcg of selenium, combined with 2,000 IU of retinol, 120 mg of ascorbic acid, and 30 IU of α-tocopherol, increased total plasma antioxidant status after exercise.[41] Nonetheless, because little data are available and excess selenium is toxic, people who exercise should consume no more than the DRI for selenium and should never exceed the UL. The selenium content of food can vary greatly with the soil content. Good sources of selenium are listed in Table 5.3.

Table 5.3 Trace Mineral Needs for Athletes and Respective Food Sources

Mineral	Effect of Exercise on Requirements	Recommended Intake for Athletes	Food Sources	Comments
Copper	Exercise does not seem to increase copper needs	RDA	Red meat, fish, soy products, mushrooms, sweet potatoes	
Fluoride	Exercise does not seem to increase fluoride needs	Adequate Intake	Fluoridated water, fish, tea	
Iodide	Exercise does not seem to increase iodide needs	RDA	Eggs, milk, strawberries, mozzarella cheese, cantaloupe	
Iron	Exercise may increase iron requirements	Recommended Dietary Allowances (RDA); may need more if iron depleted or iron-deficient anemic	Clams, red meat, oysters, egg yolks, salmon, tofu, raisins, whole grains	May have an ergogenic effect if the athlete is iron depleted or iron-deficient anemic; may impact thyroid hormone function if iron deficient
Manganese	Exercise does not seem to increase manganese needs	RDA	Liver, kidneys, wheat germ, legumes, nuts, black tea	
Selenium	Despite antioxidant properties, exercise does not seem to increase selenium needs	RDA	Fish, meat, poultry, cereal, grains, mushrooms, asparagus	
Zinc	Exercise does not seem to increase zinc needs; however, transient losses are often observed	RDA	Oysters, red meat, poultry, fish, wheat germ, fortified cereals	May have ergogenic effects, but not definitive; may impact thyroid hormone function if zinc deficient

SULFUR

The mineral sulfur is present in the body in a nonionic form and is a constituent of some vitamins (eg, thiamin and biotin), amino acids (eg, methionine and cysteine), and some proteins. Sulfur also helps maintain acid-base balance in the blood. If protein needs are met, sulfur is not required in the diet because it is present in protein foods.[2]

Sulfur is part of a number of proteins, so the small body of research examining its effects on exercise performance is limited to sulfur-containing amino acids. It has been established that dietary sulfur-containing amino acids affect glutathione synthesis; however, their acute effect under conditions of oxidative stress, such as exercise, is not understood. Aoi and colleagues investigated the effects of oral glutathione supplementation on muscle metabolism and fatigue in mice and humans. Results showed that all mice, those who were supplemented with glutathione and the control group, had significantly reduced interstitial pH levels in muscle following exercise ($P < .001$). However, the mice supplemented with glutathione had significantly higher pH ($P < .05$) than those in the control group, demonstrating an improved pH buffering system in the muscle, which may lead to improved performance. These results were replicated in human participants as well. After glutathione supplementation, participants who performed an exercise bout exhibited a decrease in intermuscular pH following exercise. This was shown by increased blood lactate concentrations following exercise. The supplemented participants also reported significantly improved rating of perceived exertion ($P < .05$), a psychological parameter of fatigue, compared with the placebo group.[42] Additional research is needed to validate these results before recommendations may be warranted. Those who consume the proper amount of complete protein in their diet will be consuming adequate amounts of sulfur. Vegans can combine grains and legumes to obtain all of the essential amino acids. See Table 5.4 (page 90) for dietary sources of sulfur.

MANGANESE

Manganese is a trace mineral and an essential cofactor for many enzymes in the body. Manganese plays an essential role as an antioxidant as part of superoxide dismutase.[2] No data show that people who exercise require more manganese in their diet or that manganese contributes as an ergogenic aid. Due to the lack of current research and the risk of toxicity,[17] athletes should not increase manganese consumption. Dietary sources of manganese are listed in Table 5.3.

Bone Health and Development in Athletes

Bone health is critical for the health and physical performance of athletes. Bone is capable of being resorbed and remodeled in response to hormonal and mechanical changes. Weight-bearing exercise and hormonal activity determine quantity and location of resorption and reformation. Certain vitamins and minerals are crucial for health and development. The following sections will review the vitamins and minerals essential for bone health and examine the relationship to athletes.

CALCIUM

Calcium is the fifth most common element in the human body.[9] Ninety-nine percent of calcium exists in the bones and teeth, and the remaining 1% is distributed in extracellular fluids, intracellular structures, cell membranes, and various soft tissues.[9,17] The major functions of calcium include bone metabolism, blood coagulation, neuromuscular excitability, cellular adhesiveness, transmission of nerve impulses, maintenance and functionality of cell membranes, and activation of enzymatic reactions and hormonal secretions.[17]

Calcium Homeostasis: Serum calcium concentrations are tightly controlled within a range of 8.8 to 10.0 g/dL (2.2 to 2.5 mmol/L) by the calcitotropic hormones: parathyroid hormone (PTH), vitamin D, and calcitonin.[9,17] When serum calcium concentrations decrease to below 8.8 mg/dL, PTH responds by increasing the synthesis of calcitriol (the most active form of vitamin D) in the kidney.[17] Calcitriol responds by increasing calcium reabsorption in the kidneys, increasing calcium absorption in the intestines, and increasing osteoclastic activity in the bone (releasing calcium from the bone into circulation and decreasing bone mineral density). When serum calcium concentrations are above 10 mg/dL, the hormone calcitonin responds by increasing renal excretion of calcium, decreasing calcium absorption in the intestines, and increasing osteoblastic activity by placing more calcium into the bone.[9,17]

Average Calcium Intakes: Although serum calcium concentrations are easy to identify, precise levels of calcium intake are more difficult to determine. Serum calcium concentrations do not accurately correlate with calcium intake concentrations, primarily due to poor precision in dietary records and varying amounts of calcium in foods.[43] Women tend to consume less calcium than men, and teenage girls and adult women tend to consume less calcium than teenage and adult males. Female athletes older than 50 years consume approximately 79% of the recommended intake.[44]

Table 5.4 Major Mineral Needs for Athletes and Respective Food Sources

Mineral	Effect of Exercise on Requirements	Recommended Intake for Athletes	Food Sources	Comments
Calcium	Individuals who consistently exercise in the heat may have greater calcium requirements	Recommended Dietary Allowances (RDA); those who exercise in the heat should consume more than the Dietary Reference Intakes but below the Tolerable Upper Intake Level	Milk, cheese, yogurt, tofu processed with calcium, kale, almonds, collard greens, spinach, canned salmon with bones, bok choy, soy milk fortified with calcium	Higher calcium intakes may also be related to fat loss; important for athletes in sports with weight categories or aesthetic sports (eg, wrestling, gymnastics, lightweight rowers, jockeys)
Chloride	Exercise typically results in increased chloride needs, especially for those who exercise in the heat	Adequate Intakes (AIs)	Foods with high sodium; also found in salt substitutes with potassium chloride	
Magnesium	Exercise does not seem to increase magnesium needs; however, those exercising in hot environments may have increased magnesium needs	AI	Peanuts, tofu, broccoli, spinach, Swiss chard, tomato paste, nuts, seeds	No ergogenic effects established
Phosphorus	Exercise does not seem to increase phosphorus needs	RDA	Milk, cheese, yogurt, nuts, oatmeal, sardines, asparagus	Phosphate loading has not been researched enough; may be more harmful than helpful
Potassium	Exercise does not seem to increase potassium needs; however, individuals with a high sweat rate may need more	RDA	Oranges, bananas, tomatoes, sardines, flounder, salmon, potatoes, beans, blackstrap molasses, milk	No ergogenic effects observed at this time
Sodium	Exercise typically results in increased sodium needs, especially for those who exercise in the heat and who sweat a lot of salt	AI	Bread, milk, beets, celery, carrots, spinach, chard, lean meats	
Sulfur	Exercise does not seem to increase sulfur needs	RDA; vegans need to ensure that they consume adequate sulfur	Garlic, legumes, nuts, seeds, red meat, eggs, asparagus	

Physically active people should strive to consume at least the DRI for calcium. Barry and colleagues sought to diminish the exercise-induced calcium homeostasis disruption via calcium supplementation in 20 healthy adult male, endurance-trained cyclists and triathletes. Participants consumed either a calcium-fortified sports drink (100 mg/L of calcium) or placebo. The researchers measured exercise-induced increases in PTH, a response to calcium loss. The athletes who consumed the calcium-supplemented drink before exercise had attenuated concentrations of PTH relative to those who consumed the placebo ($P = .04$); however, this change was not observed when calcium was supplemented during or after exercise.[45] Limited data are available to validate calcium changes during exercise; therefore, it is difficult to determine if athletes need to consume more calcium than their sedentary counterparts. Based on the limited research at this time, it would be safe to recommend that athletes strive to consume the DRI for calcium.

Calcium has been studied for its possible effects on decreasing body weight.[46] This could be of significant value, especially for athletes in sports in which body weight is a concern (eg, wrestlers, jockeys, gymnasts, figure skaters, lightweight rowers). Results from numerous research studies on calcium and weight loss have been equivocal.

Some of the first studies on calcium and weight loss were conducted in animals. Since then, others have reported that increased calcium intake is associated with weight loss in humans as well.[46-53] In a cross-sectional study, Huang and colleagues reported that dietary calcium intake, but not elemental calcium from supplements, had beneficial effects for maintaining body composition and abdominal obesity.[47] Others have reported similar results of calcium intake and decreases in body weight in adults. For example, Skinner and colleagues reported that higher calcium intakes correlated with a lower percent body fat in healthy white men and women aged 18 to 28 years.[50]

Although these results indicate a positive relationship between calcium intake and improved body composition, many researchers have failed to confirm this relationship.[54-56] For example, Palacios and colleagues conducted a 21-week randomized trial in 30 Puerto Rican adults (21 to 50 years old) who were obese to determine the connection between dairy calcium intake/calcium supplementation and change in body composition. The participants were randomized into three groups receiving one of the following interventions: high dietary dairy intake (~1,300 mg calcium per day) through the consumption of four servings of dairy products per day in place of other food groups; high elemental calcium (~1,300 mg calcium per day) from a combination of dietary dairy intake (~700 mg calcium per day) and a daily calcium carbonate supplement (600 mg); or a control group instructed to consume their usual diet. All participants were instructed to consume an isoenergetic diet throughout the intervention to prevent restricted energy intake from influencing body composition change. Although calcium intake increased throughout the trial in the two intervention groups, the researchers found no significant differences between the groups in body weight ($P = .77$), body mass index ($P = .71$), total lean body mass ($P = .85$), or total body fat mass ($P = .71$), indicating that the type of calcium consumed (elemental supplement or dietary) does not significantly affect weight and body composition outcomes.[55]

Although the type of calcium consumed does not influence body weight and composition, the source of the dietary calcium consumed does affect bioavailability of the element within the body. Dairy sources have the highest bioavailable form of calcium. If a person is not consuming enough dietary calcium, supplementation with calcium citrate or calcium carbonate is recommended due to the increased bioavailability of these supplements. People should avoid calcium supplements containing bone meal, oyster shell, and shark cartilage because of the increased lead content in these supplements, which can be toxic. Calcium supplements are best absorbed if taken in doses of 500 mg or less and when taken between meals. Thus, if a person requires 1,000 mg calcium per day in the form of supplements, taking 500 mg in the morning and 500 mg in the evening would enhance absorption. Calcium supplements should be taken with vitamin D (contained within the supplement or separately) because vitamin D promotes calcium absorption. Persons older than 60 years may have a difficult time absorbing calcium citrate with meals, especially if they suffer from achlorhydria (lack of hydrochloric acid production in the stomach).[2]

Although a conclusive recommendation regarding calcium intake to maintain body composition has not been determined through research, it would be prudent to encourage athletes to consume the DRI for calcium through food to maintain bone health and integrity. Factors affecting calcium absorption will be discussed later in this chapter. Various sources of calcium are listed in Table 5.4.

VITAMIN D

Vitamin D is considered both a hormone or secosteroid and a fat-soluble vitamin. Its well-established roles in maintaining calcium homeostasis and in bone remodeling are discussed later in this chapter. The best form of vitamin D is obtained from sunlight, by which 7-dehydrocholesterol is converted to pre–vitamin D-3 in the skin. Conversion of vitamin D to its more active forms begin in the liver, where 25-α-hydroxylase adds a hydroxyl (OH) group to the 25th position on vitamin D to form 25-hydroxyvitamin D or calcidiol. The second hydroxylation of vitamin D occurs in the kidney, where 1-α-hydroxylase adds another hydroxyl group to the first position of calcidiol to form 1,25-dihydroxyvitamin D-3, also known as calcitriol, the most active form of vitamin D. The effects of calcitriol on calcium metabolism are discussed in more detail in the section on calcium.

Vitamin D deficiency is fairly widespread. Certain people may be at higher risk for developing vitamin D deficiencies. For example, those aged 65 years and older are at high risk for developing vitamin

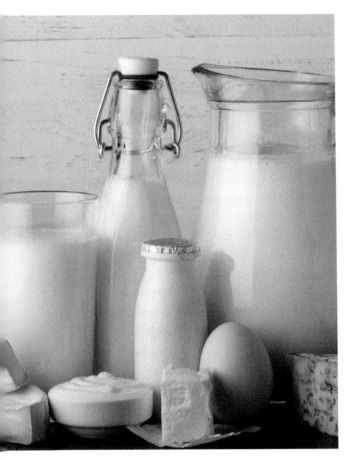

D deficiency, possibly due to low sunlight exposure from decreased time outdoors, decreased ability of older skin to synthesize vitamin D, or low intake of dietary vitamin D.[57] Additionally, those who live at or north of 42° latitude (eg, the northern United States and Canada) may require more vitamin D during the winter months to prevent increases in PTH secretion and decreased bone mineral density.[58] Kroll and colleagues used laboratory results (from the Quest Diagnostic database) to retrospectively determine the weekly mean concentrations of calcidiol and PTH of nearly 3.8 million adults aged 20 to 99 years. The researchers reported variations in vitamin D status for men and women that changed seasonally; the highest vitamin D concentrations were reported in September and the lowest in March. The researchers also reported vitamin D deficiencies, even in those taking vitamin D supplements.[59]

Researchers in the United Kingdom reported that 62% of adult athletes studied (rugby players, soccer players, flat jockeys, and hunt jockeys) had low serum calcidiol concentrations (<20.0 nmol/L or 8 ng/mL) compared with 73% of healthy nonathlete adult control subjects.[60] The high percentage of participants, athletes and nonathletes alike, with low vitamin D concentrations reiterates the overall low vitamin D status Kroll and colleagues[59] found in the general population.

Leventis and colleagues also investigated the difference between intramuscular vitamin D-2 injections (300,000 IU) compared with oral vitamin D-3 supplementation (300,000 IU) in 69 participants with insufficient vitamin D (calcidiol <40 nmol/L [16 ng/L]). The researchers determined that an oral vitamin D-3 supplement significantly increased calcidiol levels at 6 and 12 weeks ($P<.0001$ and $P<.0001$, respectively) compared with baseline. In contrast, participants who were given vitamin D-2 supplements via injection had modest but not significant increases in calcidiol.[61]

Lehmann and colleagues studied the difference between 50 mcg/day of oral vitamin D-2 and D-3 supplementation in healthy participants compared with a placebo.[62] Their results were similar to those of Leventis and colleagues.[61] Lehmann and colleagues found that total serum calcidiol concentrations remained significantly higher ($P<.001$) in participants supplemented with vitamin D-3 after 4 and 8 weeks of supplementation compared with participants receiving vitamin D-2 or placebo.[62]

Research shows that vitamin D is necessary for optimal bone growth. Emerging research suggests that vitamin D deficiency increases the risk of autoimmune diseases and nonskeletal chronic diseases, and it can affect muscle function and inflammation.[63] Some suggest that exercise performance may be influenced by vitamin D status due to its wide functionality in the body; a key symptom of vitamin D deficiency is muscle weakness. Forney and colleagues investigated the relationship between calcidiol and fitness levels in 40 physically active college students (20 men and 20 women). Serum vitamin D concentrations were designated as low or high, that is, below or above the adequate serum concentrations of 35 ng/mL (14 nmol/L). The researchers did not find a significant difference in aerobic capacity (measured by VO_2 max) based on vitamin D status in women participants. They did, however, report a significantly higher VO_2 max ($P < .01$) in men in the high vitamin D group compared with those in the low vitamin D group. Nonetheless, this difference was not seen when measuring anaerobic power output ($P = .34$). These results indicate that male participants with high vitamin D concentrations may have improved aerobic capacity compared with men with lower vitamin D concentrations. Incidentally, the researchers also found that 20 of the 39 participants (1 female participant was not included in data analyses) presented with low concentrations of serum vitamin D.[64]

Sources of naturally occurring foods containing vitamin D are limited. The best dietary sources include fatty fish and fortified foods, such as milk, breakfast cereal, and orange juice. With the addition of fortified foods, it is possible to achieve adequate vitamin D intake from food alone [2] (see Table 5.2 for more foods rich in vitamin D). Furthermore, exposing the face and arms to 15 minutes of sunlight per day in light-skinned persons and 30 minutes per day in dark-skinned persons will result in sufficient amounts of vitamin D. However, confinement to indoors, geographic location, or use of sunscreen may make it difficult for some to acquire the necessary sunlight exposure on the skin to ensure vitamin D conversion. Because of the ubiquitous nature of vitamin D deficiency, athletes should aim to consume foods rich in vitamin D and obtain the appropriate amount of sun exposure. If a vitamin D deficiency is found, then taking a vitamin D-3 supplement would be warranted as it is well documented that vitamin D-3 has higher bioavailability than vitamin D-2.[61,62]

PHOSPHORUS

Phosphorus is the second most abundant mineral in the body; approximately 85% of total body phosphorus is found in bone, mainly as hydroxyapatite crystals.[9] Phosphate is important in bone mineralization in animals and humans. Even in the presence of high amounts of calcitriol in the blood, hypophosphatemia can disrupt the negative feedback loops regulating blood phosphate levels and result in bone matrix breakdown, which may lead to rickets in children and osteoporosis in adults. Although phosphorus is required for bone growth, excessive amounts may actually harm the skeleton, especially when accompanied by a low calcium intake. Excessive phosphorus intakes have been negatively correlated with bone mineral density in the radius.[60]

High phosphorus intakes reduce serum calcium concentrations, especially when calcium intake is low, because phosphorus carries calcium with it into soft tissues. The resulting hypocalcemia activates PTH secretion, which results in increased bone loss (resorption) to maintain serum calcium homeostasis. High phosphorus intakes can also decrease active vitamin D production, further reducing calcium absorption and producing secondary hyperparathyroidism.[65,66] Because of its ubiquitous nature, phosphorus intakes are usually higher than the recommended intakes.[67]

Because most people consume enough phosphorus in their diets, overconsumption is usually the concern. A special concern is the amount of soft drinks consumed because many contain high amounts of phosphate. Children and teenagers pose a particular problem because soft drinks often replace milk in their diet. Researchers have reported that the greater the consumption of carbonated beverages, especially cola beverages, the greater the risk of fracture.[68,69] This association was strongest in women and girls. Additionally, the intake of phosphorus-containing food additives may lead to hyperphosphatemia and may disrupt bone mineral density.[70]

Phosphate loading is another way many people, especially competitive athletes, consume excessive amounts of phosphorus. Phosphate loading is thought to decrease the buildup of hydrogen ions that increase during exercise and negatively affect energy production. Although research on phosphate loading as an ergogenic aid has shown equivocal results, Bremner and colleagues reported a 30% increase in plasma inorganic phosphate concentrations with a 25% increase in erythrocyte 2,3-bisphosphoglycerate concentrations after 7 days of phosphate loading in healthy people. They concluded that phosphate loading increased plasma and erythrocyte phosphate pools but that the increase in erythrocyte 2,3-bisphosphoglycerate was probably a result of the increase in cell inorganic phosphate. These researchers did not assess the effect of phosphate loading on exercise performance.[71] Brewer and colleagues, however, assessed sodium phosphate supplementation on short-duration (< 15 minutes), high-intensity exercise performance. Competitive male cyclists were randomized into a sodium phosphate or a placebo group and evaluated 1 and 8 days after supplementation. The researchers found no significant differences in time to completion of exercise, mean power output, or VO_2 max.[72] The long-term negative consequences of phosphate loading on bone-mineral density have not been documented and should be considered before an athlete adopts this practice. Furthermore, research in this area is limited, and, thus, the risk-benefit ratio of phosphate loading has not been established. Table 5.4 (page 90) lists some food sources of phosphorus.

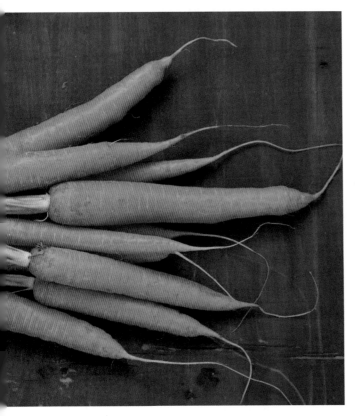

VITAMIN A

An in-depth discussion of vitamin A was provided earlier in this chapter; however, it should be noted that excessive serum vitamin A concentrations may be detrimental to bone health. It is often difficult to accurately assess vitamin A status in research participants. Barker and colleagues reviewed the methods and results of several animal and human studies. Although they discussed several findings in their extensive review, including a correlation between serum vitamin A concentrations and increased rate of bone resorption, ossification of cartilage, hypercalcemia, extraosseous calcification, and suppressed parathyroid hormone concentrations and fractures, they also found the quality of the reviewed work to be inadequate. This review emphasized that the current state of research in vitamin A and bone interaction is limited due to inaccurate assessments of vitamin A intake and varying definitions of intake thresholds.[73] Although the current research is limited, it underscores the fact that vitamin A intakes of more than the UL can have detrimental effects on the body.

Red Blood Cell Function

The primary function of erythrocytes (red blood cells) is to deliver oxygen through the blood to the cells of the body. Because athletes have increased oxygen demands, the proper formation and function of red blood cells is critical for health and performance. In the next sections, the role of several vitamins and minerals involved in the formation of red blood cells will be discussed.

VITAMIN B-12 AND FOLATE

Vitamin B-12 (cyanocobalamin) and folate (folic acid) are both necessary for DNA synthesis[9] and are interrelated in their synthesis and metabolism. Both vitamins are required for normal erythrocyte synthesis; creation of normal red blood cells is the function by which these two vitamins may affect exercise.[14] There is no evidence, however, to suggest that exercise increases the need for either of these vitamins. Lukaski states that, although there are limited data assessing blood biochemical measures of folate status in physically active people, physical performance did not improve in athletes who were folate deficient and received folate supplementation. A clinically normal blood concentration of vitamin B-12 is between 200 and 900 pg/mL. Normal blood concentrations of folate range from 2.7 to 17.0 ng/mL. However, inadequate intakes of both vitamins may lead to megaloblastic anemia.[1]

Although injections of vitamin B-12 are used clinically for persons diagnosed with megaloblastic anemia, oral supplementation is sufficient if frank anemia has not been diagnosed. A multivitamin and mineral supplement that includes 500 to 1,000 mg of vitamin C may decrease vitamin B-12 bioavailability from food and may lead to vitamin B-12 deficiency.[14] Vitamin B-12 deficiency can be masked by high folate intakes; thus, if vitamin B-12 deficiency is suspected, dietary intake will need to be assessed, especially if biochemical tests are negative for vitamin B-12 deficiency. These nutrients are important for vegan athletes and are discussed later in this chapter.

Athletes who consume adequate amounts of vitamin B-12 and folate in their diets are probably not at risk for vitamin B-12 or folate deficiencies. Nonetheless, vitamin B-12 or folate deficiencies can lead to increased serum homocysteine concentrations, a risk factor for cardiovascular disease.[74] Normal blood homocysteine concentrations range between 4 and 15 nmol/L, with optimal concentrations below 10 to 12 nmol/L. The risk of hyperhomocysteinemia (> 15 nmol/L) demonstrates that people who exercise need to be concerned not only about nutrition and performance but also about overall health.

To conceptualize the effects of exercise intensity on homocysteine concentrations Iglesias-Gutiérrez and colleagues studied changes in serum homocysteine concentrations in eight sedentary males during and after low- and high-intensity interval exercises. Their findings indicate that high-intensity exercise raises serum homocysteine concentrations more quickly than lower-intensity exercise. Incidentally, the researchers also reported that serum concentrations of vitamin B-12, folate, and vitamin B-6 all significantly increased ($P < .05$) after both high- and low-intensity exercise.[75]

König and colleagues also sought to identify changes in blood homocysteine concentrations in response to exercise. Their findings reiterate that serum homocysteine concentrations increase in response to exercise; however, the timing of the alteration in concentration is not well defined.[76]

Herrmann and colleagues had previously explored the relationship of exercise to homocysteine concentrations, and, contrary to the findings of König and colleagues, he found that serum homocysteine concentrations increased during, not after, the bout of exercise.[77] However, both researchers agreed that homocysteine concentrations remained elevated following exercise cessation and continued to remain above normal throughout the 5-day recovery training period. They also found that serum vitamin B-12 concentrations were unchanged during training but decreased during the recovery phase, indicating a delayed response to the training. Serum folate concentrations, however, decreased during training but returned to normal by the end of the recovery period.[76,77]

Because vitamin B-12 and folate are metabolically interrelated, the changes in one and not the other at different times of exercise and recovery may indicate an adaptive response by each to protect the other. It is important for those who exercise to consume adequate amounts of vitamin B-12 and folate despite evidence that supplementation may only improve performance if a nutritional deficit is present.[1] Dietary sources of vitamin B-12 and folate are shown in Table 5.1.

IRON

The vital role iron plays in oxygen delivery is paramount to overall exercise performance, yet iron-deficiency anemia affects one quarter of the world's population.[78] For athletes in particular, iron-deficiency anemia may negatively affect exercise performance. Iron-deficiency anemia negatively affects the oxidative production of adenosine triphosphate in skeletal muscle.[79] It is therefore understandable that iron-deficiency anemia has been shown to decrease overall aerobic capacity and, thus, overall athletic performance[79-81]

Iron Supplementation: Persons with iron-deficiency depletion or anemia find that iron supplementation is the most prudent way to increase iron stores and prevent adverse physiological effects.[82] Ferrous sulfate or gluconate are the least expensive and most widely used forms of iron supplementation[82,83]; however, ferrous chelate and polysaccharide have been shown to be more bioavailable.[84] For adults diagnosed with iron-deficiency anemia, a daily dose of 100 to 150 mg of elemental iron taken between meals is recommended.[82]

Supplementation is also warranted for athletes with iron depletion (low serum ferritin levels) without iron-deficiency anemia to prevent full-blown iron-deficiency anemia from developing. DellaValle and Haas assessed the effect of iron supplementation on 4-km run performance, VO_2 peak, energy expenditure, lactate response, and iron stores (serum ferritin concentrations) in 40 female rowers (~19 years old). Their goal was to show a relationship between iron depletion without anemia and physical performance. In this double-blind, placebo-controlled study, rowers received either a ferrous sulfate supplement (100 mg/day) or a placebo for 6 weeks. At baseline, rower characteristics did not differ; however, after supplementation, iron-supplemented rowers had a delayed lactate response during the first half of exercise ($P = .05$) and increased energy expenditure after 6 weeks of training ($P = .03$) compared with the rowers who received the placebo.[85] These results suggest that because iron depletion may impair aerobic exercise performance and possibly diminish the effects of exercise, practitioners need to understand the importance of treating iron depletion in addition to iron-deficiency anemia, in athletes. For adults with iron depletion stage 1 (serum ferritin levels < 20 ng/mL), a daily dose of 25 to 65 mg of elemental iron taken between meals is recommended; and 65 to 130 mg of elemental iron is recommended for iron depletion stage 2.[82]

Factors Affecting Iron Absorption: Several factors inhibit or enhance iron absorption. Factors that inhibit iron absorption include phytates and oxalates, tannins in tea and coffee, adequate iron stores, excessive intake of other minerals (eg, zinc, calcium, and manganese), reduced gastric acid production, and certain antacids. Factors that enhance iron absorption include heme iron, meat protein factor, ascorbic acid, low iron stores, normal gastric acid secretion, and a high demand for red blood cells, such as occurs with blood loss, exercise training (especially at altitude), and pregnancy.[2] Consuming foods or beverages that contain vitamin C with meals and consuming tea or coffee at least an hour before or after a meal rather than with a meal will enhance dietary iron absorption of iron. Table 5.3 (page 88) lists some examples of dietary sources of iron.

Immune System

The extreme physiological stress athletes impose on their bodies is associated with immunosuppression and increased risk of infection. Intense exercise exposes the body to stress-induced hormones, such as cortisol, and increased levels of oxidative stress. Elements of the immune system appear to be temporarily depressed following bouts of exercise, leading to susceptibility to infection.[86] Certain vitamins and minerals may alleviate the stress to the immune system associated with exercise.

VITAMIN C

Vitamin C is a well-known antioxidant that was discussed earlier in this chapter. Some people supplement with vitamin C in very high doses ($\geq 1,000$ mg/day) because they believe it may prevent or reduce the severity and duration of common colds[30]; however, this conclusion remains uncertain. Most of the existing data from supplementation and dietary studies do not support the concept that athletes require an increased amount of vitamin C for a variety of reasons.[29] Hemilä and Chalker conducted a meta-analysis to assess the risk and duration of the common cold in placebo-controlled trials. One criterion of the studies they selected was that the researchers administered 2 g/d or more of vitamin C to their participants. They determined that, among the general population, high-dose vitamin C supplementation does not reduce the occurrence of the common cold, but it does reduce the length of cold symptoms. Additionally, the researchers determined that athletes (n = 598) undergoing short periods of extreme physical stress (marathon runners and skiers) in five separate studies presented with nearly half the risk of developing the common cold compared with the general population, indicating that exercise itself, although a stressor, can be protective in developing the common cold.[30]

Athletes and sedentary persons generally do not require different amounts of vitamin C. Some researchers have reported a similar vitamin C intake between athletes and sedentary control subjects. Furthermore, there does not appear to be a strong association between blood concentrations of ascorbic acid and dietary intake of vitamin C. In addition, no difference has been reported between athletes and nonathletes in the excretion of ascorbic acid in urine, which is an assessment of the utilization of vitamin C within the body.[29] However, people who consistently exercise may require at least 100 mg/day of vitamin C, which can be easily obtained from food, to maintain normal vitamin C status and protect the body from oxidative damage caused by exercise. Athletes competing in ultraendurance events may require up to 500 mg/day or more of vitamin C,[14] likely obtained from foods and supplements combined. Nonetheless, athletes should not exceed the UL for vitamin C (2,000 mg/day in adults aged 19 years and older). Dietary sources of vitamin C are shown in Table 5.1 (page 83).

ZINC

Zinc exists in all organs, tissues, fluids, and secretions. Approximately 60% of total body zinc is present in muscle, 29% in bone, and roughly 1% in each of the following: gastrointestinal tract, skin, kidney, brain, lung, and prostate.[87] Zinc plays a role in more than 300 metabolic reactions in the body. Alkaline phosphatase, carbonic anhydrase, and zinc-copper superoxide dismutase are just a few of the zinc metalloenzymes.[2] Low zinc status can also impair immune function,[88] which can be detrimental to exercise and overall health.

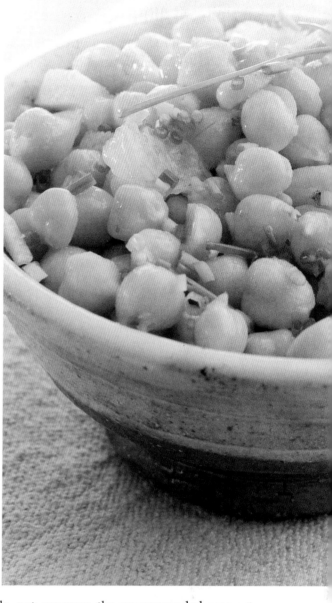

Many athletes, like many people in the United States, do not consume the recommended amount of zinc both in and out of the training season.[89-91] In a crossover study, Volpe and colleagues used stable isotopes of zinc to evaluate the effect of acute exhaustive exercise compared with rest on short-term zinc kinetics in 12 healthy, sedentary men aged 25 to 35 years. They reported a significant decrease ($P<.05$) in plasma zinc concentrations after exercise. From the stable isotope data, they reported a shift of plasma zinc into the liver and interstitial fluid after exercise, likely demonstrating the acute stress response of exhaustive exercise.[92] It is not clear whether these changes in zinc are transient or continue after exercise. More research is required to assess athletes' zinc status, but it would be prudent for athletes to consume the DRI for zinc. See Table 5.3 (page 88) for dietary sources of zinc.

RISK FACTORS AFFECTING VITAMIN AND MINERAL NEEDS

Training in Heat and Humidity

Athletes who exercise in excessive heat and humidity face challenges to replenish fluid and electrolytes lost through sweat. The loss of electrolytes (sodium, potassium, calcium, and magnesium) are extensively covered in Chapter 6. Table 5.4 lists some food sources of these nutrients.

Training at Altitude

Training at altitude, where oxygen concentrations are considerably lower, allows an athlete to increase red blood cell volume and, in turn, increase oxygen delivery to muscles. Such blood alterations allow for

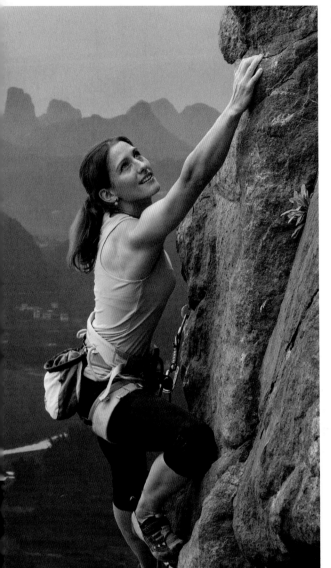

increased aerobic activity and improved performance.[93,94] Certain vitamins and minerals are crucial in the adaptations associated with altitude training.

Iron, which was discussed earlier in this chapter, is a crucial mineral for altitude acclimation. Many athletes follow the live high, train low protocol to increase hemoglobin mass and, in turn, increase oxygen delivery to improve athletic performance. Govus and colleagues assessed hematologic data of 178 endurance athletes who were exposed to high-altitude training and discovered that daily oral ferrous sulfate supplements containing 210 mg of elemental iron slowed the decrease of serum ferritin concentrations that occurs after exposure to altitude compared with athletes who did not receive iron supplements.[95] Thus, athletes who may be new to training or competing at high altitude should consider iron supplementation, especially if they have low serum ferritin concentrations when they begin training.

Exposure to altitude also increases the production of reactive oxygen species and decreases plasma antioxidant concentrations. Pialoux and colleagues reported that antioxidant status remained low following simulated altitude training.[96] Antioxidants were discussed in more detail earlier in this chapter.

Nutritional Needs for Female Athletes

Female athletes require a complete and healthy diet to support their needs and recover from the physical stress of exercise. It is vital for female athletes to achieve proper nutrition as inadequate nutrition may lead to particular nutrient deficiencies.[46] Common micronutrients important to female athletes will be discussed in the following sections.

IRON

Some researchers have reported that as many as 60% of female athletes may have some degree of iron depletion. This is especially common in female athletes who participate in endurance sports.[97] Female athletes typically do not consume adequate amounts of dietary iron as a result of restricted energy consumption and a reduction in heme iron content of the diet. These dietary patterns, paired with additional losses in the body (sweat, menstruation, intravascular hemolysis, or foot strike hemolysis in runners), may contribute to suboptimal iron content in the body.[79]

CALCIUM AND VITAMIN D

As previously mentioned, calcium and vitamin D are important nutrients for developing and maintaining strong, healthy bones. For female athletes, it is especially important to consume adequate amounts of calcium and vitamin D as deficiencies are not uncommon. Nationwide median calcium intakes of female athletes are below recommended amounts,[98] and approximately one-third of female athletes are deficient in vitamin D.[14] All athletes, especially female athletes, should be encouraged to consume adequate amounts of calcium and vitamin D in their diet to maintain healthy bones. Female athletes with low energy availability should have their calcium and vitamin D status assessed and addressed.[99,100] Table 5.3 lists some dietary sources of calcium and vitamin D. See earlier sections of this chapter for more detailed information on each of these nutrients.

VITAMIN K

Vitamin K, a group of three related substances, is a fat-soluble vitamin. Phylloquinone, also known as phytonadione (vitamin K-1) is found in plants; menaquinone (vitamin K-2) is produced by bacteria in the intestines that supply an undetermined amount of the daily requirement of vitamin K-2 ; and menadione (vitamin K-3) is the synthetic form of vitamin K. All vitamin K variants are fat soluble and stable to heat. Alkalis, strong acids, radiation, and oxidizing agents can destroy vitamin K. It is absorbed from the upper small intestine with the help of bile or bile salts and pancreatic juices and then carried to the liver for the synthesis of prothrombin, a key blood-clotting factor.[2]

Much of the vitamin K research in athletes is focused on the interaction of vitamin K with estrogen and bone metabolism. Female athletes, especially those with abnormal menstrual cycles and those who are postmenopausal, are particularly vulnerable to bone metabolism disorders due to decreased circulating estrogen.[101] Braam and colleagues studied the effects of estrogen and vitamin K supplementation on bone loss in female endurance athletes. Based on their menstrual-cycle status, 115 participants were assigned to one of three groups: (1) athletes with amenorrhea (no menstrual cycles per year) or oligomenorrhea (scanty/few menstrual cycles per year); (2) athletes with eumenorrhea (normal menstruation); and (3) athletes who used oral contraceptives (estrogen supplemented). The participants in each group were then randomized for treatment with either 10 mg vitamin K-1 per day or a placebo. All three groups and subgroups showed significant decreases in femoral neck bone mineral density after 2 years of supplementation or placebo. Athletes who were amenorrheic/oligomenorrheic had the most bone loss compared with those who were eumenorrheic and those who supplemented with estrogen. The researchers found that neither estrogen nor vitamin K supplementation helped slow the rate of bone mineral density decline over the 2-year period in any of the groups.[102] These results are concerning considering the rate of bone mineral density loss in all participants. Although vitamin K supplementation was not shown to prevent or reverse the loss of bone mineral density, it is important for athletes to consume adequate amounts of vitamin K in their diets.

An average diet usually provides at least 75 to 150 mcg/day of total vitamin K (the suggested minimum intake); although, 300 to 750 mcg/day may be optimal. Absorption of vitamin K ranges from 20% to 60% of total intake.[103] Vitamin K deficiency is more common than previously thought. Western diets high in sugar and processed foods, intake of vitamins A and E higher than the ULs, and use of antibiotics may contribute to a decrease in intestinal bacterial function, resulting in a decrease in the production and/or metabolism of vitamins K-1 and K-2.[17] The best dietary sources of vitamin K are listed in Table 5.2 (page 87).

VITAMINS AND MINERALS OF CONCERN DUE TO DIETARY INTAKE

Athletes who restrict certain foods or food groups may be at higher risk for deficiencies over those who eat a wide variety of foods. The following sections will touch on certain diets and how they may affect athletes.

Vegetarians and Vegans

According to the Academy of Nutrition and Dietetics, "appropriately planned vegetarian, including vegan, diets are healthful, nutritionally adequate and may provide health benefits for the prevention and treatment of certain diseases."[104] However, due to the increased demand placed on athletes, vegetarian and vegan athletes may be at higher risk for certain nutrient deficiencies. While vegetarian and vegan diets provide high levels of antioxidants necessary to attenuate the oxidative stress of exercise, avoidance of meat and poultry decreases intake of certain nutrients, namely vitamin B-12, iron, and zinc.[3]

Adequate intake of vitamin B-12 is of special concern in vegan athletes because vitamin B-12 is almost exclusively found in animal products.[3,14] Vegetarians who consume dairy products or eggs are likely to have adequate intakes of vitamin B-12, but vegan athletes need to regularly consume foods fortified with vitamin B-12 or B-12 supplements.[14,105]

Iron absorption depends on the type of iron consumed from the diet. Heme iron, found in animal products, is highly bioavailable; whereas nonheme iron, found in plant foods, is less bioavailable because it is affected by factors within the gastric lumen. Additionally, some plant foods contain inhibitors, such as phytates and oxalates, that further restrict the bioavailability of all iron types, especially nonheme iron.[105] The combination of a less absorbable iron and inhibitors found in plants places vegetarians and vegans at higher risk of developing iron depletion or iron-deficiency anemia.

Zinc is another mineral that should be of concern to vegetarians and vegans. Zinc is highly available from animal products but is not readily absorbed from plant foods, especially foods containing phytates, which inhibit zinc absorption. Vegans should consider including high-zinc foods into their diet, such as pumpkin and hemp seeds (each contains 5 mg of zinc per half cup) or supplement with zinc.[106] Additional information on vegetarian and vegan diets can be found in other chapters of this text.

High- and Low-Carbohydrate Diets

There seems to be a strong correlation between high carbohydrate intakes, physical activity, and thiamin requirements.[14] This may be a concern for people who exercise because a high-carbohydrate diet is recommended for athletes; however, there is no clear evidence indicating that people who exercise require more thiamin in their diets than those who are sedentary. Nonetheless, it is prudent to recommend that people who exercise obtain at least the DRI for thiamin to prevent depletion. Additionally, high carbohydrate intakes, paired with low protein and fat intakes, have led to suboptimal zinc intakes in 90% of all athletes.[106]

Low-carbohydrate diets may introduce different nutrient deficiencies. Zhang and colleagues compared macronutrient and micronutrient intakes across several traditional diets (Chinese, Mediterranean/Italian, Japanese, and American). The researchers used dietary data derived from the China National Nutrition and Health Monitoring Survey (2010 to 2012) to compare nutrient intake to those of other countries. Dietary data from other countries were obtained from the third National Food Consumption Survey in Italy, the National Health and Nutrition Survey in Japan, and the National Health and Nutrition Examination Survey (NHANES 2009 to 2010) in the United States. The Chinese data were collected from three consecutive 24-hour dietary recalls of 2,659 Chinese participants (1,274 males; 1,385 females), age 2 to 89 years, in the Zhejiang province. The researchers found that Chinese persons consuming diets with the lowest percentage of energy from carbohydrates consumed significantly lower ($P < 100.04$) amounts of vitamins B-1, B-2, A, and C than those who consumed the other diets studied.[107] Although Zhang and colleagues did not conduct this study in athletes, the findings suggest that low-carbohydrate diets can lead to nutrient deficiencies, ultimately affecting athletic performance and overall health.

Energy-Restricted Diets

Athletes may consume an energy-restricted diet for many reasons. Elite athletes may have an idealized perception of a particular body type for their specific sport, may believe perceived energy restriction has performance benefits, and may feel social and cultural pressures toward thinness or a certain body shape.[108] Energy restriction is a common, albeit unhealthy, practice among athletes, especially those in weight-dependent sports, such as wrestling, gymnastics, jockeying, and rowing. Hinton and colleagues assessed the dietary intakes and behaviors of male and female collegiate athletes (n = 345) at National Collegiate Athletic Association Division I universities. The researchers reported that, on average, the athletes consumed only 15% of the recommended carbohydrates and 26% of the recommended protein. They also noted that more than half of the female athletes (62%) reported a desire to lose at least 5 lb. This desire was associated with decreased energy and macronutrient consumption, but, surprisingly, their micronutrient intake was within the recommended ranges.[109]

The desire to lose weight or exhibit an idealized body type drives many athletes to restrict food intake. El Ghoch and colleagues examined how restrictive eating disorder behaviors affected athletic performance. Although athletes who lost weight from restricted eating behaviors demonstrated improved physical performance initially, long-term effects of glycogen depletion, increased muscular pain, dehydration, and loss of lean body mass were all detriments of energy restriction.[110] Additionally, low energy availability can significantly compromise immune function.[111] Although restrictive diets are common among athletes, the long-term detriments can compromise overall athlete performance, and athletes need to be taught proper dietary intake to optimize performance and overall long-term health.

SUMMARY

Special attention must be given to persons who are physically active to assess their micronutrient needs. Consider the following: frequency, intensity, duration, and type(s) of physical activity; environment (hot or cold) in which exercise is performed; sex; and dietary intakes and food preferences. It is particularly important to evaluate usual dietary intakes of calcium and iron in female athletes.

Proper assessment will help practitioners counsel those who are physically active to consume adequate amounts of micronutrients for optimal health and performance. In particular, athletes should be encouraged to consume adequate total energy. If they do so, they will typically consume adequate vitamins and minerals as well. Encouraging those who exercise to consume sufficient fruits, vegetables, and animal products will also help to ensure that they will obtain the adequate amounts of vitamins and minerals needed for overall health and optimal performance.

A general summary of all the vitamins and minerals discussed in this chapter, including the effect of exercise on vitamin and mineral requirements, recommended intakes for athletes, general food sources, and possible ergogenic effects, is provided in Tables 5.1 through 5.4, which can be used as a quick reference guide for nutrition and dietetics practitioners. Box 5.1 contains some helpful vitamin and mineral resources.

Box 5.1 Online Resources of Vitamins and Minerals

Food and Nutrition Board of the Institute of Medicine

https://iom.nationalacademies.org/About-IOM/Leadership-Staff/IOM-Staff-Leadership-Boards/Food-and-Nutrition-Board.aspx

"Established in 1940, the Food and Nutrition Board studies issues of national and global importance on the safety and adequacy of the United States food supply; establishes principles and guidelines for good nutrition; and provides authoritative judgment on the relationships among food intake, nutrition, and health maintenance and disease prevention."

Institute of Medicine Dietary Reference Intakes

http://iom.edu/Activities/Nutrition/SummaryDRIs/DRI-Tables.aspx

Tables of Dietary Reference Intakes, as well as summaries and full reports, can be found at the Institute of Medicine website.

National Institutes of Health Office of Dietary Supplements

https://ods.od.nih.gov

"The mission of Office of Dietary Supplements is to strengthen knowledge and understanding of dietary supplements by evaluating scientific information, stimulating and supporting research, disseminating research results, and educating the public to foster an enhanced quality of life and health for the U.S. population."

Food and Nutrition Information Center

http://fnic.nal.usda.gov

"The Food and Nutrition Information Center provides credible, accurate, and practical resources for nutrition and health professionals, educators, government personnel, and consumers."

KEY TAKEAWAYS

Overall, the vitamin and mineral needs of people who are physically active are similar to the requirements for all healthy people.

If dietary intakes are adequate (ie, meet 70% or more of the DRI for nutrients), supplementation is unnecessary.

Sweat losses may require some people to consume higher amounts of some micronutrients, quantities that can be obtained with a varied diet of properly selected foods.

Supplementation may be necessary when intake is inadequate or there is a deficiency in status. Care must be taken so that people do not exceed the UL, which could impair exercise performance and health.

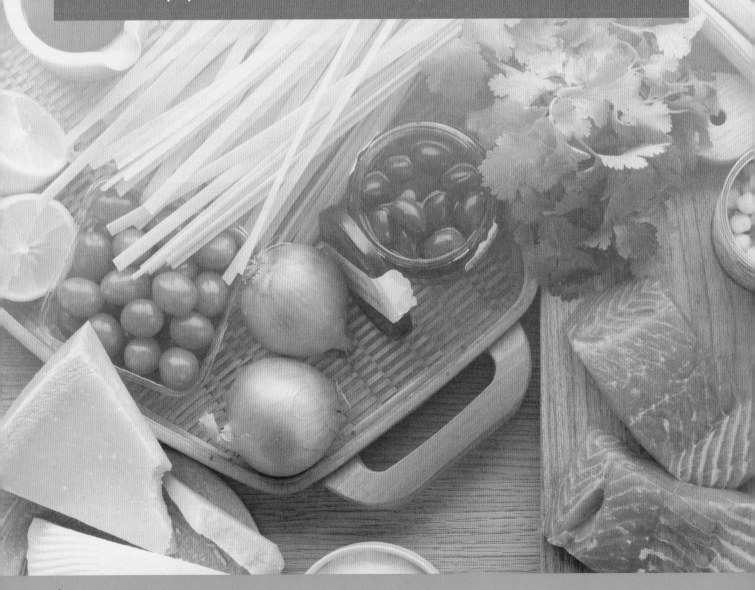

REFERENCES

1. Lukaski HC. Vitamin and mineral status: effects on physical performance. *Nutrition.* 2004;20(7-8): 632-644.

2. Byrd-Bredbenner C, Moe G, Beshgetoor D, Berning J. *Wardlaw's Perspectives in Nutrition.* 9th ed. Boston, MA: McGraw-Hill; 2013.

3. Burke L, Deakin V. *Clinical Sports Nutrition.* 4th ed. Sydney, Australia: McGraw-Hill; 2009.

4. Kimura N, Fukuwatari T, Sasaki R, Hayakawa F, Shibata K. Vitamin intake in Japanese women college students. *J Nutr Sci Vitaminol (Tokyo).* 2003;49(3):149-155.

5. Institute of Medicine, Food and Nutrition Board. *Dietary Reference Intakes for Calcium and Vitamin D.* Washington, DC: National Academies Press; 2011.

6. Barr SI. Introduction to Dietary Reference Intakes. *Appl Physiol Nutr Metab.* 2006;31(1):61-65.

7. Collins AC, Ward KD, Mirza B, Slawson DL, McClanahan BS, Vukadinovich C. Comparison of nutritional intake in US adolescent swimmers and non-athletes. *Health.* 2012; 4(10):873-880.

8. Vaz M, Paulin M, Unni US, et al. Micronutrient supplementation improves physical performance measures in Asian Indian school-age children. *J Nutr.* 2011;141(11):2017-2023.

9. Erdman JW Jr, Macdonald IA, Zeisel SH. *Present Knowledge in Nutrition.* 10th ed. Oxford, UK: Wiley-Blackwell; 2012.

10. Woolf K, Manore MM. B-vitamins and exercise: does exercise alter requirements? *Int J Sport Nutr Exerc Metab.* 2006;16(5):453–484.

11. Kim YN, Choi JY, Cho YO. Regular moderate exercise training can alter the urinary excretion of thiamin and riboflavin. *Nutr Res Pract.* 2015;9(1):43-48.

12. Sato A, Shimoyama Y, Ishikawa T, Murayama N. Dietary thiamin and riboflavin intake and blood thiamin and riboflavin concentrations in college swimmers undergoing intensive training. *Int J Sport Nutr Exerc Metab.* 2011;21(3):195-204.

13. Bronkhorst I, Silva L, Freitas L, Martins M, Martins H, Malfatti C. Vitamin B6 and maltodextrin sports drink modify glucose levels of elite mountain biking athletes. *J Exerc Physiol Online.* 2014;17(4):113-121.

14. Wolinsky I, Driskell JA. *Sports Nutrition: Energy Metabolism and Exercise.* 2nd ed. Boca Raton, FL: CRC Press; 2007.

15. Manore M. Effect of physical activity on thiamine, riboflavin, and vitamin B-6 requirements. *Am J Clin Nutr.* 2000;72(2)(suppl):598S-606S.

16. Wall BT, Stephens FB, Marimuthu K, Constantin-Teodosiu D, Macdonald IA, Greenhaff PL. Acute pantothenic acid and cysteine supplementation does not affect muscle coenzyme A content, fuel selection, or exercise performance in healthy humans. *J Appl Physiol (1985).* 2012;112(2):272-278

17. Ross CA, Cabalero B, Cousins RJ, Tucker KL, Ziegler TR. *Modern Nutrition in Health and Disease.* 11th ed. Philadelphia, PA: Wolters Kluwer Health/Lippincott Williams & Wilkins; 2014.

18. Penry JT, Manore MM. Choline: an important micronutrient for maximal endurance-exercise performance? *Int J Sport Nutr Exerc Metab.* 2008;18(2):191-203.

19. Dunford M, Doyle JA. *Nutrition for Sport and Exercise.* 3rd ed. Gaithersburg, MD: Aspen Publishers; 2012.

20. Lee EC, Maresh CM, Kraemer WJ, et al. Ergogenic effects of betaine supplementation on strength and power performance. *J Int Soc Sports Nutr.* 2010;7:27.

21. Hoffman JR, Ratamess NA, Kang J, Rashti SL, Faigenbaum AD. Effect of betaine supplementation on power performance and fatigue. *J Int Soc Sports Nutr.* 2009;6:7.

22. McCarthy CG, Farney TM, Canale RE, Dessoulavy ME, Bloomer RJ. High-fat feeding, but not strenuous exercise, increases blood oxidative stress in trained men. *Appl Physiol Nutr Metab.* 2013;38(1):33-41.

23. Sies H, Stahl W, Sevanian A. Nutritional, dietary and postprandial oxidative stress. *J Nutr.* 2005;135(5):969-972.

24. Fisher-Wellman K, Bloomer RJ. Acute exercise and oxidative stress: a 30 year history. *Dyn Med.* 2009;8:1.

25. Djordjevic DZ, Cubrilo DG, et al. Comparison of blood pro/antioxidant levels before and after acute exercise in athletes and non-athletes. *Gen Physiol Biophys.* 2012;31(2):211-219.

26. Bloomer RJ. Effect of exercise on oxidative stress biomarkers. *Adv Clin Chem.* 2008;46:1-50.

27. Ferreira LF, Reid MB. Muscle-derived ROS and thiol regulation in muscle fatigue. *J Appl Phys (1985).* 2008;104(3):853-860.

28. Slattery K, Bentley D, Coutts AJ. The role of oxidative, inflammatory and neuroendocrinological systems during exercise stress in athletes: implications of antioxidant supplementation on physiological adaptation during intensified physical training. *Sports Med.* 2015;45(4):453-471.

29. Peake JM. Vitamin C: effects of exercise and requirements with training. *Int J Sport Nutr Exerc Metab.* 2003;13(2):125-151.

30. Hemilä H, Chalker E. Vitamin C for preventing and treating the common cold. *Cochrane Database Syst Rev.* 2013;1:CD000980.

31. Robson PJ, Bouic PJ, Myburgh KH. Antioxidant supplementation enhances neutrophil oxidative burst in trained runners following prolonged exercise. *Int J Sport Nutr Exerc Metab.* 2003;13(3):369-381.

32. Gomez-Cabrera MC, Domenech E, Romagnoli M, et al. Oral administration of vitamin C decreases muscle mitochondrial biogenesis and hampers training-induced adaptations in endurance performance. *Am J Clin Nutr.* 2008;87(1):142-149.

33. Mullins VA, Houtkooper LB, Howell WH, Going SB, Brown CH. Nutritional status of US elite female heptathletes during training. *Int J Sport Nutr Exerc Metab*. 2001;11(3):299-314.

34. Braakhuis AJ, Hopkins WG, Lowe TE. Effect of dietary antioxidants, training, and performance correlates on antioxidant status in competitive rowers. *Int J Sports Physiol Perform*. 2013;8(5):565-572.

35. Garelnabi M, Veledar E, White-Welkley J, et al. Vitamin E differentially affects short term exercise induced changes in oxidative stress, lipids, and inflammatory markers. *Nutr Metab Cardiovasc Dis*. 2012;22(10):907-913.

36. Bryant RJ, Ryder J, Martino P, Kim J, Craig BW. Effects of vitamin E and C supplementation either alone or in combination on exercise-induced lipid peroxidation in trained cyclists. *J Strength Cond Res*. 2003;17(4):792-800.

37. Avery NG, Kaiser JL, Sharman MJ, et al. Effects of vitamin E supplementation on recovery from repeated bouts of resistance exercise. *J Strength Cond Res*. 2003;17(4):801-809.

38. Young AJ, Lowe GM. Antioxidant and prooxidant properties of carotenoids. *Arch Biochem Biophys*. 2001;385(1):20-27.

39. Aguiló A, Tauler P, Pilar Guix M, et al. Effect of exercise intensity and training on antioxidants and cholesterol profile in cyclists. *J Nutr Biochem*. 2003;14(6):319-325.

40. Vassilakopoulos T, Karatza MH, Katsaounou P, Kollintza A, Zakynthinos S, Roussos C. Antioxidants attenuate the plasma cytokine response to exercise in humans. *J Appl Physiol*. 2003;94:1025-1032.

41. Margaritis I, Palazzetti S, Rousseau AS, Richard MJ, Favier A. Antioxidant supplementation and tapering exercise improve exercise-induced antioxidant response. *J Am Coll Nutr*. 2003;22(2):147-156.

42. Aoi W, Ogaya Y, Takami M, et al. Glutathione supplementation suppresses muscle fatigue induced by prolonged exercise via improved aerobic metabolism. *J Int Soc Sports Nutr*. 2015;12:7.

43. Deldicque L, Francaux M. Recommendations for healthy nutrition in female endurance runners: an update. *Front Nutr*. 2015;2:17.

44. Beshgetoor D, Nichols JF. Dietary intake and supplement use in female master cyclists and runners. *Int J Sport Nutr Exerc Metab*. 2003;13(2):166-172.

45. Barry DW, Hansen KC, Van Pelt RE, Witten M, Wolfe P, Kohrt WM. Acute calcium ingestion attenuates exercise-induced disruption of calcium homeostasis. *Med Sci Sports Exerc*. 2011;43(4): 617-623.

46. Moyad MA. The potential benefits of dietary and/or supplemental calcium and vitamin D. *Urol Oncol*. 2003;21(5):384-391.

47. Huang L, Xue J, He Y, et al. Dietary calcium but not elemental calcium from supplements is associated with body composition and obesity in Chinese women. *PLoS One*. 2011;6(12):e277703.

48. Zemel MB, Shi H, Greer B, Dirienzo D, Zemel PC. Regulation of adiposity by dietary calcium. *FASEB J*. 2000;14(9):1132-1138.

49. Samadi M, Sadrzadeh-Yeganeh H, Azadbakht L, Feizi A, Jafarian K, Sotoudeh G. Dietary calcium intake and risk of obesity in school girls aged 8-10 years. *J Res Med Sci*. 2012;17(12):1102-1107.

50. Skinner ML, Simpson JA, Buchholz AC. Dietary and total calcium intakes are associated with lower percentage total body and truncal fat in healthy adults. *J Am Coll Nutr*. 2011;30(6):484-90.

51. Lorenzen JK. Mølgaard C. Michaelsen KF. Astrup A. Calcium supplementation for 1 y does not reduce body weight or fat mass in young girls. *Am J Clin Nutr*. 2006;83(1):18-23.

52. Melanson EL, Sharp TA, Schneider J, Donahoo WT, Grunwald GK, Hill JO. Relation between calcium intake and fat oxidation in adult humans. *Int J Obes Relat Metab Disord*. 2003;27(2):196-203.

53. Shapses SA, Heshka S, Heymsfield SB. Effect of calcium supplementation on weight and fat loss in women. *J Clin Endocrinol Metab*. 2004;89(2):632-637.

54. Murakami K, Okubo H, Sasaki S. No relation between intakes of calcium and dairy products and body mass index in Japanese women aged 18 to 20 y. *Nutrition*. 2006;22(5):490-495.

55. Palacios C, Bertrán JJ, Rios RE, Soltero S. No effects of low and high consumption of dairy products and calcium supplements on body composition and serum lipids in Puerto Rican obese adults. *Nutrition*. 2011;27(5):520-525.

56. Gunther CW, Legowski PA, Lyle RM, et al. Dairy products do not lead to alterations in body weight or fat mass in young women in a 1-y intervention. *Am J Clin Nutr*. 2005;81(4):751-756.

57. Wicherts IS, van Schoor NM, Boeke JP, V et al. Vitamin D status predicts physical performance and its decline in older persons. *J Endocrinol Metab*. 2007;92(6):2058-2065.

58. Cashman KD, Hill TR, Lucey AJ, et al. Estimation of the dietary requirement for vitamin D in healthy adults. *Am J Clin Nutr*. 2008;88(6):1535-1542.

59. Kroll MH, Bi C, Garber CC, et al. Temporal relationship between vitamin D status and parathyroid hormone in the United States. *PLoS One*. 2015;10(3):1-13.

60. Metz JA, Anderson JJ, Gallagher PN Jr. Intakes of calcium, phosphorus, and protein, and physical-activity level are related to radial bone mass in young adult women. *Am J Clin Nutr*. 1993;58(4):537-542.

61. Leventis P, Kiely DW. The tolerability and biochemical effects of high-dose bolus vitamin D-2 and D-3 supplementation in patients with vitamin D insufficiency. *Scand J Rheumatol*. 2009;38(2):149-153.

62. Lehmann U, Hirche F, Stangl GI, Hinz K, Westphal S, Dierkes J. Bioavailability of D2 and D3 in healthy volunteers, a randomized placebo-controlled trial. *J Clin Endocrinol Metab.* 2013;98(11):4339-4345.

63. Willis KS, Peterson NJ, Larson-Meyer DE. Should we be concerned about the vitamin D status of athletes? *Int J Sport Nutr Exerc Metab.* 2008;18(2):204-224.

64. Forney LA, Earnest CP, Henagan TM, Johnson LE, Castleberry TJ, Stewart LK. Vitamin D status, body composition, and fitness measures in college-aged students. *J Strength Cond Res.* 2014;28(3):814-824.

65. Moe SM. Disorders involving calcium, phosphorus, and magnesium. *Prim Care.* 2008;35(2):215-237. doi:10.1016/j.pop.2008.01.007.

66. Penido MG, Alon US. Phosphate homeostasis and its role in bone health. *Pediatr Nephrol.* 2012;27(11):2039-2048. doi:10.1007/s00467-012-2175-z.

67. Institute of Medicine Standing Committee on the Scientific Evaluation of Dietary Reference Intakes. *Dietary Reference Intakes for Calcium, Phosphorus, Magnesium, Vitamin D, and Fluoride.* Washington, DC: National Academies Press; 1997. www.ncbi.nlm.nih.gov/books/NBK109825/. doi: 10.17226/5776. Accessed January 5, 2016.

68. Wyshak G. Teenaged girls, carbonated beverage consumption, and bone fractures. *Arch Pediatr Adolesc Med.* 2000;154(6):610-613. doi:10.1001/archpedi.154.6.610.

69. Tucker KL, Morita K, Qiao N, Hannan MT, Cupples LA, Kiel DP. Colas, but not other carbonated beverages, are associated with low bone mineral density in older women: the Framingham Osteoporosis Study. *Am J Clin Nutr.* 2006;84(4):936–942.

70. Gutiérrez OM, Luzuriaga-McPherson A, Lin Y, Gilbert LC, Ha SW. Beck GR Jr. Impact of phosphorus-based food additives on bone and mineral metabolism. *J Clin Endocrinol Metab.* 2015;100(11):4264-4271.

71. Bremner K, Bubb WA, Kemp GJ, Trenell MI, Thompson CH. The effect of phosphate loading on erythrocyte 2,3-bisphosphoglycerate levels. *Clin Chim Acta.* 2002;323(1-2):111-114.

72. Brewer CP, Dawson B, Wallman KE, Guelfi KJ. Effect of sodium phosphate supplementation on cycling time trial performance and VO$_2$ 1 and 8 days post loading. *J Sports Sci Med.* 2014;13(3):529-534.

73. Barker ME, Blumsohn A. Is vitamin A consumption a risk factor for osteoporotic fracture? *Proc Nutr Soc.* 2003;62(4):845-850.

74. Veeranna V, Zalawadiya SK, Niraj A, Pradhan J, Ference B, Burack RB, et al. Homocysteine and reclassification of cardiovascular disease risk. *J Am Coll Cardiol.* 2011;58(10):1025-1033.

75. Iglesias-Gutiérrez E, Egan B, Díaz-Martinez AE, Peñalvo JL, González-Medina A, Martinez-Camblor P, et al. Transient increase in homocysteine but not hyperhomocysteinemia during acute exercise at different intensities in sedentary individuals. *PLoS One.* 2012; 7(12):e51185.

76. König D. Bisse E. Deibert P. Müller HM. Wieland H, Berg A. Influence of training volume and acute physical exercise on the homocysteine levels in endurance-trained men: interactions with plasma folate and vitamin B12. *Ann Nutr Metab.* 2003;47(3-4):114-118.

77. Herrmann M, Wilkinson J, Schorr H, et al. Comparison of the influence of volume-oriented training and high-intensity interval training on serum homocysteine and its cofactors in young, healthy swimmers. *Clin Chem Lab Med.* 2003;41911):1525-1531.

78. McLean E, Cogswell M, Egli I, Wojdyla D, de Benoist B. Worldwide prevalence of anaemia, WHO Vitamin and Mineral Nutrition Information System, 1993-2005. *Public Health Nutr.* 2009;12(4):444–454

79. Haymes EM. Iron. In: Driskell JA, Wolinsky I, eds. *Sports Nutrition: Vitamins and Trace Elements.* 2nd ed. New York, NY: CRC/Taylor & Francis; 2006:203-216.

80. Woolf K, St Thomas M, Hahn N, Vaughan LA, Carlson AG, Hinton P. Iron status in highly active and sedentary young women. *Int J Sport Nutr Exerc Metab.* 2009;19:519-535

81. Di Santolo M, Stel G, Banfi G, Gonano F, Cauci S. Anemia and iron status in young fertile non-professional female athletes. *Eur J Appl Physiol.* 2008;102(6):703-709.

82. Hueglin S. A practical approach for developing an iron protocol for athletes. *SCAN's PULSE.* 2016;35(2):10-13.

83. Cook JD. Diagnosis and management of iron-deficiency anaemia. *Best Pract Res Clin Haematol.* 2005;18(2):319-332.

84. Ashmead HD. The absorption and metabolism of iron amino chelate. *Arch Latinoam Nutr.* 2001;51(1 suppl 1):13-21.

85. DellaValle DM, Haas JD. Iron supplementation improves energetic efficiency in iron-depleted female rowers. *Med Sci Sports Exerc.* 2014;46(6):1204-1205.

86. Jin CH, Paik IY, Kwak YS, Jee YS, Kim JY. Exhaustive submaximal endurance and resistance exercises induces immunosuppression via physical and oxidative stress. *J Exerc Rehabil.* 2014;11(4):198-203.

87. Cunnane SC. *Zinc: Clinical and Biochemical Significance.* Boca Raton, FL: CRC Press; 1988.

88. Gleeson M, Nieman DC, Pedersen BK. Exercise, nutrition and immune function. *J Sports Sci.* 2004;22(1):115-125.

89. Micheletti A, Rossi R, Rufini S. Zinc status in athletes: relation to diet and exercise. *Sports Med.* 2001;31(8):577-582.

90. Nikić M, Pedišić Ž, Šatalić Z, Jackovljević S, Venus D. Adequacy of nutrient intakes in elite junior basketball players. *Int J Sports Nutr Exerc Metab*. 2014;24(5):516-523.

91. Giolo De Carvahlo F, Rosa FT, Marques Miguel Suen V, Freitas EC, Padovan GJ, Marchini JS. Evidence of zinc deficiency in competitive swimmers. *Nutrition*. 2012;28(11-12):1127-1131.

92. Volpe SL, Lowe NM, Woodhouse LR, King JC. Effect of maximal exercise on the short-term kinetics of zinc metabolism in sedentary men. *Br J Sports Med*. 2007;41(3):156-161.

93. Wehrlin JP, Zuest P, Hallén J, Marti B. Live high-train low for 24 days increases hemoglobin mass and red blood cell volume in elite endurance athletes. *J Appl Physiol*. 2006;100(6):1938-1945.

94. Neya M, Enoki T, Ohiwa N, Kawahara T, Gore CJ. Increased hemoglobin mass and VO2max with 10 h nightly simulated altitude at 3000 m. *Int J Sports Physiol Perform*. 2014;8(4):366-372.

95. Govus AD, Garvican-Lewis LA, Abbiss CR, Peeling P, Gore CJ. Pre-altitude serum ferritin levels and daily oral iron supplement dose mediate iron parameter and hemoglobin mass responses to altitude exposure. *PLoS One*. 2015;10(8):e0135120.

96. Pialoux V, Mounier R, Rock E, et al. Effects of acute hypoxic exposure on prooxidant/antioxidant balance in elite endurance athletes. *Int J Sports Med*. 2009;30(2):87-93.

97. Cowell BS, Rosenbloom CA, Skinner R, Summers SH. Policies on screening female athletes for iron deficiency in NCAA Division I-A institutions. *Int J Sport Nutr Exerc Metab*. 2003;13(3):277-285.

98. Holick MF, Binkley NC, Bischoff-Ferrari HA, et al. Evaluation, treatment, and prevention of vitamin D deficiency: an Endocrine Society clinical practice guideline. *J Clin Endocrinol Metab*. 2011;96(7):1911-1930.

99. De Souza MJ, Nattiv A, Joy E, et al; Expert Panel. 2014 Female Athlete Triad Coalition Consensus Statement on Treatment and Return to Play of the Female Athlete Triad: 1st International Conference held in San Francisco, California, May 2012, and 2nd International Conference held in Indianapolis, Indiana, May 2013. *Br J Sports Med*. 2014;48(4):289.

100. Mountjoy M, Sundgot-Borgen J, Burke L, et al. The IOC consensus statement: beyond the Female Athlete Triad—Relative Energy Deficiency in Sport (RED-S). *British J Sports Med*. 2014;48(7):491-497.

101. Niemitz E. Estrogen and bone loss. *Nat Genet*. 2007;39(10):1195.

102. Braam LA, Knapen MH, Geusens P, Brouns F, Vermeer C. Factors affecting bone loss in female endurance athletes: a two-year follow-up study. *Am J Sports Med*. 2003;31(6):889-895.

103. Booth SL, Suttie JW. Dietary intake and adequacy of vitamin K. *J Nutr*. 1998;128(5):785-788.

104. Melina V, Craig W, Levin S. Position of the Academy of Nutrition and Dietetics: vegetarian diets. *J Acad Nutr Diet*. 2016:116(12):1970-1980.

105. Fuhrman J, Ferreri DM. Fueling the vegetarian (vegan) athlete. *Curr Sports Med Rep*. 2010;9(4):233-241.

106. Micheletti A, Ross R, Rufini S, Zinc status in athletes: relation to diet and exercise. *Sports Med*. 2001;31(8):577-582.

107. Zhang R, Wang Z, Fei Y, et al. The difference in nutrient intakes between Chinese and Mediterranean, Japanese and American Diets. *Nutrition*. 2015;7(6):4661-4688.

108. Sundgot-Borgen J, Torstveit MK. Aspects of disordered eating continuum in elite high-intensity sports. *Scand J Med Sci Sports*. 2010;20(suppl 2):112-121.

109. Hinton PS, Sanford TC, Davidson MM, Yakushko OF, Beck NC. Nutrient intakes and dietary behaviors of male and female collegiate athletes. *Int J Sport Nutr Exerc Metab*. 2004;14(4):389-405.

110. El Ghoch M, Soave F, Calugi S, Grave RD. Eating disorders, physical fitness and sport performance: a systematic review. *Nutrients*. 2013;5(12):5140-5160.

111. Nazem TG, Ackerman KE. The female athlete triad. *Sports Health*. 2012;4(4):302-311. doi:10.1177/1941738112439685.

ONLINE RESOURCES

- Nutrion.gov: http://nutrition.gov
- National Academy of Medicine: https://nam.edu/
- Vitamin D Council: www.vitamindcouncil.org
- Food and Nutrition Information Center, US Department of Agriculture: http://fnic.nal usda.gov
- Office of Dietary Supplements: https://ods.od.nih.gov/

CHAPTER 6

FLUID, ELECTROLYTES, AND EXERCISE

Bob Murray, PhD, FACSM, and Kris Osterberg, PhD, RD, CSSD

INTRODUCTION

Staying well hydrated during physical activity can help delay the onset of fatigue as well as protect health and well-being by preventing the physiologically deleterious effects of dehydration. In fact, even a slight amount of dehydration (eg, 1% loss of body weight, which is 1.5 lb [0.7 kg] in a 150-lb [68-kg] athlete) can adversely affect the body's ability to cope with physical activity, particularly when that activity occurs in a warm environment.[1,2] That is not to say that dehydration always impairs performance or negatively impacts health, because that is clearly not the case. There are many occasions when temporary mild dehydration has no deleterious consequences. However, during physical activity and heat exposure, it is always better to be euhydrated (normal hydration) than hypohydrated (dehydrated), simply because euhydration helps sustain critical cardiovascular and thermoregulatory functions. The physiological consequences of dehydration during physical activity are comprehensively reviewed in the scientific literature.[3-6] But when educating coaches and athletes, the emphasis is better placed on the physiological and performance benefits of hydration,[7-9] along with practical advice for keeping athletes well hydrated.

This chapter focuses on how consuming adequate amounts of fluid and electrolytes before, during, and after physical activity affects physiological function, safeguards health, and improves performance. The information in this chapter is gleaned from decades of research on the physiological and performance-related responses to changes in hydration status. In addition, numerous position stands on the topic of hydration and exercise have been published by a variety of professional organizations,[10-20] and key points from those documents are included in this chapter.

For individuals who engage in vigorous physical activity or who spend considerable time in warm environments, daily water and electrolyte losses can be prodigious, increasing the prevalence of dehydration. Even on days when no sweating occurs, it is not unusual for people to remain slightly dehydrated, a potential risk factor for the development of kidney stones and other ailments.[21] For those reasons, it is important for sports health professionals to have a fundamental understanding of daily fluid and electrolyte balance, beginning with the unique—some might say weird—characteristics of the simple water molecule.

THE UNIQUENESS OF WATER

To understand why the hydration status of the human body has such a great impact on virtually every physiological function, it is essential to first appreciate the fact that water is the most biologically active molecule in the body. No other nutrient is as essential or is needed in as great an amount on a daily basis. Water's central role in life is not just because it is a solvent but because water also acts as solute, reactant, product, carrier, lubricant, shock absorber, coolant, catalyst, ionizing agent, messenger, and controller, as well as the primary volumetric constituent of most cells. It is this compendium of unique characteristics that makes water the most important molecule in biology.

Yet, until recent decades, water has been a somewhat neglected molecule in biology. After all, water molecules are rarely portrayed in structural drawings of other biological molecules, yet without water, those molecules could not function.[22] Water is a small molecule: 1 L of water at room temperature contains a septillion molecules (10^{24}); in other words, a million, million, million, million molecules. Most water on earth is in liquid or solid (ice) form, even though the water molecule (H_2O) is smaller and lighter than gases such as oxygen (O_2) and carbon dioxide (CO_2). The reason that water molecules prefer to remain in liquid form has to do in large part with the structure of H_2O. Picture an individual water molecule as a plump sphere where one portion bears a negative charge while the other portion is positively charged. That bipolar charge characteristic is what attracts one water molecule to the next, allowing water to exist mostly in liquid or solid form rather than as a gas. The bipolar charge also governs water's interactions with all other elements and compounds.

In cells, water molecules not only allow proteins to form three-dimensional shapes but are also indispensable for allowing proteins such as enzymes to perform their various functions.[22] For example, it is now thought that within cells, the enzymatic pathways, water, and ions are organized into various clusters associated with membranes and the cytoskeleton. That arrangement allows metabolites to be channeled through these clusters (referred to as metabolons) rather than randomly circulating as free solutes in solution, which has been the traditional vision of how the cytoplasm was organized.[23]

Among water's unique properties is a high heat capacity, a high thermal conductivity, and a high latent heat of evaporation, all of which help keep the body and its various parts (most of which have a high water content) from overheating during exercise and heat exposure. For example, the unique thermal characteristics of water prevent a runner's leg muscles from being destroyed by local overheating, allowing the heat produced by muscles to be quickly transferred, with the help of circulating blood, away from active muscle and distributed throughout the body for eventual loss to the environment through the evaporation of sweat and through radiation, convection, and conduction to cooler surroundings.

DAILY FLUID AND ELECTROLYTE BALANCE

Control of Fluid Balance

Considering the central importance of water to every aspect of life, it should be no surprise that the human body is endowed with intricate physiological systems responsible for maintaining water balance within a fairly narrow range of normal. For example, at rest in thermoneutral conditions—which refer to environmental temperatures and activity levels in which the body can maintain a normal temperature—body fluid balance is maintained at $\pm 0.2\%$ of total body weight,[24-25] a very narrow tolerance befitting the critical importance of hydration status to physiological function, even in nonexercise conditions. Under thermoneutral, sedentary conditions, the daily intake of fluid usually matches or exceeds the volume of fluid lost in urine, feces, and sweat; through respiration; and via transcutaneous water loss (Table 6.1). In other words, over 24 hours people usually consume enough fluid from foods and beverages to replace fluid losses—although that is certainly not always the case.

Maintaining fluid balance requires the constant integration of input from hypothalamic osmoreceptors (to gauge the osmolality of the

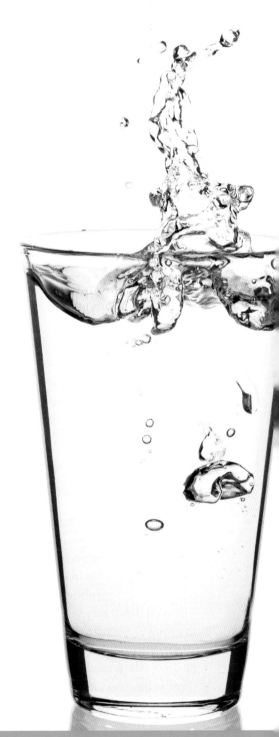

blood) and vascular baroreceptors (to gauge the pressure within major vessels) so that fluid intake matches or modestly exceeds fluid loss. In this regard, the combination of thirst-driven and spontaneous drinking is such that fluid balance is normally maintained in most people over the course of a day. Interestingly, thirst-driven fluid intake accounts for only a small percentage of daily fluid intake; most fluid is spontaneously consumed with meals or snacks during the day and not directly in response to being thirsty.[21]

When sweating occurs, body fluid balance is further regulated by mechanisms that reduce urinary water and sodium excretion and stimulate thirst. Sweat loss is accompanied by a decrease in plasma volume and an increase in plasma osmolality (because more water than salt is lost in sweat, the sodium and chloride concentrations in blood plasma increase). These changes are sensed by vascular pressure receptors (baroreceptors), which respond to a drop in blood volume, and hypothalamic osmoreceptors, which respond to an increase in plasma sodium concentration (ie, increased plasma osmolality). In response to dehydration, integrated input from baroreceptors and osmoreceptors results in an increase in vasopressin (antidiuretic hormone) release from the pituitary gland and in renin release from the kidneys (see Figure 6.1, page 110). These hormones, including angiotensin II and aldosterone, which result from an increase in plasma renin activity, increase water and sodium retention by the kidneys and provoke an increase in thirst.[26]

Table 6.1 Typical Daily Fluid Losses in mL for a 70-kg Athlete[a]			
Insensible loss	Normal Weather (68°F/20°C)	Warm Weather (85°F/29°C)	Exercise in Warm Weather (85°F/29°C)
Skin	350	350	350
Respiratory tract	350	250	650
Urine	1,400	1,200	500
Feces	100	100	100
Sweat	100	1,400	5,000
TOTAL	2,300	3,300	6,600

[a] Daily fluid loss varies widely among athletes and can exceed 10 L/d under some circumstances.

Adapted from Guyton AC, Hall JE. *Textbook of Medical Physiology*. 10th ed. Philadelphia, Pa: WB Saunders Co; 2000, with permission from Elsevier. Copyright © 2000, Elsevier, Inc.

During the course of a day, ingesting adequate water and electrolytes in foods and beverages eventually restores plasma volume and osmolality to normal levels, and whenever too much fluid is ingested, the kidneys excrete the excess. However, for physically active people, body fluid balance is often compromised because the human thirst mechanism is an imprecise gauge of immediate fluid needs and because it is sometimes difficult to ingest enough fluid to offset the large volume of sweat lost during physical activity.[27]

Daily Fluid Needs

Some people are confused by well-intended but errant hydration recommendations such as that everyone should consume eight 8-oz glasses of water per day to maintain proper hydration.[28] Although the genesis of this advice is a matter of debate, it is interesting that eight, 8-oz servings amount to 2 L (approximately 2 qt), the volume that has been often cited as the daily fluid requirement for sedentary adults.[29] In fact, there is no one fluid-intake recommendation that will suffice for everyone because of the wide disparity in daily

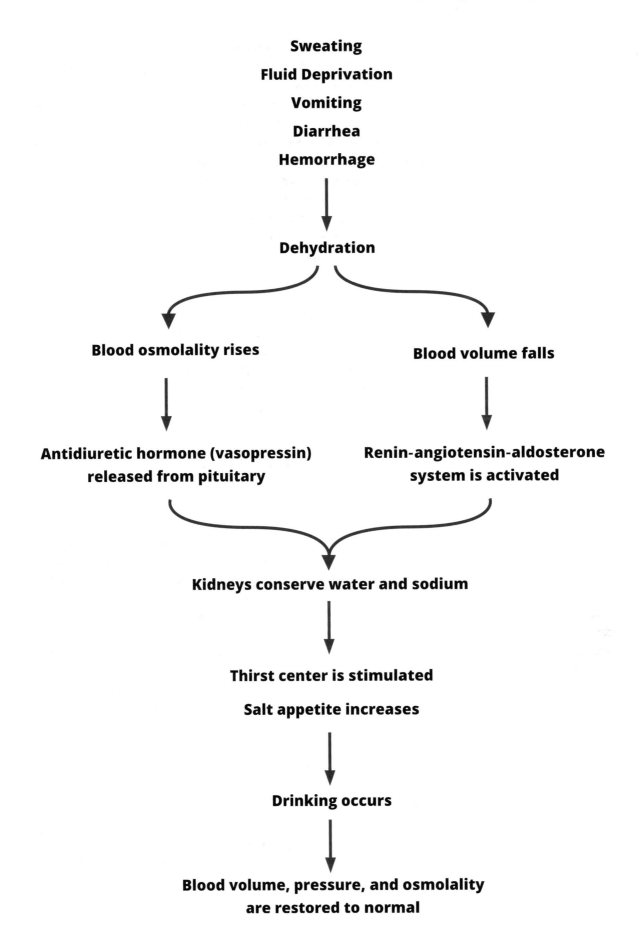

FIGURE 6.1 Dehydration and Thirst, Simplified

fluid needs created by differences in body size, body composition, physical activity, and environmental conditions.[21,30] For a small, elderly, sedentary individual, 2 L per day might be too much fluid, but for a young, relatively large, and physically active person, 2 L might represent the fluid needs of just 1 hour of activity. The 2004 Dietary Reference Intake (DRI) recommendations for water and electrolytes identify the adequate intake (AI) for water as 3.7 L/d in men (130 oz/d; the equivalent of 16 cups/d of fluid) and 2.7 L/d for women (95 oz/d; about 12 cups/d).[21] The AI is an estimate of the daily nutrient intake assumed to be adequate for most people. In other words, there is a low probability of inadequacy if sedentary women and men ingest between 2.7 and 3.7 L/d of fluid. The AI volumes are median values from the Third National Health and Nutrition Examination Survey, 1988-1994, (NHANES III) data for adults ages 19 and older; AI values for children and adolescents range from 1.3 to 3.3 L/d. In Europe, the recommended values for daily fluid intake are 2.5 L for men and 2.0 L for women.[31]

The 12 cups of fluid per day that represent the AI for water intake in adult women does not mean that women should literally drink at least 12 cups of water each day. Rather, it means that a total of 12 cups of fluid from all sources will meet the hydration needs of most adult women. This important distinction should be stressed when educating and counseling people about their hydration needs. Regardless of the extent of daily water needs, water can be supplied by a variety of foods and fluids such as fruits and vegetables, milk, soft drinks, fruit juices, sports drinks, coffee, tea, and soups. Approximately 80% of daily water needs are provided by fluids ingested during the day, and the remaining 20% comes from water found in food.[21] For example, bananas are roughly 75% water by weight, a chicken breast 65%, and a hot dog 50%. In brief, the prevailing scientific consensus is that sedentary individuals living in temperate environments can rely on the combination of thirst and spontaneous drinking to successfully maintain daily fluid balance, whereas physically active people and those living in warm environments often find it difficult to keep pace with their daily fluid needs.

Control of Electrolyte Balance

The concentrations of electrolytes across cell membranes must be tightly regulated to ensure proper function of cells throughout the body. In the case of cardiac muscle, for example, an electrolyte imbalance such as hyperkalemia can have fatal consequences if plasma potassium concentration increases just a few millimoles per liter. For this and other reasons, the kidneys are well equipped to maintain electrolyte balance by conserving or excreting minerals such as sodium, chloride, potassium, calcium, and magnesium.

Although an appetite for sodium chloride does exist in humans,[32] there is no evidence to suggest that the intake of other minerals is governed similarly. In most individuals, when dietary energy intake is adequate, mineral intake is usually in excess of mineral needs, ensuring positive mineral balance. However, repeated days of profuse sweating can result in substantial electrolyte loss, especially sodium and chloride, the two minerals found in greatest concentrations in sweat. When dietary mineral intake (especially sodium intake) is not sufficient to compensate for such large losses, severe muscle cramping or hyponatremia might result.[33,34]

Daily Electrolyte Needs

Electrolytes (minerals such as sodium, potassium, calcium, and magnesium) are lost in urine and sweat. Some athletes, soldiers, and workers lose large volumes of sweat daily (eg, 4 to 10 L or more), and that loss is accompanied by a similarly large electrolyte loss. As shown in Table 6.2 (page 112), the concentrations of potassium, magnesium, and calcium in sweat are low and relatively constant compared with the higher, more variable concentrations of sodium and chloride. The fact that sodium concentration in sweat varies widely among individuals means that some athletes will be prone to large sodium losses, whereas others will not. Large salt loss in sweat is often characterized by dry, white residue on the skin and clothing after the sweat dries. Increased risk of heat-related problems, hyponatremia, and muscle cramps has been linked to large sodium chloride losses.[33-35]

Table 6.2 Mineral (Electrolyte) Losses in Sweat

Mineral	Concentration in Sweat, mmol/L (mg/L)	AI[a] Values, mg/d	Possible AI Lost in Sweat, %AI/L
Sodium	20–80 (460–1,840)	1,300	35–140
Chloride	20–80 (710–2,840)	1,300	35–140
Potassium	4–8 (160–320)	4,700	3–8
Magnesium	0–1.5 (0–36)	240–420	0–15
Calcium	0–3 (0–120)	1,000–1,300	0–12

[a] AI = adequate intake.

Adapted from Shirreffs SM, Maughan RJ. Whole body sweat collection in humans: an improved method with preliminary data on electrolyte content. *J Appl Physiol*. 1997;82(1):336-341.

POSITION STANDS ON FLUID AND ELECTROLYTE REPLACEMENT

There are numerous position stands published by professional organizations that address fluid and electrolyte replacement before, during, and after physical activity.[10-20] Table 6.3 summarizes the key recommendations from those documents. The recommendations vary and have evolved over time, although the differences among the recommendations are relatively small; the central intent of each is to ensure that physically active individuals remain well hydrated. The common message among these positions is that proper hydration practices help reduce the risk of dehydration and heat illness, maintain cardiovascular and thermoregulatory function, and improve performance during vigorous physical activity.

Table 6.3 Recommendations for Fluid and Electrolyte Replacement When Exercising

Position Stand	Before Exercise	During Exercise	After Exercise	Electrolyte Replacement
American College of Sports Medicine Position Stand: Exercise and Fluid Replacement (2007)[11]	Drink 5–7 mL/kg body weight (BW) at least 4 h before exercise. If needed, drink 3–5 mL/kg BW 2 h before.	Follow a customized fluid replacement program to prevent excessive dehydration (ie, >2% loss of BW).	Fully replace fluid and electrolyte deficits. For rapid rehydration, drink 1.5 L of fluid (with electrolytes) per kilogram of BW loss.	Consume snacks and beverages with sodium to help stimulate thirst and retain fluids.
American College of Sports Medicine Roundtable on Hydration and Physical Activity: Consensus Statements (2005)[20]	No recommendation.	Replace but do not exceed sweat losses. Limit fluid deficits to <2% loss of BW.	Rehydration within 6 h of exercise requires drinking 125%–150% of BW loss. Fluids should contain sodium. If 24 h before next exercise, rely on normal food and fluid intake.	Rely on salty foods, fluids, and sports drinks.

Continued on next page

Position Stand	Before Exercise	During Exercise	After Exercise	Electrolyte Replacement
National Athletic Trainers Association (2000)[13]	Consume approximately 500–600 mL (17–20 oz) of water or sports drink 2–3 h before exercise and 200–300 mL (7–10 oz) 10–20 min before exercise.	Fluid replacement should approximate sweat and urine losses, with the goal of keeping weight loss < 2% body mass. Example: 200–300 mL (7–10 oz) every 10–20 min, but individualized recommendations should be followed.	To ensure hydration within 4–6 h after exercise, drink about 25%–50% more than existing weight loss.	Adding a modest amount of salt (0.3–0.7 g/L) is acceptable to stimulate thirst, increase voluntary fluid intake, and decrease the risk of hyponatremia.
American Academy of Pediatrics (2000)[14]	Before prolonged physical activity, the child should be well hydrated.	Periodic drinking should be enforced, even if a child is not thirsty. Example: for a child weighing 40 kg (88 lb), drink 150 mL of water or a flavored, salted beverage every 20 min.	No recommendation.	Make water or a flavored, salted beverage available for active children.
Academy of Nutrition and Dietetics, Dietitians of Canada, and the American College of Sports Medicine (2016)[15]	To achieve euhydration, drink 5–10 mL/kg BW 2–4 h before exercise.	Fluid intake depends on sweat rate, but general guideline is 0.4–0.8 L/h.	Drink 1.25–1.5 L fluid for every 1 kg BW lost.	Ingest sodium during exercise when large sweat sodium losses occur.
3rd International Exercise-Associated Hyponatremia Consensus Development Conference (2015)[17]	Do not overconsume fluids.	Drink to thirst but have an idea of individual fluid needs.	For those with asymptomatic hyponatremia, consume hypertonic saline solutions to reduce the risk of symptomatic hyponatremia.	Foods and beverages containing sodium should be available at marathon aid stations.
Inter-Association Task Force on Exertional Heat Illnesses (2003)[18]	Athletes should begin exercise properly hydrated.	Fluid intake should nearly approximate fluid losses. Individualized recommendations must be followed.	No recommendation.	Hydrating with a sports drink containing carbohydrates and electrolytes before and during exercise is optimal to replace losses and provide energy. Replacing lost sodium after exercise is best achieved by consuming food, in combination with a rehydration beverage.

Continued on next page

Position Stand	Before Exercise	During Exercise	After Exercise	Electrolyte Replacement
USA Track & Field Advisory (2003)[19]	Consume approximately 500–600 mL (17–20 oz) of water or sports drink 2–3 h before exercise and 300–360 mL (10–12 oz) 0–10 min before exercise.	During the race, drink no more than 1 cup (8–10 oz) every 15–20 min.	Drink about 25% more than sweat loss to ensure optimal hydration 4–6 h after the event.	Adding modest amounts of sodium (0.5–0.7 g/L) can offset sodium lost in sweat and may minimize medical events associated with electrolyte imbalances (eg, muscle cramps, hyponatremia).

Fluid and Electrolyte Replacement Before Exercise

Adequate hydration before physical activity helps ensure optimal physiological and performance responses. For example, laboratory subjects who ingest fluid in the hour before exercise exhibit lower core temperatures and heart rates during exercise than when no fluid is ingested.[36] Unfortunately, many athletes enter training sessions and competitive events already dehydrated. For example, Volpe and colleagues reported that over 60% of the college athletes (n = 174) participating in their study had prepractice urine specific gravity measures indicative of hypohydration.[37] Palmer and Spriet noted similar findings in half of the ice hockey players they studied (n = 44).[38]

Clearly, athletes who enter competition in a dehydrated state are often at a competitive disadvantage.[6] For example, in a study by Armstrong and colleagues, subjects performed runs of 5,000 m (approximately 19 minutes) and 10,000 m (approximately 40 minutes) in either a normally hydrated or dehydrated condition. When dehydrated by approximately 2% of body weight (by a diuretic given before exercise), their running speeds decreased by 6% to 7% in both events.[39] To make matters worse, exercise in the heat exacerbates the performance-impairing effects of dehydration.[1,40]

When people live and are physically active in warm environments, voluntary fluid intake is often insufficient to meet fluid needs, as verified by a study conducted with soccer players in Puerto Rico. The athletes were studied during 2 weeks of training. When the players were allowed to drink fluids throughout the day as they wished (average intake equaled 2.7 L/d), their total body water at the end of 1 week was approximately 1.1 L less than when they were mandated to drink 4.6 L of fluid per day.[41] In other words, voluntary fluid consumption did not match fluid losses and caused the players to enter training and competition already dehydrated.

Fluid and Electrolyte Replacement During Exercise

Recent research has shown that cardiovascular, thermoregulatory, and performance responses are optimized by replacing sweat loss during exercise.[2,9,42,43] These and similar research findings are reflected in the various recommendations for fluid and electrolyte intake during exercise.

For example, the American College of Sports Medicine recognizes the physiological and performance benefits of minimizing dehydration by simply recommending that "Individuals should develop customized fluid replacement programs that prevent excessive (>2% body weight reductions from baseline body weight) dehydration."[11] In some cases, minimizing dehydration during exercise may require little more than athletes drinking whenever they are thirsty[44]; in most cases, however, athletes are best advised to create a personal hydration plan to guide the frequency and volume of their fluid intake during exercise. Developing a personal hydration plan requires that athletes periodically record body weights before and after activity. Using the simplest approach, weight loss indicates inadequate drinking, while weight gain indicates excessive drinking (see Table 6.4).[45] That basic feedback is often all athletes need to fine-tune their hydration practices. For athletes who continue to struggle with dehydration, calculations based on preexercise and postexercise body weights, fluid intake, and urine output can be used to prescribe the volume and frequency of fluid intake required to minimize dehydration. Such measurements should be made periodically throughout the season to adjust for changes in environment, training intensity, fitness, and acclimation. Beginning activity with a comfortable volume of fluid already in the stomach, followed by additional fluid intake at 10- to 30-minute intervals (depending on sweat rate) will help assure a rapid gastric emptying rate by maintaining gastric volume, an important driver of gastric emptying during exercise.[46]

Table 6.4 Calculating Sweat Rates

Drinking fluid during exercise to keep pace with sweat loss goes a long way toward helping fitness enthusiasts, athletes, and workers feel good and work hard. Because sweat rates can vary widely, it is important to be aware of how much sweat is lost during physical activity. Knowing how much fluid is typically lost through an hour of activity becomes a goal for fluid replacement. Here are some simple steps to take to determine hourly sweat rate. In the example given at the bottom, Shelby F. should drink about 1 liters (32 oz) of fluid during each hour of activity to remain well hydrated

A	B	C	D	E	F	G	H	I	J
		Body Weight (kg)					Sweat		Sweat
Name	Date	Before Exercise	After Exercise	Δ BW[a], g (C − D)	Drink Volume, mL	Urine Volume, mL[b]	Loss, mL (E + F − G)	Exercise Time, min	Rate, mL/min (H/I)
Shelby F.	9/15	61.7 kg	60.3 kg	1,400 g	420 mL	90 mL	1,730 mL	90 min	19 mL/min
		(lb/2.2)	(lb/2.2)	(kg × 1,000)	(oz × 30)	(oz × 30)	(oz × 30)	(h/60)	(mL/h x 60)
		kg	kg	g	mL	mL	mL	min	mL/min
		(lb/2.2)	(lb/2.2)	(kg × 1,000)	(oz × 30)	(oz × 30)	(oz × 30)	h	mL/h
		kg	kg	g	mL	mL	mL	min	mL/min
		(lb/2.2)	(lb/2.2)	(kg × 1,000)	(oz × 30)	(oz × 30)	(oz × 30)	h	mL/h
		kg	kg	g	mL	mL	mL	min	mL/min
		(lb/2.2)	(lb/2.2)	(kg × 1,000)	(oz × 30)	(oz × 30)	(oz × 30)	h	mL/h

[a] Δ BW = change in body weight

[b] Weight of urine should be subtracted if urine was excreted prior to postexercise body weight.

Reproduced with permission from Murray R. Fluid replacement: the American College of Sports Medicine position stand. *Sports Sci Exch.* 1996;9(63):6.

Not surprisingly, most humans prefer—and drink more of—beverages that are flavored and sweetened.[47] This is an important consideration in preventing dehydration because any step that can be taken to increase voluntary fluid intake will help reduce the risk of health issues associated with dehydration and heat stress. In addition to having palatable beverages available for athletes to drink, it is also important for athletes to periodically record body weights before and after vigorous physical activity as a way to assess the effectiveness of fluid intake and as a reminder of the importance of drinking adequate volumes of fluid during exercise.[48,49] Consuming sufficient fluid during exercise has well-established benefits that should be emphasized when speaking to coaches and athletes about hydration strategies (see Table 6.5).

Table 6.5 Beneficial Responses to Adequate Fluid Intake During Exercise[2,9,42,43]

Characteristic	Response
Heart rate	Lower
Stroke volume	Higher
Cardiac output	Higher
Skin blood flow	Higher
Core temperature	Lower
Perceived exertion	Lower
Performance	Better

Fluid and Electrolyte Replacement After Exercise

When hypohydration occurs after physical activity, it is often important to rehydrate quickly. An afternoon of working in the yard, two-a-day football practices, a day-long sports tournament, and 8 hours of manual labor are all examples of activities in which hypohydration is likely. Fluid and electrolyte intake after physical activity is a critical factor in helping people recover quickly—both physically and mentally. Maughan and colleagues concluded that ingesting plain water is ineffective at restoring euhydration because water absorption causes plasma osmolality to decrease, suppressing thirst and increasing urine output.[50] When sodium is provided in fluids or foods, the osmotic drive to drink is maintained,[51,52] and urine production is decreased.

Plain water is a good thirst quencher but not an effective rehydrator. In short, consuming plain water turns off the thirst mechanism and turns on urine production. Only when water is ingested in combination with foods that contain sodium, chloride, and other minerals will sufficient water be consumed and retained to promote complete rehydration. Low-fat foods and beverages containing ample sodium include tomato juice, baked potato chips, pretzels, pickles, and crackers. These can be consumed as snacks on days when large sweat sodium losses are expected.

Maughan and colleagues also emphasized the importance of ingesting fluid in excess of the deficit in body weight to account for obligatory urine losses.[50] In other words, the advice sometimes given athletes— drink a pint [454 mL] of fluid for every pound [454 grams] of body weight deficit—should be amended to drink *at least* a pint of fluid for every pound of body weight deficit. Ideally, fluids and foods consumed after exercise should contain sodium, chloride, and other minerals required for complete rehydration. More precise recommendations for how much fluid athletes should ingest to ensure rapid and complete rehydration will evolve from future research; existing data indicate that ingesting 125% to 150% of weight loss is required to achieve normal hydration within 6 hours after exercise.[51]

Finally, when rapid rehydration is the goal, consumption of alcoholic beverages is contraindicated because of alcohol's diuretic properties. Caffeine is, by comparison, a much milder diuretic and, in those who regularly ingest caffeine, might not be much of a diuretic at all.[21,30] The 2004 DRI recommendations conclude that, "While consumption of beverages containing caffeine and alcohol have been shown in some studies to have diuretic effects, available information indicates that this may be transient in nature, and that such beverages can contribute to total water intake and thus can be used in meeting recommendations for dietary intake of total water."[21] However, when rapid rehydration is required, athletes should rely on noncaffeinated and nonalcoholic beverages. Education efforts with athletes should reflect the reality that many individuals will choose to consume alcoholic and caffeinated beverages. For those who do drink coffee, colas, beer, and similar beverages, the best advice is to do so in moderation, avoiding such drinks in the first few hours after physical activity.

Fluid and Electrolyte Balance at Environmental Extremes

The environment has a major impact on fluid and electrolyte balance.[53] Exposure to extreme heat, high humidity, prolonged cold, water immersion, altitude, and reduced gravity increases the need for water and electrolytes to match the increased losses that occur in those circumstances.[54] In extreme dry heat, combined water loss from sweating, respiration, and transcutaneous routes can increase water and salt needs to high levels, often exceeding 10 L and 20 g, respectively. Not surprisingly, a high proportion of children who live in hot and arid environments were found to be in a state of moderate to severe dehydration.[55] Although respiratory water loss is minimal during exposure to wet heat, sweating is profuse as the body struggles to lose heat through the evaporation of sweat from the skin. This can be particularly troublesome for unacclimated individuals exposed to high humidity; the inability of the sweat glands to respond maximally to environmental heat and humidity imposes a limit on both thermal comfort and the physiological capacity to sustain even mild exercise. During physical activity in cold environments, respiratory water loss increases due to the low humidity and increased ventilation rate, and it is also possible for sweat rates to exceed 1 L/h due to the warm, humid microenvironment created underneath the clothing. Being immersed in water increases urine production because the increase in plasma volume that accompanies immersion triggers high-pressure baroreceptors. It should be noted that competitive swimmers can sweat during tough workouts whenever internal body temperature exceeds the sweat threshold. Physical activity at altitude provokes the same responses as activity in the cold, with additional challenges to hydration posed by an altitude-induced reduction in food and fluid intake and increased urinary water and salt loss.[56] Astronauts who spend days in zero-gravity conditions lose considerable water and salt from the inevitable diuresis that occurs. All of these conditions promote fluid loss and increase the risk of dehydration.

Diarrheal disease also promotes rapid dehydration and has claimed the lives of millions of people worldwide. Each year in the United States, diarrheal illnesses in children result in roughly 3 million physician visits, 220,000 hospitalizations, and about 400 deaths.[57] The World Health Organization and various medical bodies recommend the use of oral rehydration solutions—simple concoctions of carbohydrates and electrolytes—to combat diarrheal fluid loss and save lives.[58] As is the case with sports drinks, a small amount of carbohydrate stimulates rapid water absorption in the small intestine, with sodium, chloride, and potassium replacing electrolytes lost in diarrhea and thereby helping sustain fluid balance. Oral rehydration is as effective as intravenous rehydration and is a home remedy that can be administered at a much lower cost and risk. Interestingly, fluid replacement during diarrheal disease does not reduce disease duration; fluid replacement saves lives by maintaining body fluid balance until the disease runs its course.[59]

HYDRATION Q&A

How Much of the Human Body is Water?

Between 45% and 75% of body weight is water, a value that varies inversely with fat mass.[21] Regardless of the volume of total body water, maintenance of fluid balance in physically active people can be an ongoing challenge. Fluid is constantly lost from the body by way of the kidneys (urine), gastrointestinal tract (feces), respiratory tract (exhaled air is saturated with water vapor), and skin (the latter two routes represent insensible water loss). Water and electrolytes are also periodically lost from the eccrine sweat glands during exercise and heat exposure.[4,5,21,60] Eccrine sweat glands are responsible for secreting sweat onto the skin in response to physical activity and heat stress. Apocrine glands are found in the armpits and are not part of the thermoregulatory response.

What Determines Daily Fluid Loss?

The total volume of fluid lost from the body daily is determined by a combination of factors, including environmental conditions, the size (and surface area) of the individual, the individual's metabolic rate, physical activity, sweat loss, composition of the diet, and the volume of excreted fluids. Insensible water loss via the skin is relatively constant (see Table 6.1, page 109),[29,61] but water loss via the respiratory tract is affected by the ambient temperature, relative humidity, and ventilatory volume. Inhaled air is humidified during its passage through the respiratory tract, and, as a result, exhaled air has a relative humidity of 100%. Inhaling warm, humid air reduces insensible water loss because the inhaled air already contains substantial water vapor. Athletes and workers experience more insensible water losses via the respiratory tract because of the overall increase in breathing that accompanies physical activity. The air inhaled during cold-weather activity contains relatively little water vapor, so as it is warmed and humidified during its transit through the respiratory tract, additional water loss occurs. For this reason, during cold-weather activity, especially when conducted at altitude, transcutaneous and respiratory water loss can be quite high, at times exceeding 1 L/d.[21-61]

What Is the Absolute Minimum Daily Water Need for a Sedentary Individual?

A minimum daily water need is difficult to accurately discern, but it is likely to be no less than 1 L/d. The reasoning for this is that minimum urine flow is approximately 500 mL/d, transcutaneous water loss is approximately 400 mL/d, and respiratory loss is a minimum of 200 mL/d. Keep in mind that this minimum value would apply only to someone who was completely sedentary for the entire day in a thermoncutral environment. Current thinking is that the water requirement in most minimally active adults ranges between 3 and 4 L/d due to the transcutaneous, respiratory, and urinary water loss that accompanies normal daily living.[32]

What Are Typical Daily Water Needs Among Athletes?

When individuals work, train, and compete in warm environments, their daily water needs can be considerably larger than those for sedentary individuals and might increase to more than 10 L/d.[60] For example, an athlete who trains 2 hours each day can easily lose an additional 4 L of body fluid, resulting in a daily fluid requirement in excess of 7 to 8 lL. Some people are active more than 2 hours each day, further increasing their fluid needs. Such losses can strain the capacity of the fluid regulatory system such that thirst becomes an inadequate stimulus for fluid intake and, coupled with limited opportunities for spontaneous drinking, persistent dehydration (hypohydration) can occur.

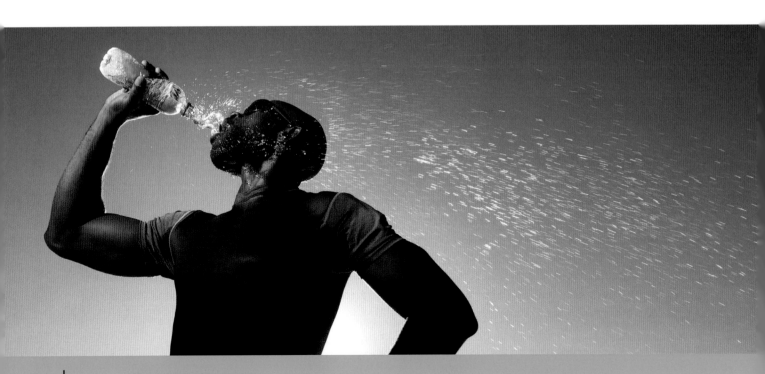

To put these volumes of fluid loss in perspective, consider that the body of a 60-kg (132-lb) individual contains approximately 36 kg water (60% of body weight). That same 36 kg of water is equivalent to 36 L of water. If that person remains sedentary in a moderate environment, daily fluid requirements will be approximately 3 L or 8.3% of total body water each day: [3 L/day ÷ (36 kg ÷ 1 kg/L) × 100% = 8.3% per day]. In other words, every 12 days that person's body water will completely turn over. Now consider an 80-kg (176-lb; estimated total body water [TBW] = 48 L) American football player who sweats profusely during two-a-day practices in the summer heat. His water needs might be 8 L/d (about 17% of his total body water), resulting in a complete turnover of body water in 6 days. If such large sweat volumes seem unreasonably high, consider that most athletes engaged in vigorous exercise will lose between 1 and 2 L of sweat per hour of exercise, and some people are capable of sweating more than 3 L/h.[5,6,21,60] As one example, Palmer and Spriet reported an average sweat loss of 1.8 L/h in competitive ice hockey players during a training session. Three of the 44 players lost less than 1 L/h, while 12 players lost in excess of 2 L/h.[38]

How Does Urine Production Figure into Water Balance in Athletes?

During physical activity, urine production is reduced as the kidneys attempt to conserve water and sodium to offset losses due to sweating. When fluid intake is limited and dehydration occurs, the kidneys are capable of concentrating the urine to four to five times the concentration of blood. However, some renal fluid loss (approximately 500 mL/d) is obligatory for waste removal. Daily urine losses in some athletes and workers tend to be less than in sedentary individuals, a trend that is exacerbated by warm weather as the body strives to conserve fluid. However, most athletes consume large volumes of fluid during the day and, as a result, produce more urine than their sedentary counterparts. Reduced urine volume in physically active individuals usually indicates inadequate fluid intake. In general, urine volumes tend to be 800 to 1,500 mL/d in sedentary individuals and can exceed 4 L/d in physically active individuals who ingest large volumes of fluid.

Does Diet Composition Impact Daily Water Needs?

The primary components of the diet that influence daily water needs are protein and sodium, specifically excess protein and sodium. For sedentary individuals consuming a high-protein diet (eg, > 2.0 g/kg/d), the water required to excrete urea nitrogen from protein (amino acid) degradation and to excrete excess sodium intake can represent a meaningful increase in daily water needs. For example, ingesting an excess 3 g of sodium requires an additional liter of water intake.[6] However, for physically active people who already have an increased water requirement, the effect of protein and salt intake on overall water needs is usually quite small. For example, to excrete the urea produced from the degradation of 100 g of protein requires approximately 700 mL water to be excreted from the body.[29] Healthy kidneys are well equipped to excrete excess dietary components, such as the urea from proteins and excess electrolytes, from the diet. In fact, this is one reason why adequate daily fluid intake is important.

How Much Water Does the Oxidation Of Macronutrients Contribute?

This volume is relatively small—approximately 130 mL/1,000 kcal in a mixed diet[21]—and is relatively inconsequential for individuals consuming more than 2 L of fluid per day. To be more specific, the oxidation of carbohydrate, fat, and protein produces 15, 13, and 9 mL of water per 100 kcal of oxidized substrate, respectively.[21]

Why Is Thirst Often an Unreliable Regulator of Fluid Needs During Exercise?

There are at least three reasons why thirst is an unreliable regulator of fluid needs during exercise. The first is behavioral; there are often many distractions during physical activity, so thirst signals can easily be missed or disregarded. The second reason is that fluid is often not readily available, so even if thirst is perceived, it might not be convenient to act on it. The third reason is rooted in the physiology of the thirst mechanism. Consider that the plasma osmolality of a well-hydrated (euhydrated) person is 285 mOsm/kg H_2O. The thirst threshold is the plasma osmolality above which thirst is triggered, and this is thought to be 293 mOsm/kg (this varies among people, but usually falls within 290 to 295 mOsm/kg).[21] A simple calculation relying on TBW (represented in liters) illustrates the volume of fluid that has to be lost from the body before thirst is stimulated: $V^{thirst} = TBW - [(TBW \times 285)/293]$. For example, if TBW is 36 L, then 1 L of water must first be lost from the body for thirst to be initiated: [36 L – [(36 L × 285 mOsm/kg) / 293 mOsm/kg] = ~1 L]. This is the scientific rationale for the admonition that by the time thirst is perceived, some dehydration has already occurred.

One of many examples of the inadequacy of the human thirst mechanism during exercise can be found in the study by Passe and colleagues. Experienced runners participated in a 10-mile race conducted on a 400-meter track. The environmental conditions were moderate (69°F, 77% relative humidity) but sufficient for ample sweating to occur. Every 2 miles, the runners had the opportunity to grab a 24-oz sports bottle containing a commercial sports drink. They could drink from the bottle ad libitum; when they desired no more, the runners tossed the bottles onto the infield where the bottles were collected, part of a measurement system whereby drink volumes for each runner were calculated. As in a road race, if the runners chose not to drink, they had to wait until the next 2-mile opportunity. After the race, each runner completed a questionnaire so that their impressions of the adequacy of their fluid intake could be recorded. On average, the runners replaced only 30% of sweat loss (range from 5% to 67%), even though the conditions for fluid intake were purposefully optimized.[62] Had thirst been an adequate stimulus for fluid intake, the runners would have done a better job hydrating. The fact they did not is evidence that other factors often conspire to produce the voluntary dehydration that is so often reported in the literature.[24,27] The postrun questionnaires revealed that the runners grossly underestimated the extent of their sweat loss while accurately estimating their fluid intake. These results led the investigators to conclude that the inability to accurately estimate sweat loss contributed to the runners' inadequate fluid intake. For those reasons, there are numerous steps athletes can take to help ensure that they consume enough fluid during exercise to minimize dehydration (see Box 6.1).

Box 6.1 **Tips for Encouraging Drinking Before, During, and After Sweaty Physical Activity**

Preparation
- Know the warning signs of dehydration (thirst, unusual fatigue, light-headedness, headache, dark urine, dry mouth, infrequent urination, unusually rapid heartbeat).
- Know where to find fluid (water fountains, stores, neighbors, etc).
- Freeze fluid bottles overnight to allow the drink to stay cold longer during workouts.
- Ideally, have a variety of beverage flavors to choose from.
- Prehydrate to produce a light-colored urine.

Training
- When sweating is anticipated, start activity with a stomach comfortably full of fluid.
- Practice drinking during training.
- Take fluid with you. Wear a bottle belt or fluid pack; take along a cooler full of drinks.
- Keep a comfortably full stomach during activity.
- Train yourself to drink more during exercise.
- One medium mouthful of fluid = about 1 oz.
- Always carry money to buy drinks.
- Periodically record your body weight before and after activity.
- Complete rehydration requires full replacement of fluid and sodium losses.
- After activity, drink 24 oz for every pound of weight lost during activity.

Competition
- Better hydration means better performance—plan to drink during competition.
- When sweating, drink early and often, but do not overdrink.
- In distance running, stop to drink if that is what it takes to ensure adequate intake. Runners will more than make up the time by staying well-hydrated.
- During a road race, pinch the top of the drink cup to form a spout that will make drinking easier.
- Carry fluid with you during a road race by folding the top of the cup over, keeping the fluid from spilling.
- Put more in your stomach than on your head. Pouring water over your head does nothing to lower body temperature.
- If prone to dehydration, drink by schedule—not by thirst.

Are There Circumstances Where Thirst Might Be an Adequate Gauge of Fluid Needs During Physical Activity?

Undoubtedly there are. For example, it is relatively easy to drink during long-duration, low-intensity activity, such as slow marathon runs lasting more than 4 hours, ultraendurance biking and running, hiking and backpacking, military marches, and similar activities. Under those circumstances, thirst may be an adequate stimulus for fluid intake in many people because there is ample opportunity to sense the presence of thirst and to drink accordingly. However, perceptions of thirst can also be inadequate in these circumstances, leading to dehydration and volume depletion in some participants and hyperhydration and hyponatremia in others.

How prevalent is Dehydration Among Children?

A number of studies have reported inadequate hydration among children and adolescents, associated with decrements in cognitive performance and mood.[63-65] Using NHANES data from 2009 to 2012, researchers collected hydration-related information on 4,134 participants, ages 6 to 19.[66] Over half (54.5%) showed signs of inadequate hydration (> 800 mOsm/kg). The risks were higher in boys and black children. In addition, one out of four participants reported drinking no plain water during the day. The authors recommended that improving access to drinking water during the school day and encouraging students to drink may help reduce the risk of inadequate hydration. It should be noted that inadequate hydration may not be the same as dehydration; it is possible that some of the children with high urine osmolality were not dehydrated. In addition, it has not yet been determined if such levels of inadequate hydration have a meaningful effect on physiological response, mental function, or general health.

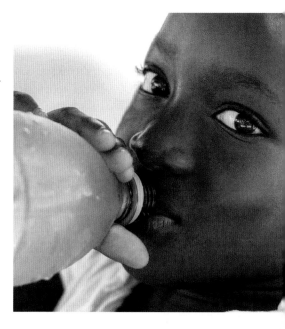

When Is Sodium Replacement During Exercise Recommended?

Box 6.2 (page 123) includes recommendations about sodium intake during exercise as a way to improve beverage palatability, promote rehydration, and reduce the risk of hyponatremia and severe muscle cramps. Electrolyte intake becomes important whenever sweat loss is greater than 4 L/d, as commonly occurs during two-a-day practices and prolonged training or competition. Sweat contains more sodium and chloride than other minerals, and although the sodium content of sweat is normally substantially less than the plasma value (plasma = 138 to 142 mmol/L; sweat = 20 to 80 mmol/L), large sweat losses can result in considerable salt loss (refer to Table 6.2, page 112). Normally, sodium deficits are uncommon among athletes and military personnel, in large part because a normal diet often provides more than enough salt to replace that lost in sweat.[67]

However, persistent sodium losses can present problems, as illustrated by Bergeron in a case study of a nationally ranked tennis player who suffered from frequent muscle cramps. A high sweat rate (2.5 L/h), coupled with a higher-than-normal sweat sodium concentration (90 mmol/L), predisposed the player to severe cramping. The cramps were eliminated when the player increased his daily dietary intake of sodium chloride from less than 10 g/d to 15 to 20 g/d, relied on a sports drink during practices and games, and increased his daily fluid intake to assure adequate hydration.[68] A link between sweat sodium loss and cramping has also been reported in American football players.[69]

It is important to understand that ingesting sodium chloride in a beverage consumed during physical activity not only helps ensure adequate fluid intake but also stimulates more complete rehydration after activity.[50,70] Both of these responses reflect the critical role that sodium plays in maintaining the osmotic drive to drink and in providing an osmotic stimulus to retain fluid in the extracellular space, including in the plasma and interstitial fluid compartments. The carbohydrate and electrolyte content of sports drinks can vary widely, so product nutrition labels should be carefully read before recommending specific beverages or foods.

The sodium content of a fluid-replacement beverage does not directly affect the rate of fluid absorption.[71] This is because the amount of sodium that can be included in a beverage is small compared with the amount of sodium that can be provided from the bloodstream. Whenever fluid is ingested, sodium diffuses from plasma into the gut, driven by an osmotic gradient that strongly favors sodium influx. In brief, sodium chloride is an important constituent of a properly formulated sports drink because it improves beverage palatability, helps maintain the osmotic drive for drinking, reduces the amount of sodium that the blood has to supply to the intestine prior to fluid absorption, helps maintain plasma volume during exercise, and serves as the primary osmotic impetus for restoring extracellular fluid volume after exercise.[50,51]

How Does Sodium Ingestion During Exercise Affect Thirst and Fluid Intake?

A good example of the effect that beverage composition has on voluntary fluid intake is demonstrated by the work of Wilk and Bar-Or. Preadolescent boys (ages 9 to 12 years) completed 3 hours of intermittent exercise in the heat, during which time they could drink one of three beverages ad libitum. The beverages tested included water, a sports drink, and a placebo (a flavored, artificially sweetened replica of the sports drink). The boys drank almost twice as much sports drink as they did water, whereas consumption of the placebo fell in between. Flavoring and sweetness increased voluntary fluid intake (more intake with placebo vs water), and the presence of sodium chloride in the sports drink further increased consumption (the subjects drank more sports drink than placebo).[72]

These results are consistent with the physiology of the thirst mechanism. In humans, the sensation of thirst is a function of changes in plasma sodium concentration (plasma osmolality) and of changes in blood volume.[26,27,60] Drinking plain water removes the osmotic drive to drink (by quickly diluting the

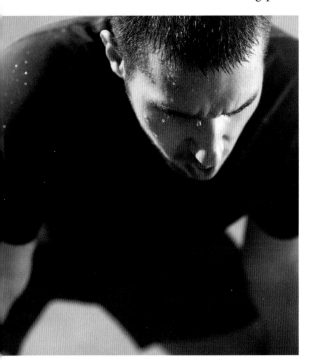

sodium concentration of the blood) and reduces the volume-dependent drive (by partially restoring blood volume), causing the premature satiation of thirst. Unfortunately, the resulting decrease in fluid intake occurs before adequate fluid has been ingested. As the Wilk and Bar-Or research demonstrated, the osmotic drive for drinking can be maintained by the presence of low levels of sodium chloride in a beverage, resulting in greater fluid intake.[52] This application of basic physiology is nothing new. For centuries, bartenders have known that salty foods and snacks help sustain fluid intake among their patrons.

What Is the Composition of Sweat?

In addition to sodium, potassium, and chloride, human sweat contains small amounts of dozens of organic and inorganic substances, including amino acids, urea, lactic acid, and the minerals calcium, magnesium, and iron.[59] Even when sweat losses are large, it is unlikely that minerals such as magnesium, iron, and calcium will be lost in sufficient quantities in sweat to provoke a mineral imbalance in most people. However, for some individuals, such losses could constitute an additional dietary challenge, as might be the case with sweat calcium losses in physically active females (see Table 6.2, page 112). For example, a female athlete who loses 3 L of sweat in a day could lose up to 120 to 360 mg calcium. Although this amount of calcium can be easily replaced by consuming a cup of milk, sweat calcium loss does increase the dietary calcium needs of active males and females.

How Much Sodium Chloride Is Actually Lost in Sweat?

For some individuals, the amount of sodium chloride lost in sweat is not trivial. Consider, for example, a football player who practices for 5 h/d, during which time he loses 8 L of sweat (average sweat loss of 1.6 L/h). If his sweat contains 50 mmol of sodium per liter, his total sodium loss will be 9,200 mg sodium (23 g NaCl). This sodium loss, which does not include the 50 to 200 mmol (1,150 to 4,600 mg) of sodium that is typically lost in urine, makes it apparent that physically active people often require a large salt intake to replace losses in sweat. The 2004 DRI recommendations indicate that Americans and Canadians should restrict their daily sodium intake to only 1.5 g/d (3.8 g salt per day), with a tolerable upper intake level for salt of 5.8 g/d (2.3 g sodium per day).[21]

The basis of this recommendation is that a reduction in dietary sodium intake can blunt the age-related increase in blood pressure. Clearly, these stringent dietary recommendations are inadequate for athletes, fitness enthusiasts, and workers who lose considerably more salt in their sweat. However, this discrepancy is recognized in the DRI report: "This [recommendation] does not apply to highly active individuals … who lose large amounts of sweat on a daily basis."[21]

Should Current Hydration Recommendations Be Revised to Protect Athletes Against Hyponatremia?

Some individuals mistakenly interpret the current recommendations for fluid intake to mean that dehydration is to be avoided at all costs and that there is no such thing as drinking too much fluid. This is certainly not true. Excessive water intake, even at rest, can result in life-threatening hyponatremia. Ingesting too much water, beer, or other low-sodium fluid can quickly dilute the plasma sodium concentration. When this occurs, the osmotic balance across the blood-brain barrier is disrupted and water enters the brain, causing swelling that can lead to seizures, coma, and even death.[73] In similar fashion, excessive drinking during prolonged exercise can also result in hyponatremia.[74] For that reason, physically active individuals should be counseled to limit their fluid intake to no more than is needed to minimize dehydration and to ingest sodium in food or drink during prolonged exercise (>2 hours) (see Boxes 6.2 and 6.3, pages 125-126).[60]

Some sports scientists have argued that current hydration recommendations have increased deaths from hyponatremia and that hydration recommendations should be changed to encourage people to drink only when thirsty during exercise.[16,17] This argument defies logic, common sense, and the existing evidence. Symptomatic hyponatremia remains a very rare disorder, which suggests that current hydration recommendations are not the cause of the problem.[74,75] In addition, drinking to thirst obviously failed those who suffer from exercise-associated hyponatremia. There is a large body of evidence demonstrating that those who drink enough fluid during exercise to minimize dehydration suffer no ill consequences and benefit from better cardiovascular and thermoregulatory function.[2,4,5,11,60]

What Are the Physiological Implications of Dehydration in Athletes?

The effects of dehydration on various types of physical performance have been well documented.[4,6,9,21,60] Because dehydration results in a loss of blood volume, numerous cardiovascular and thermoregulatory responses are adversely affected. The greater the level of dehydration and the hotter the environment, the greater the overall negative impact on physiological function.[9] For instance, Canadian researchers studied the effects of dehydration (–2% to –3% body weight) during 2 hours of cycling at 65% VO_2 peak and reported that carbohydrate oxidation, heart rate, core temperature, perceived exertion, and muscle glycogen use were all greater when the subjects were allowed to dehydrate during exercise.[42,43]

Impaired physiological function often translates to impaired performance. Cross-country runners who were dehydrated by less than 1% of their body weight by overnight fluid restriction experienced a 3% reduction in 10-K running performance, even though heart rate and core temperature were not different between trials.[76] The runners rated their perceived exertion as greater during dehydrated treatment, indicating that their effort felt more difficult even though they were running more slowly.

Does Dehydration Always Impair Performance?

The simple answer is no. There are likely many circumstances when dehydration has minimal or no impact on performance. Of course, in science, simple answers rarely suffice, and in this case, the extent

Box 6.2 Drinking Dos and Don'ts

Dehydration is the most common performance-sapping mistake, but it is also the most preventable. Here are some guidelines to help physically active people stay well-hydrated.

DO	DON'T
Do start exercise well-hydrated. When heavy sweating is expected, drink 2–3 cups (475–700 mL; ~7 mL/kg body weight or ~1 oz/10 lb body weight) of fluid 4 h before exercise to allow excess fluid to be lost as urine. If urine output is still low 2 h before exercise, drink 5–12 oz (150–300 mL; ~3–5 mL/kg body weight or ~0.6 oz/10 lb body weight). There is no benefit to hyperhydration, so do not drink excessively.	**Don't rely solely on water.** If sweating lightly, water is an acceptable fluid replacement beverage. For heavier sweating (eg, >0.5 L/h), sports drinks help replace the electrolytes lost in sweat and supply performance-boosting carbohydrates to aid exercise performance. Excessive drinking of low-sodium beverages can lead to dangerous electrolyte disturbances (hyponatremia).
Do weigh yourself. The best way to determine if you had enough to drink during a workout is to check to see how much weight you have lost. Minimal weight loss (eg, <1 lb; ~0.5 kg) means that you have done a good job staying hydrated. Remember that weight loss during an exercise session is water loss, not fat loss, and must be replaced.	**Don't overdrink.** Water is definitely a good thing, but you can get too much of a good thing. Drinking large amounts of fluid is not only unnecessary but can be downright dangerous. A bloated stomach, puffy fingers and ankles, a bad headache, and confusion are warning signs of hyponatremia.
Do drink during exercise. When sweating, drink every 10–20 min during a workout. Those who sweat heavily can benefit from drinking more often (eg, every 10 min) whereas individuals who sweat lightly should drink less often (every 20+ min).	**Don't gain weight during exercise.** If you weigh more after exercise than you did before, that means that you drank more than you needed. Be sure to cut back the next time so that no weight is gained.
Do ingest sodium during exercise. The best time to begin replacing the sodium lost in sweat is during exercise. That is one reason why a good sports drink is better than plain water. Sodium intake of 1 g/h is recommended during prolonged exercise where heavy sweat loss is expected.	**Don't restrict salt in your diet.** Ample salt (sodium chloride) in the diet is essential to replace the salt lost in sweat. Because athletes sweat a lot, their need for salt is often much more than for nonathletes.
Do follow your own plan. Everyone sweats differently, so every athlete should have a drinking plan tailored to his or her individual hydration needs.	**Don't use dehydration to lose weight.** Restricting fluid intake during exercise impairs performance and increases the risk of heat-related problems. Dehydration should be kept to a minimum by following an individualized fluid-replacement plan.
Do drink plenty during meals. If you were not able to drink enough during practice to keep from losing weight, be sure to drink enough before the next practice. Mealtime makes it easy to drink and to consume the sodium that comes along with food. When rapid rehydration is required, drink 50% more than the existing fluid deficit (eg, if a 2-lb [~1-kg] fluid deficit exists, drink 48 oz [1,500 mL] of fluid to catch up).	**Don't delay drinking during exercise.** Stick to a drinking schedule so that you avoid dehydration early in exercise. Once dehydrated, it is next to impossible to catch up to what your body needs because dehydration actually slows the speed at which fluid exits the stomach.

Adapted with permission from Murray R, Stofan J, Eichner ER. Hyponatremia and exercise. *Sports Sci Exch.* 2003;16:1-6.

of dehydration, the environmental conditions, the person's level of fitness and heat acclimation, and the intensity and duration of exercise combine to determine the impact of dehydration on exercise performance. And there are studies that report no effect of dehydration on performance. However, the preponderance of evidence collected over many decades demonstrates that even low levels of dehydration (−1% body weight) can negatively affect physiological and performance responses, including aerobic capacity, anaerobic power and capacity, muscle endurance, and strength.[2,5,21,60]

Can Dehydration Affect Driving Performance?

Even low levels of dehydration may impair everyday tasks such as driving, although scientific literature is far from conclusive because so few studies have been done. In a 2015 study from the United Kingdom, 11 male subjects (22 ± 4 y) were studied to determine how their hydration status affected driving skills during a 2-hour session in a driving simulator. Restricting fluid intake on the day before the trial and at a breakfast prior to the trial resulted in a modest 1% loss of body weight. During the simulated drive, subjects consumed 200 mL of fluid each hour during the euhydrated trial and 25 mL during the dehydrated trial. The frequency of minor driving errors (eg, lane drifting, late braking) was significantly greater during the fluid restriction trial (101 ± 84 errors) compared with the euhydrated trial (47 ± 44 errors). The researchers noted that the magnitude of the decline in driving skill was similar to that previously reported after alcohol ingestion sufficient to produce a blood alcohol content of 0.08% or after sleep deprivation.[77] Mild dehydration is known to impair mood state and reduce alertness, concentration, and short-term memory, and such changes could explain the increase in driving errors in the dehydration trial.[78,79]

What Role Does Potassium Loss Play in the Etiology of Muscle Cramps?

Some people mistakenly believe that potassium loss causes muscle cramps and suggest eating oranges and bananas to replace the potassium lost in sweat. However, potassium loss is not the culprit. Potassium is lost in sweat (see Table 6.2),[21,60] but the concentration of potassium in sweat, usually less than 10 mmol/L, is far less than that of sodium, 20 to more than 100 mmol/L. In addition, the amount of potassium lost in even a large volume of sweat represents a small fraction of total body potassium content, whereas sweat sodium losses in a single 2-hour training session can approximate 20% of total body sodium content.

How Do Individuals Know When They Are Adequately Hydrated?

This simple question continues to perplex scientists and clinicians because there is no one method that can accurately and reliably determine adequate hydration status. Measuring plasma osmolality is considered the gold standard for assessing hydration status and is commonly used in laboratory settings, but a blood sample and expensive equipment are required. The specific gravity of urine from the first void after awaking in the morning can provide useful information about hydration status, but some equipment is needed, such as a refractometer or a hydrometer. The cost of such equipment is typically less than $200.

Noting the color and volume of urine is a practical way to help physically active people subjectively assess their hydration status. Darkly colored urine of relatively small volume is an indication of dehydration, a signal to ingest more fluid before activity. Monitoring urine output is a common recommendation in occupational settings, such as the mining industry, in which the workers are constantly exposed to conditions of high heat and humidity. In addition to measuring body weight after awaking, the use of some measure of urine concentration (specific gravity, osmolality, or color) will often allow for the detection of dehydration.[11,60,80] It should be noted that the intake of B vitamin supplements, specifically riboflavin, can cause brightly colored urine, even when an individual is well hydrated.

Does Hyperhydration Confer Any Physiological or Performance Benefits?

Ingesting a glycerol solution before physical activity in the heat might confer cardiovascular and thermoregulatory advantages resulting from hyperhydration. In fact, ingesting glycerol solutions before exercise does result in a reduction in urine production and in the temporary retention of fluid.[81] Glycerol-induced hyperhydration is accompanied by temporary weight gain proportional to the amount of water retained (usually approximately 0.5 to 1 kg). Fluid retention occurs because the presence of glycerol molecules after they are absorbed and distributed throughout the body water (with the exception of the aqueous-humor and the cerebral-spinal fluid compartments) provokes a transient increase in plasma osmolality, prompting a temporary decrease in urine production. As glycerol molecules are removed from the body water in subsequent hours, plasma osmolality decreases, urine production increases, and excess water is excreted.

There are several reasons why it is unwise to recommend glycerol-induced hydration to athletes:

1. Athletes pay a metabolic cost for carrying extra body weight.
2. There is no compelling evidence that glycerol-induced hyperhydration results in a physiological benefit.[36]
3. The side effects of ingesting glycerol can range from mild sensations of bloating and light-headedness to more severe symptoms of headaches, dizziness, and nausea.[82]
4. Glycerol-induced hyperhydration can cause blood sodium levels to decrease,[83] possibly predisposing to hyponatremia.
5. Glycerol is on the World Anti-Doping Agency list of prohibited substances out of concern that glycerol loading could be used to mask doping.[84]

What Are the Current Recommendations Regarding Fluid Intake for Athletes?

As noted in Table 6.3 (page 113), there are several similar recommendations for fluid intake before exercise where heavy sweating is anticipated, but a general recommendation is this: Drink approximately 5 to 7 mL/kg body weight (about 1 oz/10 lb body weight) of water or sports drink 4 hours before exercise. This will allow ample time for excess fluid to be excreted or for additional fluid to be consumed. If profuse sweating is expected, as would be the case with a vigorous workout in a warm environment, drink an additional 3 to 5 mL/kg body weight (0.6 oz/10 lb body weight) about 2 hours before exercise.[11] For example, a 70-kg (154-lb) individual would ingest 500 mL (about 16 oz) of fluid 4 hours before exercise and an additional 200 to 350 mL (7 to 12 oz) 2 hours before exercise. There is no need to drink large volumes of fluid immediately before exercise. In fact, doing so can lead to gastrointestinal discomfort and an increased risk of hyponatremia, a dangerously low blood sodium level that can be prompted by excessive fluid intake.

There is currently no specific recommendation regarding electrolyte intake before physical activity, although some football players, tennis players, endurance athletes, and workers have learned to stave off muscle cramps and reduce the risk of hyponatremia by consuming salty food or drink before exercise. Individuals who excrete large volumes of salty sweat (skin and clothing caked in the white residue of salt after exercise) are advised to take steps to ensure adequate salt intake throughout the day.[11,35] Some endurance athletes rely on salt tablets to help ensure adequate sodium replacement during long training sessions and competition. If used judiciously and taken with ample fluid, salt tablets can be an acceptable way to replace sodium. However, the main risk is that insufficient fluid is ingested with the tablets. Doing so will cause a concentrated saline solution to be introduced into the small intestine, prompting the movement of water from the bloodstream into the intestinal lumen to dilute the saline solution as it empties from the stomach. To prevent such an occurrence, a salt tablet that contains 180 mg sodium should be consumed with at least 8 oz (240 mL) of water or sports drink. Salty foods, such as pretzels, tomato juice, and various soups, can also serve as additional sources of dietary sodium. Figure 6.2 provides general guidelines for fluid and sodium ingestion across a variety of activity levels.

When Is a Sports Drink Better Than Plain Water?

When performance is a key consideration in a workout or competition, a sports drink has well-documented advantages over plain water. Carbohydrate is an important component of a fluid-replacement beverage because it improves palatability by conferring sweetness, provides a source of fuel for active muscles, and stimulates fluid absorption from the intestine.[60,85,86] The performance benefits of carbohydrate feeding during physical activity are covered in more detail in other chapters. Although it is clear that carbohydrate feeding benefits performance,[11,13,15,60,85] more carbohydrate in a beverage is not necessarily better. Research has demonstrated that ingesting drinks containing more than 6% to 7% carbohydrate (14 to 17 g per 8-oz serving) will decrease the rate of gastric emptying[45,49] and fluid absorption.[87]

Does Coconut Water Make a Good Hydration Beverage?

Millions of people around the world enjoy fresh coconut water directly from coconuts. The carbohydrate and electrolyte content of coconuts depends on the species of coconut and the age of the coconut. Coconut water is high in potassium and contains sodium and other minerals such as calcium and magnesium. The carbohydrate content of a coconut less than 6 months of age is roughly 4%, with a combination of sucrose, glucose, and fructose. For those reasons, coconut water is a better hydration choice than plain water. Some sports drinks contain coconut water as part of their formulation, and, in those cases, the products often have the proper levels and types of carbohydrates and electrolytes.

What Is the Relationship Between Hydration Status and the Risk Of Disease?

The science related to hydration and disease is suggestive of benefits for some acute and chronic conditions,[21,60] but there is simply not enough evidence to draw a conclusion. Some research has concluded that being well hydrated helps decrease the risk of kidney stones, in part by ensuring adequate daily urine output. But hydration status is just one of many factors that influence the development of kidney stones; sex, age, genetics, diet, medications, dietary supplements, and obesity can all play a role in stone development.

Hydration Continuum

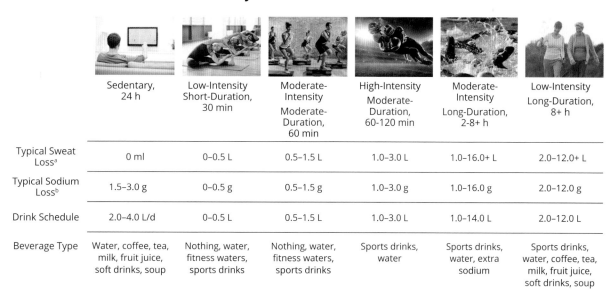

	Sedentary, 24 h	Low-Intensity Short-Duration, 30 min	Moderate-Intensity Moderate-Duration, 60 min	High-Intensity Moderate-Duration, 60-120 min	Moderate-Intensity Long-Duration, 2-8+ h	Low-Intensity Long-Duration, 8+ h
Typical Sweat Loss[a]	0 ml	0–0.5 L	0.5–1.5 L	1.0–3.0 L	1.0–16.0+ L	2.0–12.0+ L
Typical Sodium Loss[b]	1.5–3.0 g	0–0.5 g	0.5–1.5 g	1.0–3.0 g	1.0–16.0 g	2.0–12.0 g
Drink Schedule	2.0–4.0 L/d	0–0.5 L	0.5–1.5 L	1.0–3.0 L	1.0–14.0 L	2.0–12.0 L
Beverage Type	Water, coffee, tea, milk, fruit juice, soft drinks, soup	Nothing, water, fitness waters, sports drinks	Nothing, water, fitness waters, sports drinks	Sports drinks, water	Sports drinks, water, extra sodium	Sports drinks, water, coffee, tea, milk, fruit juice, soft drinks, soup

FIGURE 6.2 Hydration Continuum with Recommendations for Fluid and Sodium Intake During Various Activities
[a] Typical sweat rates for most people under most conditions; some may sweat more
[b] Assumes a loss of 1.0 g sodium per liter of sweat (43 mmol Na+/L)
Reprinted with permission from www.sportssienceinsights.com

However, with minimal risks and potentially plentiful benefits, the existing evidence supports the recommendation that we should all drink enough each day to avoid chronic dehydration. At the very least, in terms of maintaining basic physiological functions, it is always better to be well hydrated than dehydrated.

How Do Age and Sex Affect Daily Hydration Needs, as Well as Hydration Needs During Physical Activity?

As the US Dietary Guidelines indicate, daily fluid needs are lower in women, infants, children, adolescents, and older adult women compared with men over the age of 19.[21] Body size is obviously one determinant of daily fluid needs, with sweat loss being a factor that varies widely from person to person and plays a large role in determining daily hydration needs.

SUMMARY

Water is constantly lost from the body with each water-saturated breath, with the slow seeping of water through the skin, with the obligatory production of urine and feces, in substantial volumes in sweat, and, when ill, through emesis and diarrhea. Fortunately, the combination of thirst and spontaneous drinking is usually sufficient to match fluid intake to losses so that progressive, chronic dehydration is typically not an issue, even for older adults. However, for any individual who sweats profusely day after day, adequate water and salt replacement can pose a considerable challenge that can only be met by following practical yet scientifically founded recommendations for fluid and electrolyte intake.

The human body relies on an adequate volume of body water for all physiological and biochemical processes, so it should be no surprise that dehydration can adversely affect the health and performance of athletes and nonathletes. For that reason, it is essential that physically active people ingest ample fluids throughout the day to replace what is lost in sweat and urine. Two hours before a physical activity during which heavy sweating is expected, approximately 7 mL/kg body weight (about 1 oz/10 lb body weight) of water or sports drink should be consumed. During exercise, the goal is to drink enough to minimize weight loss and dehydration. Light sweaters require only modest volumes of fluid intake (< 500 mL/h [16 oz/h]), whereas heavy sweaters may have to ingest in excess of 1.5 L/h (about 50 oz/h) to minimize dehydration. To fully restore hydration status after exercise, it is necessary to ingest 150% of the existing fluid deficit. For example, if the fluid deficit is 2 lb (0.9 kg), 48 oz (1.4 L) of fluid should be consumed. For those who exercise only once per day, fluid deficits are usually corrected during the course of normal eating and drinking. Those who train more than once a day or who sweat throughout the day (eg, workers and soldiers) have to adopt a more aggressive fluid replacement plan, along with adequate salt intake, to avoid chronic dehydration.

KEY TAKEAWAYS

Water is essential for the body to function properly. Dehydration of just 1% to 2% of body weight can negatively impact performance, particularly in hot and humid climates.

Sodium is the primary electrolyte lost in sweat. Consuming sodium during and after exercise helps encourage drinking, maintain blood volume, reduce urine production, and stimulate more complete rehydration.

A practical way for athletes to monitor their hydration status is through the color and volume of their urine. A small volume of dark-colored urine likely indicates hypohydration and should signal greater fluid intake.

Diet generally has little impact on fluid requirements. However, high-protein or high-sodium diets may slightly increase fluid needs.

Daily fluid needs vary widely among and even within individuals depending on the intensity and duration of physical activity, environmental conditions, heat acclimation, and fitness.

Individual hydration plans can be established by periodically monitoring changes in body weight before and after exercise and encouraging athletes to consume enough fluid during activity to minimize postexercise weight loss.

Helpful Resources:

The Beverage Institute for Health and Wellness is a resource for health professionals on the science of beverages, hydration, and active healthy living (www.beverageinstitute.org/hydration/).

Hydration and heat illness guidelines are available from US Youth Soccer (www.usyouthsoccer.org/assets/1/15/Heat_Hydration_GuidelinesUSSF.pdf).

Hydration strategies for athletes, coaches, and families are available from USA Football. (http://usafootball.com/health-safety/hydration)

The Gatorade Sports Science Institute provides research and education on hydration for athletes (www.gssiweb.org/en).

The Korey Stringer Institute provides research and education to maximize performance, optimize safety, and prevent sudden death in active individuals. (http://ksi.uconn.edu/).

1. Cheuvront S, Carter R, Castellani JW, Sawka MN. Hypohydration impairs endurance exercise performance in temperate but not cold air. *J Appl Physiol*. 2005;99(5):1972-1976.

2. Murray R. Hydration and physical performance. *J Am College Nutr*. 2007;26(5 suppl):542S-548S.

3. Murray R. Nutrition for the marathon and other endurance sports: environmental stress and dehydration. *Med Sci Sports Exerc*. 1992;24(9 suppl):319S-323S.

4. Sawka MN. Body fluid responses and dehydration during exercise and heat stress. In: Pandolf KB, Sawka MN, Gonzalez RR, eds. *Human Performance Physiology and Environmental Medicine at Terrestrial Extremes*. Indianapolis, IN: Benchmark Press; 1988:227-266.

5. Savoie FA, Kenefick RW, Ely BR, Cheuvront SN, Goulet ED. Effect of hypohydration on muscle endurance, strength, anaerobic power and capacity and vertical jumping ability: a meta-analysis. *Sports Med*. 2015;45(8):1207-1227.

6. Sawka MN. Physiological consequences of dehydration: exercise performance and thermoregulation. *Med Sci Sports Exerc*. 1992;24(6):657-670.

7. Below PR, Mora-Rodríguez R, González-Alonso J, Coyle EF. Fluid and carbohydrate ingestion ingestion independently improve performance during 1 h of intense exercise. *Med Sci Sports Exerc*. 1995;27:200-210.

8. Coyle EF, Montain SJ. Benefits of fluid replacement with carbohydrate during exercise. *Med Sci Sports Exerc*. 1992;24(9 suppl):324S-330S.

9. Montain SJ, Coyle EF. The influence of graded dehydration on hyperthermia and cardiovascular drift during exercise. *J Appl Physiol*. 1992;73(4):1340-1350.

10. American College of Sports Medicine position stand on the prevention of thermal injuries during distance running. *Med Sci Sports Exerc*. 1987;19(5):529-533.

11. American College of Sports Medicine, Sawka MN, Burke LM, et al. American College of Sports Medicine position stand. Exercise and fluid replacement. *Med Sci Sports Exerc*. 2007 Feb;39(2):377-90.

12. Armstrong LE, Epstein Y., Greenlead JE. American College of Sports Medicine position stand on heat and cold illnesses during distance running. *Med Sci Sports Exerc*. 1996;28(12):i-x.

13. Casa DJ, Armstrong LE, Hillman SK, et al. National Athletic Trainers' Association position statement: fluid replacement for athletes. *J Athl Train*. 2000;35(2):212-224.

14. American Academy of Pediatrics, Committee on Sports Medicine and Fitness. Climatic heat stress and the exercising child and adolescent. *Pediatrics*. 2000;106(1 pt 1):158-159.

15. Thomas DT, Erdman KA, Burke LM. Position of the Academy of Nutrition and Dietetics, Dietitians of Canada, and the American College of Sports Medicine: nutrition and athletic performance. *J Acad Nutr Diet*. 2016;116(3):7501-7528.

16. Noakes T. IMMDA advisory statement on guidelines for fluid replacement during marathon running. *Clin J Sports Med*. 2003;13:309-318. www.usatf.org/groups/coaches/library/2007/hydration/IMMDAAdvisoryStatement.pdf. Accessed June 12, 2016.

17. Hew-Butler T, Rosner MH, Fowkes-Godek S, et al. Statement of the Third International Exercise-Associated Hyponatremia Consensus Development Conference, Carlsbad, California, 2015. *Br J Sports Med*. 2015; 25(4):303-320.

18. Inter-Association Task Force. Exertional heat illness consensus statement. *NATA News*. 2003;6:24-29.

19. Casa DJ. Proper hydration for distance running: identifying individual fluid needs. A USA Track and Field advisory. April 2003. www.usatf.org/groups/coaches/library/2007/hydration/ProperHydrationForDistanceRunning.pdf. Accessed February 24, 2010.

20. Casa DJ, Clarkson PM, Roberts WO. American College of Sports Medicine Roundtable on Hydration and Physical Activity: consensus statements. *Curr Sports Med Reports*. 2005;4(3):115-127.

21. Institute of Medicine. *Dietary Reference Intakes for Water, Potassium, Sodium, Chloride, and Sulfate*. Washington, DC: National Academies Press; 2004. www.nap.edu. Accessed February 18, 2015.

22. Ball P. Water as an active constituent in cell biology. *Chem Rev*. 2008;108(1):74-108.

23. Shepherd VA. The cytomatrix as a cooperative system of macromolecular and water networks. *Curr Top Dev Biol*. 2006;75:171-223.

24. Phillips PA, Rolls BJ, Ledingham ML, Morton JJ. Body fluid changes, thirst and drinking in man during free access to water. *Physiol Behav*. 1984;33(3):357-363.

25. Wade CE, Freund BJ. Hormonal control of blood flow during and following exercise. In: Gisolfi CV, Lamb DR, eds. *Perspectives in Exercise Science and Sports Medicine: Fluid Homeostasis During Exercise*; Vol 3. Indianapolis, IN: Benchmark Press; 1990:207-246.

26. Booth DA. Influences on human fluid consumption. In: Ramsay DJ, Booth DA, eds. *Thirst: Physiological and Psychological Aspects*. London, UK: Springer-Verlag; 1991:53-76.

27. Greenleaf JE. Problem: thirst, drinking behavior, and involuntary dehydration. *Med Sci Sports Exerc*. 1992;24(6):645-656.

28. Valtin H. "Drink at least eight glasses of water a day?" Really? Is there scientific evidence for 8 x 8? *Am J Physiol Regul Integr Comp Physiol*. 2002;283(5):993R-1004R.

29. Guyton AC, Hall JE. *Textbook of Medical Physiology*. 10th ed. Philadelphia, PA: WB Saunders Co; 2000.

30. Grandjean AC, Reimers KJ, Buyckx ME. Hydration: issues for the 21st century. *Nutr Rev*. 2003;61(8):261-271.

31. EFSA Panel on Dietetic Products, Nutrition and Allergies. Scientific opinion on dietary reference values for water. *EFSA J*. 2010;8(3):1-48.

32. Ladell WS. Water and salt (sodium chloride) intakes. In: Edholm O, Bacharach A, eds. *The Physiology of Human Survival*. New York, NY: Academic Press; 1965:235-299.

33. Bergeron MF. Heat cramps: fluid and electrolyte challenges during tennis in the heat. *J Sci Med Sport*. 2003;6(1):19-27.

34. Montain SJ, Sawka MN, Wenger CB. Hyponatremia associated with exercise: risk factors and pathogenesis. *Exerc Sports Sci Rev*. 2001;29(3):113-117.

35. Bauman A. The epidemiology of heat stroke and associated thermoregulatory disorders. In: Sutton JR, Thompson MW, Torode ME, eds. *Exercise and Thermoregulation*. Sydney, Australia: University of Sydney; 1995:203-208.

36. Latzka WA, Sawka MN, Montain SJ, et al. Hyperhydration: tolerance and cardiovascular effects during uncompensable exercise-heat stress. *J Appl Physiol*. 1998;84(6):1858-1864.

37. Volpe SL, Poule KA, Bland EG. Estimation of prepractice hydration status of National Collegiate Athletic Association Division I athletes. *J Athl Train*. 2009;44(6):624-629.

38. Palmer MS, Spriet LL. Sweat rate, salt loss, and fluid intake during an intense on-ice practice in elite Canadian male junior hockey players. *App Physiol Nutr Metab*. 2008;33(2):263-271.

39. Armstrong LE, Costill DL, Fink WJ. Influence of diuretic-induced dehydration on competitive running performance. *Med Sci Sports Exerc*. 1985;17(4):456-461.

40. Sawka MN, Francesconi RP, Young AJ, Pandolf KB. Influence of hydration level and body fluids on exercise performance in the heat. *JAMA*. 1984;252(9):1165-1169.

41. Rico-Sanz J, Frontera WA, Rivera MA, Rivera-Brown A, Mole PA, Meredith CN. Effects of hyperhydration on total body water, temperature regulation and performance of elite young soccer players in a warm climate. *Int J Sports Med*. 1996;17(2):85-91.

42. Logan-Sprenger HM, Heigenhauser GJ, Killian KJ, Spriet LL. Effects of dehydration during cycling on skeletal muscle metabolism in females. *Med Sci Sports Exerc*. 2012;44(10):1949-1957.

43. Logan-Sprenger HM, Heigenhauser GJ, Jones GL, Spriet LL. Increase in skeletal-muscle glycogenolysis and perceived exertion with progressive dehydration during cycling in hydrated men. *Int J Sport Nutr Exerc Metab*. 2013;23(3):220-229.

44. Noakes TD. Hydration in the marathon: using thirst to gauge safe fluid replacement. *Sports Med*. 2007:37(4-5):463-466.

45. Murray R. Fluid replacement: the American College of Sports Medicine position stand. *Sports Sci Exch*. 1996;9:1-6.

46. Maughan RJ. Gastric emptying during exercise. *Sports Sci Exch*. 1993;6(5):1-6.

47. Hubbard RW, Szlyk PC, Armstrong LE. Influence of thirst and fluid palatability on fluid ingestion during exercise. In: Gisolfi CV, Lamb DR, eds. *Perspectives in Exercise Science and Sports Medicine: Fluid Homeostasis During Exercise*. Vol 3. Indianapolis, IN: Benchmark Press; 1990:39-96.

48. Broad E. Fluid requirements of team sport players. *Sports Coach*. 1996:(summer):20-23.

49. Horswill CA. Effective fluid replacement. *Int J Sport Nutr*. 1998;8(2):175-195.

50. Maughan RJ, Shirreffs SM, Leiper JB. Rehydration and recovery after exercise. *Sport Sci Exch*. 1996;9(62):1-5.

51. Shirreffs SM, Taylor AJ, Leiper JB, Maughan RJ. Post-exercise rehydration in man: effects of volume consumed and drink sodium content. *Med Sci Sports Exerc*. 1996;28(10):1260-1271.

52. Gonzalez-Alonso J, Heaps CL, Coyle EF. Rehydration after exercise with common beverages and water. *Int J Sports Med*. 1992;13(5):399-406.

53. Piantodosi CA. *The Biology of Human Survival*. New York, NY: Oxford University Press; 2003.

54. Greenleaf JE. Environmental issues that influence intake of replacement beverages. In: Marriott BM, ed. *Fluid Replacement and Heat Stress*. Washington, DC: National Academy Press; 1994:1-30.

55. Bar-David Y, Urkin J, Landau D, Bar-David Z, Pilpel D. Voluntary dehydration among elementary school children residing in a hot arid environment. *J Hum Nutr Diet*. 2009;22(5):455-460.

56. Hoyt RW, Honig A. Environmental influences on body fluid balance during exercise: altitude. In: Buskirk ER, Puhl SM. *Body Fluid Balance*. Boca Raton, FL: CRC Press; 1996;186.1277-1289.

57. Diggins KC. Treatment of mild to moderate dehydration in children with oral rehydration therapy. *J Am Acad Nurse Pract*. 2008;20(8):402-406.

58. WHO position paper on oral rehydration salts to reduce mortality from cholera. World Health Organization website. www.who.int/cholera/technical/en/index.html. Accessed August 18, 2015.

59. Atia AN, Buchman AL. Oral rehydration solutions in non-cholera diarrhea: a review. *Am J Gastroenterol.* 2009;104(10):2596-2604.

60. Baker LB, Jeukendrup AE. Optimal composition of fluid-replacement beverages. *Compr Physiol.* 2014;4(2):575-620.

61. Karppanen H, Mervaala E. Sodium intake and hypertension. *Prog Cardiovasc Dis.* 2006;49(2):59-75.

62. Passe D, Horn M, Stofan J, Horswill C, Murray R. Voluntary dehydration in runners despite favorable conditions for fluid intake. *Int J Sports Nutr Exerc Metab.* 2007:17(3):284-295.

63. Edmonds CJ, Burford D. Should children drink more water? The effects of drinking water on cognition in children. *Appetite.* 2009;52(3):776-779.

64. Benton D, Burgess N. The effect of the consumption of water on the memory and attention of children. *Appetite.* 2009;53(1):143-146.

65. Fadda R, Rapinett G, Grathwol D, et al. Effects of drinking supplementary water at school on cognitive performance in children. *Appetite.* 2012;59(3):730-737.

66. Kenney EL, Long MW, Cradock AL, Gortmaker SL. Prevalence of inadequate hydration among US children and disparities by gender and race/ethnicity: National Health and Nutrition Examination Survey, 2009-2012. *Am J Public Health.* 2015;105(8):e113-e118.

67. Armstrong LE, Costill DL, Fink WJ. Changes in body water and electrolytes during heat acclimation: effects of dietary sodium. *Aviat Space Environ Med.* 1987;58(2):143-148.

68. Bergeron MF. Heat cramps during tennis: a case report. *Int J Sport Nutr.* 1996;6(1):62-68.

69. Stofan JR, Zachwieja JJ, Horswill CA, Murray R, Anderson SA, Eichner ER. Sweat and sodium losses in NCAA football players: a precursor to heat cramps? *Int J Sports Nutr Exerc Metab.* 2005;15(6):641-652.

70. Nose H, Mack GW, Shi X, Nadel ER. Role of osmolality and plasma volume during rehydration in humans. *J Appl Physiol.* 1988;65(1):325-331.

71. Gisolfi CV, Summers RW, Schedl HP, Bleiler TL. Effect of sodium concentration in a carbohydrate-electrolyte solution on intestinal absorption. *Med Sci Sports Exerc.* 1995;27(10):1414-1420.

72. Wilk B, Bar-Or O. Effect of drink flavor and NaCl on voluntary drinking and hydration in boys exercising in the heat. *J Appl Physiol.* 1996;80(4):1112-1117.

73. Murray R, Stofan J, Eichner ER. Hyponatremia in athletes. *Sports Sci Exch.* 2003;16:1-6.

74. Eichner ER. Six paths to hyponatremia. *Curr Sports Med Rep.* 2009;8(6):280-281.

75. Hew TD, Chorley JN, Cianca JC, Divine JG. The incidence, risk factors, and clinical manifestations of hyponatremia in marathon runners. *Clin J Sport Med.* 2003;13(1):41-47.

76. Davis BA, Thigpen LK, Hornsby JH, Green JM, Coates TE, O'Neal EK. Hydration kinetics and 10-km outdoor running performance following 75% and 150% between bout fluid replacement. *Eur J Sport Sci.* 2014;14(7):703-710.

77. Watson P, Whale A, Mears SA, Reyner LA, Maughan RJ. Mild hypohydration increases the frequency of driver errors during a prolonged, monotonous driving task. *Physiol Behav.* 2015;147:313-318.

78. Adan A. Cognitive performance and dehydration. *J Am Coll Nutr.* 2012;31(2):71-78.

79. Ganio MS, Armstrong LE, Casa DJ, et al. Mild dehydration impairs cognitive performance and mood of men. *Br J Nutr.* 2011;106(10):1535-1543.

80. Cheuvront SN, Sawka MN. Hydration assessment of athletes. *Sports Sci Exch.* 2005;18:1-12.

81. Riedesel ML, Allen DY, Peake GT, Al-Qattan K. Hyperhydration with glycerol solutions. *J Appl Physiol.* 1987;63(6):2262-2268.

82. Murray R, Eddy DE, Paul GL, Seifert JG, Halaby GA. Physiological responses to glycerol ingestion during exercise. *J Appl Physiol.* 1991;71(1):144-149.

83. Freund BJ, Montain SJ, Young AJ, et al. Glycerol hyperhydration: hormonal, renal, and vascular fluid responses. *J Appl Physiol.* 1995;79(6):2069-2077.

84. World Anti-Doping Agency. The World Anti-Doping Code: The 2015 Prohibited List International Standard. www.wada-ama.org/sites/default/files/resources/files/wada-2015-prohibited-list-en.pdf. Published September 20, 2014. Accessed June 13, 2016.

85. Gisolfi CV, Duchman SD. Guidelines for optimal replacement beverages for different athletic events. *Med Sci Sports Exerc.* 1992;24(6):679-687.

86. Coyle EF, Montain SJ. Carbohydrate and fluid ingestion during exercise: are there trade-offs? *Med Sci Sports Exerc.* 1992;24(6):671-678.

87. Ryan AJ, Lambert GP, Shi X, Chang RT, Summers RW, Gisolfi CV. Effect of hypohydration on gastric emptying and intestinal absorption during exercise. *J Appl Physiol.* 1998;84(5):1581-1588.

CHAPTER 7

SUPPLEMENTS AND SPORTS FOODS

Gregory Shaw, BHSc, and Louise M. Burke, OAM, PhD, APD, FACSM

INTRODUCTION

Sports dietitians typically take a food-first approach to meeting sports nutrition goals. This is a laudable focus because of the advantages related to expense, safety, and the potential to achieve a larger range of nutritional goals and health benefits from whole foods and well-planned meals. However, to operate successfully in this field, it is necessary to have an in-depth appreciation of the large range of supplements and sports foods that are marketed to athletes and coaches. At one level, this knowledge is necessary because at least some of these products can provide benefits, which may provide a small but critical part of an athlete's performance plan. On another level, expert knowledge about supplements and sports foods is needed to gain the interest and respect of athletes and coaches because the marketing and allure around these products needs to be addressed with insight. Since there are hundreds of thousands of sports foods and supplements directed at athletes, it is impossible to undertake a summary of each. The aim of this chapter is to provide a framework that allows the sports dietitian to deal with the larger picture of this challenging area of sports nutrition.

What Is a Supplement?

Do I need to take supplements to perform at my best? Many athletes and coaches expect a simple answer to this question because companies market their supplements to closely align with what many athletes and coaches believe are their needs. Because of the incredible range of supplement products, consumers need a system that can quickly identify products that would be beneficial for use and exclude others that are of little value or may cause problems. One difficulty with achieving such a system—and of working with sports supplements in general—is finding a working definition that adequately describes these products and their characteristics. An athlete's idea of what constitutes a supplement may be different from that of a government agency regulating supplement use and can differ again from the views of a sports nutritionist. Supplements have been defined and categorized through a variety of characteristics, including the mode of action and form or function of the active ingredients, or via a regulatory definition; an overview of categorization methods is provided in Box 7.1 (page 134).

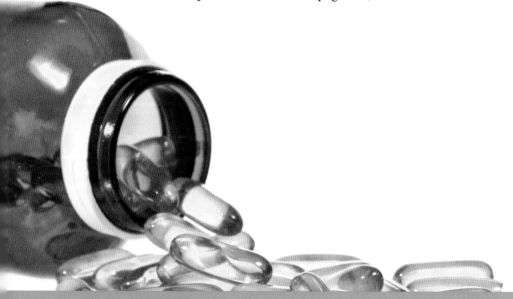

Box 7.1 Frameworks for Defining Sports Supplements

Definition	Example of categories	Comments
Official/regulatory definitions	US Food and Drug Administration (FDA) definition: "A product (other than tobacco) intended to supplement the diet that bears or contains one or more of the following dietary ingredients: a vitamin; a mineral; an herb or other botanical; an amino acid; a dietary substance for use by man to supplement the diet by increasing the total dietary intake; or a concentrate, metabolite, constituent, extract, or combination of any ingredient described previously."	Many consumers are confused by official definitions and may not recognize the role or jurisdiction of regulatory bodies such as FDA.
Form	Pills Powders Drinks Bars	Historically, this definition might have been aligned with factors that could help an athlete make a decision regarding the risks associated with a product: for example, a sports drink or a sports bar might be considered similar to everyday foods, whereas a pill might contain ingredients that are considered more unusual or risky. This distinction has become more blurred with new product development
Availability	Over-the-counter pharmacy Sports shops Supermarkets Internet and mail order Multilevel marketing	The source of a sports food or supplement may provide some level of risk assessment regarding safety and efficacy, with products sold under some supervision (eg, pharmacies) being more reputable than products sold with less oversight (eg, Internet sites). However, these distinctions have become more blurred.
Function	Weight loss Weight gain Recovery Illness prevention Fuel support	This is the way that many supplements are marketed. Many supplements of this type are multi-ingredient, with ingredients varying in their ability to achieve the claimed function. The efficacy of products cannot be judged from their claims, since many claims are not regulated or enforced.
Evidence base	Well-supported benefits Equivocal support Minimal scientific support	Products fit in these categories on a dynamic basis because the evidence around products may ebb and flow according to new research findings. The evidence base for a product is linked to a specific use, rather than universal application to all sports, all athletes, or all protocols of timing or size of dose. While this classification system may help an athlete to make some judgments about the potential use of a supplement product, it should not be the sole factor because other aspects of the product (eg, contamination risk, expense) should be included in decision making.

Regulation

In most countries or regions, there is a governing body or bodies that regulate the manufacture and marketing of foods and therapeutic agents. Such organizations provide a legal definition of a dietary supplement and regulate what can be sold as a dietary supplement and what claims can be made about the product in relation to improving health and function. Specifically, in the United States, a dietary supplement is defined by the Dietary Supplement Health and Education Act of 1994 as[1]:

a product (other than tobacco) intended to supplement the diet that bears or contains one or more of the following dietary ingredients: a vitamin; a mineral; an herb or other botanical; an amino acid; a dietary substance for use by man to supplement the diet by increasing the total dietary intake; or a concentrate, metabolite, constituent, extract, or combination of any ingredient described previously.

Such supplements fall within the jurisdiction of the Office of Dietary Supplement Programs within the US Food and Drug Administration (FDA). Recent changes within this branch have meant an increased scope and function of this division. This has led to increased resources to regulate and, in some cases, prosecute companies and products that have traditionally traded around the edges of the supplement definition.

The definition of dietary supplements is well known in the United States, but they are defined and regulated differently in Europe. The European Union defines a dietary supplement as foodstuffs the purpose of which is to supplement the normal diet and which are concentrated sources of nutrients (meaning vitamins and minerals) or other substances with a nutritional or physiological effect, alone or in combination, marketed in dose form, namely forms such as capsules, pastilles, tablets, pills and other similar forms, sachets of powder, ampoules of liquids, drop dispensing bottles, and other similar forms of liquids and powders designed to be taken in measured small unit quantities[2]:

These food supplements cannot claim the ability to cure or treat a disease but may claim to affect a physiological function. For example, a food supplement cannot claim to cure heart disease but may claim to reduce cholesterol.

In contrast, the definition of a dietary supplement in Australia is based on the form and proposed purpose of the product rather than the specified ingredients or components. Products are regulated by two bodies, which separate them into foods and therapeutic agents. Formulated sports foods are regulated by the Food Standards Australia and New Zealand, and other dietary supplements are considered therapeutic goods taken for the purpose of preventing, curing, or alleviating a disease, ailment, defect, or injury or influencing, inhibiting, or modifying a physiological process and are regulated by the Therapeutic Goods Administration (TGA).

Sports nutrition practitioners need to have an appreciation for global issues around supplement manufacture, marketing, and regulation for several reasons. First, many athletes are now seasoned international travelers and have direct access to products that can be purchased from markets outside their own countries. In addition, via the internet, athletes can purchase products that may be prohibited or unavailable in their local environments; many remain unaware of the implications of the import of such products according to their customs regulations. Finally, free-trade agreements are adding a new challenge to the availability of products in the local environment. In Australia, for example, what is recognized and sold as a dietary supplement is uniquely affected by trade agreements between Australia and its neighbor, New Zealand. In short, a product deemed a dietary supplement in Australia, due to form and composition, may be deemed a food in New Zealand due to differing interpretations of what constitutes a food source or a complementary medicine. Under trade agreements between these countries, a dietary supplement imported or manufactured as a food in New Zealand may be sold as such in Australia and bypass TGA regulation. This ambiguity has allowed products that would otherwise be considered not fit for sale within TGA guidelines to become available for purchase in Australia; some of these products have resulted in positive doping tests by athletes.[3] Although this seems trivial and unique to Australasia, recent global free-trade agreements between all countries and regions mentioned previously have meant that products flow more liberally between jurisdictions. It is now possible for products to be imported and available for on-shelf purchase before regulatory bodies become aware of their existence. This has meant that sports dietitians need to be extremely well-versed in global supplement issues.

Delivery System

Dietary supplements can be presented in a number of forms including solid foods, drinks, small-volume liquids, powders, capsules, and tablets. They can be administered via two distinct routes: oral or infusion, with the latter route including intramuscular and intravascular administration. Although supplements requiring infusion constitute only a small percentage of commercially available products, they warrant a few comments due to the riskier nature of their use, as well as the types of ingredients they often contain. Whereas some products are manufactured in such a format due to limitations of bioavailability via an oral route (eg, vitamin B-12 or iron), other more recent additions to the commercial market are likely to be targeting the perceived commercial advantages of appearing more alluring or scientific to the consumer. Indeed, there have been recent examples of the marketing of peptides, prohormones, and other forms of experimental drugs as supplements, despite the lack of evidence of the efficacy of these products or lack of approval for sale.[4] Worryingly, we note that athletes report self-administration of injectable dietary nutrients as a way of supplementing dietary sources.[5] Athletes (and their nonmedical entourage) should be clearly educated that intravascular and intramuscular injection of nutrients or other supplement compounds should be classified as a medical procedure (or pharmaceutical activity) rather than a nutritional intervention. Additionally, an increased risk of disease transmission or anaphylaxis is of concern for athletes using injectable substances and associated equipment outside of medical supervision and sterile conditions. As such, this should be done only by a trained medical professional as part of an evidence-based strategy to address a diagnosed nutrient deficiency.[6] Athletes should also be aware of current World Anti-Doping Agency (WADA) guidelines outlining the permitted use of injections, their volume, and the frequency of use.[7]

Classification

Recent evolution of the sports food industry has blurred the line between what used to be a food and dietary supplements. Typically, sports foods are considered to be specialized foods (eg, bars, drinks, and gels) with a composition, size, or presentation intended to provide a convenient and practical means of meeting a known goal of sports nutrition.[8] They were originally designed to provide a source of nutrients that might be difficult to consume, particularly around a training session or competitive event, but two significant changes have occurred. First is the increased production of multi-ingredient sports foods that contain ergogenic ingredients in the form of herbal extracts, vitamins, minerals, and chemical metabolites. Food and beverage items that fall within this group could be referred to as functional sports foods and include such examples as sports drinks containing caffeine and sports bars containing creatine. Secondly, increased scientific understanding of nutritional factors that affect performance has allowed the crossover of everyday functional foods into the athletic domain. For example, a probiotic containing specific bacteria that could alter gut microflora may be considered ergogenic because of its ability to reduce the incidence, severity, and duration of upper respiratory tract infections, thereby allowing the athlete to achieve uninterrupted training while minimizing illness.[9,10]

Although Box 7.1 shows the difficulty of producing a single classification system for real-life practice of supplement use by athletes, a system using a composite of these categories may be useful for athletes. It was the principle used in development of the Australian Institute of Sport (AIS) Sports Supplement Program/Framework.[11] This system will be covered in more detail later in this chapter.

A COST-BENEFIT ANALYSIS OF USING SUPPLEMENTS AND SPORTS FOODS

Before making a decision to use a supplement or sports food, each athlete should make a careful analysis of the risks and benefits involved. Figure 7.1 summarizes the important questions that should be answered regarding the costs, safety, efficacy, and legality of any product. While the athlete is ultimately responsible for his or her actions after undertaking this analysis, the sports dietitian may play a key role in providing expert information around the issues that factor into the decision. Sports dietitians should access information sources that provide independent risk-effectiveness assessments of supplements used in sport. Programs such as the Natural Medicines Comprehensive Database and AIS Sports Supplement Framework offer resources around safety and effectiveness that allow a practitioner to gain objective information about the pros (evidence for effectiveness) and cons (health concerns, contraindications, WADA compliance) of supplement use.[11,12]

Pros of Supplement Use

Some supplements and sports foods offer real benefits for athletic performance. Some products can be used by athletes to meet their nutrition goals and, as an indirect outcome, allow the athlete to achieve optimal health, recovery, and performance. This includes sports foods that allow the athlete to achieve the intake of key nutrients in specific amounts, especially in relation to goals for pre-, peri-, and postexercise. In some cases these effects are so well-known and easily demonstrated that beneficial uses of sports foods or supplements are clear-cut. For example, because many studies support the benefits of consuming carbohydrate during exercise or protein after exercise, the use of sports drinks and whey protein supplements by many athletes might be justified, particularly when food sources are unavailable or impractical.[13,14] In addition, when dietary supplements are used to address or prevent a nutrient deficiency that can otherwise reduce performance, the athlete may receive a performance benefit. This situation is well-known in the case of micronutrients such as iron and vitamin D.[15,16] Other products work by producing a direct performance-enhancing (ergogenic) effect. Products that enjoy a good evidence base for beneficial effects on performance include creatine, caffeine, β-alanine, bicarbonate, and beetroot juice/nitrate.[8]

The ergogenic benefits of all these products are related to their correct use. This requires that athletes follow an appropriate protocol in which they address a nutritional goal or physiological limitation to performance. Therefore, education about specific situations and strategies for the use of supplements and sports

THINKING OF TAKING A NEW SUPPLEMENT? ASK YOURSELF THESE IMPORTANT QUESTIONS.

IS IT SAFE?
- Do I recognize all the ingredients on the label and know them to be safe?
- Is it produced by a manufacturer with a good reputation?
- Am I intending to take the recommended dose?
- Have I checked with a sports nutrition expert?
- Will it negatively effect my health in any way?

IS IT LEGAL?
- Is this product and its ingredients permitted for sale in my country?
- Are any of the ingredients of this product banned for use in sport?
- Is it produced by a manufacturer with a good reputation?
- Have I checked with appropriate anti-doping experts?

IS IT EFFECTIVE?
- Does this product have good evidence to show that it can help me to meet my nutrition goals or specifically assist performance of my event?
- Am I intending to take the recommended dose?
- Have I checked with a sports nutrition expert?

CAN I AFFORD IT?
- How much will it cost me and does it fit into my budget?
- Is there a lower cost food choice that I can use instead or for some scenarios?
- Are there other resources or activities that I should be investing in to improve my sports performance?

FIGURE 7.1 Risk: Benefit Analysis to Be Undertaken When Evaluating Whether to Use a Sports Food or Supplement Safely

foods is just as important as the formulation of the product and should be a key component of any supplement program. When products are used in this way, the measureable benefit to performance of the targeted sporting event or exercise protocol is typically in the range of 1% to 3%.[17-21] While this may seem small (and may be difficult to detect with the statistical power available in many traditional studies involving sports science), it is often worthwhile in the competitive world of sport where small margins delineate the winners, and the coefficient of variation (CV) for elite athletes' performance is of a similar magnitude to the performance improvement.[22]

An additional and often misunderstood benefit of supplements and sports foods is the placebo effect, defined as a favorable outcome that arises simply from an individual's belief that her or she has received a beneficial treatment; in a clinical setting, it is often seen when a patient who has a need to receive a therapy responds positively to a sham or inactive substance or treatment. In a sports setting, an athlete who receives enthusiastic marketing material about a new supplement or hears glowing testimonials from other athletes who have used it is more likely to report a positive experience. This effect can often be associated with the hype around products lacking scientific support and is dismissed as lacking robustness or importance. Yet, several studies related to sport have shown that the placebo effect has a significant and measurable effect, which could be added to either real or nonsupported nutrition practices. For example, one study investigated the effect of carbohydrate on a 1-hour cycling time when athletes were given either a sports drink or a sweetened placebo during trial and were provided with different information about what they received.[23] The placebo effect caused by thinking they were receiving a carbohydrate drink allowed the subjects to achieve a small but worthwhile increase in performance, regardless of intake. Being unsure of which treatment was being received increased the variability of performance, illustrating that the greatest benefits from supplement use occur when athletes are confident they are receiving a useful product. Another study found that performance of a 10-km cycling time trial (CV 2.7%) was altered in a dose-response relationship according to subjects' beliefs about how much caffeine they had consumed before their performance.[24] Although no caffeine was actually consumed in any trial, mean power outputs were reduced by 1.4% compared with baseline testing in a trial in which subjects believed they had received a placebo treatment, and mean power increased by 1.3% and 3.1%, respectively, when they believed they had consumed small or large doses of caffeine. Although only the large-dose trial exceeded the CV for power output, the use of magnitude-based statistics suggested a likely dose-response relationship between perceived caffeine ingestion and power output across all trials. Clearly this is an area that requires more study, but it should be harnessed within the way that athletes are educated about the use of supplements and sports foods.

Cons of Supplement Use

Expense is an obvious concern around supplement use, especially when it involves young athletes with limited resources or is compounded for teams and sports programs that have to supply the needs of a group of athletes. This is a particular issue in the case of products that have little scientific evidence of benefits to health or performance. Even where benefits do exist, athletes must acknowledge and prioritize the cost of supplements or sports foods appropriately within their total budget.[8] At times, the expense may be justified, particularly when the product provides the most practical and palatable way to achieve a nutrition goal or when the ergogenic benefits have been well documented. On other occasions, the athlete may choose to limit the use of sports foods, which are more costly than everyday foods, to the most important events or training periods. There are often lower-cost alternatives that can be used, particularly on less critical occasions; for example, a fruit smoothie fortified with milk powder is a less expensive choice to supplement energy and protein intake than many protein powders, while fruit cereal bars or normal confectionery may be a switch for sports bars or sports confectionery.

A less universal but more serious problem associated with the use of supplements and sports is the risk of side effects or unintended health or nutritional consequences. Even the most well-supported sports foods can cause concerns when they are overused or used improperly, with the most recognizable problems being overconsumption of energy.[11] Supplements can be more problematic due to the potential presence of various toxic chemicals as ingredients, undeclared ingredients within proprietary formulas, or contaminants.

Problems arise because consumers are unaware of these ingredients (either in terms of their presence or their toxicity) or because their self-medication or polypharmacy practices mean that they inadvertently consume unsafe amounts or combinations of chemicals. In particular, multi-ingredient supplements targeted at preworkout activation, weight loss, or muscle gain may contain dangerous stimulants or steroid-like chemicals. Products containing ephedra caused a number of medical concerns, including death in susceptible individuals, before they were banned by the FDA in 2004.[25] Most recently, serious health incidents, also including deaths, have been associated with the use of supplements containing the stimulant dimethylhexanamine (also known as DMAA), and the popular weight-loss supplements Hydroxycut and OxyElite Pro have been implicated in cases of severe liver toxicity.[26,27] Table 7.1 provides the caffeine content of a sample of commercial supplements.

Table 7.1 Caffeine Content for Sample of Commercial Supplements

		Caffeine content		
Product name	Serving size, g	Stated on label, mg	Measured, mg	Other stimulants listed in ingredients
Legion Pulse	25.0	350	330.0	
Optimum Nutrition Platinum Pre	8.0	200	217.6	
Vintage Blast	15.0	150	220.4	Synephrine
Citadel Nutrition Tier 1	12.5	200	231.4	
Sheer Strength Pre-Workout	11.9	125	131.3	
MyProtein MyPre Pre-Workout	16.0	200	225.6	
Evlution Nutrition ENGN	8.4	PB[a]	260.6	Picamilon
Top Secret Nutrition Pump Igniter	7.0	300	265.4	Higenamine, picamilon
Ubervita ROCT Workout Ignitor	4.8	PB	200.8	
Six Star Pro Nutrition Pre-Workout N.O. Fury	14.0	185	235.7	
MusclePharm Assault	14.5	250	197.8	
BSN N.O.-XPLODE 2.0	22.5	275	237.3	
MuscleTech Nano Vapor	13.0	130	145.1	
Blackstone Labs Resurgence	11.0	0	0.0	
MRM Driven	12.5	125	121.63	
XPI Oxypump	9.4	PB	122.6	

Continued on next page

Product name	Serving size, g	Stated on label, mg	Measured, mg	Other stimulants listed in ingredients
Vega Sports Pre-Workout Energizer	17.0	100	115.4	
Optimum Nutrition Gold Standard Pre-Workout	10.0	175	159.3	
MusclePharm Arnold Schwarzenegger Iron Pump	6.0	PB	250.0	
Gaspari Nutrition SuperPump Max	16.0	PB	204.2	
SEI Performance Series ReFUEL-RSQ 5.0	5.0	-	-	
VPX Shotgun 5X	20.5	PB	191.7	Hordenine HCL[b]
Professional Supplements Mr. Hyde	7.5	419	78.9	Hordenine HCL, yohimbine, picamilon
Universal Nutrition Shock Therapy	20.0	PB	191.4	
iSatori Pre-Gro	8.0	175	157.2	Hordenine HCL
SNI Hardcore Series Nitric Shock	20.0	-	-	
Cellucor C4 Extreme	5.7	150	142.9	Synephrine
BSN Hyper FX	9.3	PB	212.2	
Red Leaf Pre-Workout Energizer	5.7	40	58.9	
Hi-Tech Pharmaceuticals N.O. Overload	8.0	-	-	
USP Labs Jack3d	5.1	100	118.3	Yohimbine
Muscle Warfare Napalm	5.5	PB	170.9	Hordenine
BPI Sports 1.M.R.	5.0	PB	255.9	Yohimbine
Gaspari Nutrition SuperDrive	6.0	PB	247.6	
Six Star Pro Nutrition Pre-Workout Ignition	6.0	PB	107.9	
Total Body Nutrition 1,3D NOX	6.0	PB	298.1	Hordenine, dendrobium

Continued on next page

Table 7.1: Caffeine Content for Sample of Commercial Supplements (Continued)

Product name	Serving size, g	Stated on label, mg	Measured, mg	Other stimulants listed in ingredients
MuscleMeds No Bull	12.0	PB	352.8	
Cobra Labs The Curse Pre-Workout	5.0	155	71.9	
Metabolic Nutrition E.S.P. Pre-Workout	3.3	PB	141.0	
Nutrex Research OutLift Pre-Workout	25.9	350	376.6	
Lecheek Nutrition Speed X3 Test	8.3	PB	212.6	Hordenine HCL
Nutrex Research Hemo Rage Black	8.6	PB	311.6	Synephrine
Naturo Nitro Octane	6.7	PB	260.2	Picamilon, hordenine HCL, dendrobium
Human Evolution Extreme OverRide	6.15	PB	307.3	Hordenine HCL
Betancourt Bullnox Androrush	18.1	PB	118.4	Synephrine
Train Critical FX	5.0	PB	129.5	Hordenine HCL, synephrine, octapamine, yohimbine, higenamine, beta-methylphenethylamine

a PB = proprietary blend
b HCL = hydrochloride

Another pressing problem for athletes is the potential for supplements to contain ingredients that are prohibited by the anti-doping codes of WADA and other sports bodies. These include prohormones (steroid-related compounds such as androstenedione, dehydroepiandrosterone [DHEA], and 19-norandrostene-dione), stimulants (eg, ephedrine, DMAA, sibutramine), and peptide hormones (eg, growth hormone releasing peptide-2, or GHRP-2). Drug education programs highlight the need for athletes to read the labels of supplements and sports foods carefully to ensure that they do not contain such banned substances. This is a responsibility that athletes must master to reduce the risk of an inadvertent antidoping rule violation (ADRV). However, many athletes and their support staff are either not aware of the problem or are convinced it is a problem that only occurs for other people. Because this problem has increased in recognition if not prevalence in the last decade, it will receive further attention at the end of this chapter.

THE SPORTS SUPPLEMENT PROGRAM/FRAMEWORK OF THE AUSTRALIAN INSTITUTE OF SPORT

Some sporting organizations (eg, the National Collegiate Athletic Association) or institutions (eg, the English Institute of Sport) make policies or programs for supplement use on behalf of athletes within their care. The experiences of the Sports Supplement Program of the AIS provide a case history of the management of the use of supplements and sports foods within a high-performance sport environment. The AIS program was initiated in 2000 to manage the supplement use of high-performance athletes within the AIS's scholarship program after an assessment of unsound practices within this population. It was developed as a multidisciplinary project and conducted under the oversight of the Sports Supplement Panel that included experts in sports nutrition, physiology, medicine, strength and conditioning, policy, and antidoping professionals from the AIS. Its activities were integrated into all aspects of the leadership roles of the AIS and the scholarship requirements of its athletes, with the following goals[8]:

- To allow its athletes to focus on the sound use of supplements and specific sports foods as part of their specific nutrition plans;
- To ensure that supplements and sports foods are used correctly and appropriately to deliver maximum benefits to the immune system, recovery, and performance;
- To give its athletes the confidence that they receive cutting-edge advice and achieve state-of-the-art nutrition practices; and
- To ensure that supplement use does not lead to an inadvertent doping offense.

Elements of the AIS Sports Supplement Program included an education arm to provide information suited to different groups within its community (sports science/medicine professionals, athletes, and coaches), a research arm to continue to develop the evidence base on which decisions about supplement use would be made, a provision arm to allow a supply of low-risk sports foods and supplements to be made available to athletes within a supervised sports nutrition program, and a governance arm to ensure that all components were managed with professionalism and transparency.

Evaluation of the impact of the AIS Sports Supplement Program suggests that not only has it gained international recognition for its categorization system and high-quality education resources, but it has also played a role in changing supplementation practices of the athletes with whom it directly worked. It should be noted that while the program educated athletes, including teaching them how to use its classification system to identify supplements lacking an evidence base, it still relied on athletes to make the final decision about their use of these products. A survey of supplement use by elite Australian swimmers, of whom AIS swimmers made up one-third of the cohort, revealed significant differences in self-reported practices.[28] Overall, 97% of swimmers reported taking supplements or sports foods over the preceding 12 months. AIS swimmers reported using a greater number of products overall, including a greater number of products considered to be performance supplements. However, they were less likely to use supplements considered to be lacking scientific support and more likely to report sports dietitians and sports physicians as advisers of their supplement use. The AIS swimmers sourced a greater percentage of their supplements from an organized program ($94\% \pm 16\%$) compared with other swimmers ($40\% \pm 32\%$) ($P < .001$) who sourced a greater percentage ($30\% \pm 30\%$) of their dietary supplements from supermarkets. These findings suggest a positive impact of the program, with the authors suggested that providing access to evidence-based supplements and sports foods was an important aspect of its implementation.[28]

Recently, the operation of the AIS Sports Supplement Program has evolved into an advisory framework with the responsibility for the use of supplements within Australia's high-performance sport environment falling under the oversight of National Sporting Organisations (NSO). The external review of many of these NSOs by government funding agencies requires the existence of a supplement policy as a key item of governance, cementing the importance of reference frameworks such as the AIS Sports Supplement Program resources. Although this is an Australian example, it highlights the importance that some national governments may be placing on the safe, effective, and legal use of supplements and sports foods in the high-performance sports environment.

A key part of the AIS Sports Supplement Program/Framework is the ABCD classification system for supplements and sports foods, a ranking system with four tiers. Each tier has a suggested level of use that would be justified within a specific sports supplement program. The program is underpinned by a risk-benefit assessment by a panel of sports nutrition, medicine, and sports science experts of the evidence base for the beneficial uses of each product. Although the hierarchy of categories was developed for long-term use, there is a regular assessment of supplements and sports foods to ensure that they are placed in the category that best fits the available scientific evidence. The hierarchical system allows the program to avoid the black-and-white assessment that any particular product works or fails to live up to claims. Rather, the available science is reviewed to place supplements into categories ranked from what is most likely to provide a benefit for little risk to what provides least benefit and a definite risk. Box 7.2 provides a summary of the AIS Sports Supplement Classification model at the time of publication of this review, with some details of the potential evidence-based uses of products within Category A detailed in Box 7.2. Further information about supplements and sports can be sourced from the framework website (www.ausport.gov.au/ais/supplements).[11]

This example clearly demonstrates that programs designed to educate athletes on supplement use combined with access to low-risk, evidence-based dietary supplements can positively influence athlete practice. A key takeaway message should be the inclusion of sports nutrition professionals as sources of objective advice and gatekeepers to the access of these products.

Box 7.2 Summary of ABCD Categories of Australian Institute of Sport Sports Supplement Framework 2016[11]

Group A Supplements

Overview of category	Subcategories	Examples
Evidence level: Supported for use in specific situations in sport using evidence-based protocols **Use within supplement programs:** Provided or permitted for use by some athletes according to best-practice protocols	**Sports foods:** Specialized products used to provide a practical source of nutrients when it is impractical to consume everyday foods	Sports drink Sports gel Sports confectionery Liquid meal Whey protein Sports bar Electrolyte replacement
	Medical supplements: Used to treat clinical issues, including diagnosed nutrient deficiencies Requires individual dispensing and supervision by appropriate sports medicine/science practitioner	Iron supplement Calcium supplement Multivitamin/mineral Vitamin D Probiotics (gut/immune)
	Performance supplements: Used to directly contribute to optimal performance Should be used in individualized protocols under the direction of an appropriate sports medicine/science practitioner While there may be a general evidence base for these products, additional research may often be required to fine-tune protocols for individualized and event-specific use.	Caffeine B-alanine Bicarbonate Beetroot juice Creatine

Continued on next page

Group B Supplements

Overview of category	Subcategories	Examples
Evidence level: Deserving of further research and could be considered for provision to athletes under a research protocol or case-managed monitoring situation **Use within supplement programs:** Provided to athletes within research or clinical monitoring situations	**Food polyphenols:** Food chemicals that have purported bioactivity, including antioxidant and anti-inflammatory activity May be consumed in food form or as an isolated chemical. **Other**	Quercetin Tart cherry juice Exotic berries (acai, goji, etc) Curcumin Antioxidants C and E Carnitine β-hydroxy β-methylbutyrate (also known as HMB) Glutamine Fish oils Glucosamine

Group C Supplements

Overview of category	Subcategories	Examples
Evidence level: Have little meaningful proof of beneficial effects **Use within supplement programs:** Not provided to athletes within supplement programs May be permitted for individualized use by an athlete where there is specific approval from (or reporting to) a sports supplement panel	Category A and B products used outside approved protocols. **The rest:** If you can't find an ingredient or product in Groups A, B, or D, it probably deserves to be here. Note that the framework will no longer name Group C supplements or supplement ingredients in this topline layer of information. This will avoid the perception that these supplements are special.	Fact sheets and research summaries on some supplements of interest belonging in Group C may be found on the A–Z of Supplements page in the AIS[a] Sports Nutrition section of the ASC[b] website (www.ausport.gov.au/ais/nutrition/supplements). The fact sheet will identify that such ingredients have been placed in the Group C category without drawing undue attention to them.

Group D Supplements

Overview of category use within AIS system	Subcategories	Examples
Evidence level: Banned or at high risk of contamination with substances that could lead to a positive drug test **Use within supplement programs:** Should not be used by athletes	**Stimulants** WADA[c] list **Prohormones and hormone boosters** WADA list	Ephedrine Strychnine Sibutramine DMAA[d] Other herbal stimulants DHEA[e] Androstenedione 19-norandrostenedione/ol Other prohormones Tribulus terrestris and other testosterone boosters Maca root powder

Continued on next page

Group D Supplements *(Continued)*

Overview of category use within AIS system	Subcategories	Examples
	GH releasers and peptides	
	WADA list	
	Technically, while these are sometimes sold as supplements (or have been described as such), they are usually unapproved pharmaceutical products.	
	Other	Glycerol used for rehyperhydration strategies—banned as a plasma expander
	WADA[e] list	
		Colostrum—not recommended by WADA due to the inclusion of growth factors in its composition

[a] AIS = Australian Institute of Sport
[b] ASC = Australian Sports Commission
[c] WADA = World Anti-Doping Agency.
[d] DMAA = dimethylhexanamine
[e] DHEA = dehydroepiandrosterone

PROBLEMS AND SOLUTIONS RELATED TO SUPPLEMENTS AND ANTI-DOPING RULE VIOLATIONS

Since the late 1990s, athletes have been warned about the risk of the presence of banned substances in dietary supplements. Education strategies promote the careful scrutiny of product labels and ingredient lists before the use of any product. However, even when athletes take such precautions, inadvertent intake of banned substances from supplements can occur. This outcome arises because some supplements contain banned products without declaring them as ingredients, typically as a result of contamination or poor labeling within lax manufacturing processes. However, there have been some cases where therapeutic doses of steroid compounds have been detected in supplements, suggesting a deliberate strategy by manufacturers to develop a following for their products as a result of testimonials that "they work."[29,30]

The initial evidence of supplement contamination was established in 2004 by a market survey from a laboratory accredited by the International Olympic Committee.[31] This study analyzed 634 supplements from 215 suppliers in 13 countries, with products being sourced from retail outlets (91%), the internet (8%), and telephone sales. Of the supplements sampled, 94 (15%) were found to contain hormones or prohormones that were not stated on the product label. The country of origin of these tainted supplements, according to the labels, included the United States, the Netherlands, the United Kingdom, Italy, and Germany; however, these products were purchased in other countries. In fact, 10% to 20% of products purchased in Spain and Austria were found to be contaminated. Just over 20% of the products made by companies selling prohormones were positive for undeclared prohormones, but 10% of products from companies that did not sell steroid-containing supplements were also positive. The supplements included amino acid and protein powders, and products containing creatine, carnitine, ribose, guarana, zinc, pyruvate, β-hydroxy β-methylbutyrate (also known as HMB), *Tribulus terrestris*, herbal extracts, and vitamins and minerals.

Since then, further reports of poor product labeling, deliberate adulteration, and contamination have continued to emerge from independent studies and from reports by commercial companies that undertake specific audits of supplement products.[30-32] Whether the risk of supplement contamination has decreased in line with increased awareness of the problem is equivocal. However, it appears that the prohibited ingredients involved in supplement-related ADRV cases are changing. More recently, stimulants have become the most prevalent cause of supplement-related ADRVs, with many national anti-doping agencies reporting an increase in cases involving DMAA.[3] Between 2010 and 2014, this product was reported on the ingredient list of dietary supplements under a number of botanical and chemical names, including dimethylhexanamine,

dimethylamylamine, dimethylpentylamine, pentylamine, geranamine, forthane, 2-amino-4-methylhexane, geranium root extract, or geranium oil.[33] The supplement products most at risk of contamination or mislabeling with stimulants are those targeting weight loss or preworkout goals.

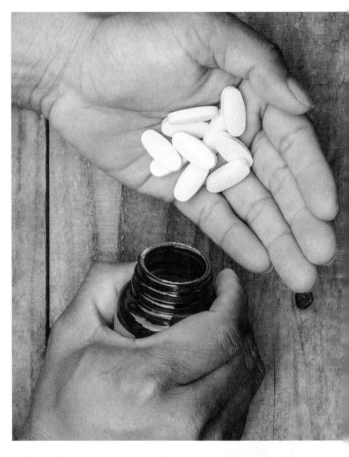

The WADA Code is built on strict liability: athletes assume responsibility for any substance found in their body, regardless of its origin. Although an ADRV is recorded in all situations where a biological specimen taken from an athlete records the presence of banned substances, sanctions arising from the outcome may differ according to the sporting authority involved, appeals through Court of Arbitration for Sport, and the detection of mitigating circumstances. In various real-life cases, sanctions have varied dramatically from a suspended sentence to a 4-year ban from participation in sport. Regardless of the sanction, however, the athlete carries the indelible reputation of having incurred an ADRV; even in cases where athletes received large financial compensation from supplement manufacturers or reduced periods of suspension from sport, they have stated that the sullying of their reputation caused overwhelming personal distress and loss of income. Therefore, the risk of the ADRV from supplement use is of major concern to sport.

Many athletes feel that doping concerns are only relevant to their elite counterparts. However, antidoping regulations cover all registered members and competitors of sporting organizations that are signatories to an antidoping code such as the WADA Code and thus apply to most sports people. While the risk of being selected to provide a biological specimen and record an analytical positive form of an ADRV is likely to be negligible in lower-level competitions, all methods of incurring an ADRV that involve evidence of the use of a banned substance are real for all levels of competitive athletes. For example, in Australia, a large percentage of the athletes currently serving sanctions for ADRV are from subelite competition levels. These infractions were noted from traditional urine and blood-based testing and from other sources, such as the seizure of imported supplements containing banned substances by customs authorities.[34]

There are now numerous programs and resources, including websites (eg, supplement411.org, run by the US Anti-Doping Agency) and smartphone applications (eg, Aegis Shield) to help athletes manage the risk associated with consuming a banned substance contained in a dietary supplement. These outline the general risks associated with supplement use and provide data or insights that allow athletes to make informed decisions about the risks associated with general or specific products. Many of these programs are built around or support activities known as third-party auditing of dietary supplements, a process whereby manufacturers submit their supply chains, manufacturing facilities, and end products for scrutiny around the presence of banned substances.[32] A commercial industry has developed around the business model of providing supplement companies with independent risk-analysis and batch testing services to enhance or confirm their quality control and provide a marketing edge of clean supplements to consumers. Certification programs around the world include Informed Sport, NSF Certified for Sport, and BSCG Certified Drug Free. Generally, such programs prior to commercial release undertake testing of samples from each supplement batch for the presence of approximately 200 substances from the WADA List of Prohibited Substances and Methods, such as S1 (anabolic agents), S3 (β2-agonists), S5 (diuretics), S6 (stimulants), P2 (β-blockers) Although these testing profiles are not as expansive as the open-ended WADA list, they include the majority of the most common banned substances and provide athletes with a credible reduction in the risk of supplement contamination, as well as a continual reminder of the issue. Athletes should be aware that there are other auditing programs with varying types of auditing activities (eg, facility testing, one-off random sampling, no ongoing testing required) and with different levels of rigor. Indeed, there is almost a need for an audit of the auditors to ensure that the level of risk assessment of supplement safety is understood by the end user. Sports dietitians can be a key information source for athletes in this area.

Activities that can be undertaken with an athlete to reduce the risk of ADRVs from supplement use include seeking continual updates on the issue, identifying low-risk products and manufacturers, and keeping a record of dietary supplement and sports food use. While no supplement or sports food can be classified as entirely risk free, appropriate choices can help minimize the risk to an acceptably low level. Keeping records of product use (product name, source of purchase, batch or product number, etc) can be useful if an antidoping rule violation does occur. In addition to allowing the source of contamination to be investigated, it can demonstrate to authorities that all due concern was taken with supplement use when the penalty for the ADRV is being decided.

SUMMARY

Sports dietitians are challenged by the excitement of athletes and coaches around the almost never-ending range of products that claim to provide benefits to enhance sports performance. The poor regulation of supplements and sports foods in many countries allows athletes and coaches to be the targets of marketing campaigns based on exaggerated claims and hype rather than documented benefits. However, there is evidence that a number of products, including sports foods, medical supplements, and performance supplements, can offer true benefits to performance or the achievement of nutritional goals. A systematic approach to educating athletes and coaches about supplements and sports foods and managing their provision to athletes and teams can allow athletes to include the successful use of these products with the activities that underpin optimal performance.

Supplements are not a shortcut to success and do not replace a well-planned periodized meal plan that meets the requirements of the athlete's training program. In a few situations where supplements may provide a performance advantage, sports dietitians are encouraged to work with athletes and coaches to ensure protocols are achievable and effective.

The definitions and categorizations of dietary supplements are broad and can include products that provide practical sources of nutrients, address medical or clinical issues related to nutrient deficiencies, or achieve indirect or direct effects on performance. Sports dietitians should be well versed in the numerous ways of classifying dietary supplements and on the intended modes of use. They should also be aware of products that are sold or promoted as dietary supplements but are more accurately defined as pharmaceutical agents.

Sports dietitians should have an in-depth understanding of the safety, legality, and effectiveness of dietary supplements, which allows them to educate athletes to make informed decisions about use of dietary supplements.

Programs that include sports dietitians and other professionals as key gatekeepers to supplement access may provide a safe and supportive environment in which athletes follow evidence-based supplement practices, as opposed to unregulated use.

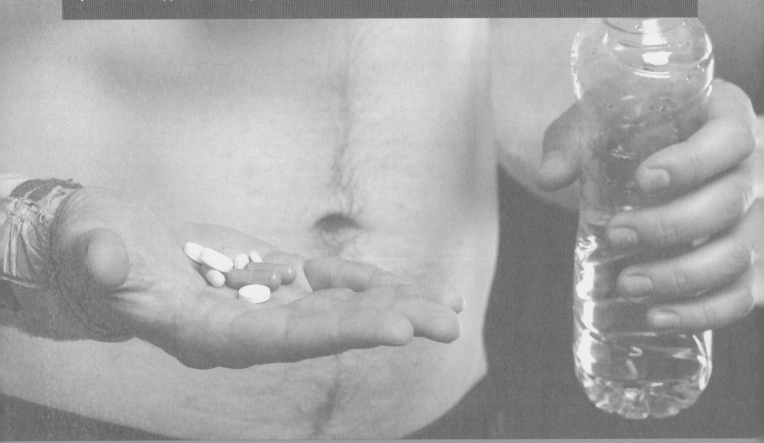

REFERENCES

1. Dietary Supplement Health and Education Act of 1994. 21 USC §321 (1994).

2. European Parliament and Council. Directive 2002/46/ec of the European Parliament and of the Council of 10 June 2002 on the approximation of the laws of the member states relating to food supplements. (2002).

3. Australian Sports Anti-Doping Authority. *Australian Sports Anti-Doping Authority, 2011-12 Annual Report.* Canberra, Australia: Australian Sports Anti-Doping Authority; 2012.

4. Australian Football League. Australian Football League, Notice of Charge Rule 1.6, Essendon Football Club. Melbourne, August 13, 2013. www.afl.com.au/staticfile/AFL%20Tenant/AFL/Files/EssendonFC-notice-of-charges.pdf. Accessed December 15, 2015.

5. Corrigan B, Kazlauskas R. Medication use in athletes selected for doping control at the Sydney Olympics. *Clin J Sport Med.* 2003;13(1):33-40.

6. Clénin GE, Cordes M, Huber A, et al. Iron deficiency in sports—definition, influence on performance and therapy: consensus statement of the Swiss Society of Sports Medicine. *Swiss Med Wkly.* 2015;145:w14196.

7. World Anti-Doping Agency. Prohibited List: January 2016. www.wada-ama.org/sites/default/files/resources/files/wada-2016-prohibited-list-en.pdf. Accessed January 1, 2016.

8. Burke LM, Cato L. Supplements and sports foods. In: Burke LM, Deakin V, ed. *Clinical Sports Nutrition.* 5th ed. Sydney, Australia: McGraw-Hill Australia; 2015:493-591.

9. West NP, Pyne DB, Cripps AW, et al. Lactobacillus fermentum (pcc®) supplementation and gastrointestinal and respiratory-tract illness symptoms: a randomised control trial in athletes. *Nutr J.* 2011;10:30.

10. Gleeson M, Bishop NC, Oliveira M, Tauler P. Daily probiotic's (lactobacillus casei shirota) reduction of infection incidence in athletes. *Int J Sport Nutr Exerc Metab.* 2011;21(1):55-64.

11. Supplements. AIS website. www.ausport.gov.au/ais/nutrition/supplements. Accessed May 23, 2016.

12. Natural Medicines Comprehensive Database website. http://naturaldatabase.therapeuticresearch.com. Accessed May 23, 2016.

13. Stellingwerff T, Cox GR. Systematic review: carbohydrate supplementation on exercise performance or capacity of varying durations. *Appl Physiol Nutr Metab.* 2014;39(9):998-1011.

14. Cermak NM, Res PT, de Groot LC, Saris WH, van Loon LJ. Protein supplementation augments the adaptive response of skeletal muscle to resistance-type exercise training: a meta-analysis. *Am J Clin Nutr.* 2012;96(6):1454-1464.

15. Deakin V, Peeling P. Prevention, detection and treatment of iron depletion and deficiency in athletes. In: Burke LM, Deakin V, ed. *Clinical Sports Nutrition.* 5th ed. Sydney, Australia: McGraw-Hill Australia; 2015:266-302.

16. Willis KS, Peterson NJ, Larson-Meyer DE. Should we be concerned about the vitamin D status of athletes? *Int J Sport Nutr Exerc Metab.* 2008;18(2):204-224.

17. Burke LM, Desbrow B, Spriet L. *Caffeine and Sports Performance.* Champaign, IL: Human Kinetics; 2013.

18. Carr AJ, Hopkins WG, Gore CJ. Effects of acute alkalosis and acidosis on performance: a meta-analysis. *Sports Med.* 2011;41(10):801-814.

19. Buford TW, Kreider RB, Stout JR, et al. International Society of Sports Nutrition position stand: creatine supplementation and exercise. *J Int Soc Sports Nutr.* 2007;4(1):6.

20. Trexler ET, Smith-Ryan AE, Stout JR, et al. International Society of Sports Nutrition Position Stand: beta-alanine. *J Int Soc Sports Nutr.* 2015;12:30.

21. Jones AM. Dietary nitrate supplementation and exercise performance. *Sports Med.* 2014;44(suppl 1):35S-45S.

22. Hopkins WG, Hawley JA, Burke LM. Design and analysis of research on sport performance enhancement. *Med Sci Sports Exerc.* 1999;31(3):472-485.

23. Clark VR, Hopkins WG, Hawley JA, Burke LM. Placebo effect of carbohydrate feedings during a 40-km cycling time trial. *Med Sci Sports Exerc.* 2000;32(9):1642-1647.

24. Beedie CJ, Stuart EM, Coleman DA, Foad AJ. Placebo effects of caffeine on cycling performance. *Med Sci Sports Exerc.* 2006;38(12):2159-2164.

25. Phillips GC. Medicolegal issues and ergogenic aids: trade, tragedy, and public safety, the example of ephedra and the Dietary Supplement Health and Education Act. *Curr Sports Med Rep.* 2004;3(4):224-228.

26. Forrester M. Exposures to 1,3-dimethylamylamine-containing products reported to Texas poison centers. *Hum Exp Toxicol.* 2013;32(1):18-23.

27. Centers for Disease Control and Prevention. Notes from the field: acute hepatitis and liver failure following the use of a dietary supplement intended for weight loss or muscle building: May-October 2013. *Morb Mortal Wkly Rep.* 2013;62(40):817-819.

28. Shaw G, Slater G, Burke L. Supplement use of elite Australian swimmers. *Int J Sport Nutr Exerc Metab.* 2016;26(3):249-258.

29. Judkins C, Prock P. Supplements and inadvertent doping—how big is the risk to athletes. *Med Sport Sci.* 2012;59:143-152.

30. Geyer H, Parr MK, Koehler K, Mareck U, Schänzer W, Thevis M. Nutritional supplements cross-contaminated and faked with doping substances. *J Mass Spectrom.* 2008;43(7):892-902.

31. Geyer H, Parr MK, Mareck U, Reinhart U, Schrader Y, Schanzer W. Analysis of non-hormonal nutritional supplements for anabolic-androgenic steroids—results of an international study. *Int J Sports Med.* 2004;25(2):124-129.

32. Judkins CM, Teale P, Hall DJ. The role of banned substance residue analysis in the control of dietary supplement contamination. *Drug Test Anal.* 2010;2(9):417-420.

33. Outram S. Doping through supplement use: a review of the available empirical data. *Int J Sport Nutr Exerc Metab.* 2015;25(1):54-59.

34. Australian Sports Anti-Doping Agency media release. Doping violation. Four-year sporting ban for Queensland Rugby player Francis Bourke. May 30, 2012. www.asada.gov.au/publications/media/media_releases/asada_release_120530_Francis_Bourke_rugby_union.pdf. Accessed February 25, 2015.

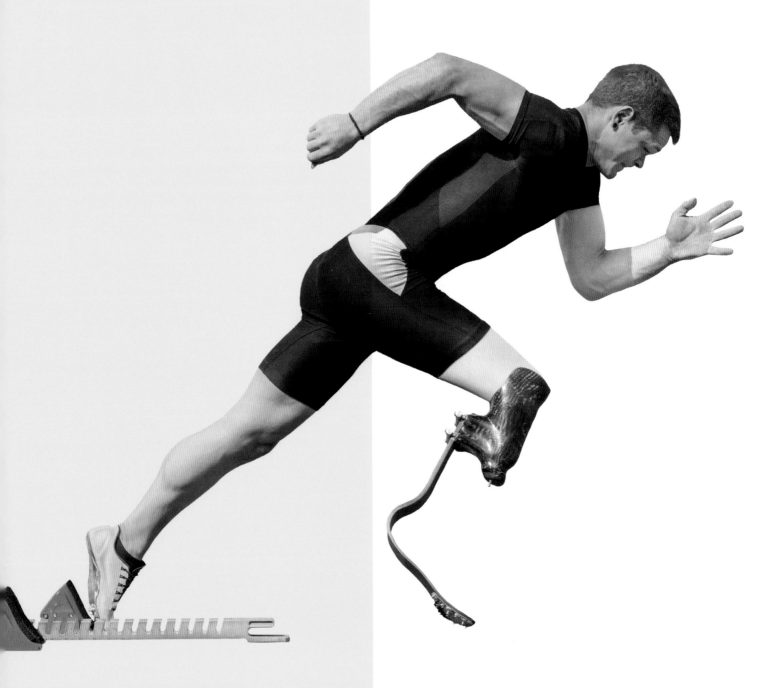

SECTION 2

Behavior change theories provide a framework for describing behaviors and barriers to change. One of the most popular is the Transtheoretical Model, which finds that change occurs over time.[5]

The sports RDN must select the appropriate assessment tools, distinguish relevant and important data from irrelevant and unimportant data, and determine the need for additional information. Once all data are obtained, the data must be analyzed and interpreted, which requires identification of the appropriate standard for comparison. The most widely accepted standards in sports nutrition are the Joint Position Statement on Nutrition and Athletic Performance and the International Olympic Committee (IOC) Consensus Statement on Sports Nutrition (see FIgure 8.1).[6,7] Once the nutrition assessment is completed, the RDN can make a nutrition diagnosis and develop a plan for nutrition intervention. Continued monitoring and evaluation will determine whether revision of the assessment and updated recommendations are required.

The following sections provide the practitioner with an overview of the various components of the nutrition assessment as applied to the athlete according to the Academy of Nutrition and Dietetics Standards of Practice and Standards of Professional Performance for Registered Dietitian Nutritionists (Competent, Proficient, and Expert) in Sports Nutrition and Dietetics.[8] The sports RDN will need to use his or her judgment as to which components to include because a complete assessment is not always necessary or practical. For example, an athlete who is referred for low levels of vitamin D may not need an evaluation of body composition. The athlete's stated primary concern should be prioritized, but the RDN must be able to read between the lines to uncover other issues that may affect health and performance. For example, an athlete who requests guidance on recovery foods may reveal disordered eating ideations during the diet history. Figure 8.1 (page 156) shows an assessment form used by the US Olympic Committee. Box 8.2 (page 159) provides a case study of the nutrition assessment of an athlete training for a marathon run.

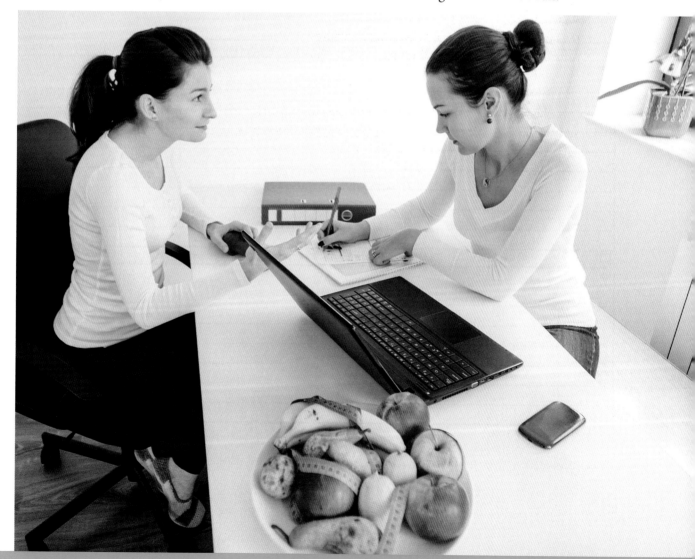

United States Olympic Committee	USA ⭕⭕⭕	Sport Nutrition Assessment Form

Athlete Demographics Sport: ___ Date: ___

Name:	DOB	Gender
Phone:	Email:	
Training location:	Coach:	

Purpose:

Anthropometry

Date	WT	HT	Σ7-8 skinfold	%BF	Method	WT class	Comp WT	Problems and Solutions

Biochemistry (e.g., iron status, vit D status, Hb & Hct, other anemias, metabolic profile, lipids, hormones)

Hx

Date	Parameter	Comments	Treatment

Clinical (e.g., illness, injury, DE/ED, MD, bone, fatigue, GI, allergies, dehydration, sleep, overtraining, physical signs)

Hx

Date	Issue	Comments	Treatment

FIGURE 8.1 United States Olympic Committee Sports Dietetics Assessment Form

Continued on next page

Clinical (e.g., Medications, Dietary/Sports Supplements)

Date	Medication/Supplement & Dosage/Brand	Risks vs Benefits?

Dietary (e.g., usual intake, FFQ)

Meal	Time	Food/Fluids	Intervention
Breakfast			
AM TR			
Lunch			
PM TR			
Dinner			
Snack			
Summary			

Food Frequency Questionnaire

PRO	red meat	poultry	game	fish	soy	eggs	yogurt	milk	cheese	Risks?
CHO	pasta	rice	potatoes	cereals	breads	tortillas	grains	legumes	panc/waff	
F/V	fruit				vegetables					
FAT	nuts/seeds	butter	olive oil	other oils	dressings	mayo	mustard	olives	hummus	
FLUIDS	soda/diet	alcohol	coffee	tea	water					
SNACKS	cookies	ice cream	candy	crackers	chips					

#meals/d	#meals out/wk	#snacks/d	#meals cooked/wk
Restaurants			

Environmental PREP PRE-COMP COMP OFF

Cycle	MON	TUE	WED	THU	FRI	SAT/SUN	Issues & Strategies: Training Nutrition
Intensity							
Intensity							
Intensity							

Peaking

Date	COMPETITION	Location	Issues & Strategies: Competition Nutrition
Overall Summary			

FIGURE 8.1 United States Olympic Committee Sports Dietetics Assessment Form (Continued)

Continued on next page

Summary and Follow Up Plan

USA

Nutrition Diagnosis (PES)

Goals & Intervention

Monitoring & Evaluation

Progress Notes

Date	
Date	
Date	
Date	
Date	
Date	
Date	

FIGURE 8.I United States Olympic Committee Sports Dietetics Assessment Form (Continued)

Box 8.2 Case Study: Female Marathoner

Athlete Description and Goals:

DW, a 22-year-old woman training for a marathon with a goal of completing it in under 4 hours

Anthropometrics,:

Height: 5′5″   Weight: 140 lb   Body mass index: 23.3

Waist circumference: 28″

Body composition as assessed with skinfold calipers: 25% body fat = 35 lb (16 kg) fat mass + 105 lb (48 kg) lean mass

Food and Nutrition-Related History:

Weight fluctuates between 135 and 140 lb. Athlete feels "lighter" at 135 lb. In the past she has reduced her intake of breads and other grains to achieve weight loss. A 24-hour recall and food frequency questionnaire were obtained. DW usually avoids food before her morning run, although she does drink a cup of coffee. She has a yogurt for breakfast once she gets to work, about 1.5 hours later. She alternates between a salad and a sandwich for lunch and will have a piece of fruit for an afternoon snack. If she is really hungry she may eat two or three cookies or a small bag of chips. Dinner is variable. She may prepare chicken or fish and vegetables or pick up items such as a burrito bowl or two slices of pizza. She drinks a glass of wine an average of three nights a week, with two glasses on Saturday nights. On weekends she will have half a bagel with butter and coffee before her long run, then pancakes with butter and syrup after. She drinks mostly water, although she does not drink during her runs. She takes a generic multivitamin and mineral supplement most days. She knows that carbohydrates are important for marathon running but also believes they lead to weight gain.

An analysis of DW's 24-hour recall indicates that she consumed 1,675 kcal, 100 g protein, and 210 g carbohydrate. Alcohol was not consumed on the day of the recall.

DW needs an estimated 1,740 kcal daily, with an additional 90 kcal for every mile she runs.[65] Her current training schedule ranges from 4 miles on short days to 11 miles on long days, requiring an additional 360 to 990 kcal for a total energy expenditure of 2,100 to 2,730 kcal.

DW had an annual physical 1 month ago. Complete blood count, lipid profile, blood glucose, vitamin D, and electrolytes were all within normal limits.

DW presents as a well-nourished, fit individual. She has a normal menstrual cycle and does not report gastrointestinal or other medical issues. She reports infrequent urination and darker urine on days of long runs than on other days of the week.

Comparison with Standards:

Energy availability (EA)[1]

Energy intake (Ein) = 1,650 kcal

Energy expenditure of exercise (EEE)= 360 kcal

EA = Ein − EEE = 1,290 kcal

Recommended EA = 30 to 45 kcal/kg fat-free mass = 30 x 48 kg = 1,440 kcal

Carbohydrate intake -= 6 to 7 g/kg body weight = 384 to 448 g for current level of training.[6] This should increase to 7 to 8 g/kg as her mileage increases.

- Current intake: 210 g carbohydrate
- Protein intake: (1.2 g/kg body weight) 77 g[6]
- Current intake: 100 g
- Fluids: Inadequate consumption before and during exercise
- Calcium intake: 600 mg   Dietary Reference Intake: 1,000 mg
- Iron intake: 12 mg   Dietary Reference Intake: 18 mg

Nutrition Diagnoses:

- Inadequate energy availability
- Inadequate carbohydrate intake
- More than adequate protein intake
- Inadequate fluid intake
- Inadequate calcium intake
- Inadequate iron intake

ANTHROPOMETRIC NUTRITION ASSESSMENT

Anthropometric measurements are used to estimate body composition. A two-compartment model estimates the percentage of fat and fat-free mass. All methods of assessing body composition in live individuals involve indirect measurements and rely on prediction equations; therefore, all contain error and should not be thought of as precise measurements.

Some sports are associated with specific body types, although there is no consensus as to optimal body fat percentages for either health or physical performance.[4] Athletes participating in power sports may benefit from a specific power-to-weight ratio, while others, such as gymnasts and figure skaters, prefer minimal body fat. The purpose of collecting anthropometric data is to evaluate the body composition and growth of the athlete. Keep in mind that, due to genetic variation, no ideal body compositions have been identified for any specific sport.

The most basic and routine anthropometric measures are a person's height and weight. Height is measured using a stadiometer or measuring tape, and weight is measured using a balance or spring scale. The sports RDN should document if equipment is unavailable and height and weight are reported by the individual rather than measured.

Body mass index (BMI) is a formula that uses an individual's measured height and weight to estimate body fatness:

$$\textbf{BMI} = \textbf{weight (kg)} / \textbf{height (m)}^2$$

The National Heart, Lung, and Blood Institute (NHLBI) website provides a BMI calculator and discusses the strengths and limitations of using BMI as a screening or diagnostic tool.[9] The Expert Panel on the Identification, Evaluation, and Treatment of Overweight and Obesity in Adults defines a healthy weight as a BMI of 18.5 to 24.9, with 25.0 and above indicating overweight or obesity.[10] BMI is not a useful tool for identifying overweight and obesity in athletes because it has been found to overestimate body fat in individuals who have a muscular build. The accuracy of BMI as an assessment of body fatness was assessed in collegiate athletes by comparing it with body fat percentage as measured using air displacement plethysmography in 226 collegiate athletes from a variety of sports.[11] Measurements were also taken from 213 nonathletes for comparison. Classifying overweight as a body fat of greater than 20% in men and 33% in women, BMI resulted in a false positive for overweight for 67% of the male athletes compared with 25% of male nonathletes and for 31% of female athletes compared with 7% of female nonathletes. Another study of men and women in their 20s also found that BMI had a limited ability to assess body fat.[12] Conversely, BMI may underestimate body fat in older individuals or others who have lost muscle mass. Although there is a positive relationship between percentage of body fat and BMI, it is not a perfect direct correlation and variations exist.[13]

BMI classification varies for children and adolescents to account for continued growth. While the same formula is used, the result is then plotted on BMI for age growth charts from the Centers for Disease Control and Prevention (CDC) and a percentile for age is obtained.[14] The CDC defines respective BMI percentile categories in these age groups as follows: less than 5th percentile, underweight; 5th through 84th percentile, healthy weight; 85th through 94th percentile, overweight; 95th percentile and above, obesity; and 99th percentile and above, severe obesity.[15]

An adult athlete whose BMI classifies him or her as overweight or obese can be further evaluated by measuring the individual's waist circumference (WC). An android fat pattern, where fat is in the abdominal region, is associated with an increased risk of chronic diseases. Measurement of abdominal or visceral fat is also useful in determining whether BMI is accurately representing an estimate of body fat. The measurement should be taken horizontally at the height of the iliac crest using a cloth tape measure with a spring-loaded handle, which reduces skin compression and improves reliability of the measurement.[4] The NHLBI recommends a WC of 40 in or less (102 cm) for men and 35 in or less (88 cm) for women. Men and women whose WC is bigger than these cutoffs and who have a BMI between 25 and 34.9 have increased obesity-associated disease risks.[16]

Body composition can be further evaluated using a variety of methods. These other measurements are designed to assess either a two-compartment (fat vs fat-free mass) model, a three-compartment (fat, fat-free mass, bone mineral) model, or a four-compartment (fat, fat-free mass, bone mineral, water) model of body composition. The two-compartment model is most frequently used. Techniques include the measurement of skinfold thickness, bioelectrical impedance analysis, dual energy x-ray absorptiometry, underwater weighing, and air displacement plethysmography. See Chapter 9 for further details on anthropometric/body composition measurements.

FOOD AND NUTRITION-RELATED HISTORY

A complete history includes not only intake but also eating patterns, diet quality, and variety of foods consumed, as well as any consumption of alcohol, caffeine, and dietary supplements. Any previous modifications to the diet should be identified. Determine whether modifications were prescribed by a physician, RDN, or other health professional or were self-selected without assessment of need. Any special dietary needs, including those related to food allergies or intolerances or medical conditions, must be clearly identified, along with any potential food-drug interactions.

Also included are knowledge, beliefs, and attitudes toward food; eating behaviors; and environmental conditions affecting food choices. Medications must be identified so their potential interactions with or impact on food can be assessed.

Diet and Weight History

The athlete should be asked about any previous dietary restrictions, the rationale behind them, and the outcome. An individual's weight history should be obtained, and, if available, current weight should be compared with previous weights. The individual should be asked whether weight is a concern and, if so, why. Is the concern performance based or appearance based? Does it arise from the athlete's own perceived need or has it been communicated by a coach or other influential person? Has the athlete experienced recent or past weight changes? If so, additional questions about whether the weight change was intentional or unintentional are necessary, and the RDN should consider whether further investigation is warranted. Intentional weight change may occur during the off-season or in preparation for the competitive season. For example, an athlete may bulk up before the competitive season or gain weight as a result of glycogen loading. Conversely, an athlete who has reduced training during the off-season may observe an unintentional and undesirable weight gain. If this has occurred, the magnitude of weight change should be ascertained. Any history of extreme weight loss related to excessive physical activity (PA) or a history of large, repeated weight fluctuations should be identified. The weight history should include the individual's minimum and maximum weight (in adults) and the athlete's perception of his or her ideal weight. Athletes should be asked if they have difficulty maintaining their weight through the competitive season.

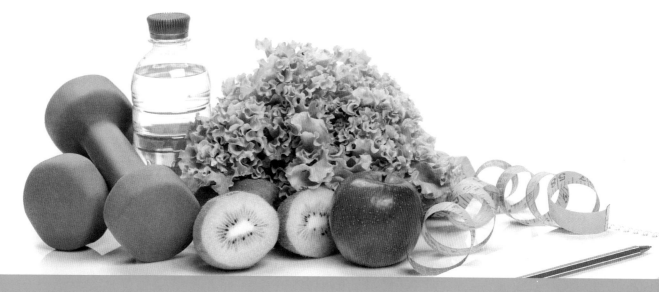

Assessment Tools

An accurate assessment of dietary intake is essential for the nutrition assessment. Data collected determine the adequacy of the diet relative to need and diagnose any nutrition related problems.[17] Components include total intake of food, fluids, sports products, alcohol, and dietary supplements.

In the absence of instruments validated for the athletic population, those developed for the general population are typically used, including a 24-hour recall, a 3- to 7-day food record, and a food frequency questionnaire (FFQ). These may be modified to include foods and sports products typically used by the athlete.[18] Data may be collected retrospectively, as with 24-hour recalls or FFQs, or prospectively as with food records. Each method has its strength and limitations.

24-HOUR RECALL

A 24-hour recall is typically conducted during the nutrition interview. The athlete is asked to describe all foods and beverages consumed the previous day or 24-hour period and to specify timing of meals and

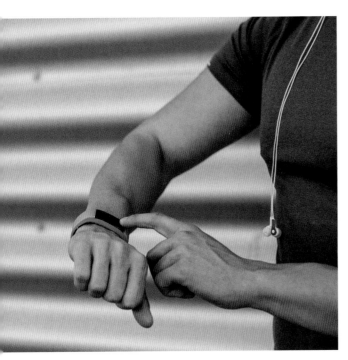

snacks. While accuracy will be limited by the respondent's ability to accurately recall all items consumed, ability to estimate portion sizes, and knowledge of all ingredients used in preparation, this method is quick and easy and can provide a useful starting point for a conversation with the athlete about dietary patterns. The relationship between the interviewer and interviewee is key to enhancing the accuracy of information provided.[19] A rapport must be developed, and negative feedback and judgments on the part of the interviewer should be avoided so the athlete feels comfortable openly discussing food behaviors during the interview. A receptive interviewer will avoid obtaining a recall altered by the athlete's perception of what may or may not be acceptable. Gentle probing can help elicit additional information.

DIETARY RECORD

Another commonly used dietary assessment method is a dietary record that is generally gathered over a 3- to 7-day period. The individual is instructed in how to accurately complete the record and estimate portion sizes. The RDN reviews the records during the interview for the purpose of filling in missing information and clarifying portion sizes. Models or pictures can be used to help the athlete estimate portion sizes. Accuracy increases with the motivation of the individual, but underreporting is commonly observed.[20] It should be noted that individuals tend to alter their food choices when keeping logs.[17]

FOOD FREQUENCY QUESTIONNAIRES

FFQs are commonly used for assessing the intake of groups but can also be used to document and monitor intake in an individual. A benefit of this method is that it can evaluate intake over a longer time than a 24-hour recall or a 3- to 7-day food log, making it a more reliable tool for assessing the intake of specific nutrients. An FFQ adapted to include sports products was used to evaluate the dietary intake of elite female athletes from a variety of sports.[18] Respondent cooperation was high, but the authors noted that this method has not been validated in athletes, results have not been compared with biological markers, and interpretation of results is difficult. Furthermore, athletes tend to change their diets according to training schedules. Because the FFQ provides a summary of foods and amounts consumed, these variations will not be evident, and content of specific meals and snacks cannot be assessed.[21]

The inaccuracy of self-reported data limits the usefulness of these methods. Pooled data from five large validation studies of FFQs and 24-hour recalls that used doubly labeled water as a biological marker for energy intake and urinary nitrogen as a marker for protein intake found low correlation coefficients. Average correlation coefficients for the FFQ were 0.21 and 0.29 for energy and protein, respectively, while correlation coefficients for a single 24-hour recall were 0.26 and 0.40 for energy and protein, respectively. This improved to 0.31 and 0.49 when averaging three 24-hour recalls. Researchers observed underreporting of 28% with an FFQ and 15% with a 24-hour recall; the underreporting was found to be related to BMI, educational level, and age. [22]

A combination of methods will improve the accuracy of data collected. A diet history combines the 24-hour recall with an FFQ and can provide a more comprehensive assessment of nutrient intake for the individual.[17]

DIRECT OBSERVATION

In some instances, such as when a sports RDN works at a school or training camp, direct observation is an option. Here the burden is placed on the RDN to accurately record all food and beverages consumed, rather than on the athlete to recall and record. While this may be helpful in validating information obtained from other methodologies, observation is generally limited to specific meals and works best when the athlete is not aware that his or her behavior is being observed so that eating behavior is not altered.

TECHNOLOGY

In recent years, practitioners have seen investments in developing technology to improve the accuracy of diet and exercise measurements.[21] The Genes, Environment and Health Initiative, a project of the National Institutes of Health, funded the development of devices and methods that would be reliable and valid, easy to use, and economically feasible for field use.[23] In another endeavor, the National Cancer Institute funded the development of an automated, self-administered 24-hour dietary recall, which is used for research purposes.

The use of diet apps on smartphones has become increasingly popular. These tools allow individuals to record food intake, from which a nutrient analysis can be derived. Many of these include a PA component. A recent survey investigated the prevalence with which these products are being used by sports RDNs and perceptions of their usefulness in assessing and tracking dietary intake.[24] While the response rate was a low 10.8%, approximately one-third of respondents reported using smartphone apps, with most finding them at least as useful as traditional assessment methods.

The use of digital photography has also been explored as a means for enhancing the accuracy of dietary records.[25] This method may appeal to some who would prefer to snap a picture rather than keep a detailed food record, but ingredients used in preparation may not be apparent, and the respondent burden remains to ensure a complete record.

Fluid and Electrolytes

Water intake must meet water loss, which is affected by body size and environmental conditions.[26] This requirement is met mostly by water in fluids and foods, with a small contribution coming from the oxidation of nutrients. The amount and type of fluid, along with electrolyte content, should be carefully evaluated. This will be best accomplished by asking the athlete to drink from measured containers rather than directly from water fountains or cups of unknown volume, which is difficult to quantify. See Chapter 6 for more on hydration.

Dietary Supplements

Athletes use dietary supplements to increase energy, build muscle, enhance athletic performance, aid in recovery, maintain health, and compensate for a poor diet.[27,28] Quality control varies, and contamination with banned substances may occur.[29] All dietary supplements should be identified along with dosing, frequency, and reason for use during the nutrition assessment to determine appropriateness of use and potential risks. See Chapter 7 for an in-depth discussion of this topic.

Environment and Access to Food

Where an individual eats, who purchases the food, access to food, access to cooking facilities, and with whom the individual eats will all affect food choices and behaviors. A college athlete living in a dormitory room may be dependent on cafeteria food, which can vary widely in quality. Some schools are in areas where fast-food restaurants and delis are more accessible than grocery stores, leading the athlete to consume more highly processed foods and fewer fruits and vegetables. Team meals may be provided. Most often, coaching staff is responsible for ordering these meals, and the focus may be on cost rather than nutrition. Time constraints are often an issue for an athlete of any age because school or work responsibilities, in addition to training time, reduce the time available for food preparation and consumption. Athletes who travel may not have access to their customary foods while on the road. The sports RDN can be instrumental in identifying foods that will be available and creating performance-enhancing menu suggestions within those limitations. The athlete's food budget should be determined and used in planning. Identification of environmental obstacles to healthy eating will enable the sports RDN to help develop strategies to overcome them.

Knowledge, Beliefs, and Attitudes

Athletes obtain nutrition information from a variety of sources, including coaches, strength and conditioning coaches, certified athletic trainers, physicians, peers, parents, the media, and the internet. The reliability of this information is highly variable.[30-32] Athletes may enter the nutrition counseling session with a firm set of beliefs based on what they have read and heard. Certain practices may be part of the culture of the sport, as in the example of dehydration to make weight for weight-class sports. It may be helpful to identify sources of knowledge, beliefs, and attitudes so that science-based recommendations can be introduced in a nonjudgmental manner. The sports RDN should determine whether educational efforts need to be directed toward key influencers.

Sports RDNs develop nutrition strategies to enhance health, fitness, and optimal physical performance.[8] For such strategies to be effective, the recipient must be open to the guidance provided and willing to make behavioral changes. Nutrition education is more likely to be effective when based on research and theory. Integrative models of health behavior change have been developed.[33] The Transtheoretical Model of health behavior change is one such model that has been used to describe the progression of change over time as occurring through a series of stages: precontemplation, contemplation, preparation, action, maintenance, and termination.[5] Planned interventions, when appropriately designed according to stage, can help move people through the stages. This model has been applied to dietary changes and found to be useful for understanding the decision-making process and designing interventions to move the individual forward.[34] Pros and cons of making behavioral changes differ in the various stages, and evidence suggests a crossover effect—a point at which the pros outweigh the cons—which occurs before the action stage where changes occur. The UCLA Center for Human Nutrition website provides a description of the six stages and a discussion of techniques effective at each stage.[35] Research is needed to evaluate the effectiveness of this approach in athletes.

Eating Behaviors

Certain behaviors related to food intake may affect the ability to achieve nutrition goals and therefore must be a part of the conversation with the athlete. The athlete should be questioned about restrictive eating, rigidity or limited food preferences, and bingeing and purging, all of which may indicate disordered eating. Other behaviors of note include pace of eating, activities performed while eating that may distract and contribute to mindless eating, and emotional eating. Behaviors that interfere with goals will need to be addressed as a part of the nutrition intervention, and pathological eating behaviors will need to be addressed with a team approach including a psychologist and physician. Disordered eating is discussed in Chapter 18.

Challenges Specific to the Dietary Assessment of the Athlete

PERIODIZED TRAINING CYCLES

An athlete's training load and, therefore, nutritional needs will vary according to whether he or she is in preparation for the competitive season, in the competitive season, or transitioning out of the competitive season. A dietary assessment specific to the training cycle will most accurately meet the athlete's needs. A reassessment should be conducted when the athlete enters a new period.

DIETARY MANIPULATION

An athlete may temporarily alter the diet in an attempt to improve performance, as in carbohydrate loading, or to change body composition before competition, as in weight-class sports. These periods of manipulation may last days or weeks and may not be indicative of the athlete's usual diet.

TRAINING DAYS VS COMPETITION DAYS

Nutritional needs and dietary intake typically vary between training days and competition days. While it is essential that nutritional needs are met on training days to promote physiological adaptations and health, the goal on competition days may be more focused on providing foods and fluids that are well tolerated by the athlete. Foods and fluids for an athlete competing in tournaments must be appropriately spaced. Variability in nutritional needs between training days and competition days requires that intake on these days be assessed independently. Because dietary intake must be interpreted relative to the needs of the athlete, a training log should be collected in parallel with the food log.[20]

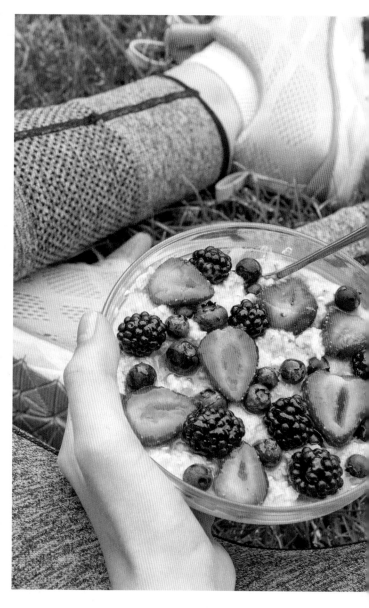

DIETARY SUPPLEMENTS, SPORTS FOODS, AND PRODUCTS

Athletes may consume sports drinks, protein shakes, gels, and other products not typically consumed by the general population. Athletes and active individuals report a variety of reasons for using dietary supplements, including improved health, increased energy, enhanced performance, and faster recovery.[27,28,36] Use of these products may be perceived as superior to or more convenient than food.[27] While research does support potential benefits for some of these products, in most cases the hype exceeds reality. The sports RDN needs to collect accurate information about supplement use and be willing to address the athlete's desire to take them.

PREEXERCISE AND POSTEXERCISE FUELING PATTERNS

While distribution of energy and nutrients throughout the day is important for anyone, this is even more critical for athletes. Questions specific to foods and fluids consumed before exercise, during exercise, and postexercise are essential.

Nutrient Analysis

Once all dietary information has been collected, the information can be entered into a nutrient analysis program. Programs vary in cost, ease of use, reports provided, and inclusion of items typically consumed by an athlete. Accurate entry is essential to prevent error.

Just about all nutrient analysis programs use the US Department of Agriculture National Nutrient Database for Standard Reference, maintained by the Nutrient Data Laboratory, Beltsville Human Nutrition Research Center (http://ndb.nal.usda.gov). A free online tool for tracking intake is available at ChooseMyPlate (www.choosemyplate.gov/tools-supertracker). Other sites, such as nutritiondata.com, sparkpeople.com, fitday.com, and calorieking.com are useful for quickly looking up the nutrient content of foods but do not provide the high-quality analyses and reports that the professional programs provide.[37] A number of programs are available for professional use, such as NutriBase Professional, Food Processor (ESHA Research), and Nutritionist Pro (Axxya Systems).

Assessment of Energy Requirements

An athlete's most basic need is for adequate energy intake to support normal body metabolism and physical activity including sport and exercise. Total daily energy expenditure is the sum of resting metabolic rate, thermic effect of food, and PA. PA includes planned exercise, as well as the energy cost of normal daily activities and involuntary muscular activity such as fidgeting and shivering.[38]

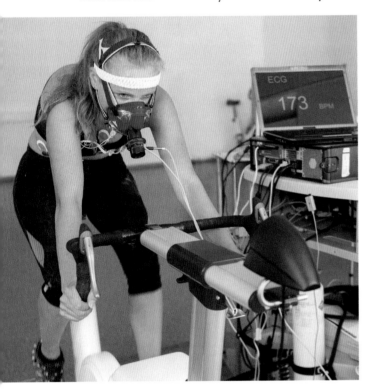

Energy requirements can be directly measured by direct calorimetry, which measures heat production using a specialized chamber or by using doubly labeled water (in which stable isotopes are ingested with water and subsequently collected in the urine and breath).[39] Energy expenditure is then calculated by analyzing the isotope turnover rate. These methods provide greater accuracy than indirect methods, but they are costly and generally reserved for research. Doubly labeled water provides a measure of energy expenditure as the individual goes about his or her normal activities but does not provide a measure of individual activities.

Indirect measurements include indirect calorimetry and movement monitors such as accelerometers and pedometers.[39] Indirect calorimetry uses the relationship between the volume of oxygen consumed (VO_2) and the respiratory quotient (RQ) to estimate energy expenditure. RQ describes the relationship between the volume of CO_2 produced and the volume of O_2 consumed; this is calculated as $RQ = (VCO_2$ produced $/ VO_2$ consumed$)$. RQ varies with the substrate used because the oxidation of carbohydrate, protein, and fat requires different amounts of oxygen. Metabolic charts used to analyze inspired and expired gases are usually programmed with the weir equation, which stipulates that the kilocalories expended per minute are equal to $([1.1 \times RQ] + 3.9) \times VO_2$.[40] In this way energy expenditure at rest and during exercise can be measured. Handheld devices using the same principle to estimate resting energy expenditure have been developed and validated and may be useful in clinical practice.[41,42]

Prediction equations are most commonly used for estimating total daily energy expenditure in clinical practice, although most have been developed using a sedentary population. A study that compared resting metabolic rate (RMR) measured in the laboratory with various equations in active men and women found the Cunningham equation to be the most accurate with the Harris-Benedict equation being the next best.[43] The Cunningham equation requires measurement of lean body mass. When this is not feasible, Harris-Benedict offers a simple, though less accurate, alternative. Once RMR has been determined, an appropriate activity factor and thermic effect of food must be added.[44] These activity factors are a crude estimation of true energy expenditure via PA. See Chapter 10 for additional details on this procedure.

As noted earlier, a training log allows for a more accurate determination of energy and nutrient needs. Training protocols typically vary daily, and nutritional needs will vary accordingly. Some athletes require considerably more fuel on training days than competition days. A swimmer, for example, may expend 5,000 kcal in training daily while their competition may involve a sprint with an energy cost of only several hundred kilocalories. Conversely, a competitive tennis athlete or triathlete needs to plan for adequate energy to delay fatigue in endurance events.

Energy availability refers to the energy left for body systems after exercise and is defined as energy intake less energy cost of exercise.[45] An assessment of energy availability will allow the practitioner to determine the adequacy of the athlete's caloric intake.

BIOCHEMICAL NUTRITION ASSESSMENT

The biochemical assessment involves the measurement of nutrient and metabolite levels in the blood and urine. A complete blood count, a comprehensive metabolic panel with a lipid profile, endocrine markers, and a urinary analysis are typically included as routine blood work to evaluate general health. Specific nutrients, such as vitamins, would be assessed only if a concern of deficiency or toxicity exists. Of particular concern in the athlete's assessment are the oxygen-carrying nutrients (iron, folic acid, and vitamin B-12) and bone-building nutrients (vitamin D and calcium) and hormones. Because dehydration can alter the results of key tests, an assessment of hydration status should be made at the time of testing (see the Fluids/Hydration section later in this chapter). The RDN should assess the adequacy of available lab work and make recommendations for additional evaluations when appropriate.

Protein

Both aerobic training and resistance training involve an upregulation of protein metabolism. Adequate dietary protein is essential for adaptations to occur. Protein status is evaluated in the laboratory using a variety of methods, including nitrogen balance, stable isotopes, and fractional synthetic rate (see Chapter 3). Key proteins, such as retinol-binding protein, prealbumin, and albumin, may be low in an athlete who is not consuming enough protein or calories. Clinical assessment of protein status is accomplished by analyzing food logs and monitoring body composition.[19]

Carbohydrate

Glucose metabolism is assessed by measuring fasting plasma glucose and hemoglobin A1c levels or by performing an oral glucose tolerance test. If an abnormal result is obtained in any of these measurements, further tests would be warranted to rule out glucose intolerance, glucose sensitivity, and type 1 or type 2 diabetes.[46]

Lipids

Lipids are generally assessed to rule out risk factors for cardiovascular disease. A basic lipid panel measures circulating levels of total cholesterol, high- and low-density lipoprotein cholesterol, and circulating levels of triglycerides in the serum.[47] Circulating levels of C-reactive protein and homocysteine levels may also be measured as additional risk factors for vascular disease.

Fluids/Hydration

Inadequate hydration can have a negative impact on aerobic exercise and can contribute to heat illness, making hydration status a critical component of the athlete's assessment. Various biomarkers can be used to assess hydration status, including plasma osmolality, urine osmolality, and urine specific gravity (USG). The choice of biomarker will vary based on whether testing will be done by a laboratory or in the field and whether it will be done by a trained technician or an athlete or coach.[48]

An athlete can assess his or her own fluid balance by monitoring daily morning weights after the first void and measuring urine concentration. Urine color and volume are simple, although subjective, ways of monitoring hydration. Darker urine indicates a greater degree of dehydration.[49] USG can be easily measured by placing a drop of urine in a refractometer or by using a reagent strip; however, this measure is prone to error, particularly during periods of fluctuating input and output of fluid.[50] When measured upon waking, USG of 1.02 or less indicates euhydration, although diet, heavy exercise, and high lean body mass can alter these results.[48,51] Due to the limitations of any one simple assessment measure, a more accurate assessment of hydration status will be provided by assessing weight, USG, and thirst.[51]

Exercise-associated hyponatremia, a potentially life-threatening condition, occurs when there is a relative excess of total body water, often as a result of drinking too much.[52] Diagnosis is made by a serum sodium concentration below 135 mEq/L accompanied by clinical symptoms, including an increase in body weight from baseline, nausea, vomiting, and altered mental status. A detailed discussion of this topic is found in Chapter 6.

Vitamin Status

Vitamin status is typically assumed based on the results of dietary intake. Athletes who consume adequate calories and eat a varied diet are unlikely to experience vitamin deficiencies. B vitamins play a vital role in the production of energy, and folate and vitamin B-12 are required for the synthesis of red blood cells and repair of damaged cells; it is possible that PA alters the need for these nutrients. A low red blood cell count, coupled with an elevated mean corpuscular volume, can indicate a deficiency of folate or vitamin B-12. While a vitamin deficiency is likely to impair athletic performance, deficiencies are rare in athletes.[53]

VITAMIN D

Vitamin D has recently been identified as a nutrient of concern for the athlete. In addition to its known effect on bone mineral density, vitamin D status has been associated with muscle strength.[54] Vitamin D status is known to vary with season because the ultraviolet B rays that trigger its activation are more plentiful in the spring and summer. Athletes who train indoors have been identified as a group at risk of inadequate vitamin D levels, as are those with dark skin, athletes who train with clothes providing little skin exposure, and athletes with higher levels of body fat.[55,56] Vitamin D status is determined by measuring serum 25(OH)D concentrations. Based on current research, a level of at least 32 ng/mL is recommended to maintain skeletal health and muscle function (see Table 8.1), although an optimal level has yet to be identified.[57] Should a thorough assessment of vitamin status be required, refer to Chapter 10, "Assessment of Vitamin Status," in the book by Driskell and Wolinsky.[58]

Table 8.1 United States Olympic Committee Protocol: Reference Ranges for Vitamin D		
	ng × mL − 1	nmol × mL − 1
Vitamin D toxicity	>150	>375
Optimal Status (bone and muscle)	40–70	100–175
Normal vitamin D status	30–80	75–200
Vitamin D insufficiency	21–29	52.5–72.5
Vitamin D deficiency	≤20	≤50

Reprinted with permission from the United States Olympic Committee.

Iron

Iron deficiency may occur with or without anemia: Either can impair performance.[59] Stage 1 iron deficiency indicates inadequate stores and is most commonly assessed by measuring serum ferritin levels. Note that ferritin is an acute-phase reactant and increases in response to vigorous PA as well as inflammation, possibly resulting in a false-negative test result.[60] There is a lack of consensus regarding the ferritin cutoff point for diagnosis of iron deficiency, although many use a level of 12 µg/mL.[61] Exercise performance may be compromised before levels reach these clinical cutoffs. The United States Olympic Committee (USOC) recommends supplementation when levels fall below 35 µg/mL in women and 4 µg/mL in men.[62] Although not as widely used, soluble transferrin receptor may be preferable in an athlete to identify low iron stores because it does not respond to inflammation.

Iron is transported through the blood to the bone marrow carried by the protein transferrin. Transferrin is generally assessed by measuring total iron-binding capacity (TIBC). Transferrin saturation is calculated by dividing serum iron by TIBC. Transferrin saturation below 16% is an indication of inadequate iron to support normal erythropoiesis.[63]

Hemoglobin and hematocrit concentrations are used to assess iron-deficiency anemia. A decrease in this value will occur only during the late stages of iron deficiency, at which point performance will clearly be diminished because it limits oxygen transport to working muscles.[60] Dehydration and inflammation, as well as deficiencies in folic acid, copper, and vitamin B-12, will affect levels of this marker.

Sports anemia may occur during the early phase of training as increased blood volume dilutes hemoglobin and results in a decline in concentration. Ferritin levels remain normal, indicating healthy iron stores, and performance is not affected. As training continues, increased erythropoiesis will lead to an increase in hemoglobin, and blood levels will normalize.

Vegetarian athletes and female athletes are at increased risk of iron depletion and deficiency. These athletes should pursue dietary strategies that will ensure the adequacy of their iron intake. Chapters 5 and 16 discuss this in detail.

Optimal levels for athletes may differ from clinical standards. Box 8.2 outlines recommended levels according to the USOC protocol.[62]

Box 8.2 United States Olympic Committee Protocol: Iron Status, Reference Ranges for Hematological Iron Status Markers [57]

Stage 1 iron depletion	<35 µg/L ferritin
	>115 g/L hemoglobin
	>16% transferrin saturation
Stage 2 iron-deficient non-anemia	<20 µg/L ferritin
	>115 g/L hemoglobin
	<16% transferrin saturation
	>total iron binding capacity >500 µg/dL
Stage 3 Iron-deficient anemia	<12 µg/L ferritin
	<115 g/L hemoglobin
	<16% transferrin saturation

Reprinted with permission from the United States Olympic Committee.

Organ Function

Biochemical tests are also used to measure organ function. Pertinent to the nutrition assessment are those organ systems involved in the digestion, absorption, metabolism, and excretion of nutrients and their end products. Included here are tests for malabsorption; sickle-cell trait or disease; endocrine studies, including sex hormones; and bone mineral density testing.

NUTRITION-FOCUSED PHYSICAL FINDINGS

These data may be collected by a member of the health care team other than the sports RDN, such as the team physician or a certified athletic trainer. Findings pertinent to assessment of nutrition status include the following:

- Clinical signs of fluid imbalance, such as skin turgor, fatigue, muscle cramps, dark urine, rapid weight change, constipation, and thirst
- Clinical signs of undernutrition or eating disorders, including muscle wasting; lanugo; hypothermia; dry, brittle, or thinning hair and nails; bradycardia; tooth erosion; bony protrusions; parotid gland enlargement; and gastrointestinal distress
- Muscularity and subcutaneous fat distribution
- Oral health, including dentition and mouth sores
- Clinical signs of digestive system impairment, such as bloating, cramping, and diarrhea

CLIENT HISTORY

Current and past medical and social histories are gathered, including age, sport and position, number of years in the sport, current or past injuries, educational level, and language, if pertinent. Any current or past medical conditions affecting the athlete or a family member that may impact nutrition should be noted. Socioeconomic factors and living situation can also be indicated.

COMPARATIVE STANDARDS

Once all data have been collected and analyzed, evidence-based standards on which the assessment will be based must be identified. The appropriate standard, or standards, will vary based on age, health status, governing bodies, and goals of the athlete. For example, the Dietary Guidelines for Americans might be appropriate for addressing the dietary adequacy of an active individual whose goal is health and fitness, while a competitive athlete may benefit from use of the Nutrition and Athletic Performance joint position paper from the Academy of Nutrition and Dietetics, the ACSM, and the Dietitians of Canada, or the IOC Consensus Statement on Sports Nutrition.[7,64] The ACSM has positions on a variety of issues relevant to nutrition assessment, including the female athlete triad, appropriate PA intervention strategies for weight loss and prevention of weight regain for adults, and exercise and fluid replacement.[48,65,66] The IOC consensus statement on relative energy deficiency in sport offers guidelines for education, detection, and treatment of this condition.[67] For school-aged athletes, the American Academy of Pediatrics offers a number of policy statements and other professional resources.[68] The National Athletic Trainers' Association and the National Strength and Conditioning Association also have several position papers on subjects of interest to the RDN, including dietary supplements, weight management, and treatment of eating disorders in athletes.[69-71]

SUMMARY

Performing a nutrition assessment on an athlete requires knowledge and skill on the part of the sports RDN. Standards of practice for RDNs in sports nutrition and dietetics delineate the skills, training, and knowledge for the competent, proficient, and expert practitioner.[8] An expert level of competency may be required for more complex issues, such as the athlete with type 1 diabetes.

Appropriate use of assessment tools, effective interviewing methods, and clear organization of data collected contribute to the usefulness of the assessment.[8] The use of standard terminology enhances communication with other members of the team. All assessment data must be carefully recorded and dated and results communicated in a timely fashion.

The experienced RDN will be able to differentiate between data that are pertinent to the situation and that which are not. For example, not all athletes will require anthropometric measurements beyond height and weight. In a healthy athlete, a complete biochemical workup may not be warranted. Conversely, the RDN may need to contact the physician or other provider to request additional tests if a specific concern exists. Athletes with an underlying health concern, such as type 1 or type 2 diabetes, celiac disease, hyperlipidemia, hypertension, or other disorder, will require more testing to determine appropriate dietary modifications. A complete discussion of medical nutrition assessment is beyond the scope of this chapter. Diabetes and exercise is thoroughly discussed in Chapter 19. The sports RDN will benefit from having an understanding of the logistics of an athlete's sport. It is important to understand the requirements of weight-class sports, periodized training protocols, and the strength, speed, and endurance needs of each athlete. After the RDN conducts a complete nutrition assessment of an athlete, the resulting nutrition diagnoses will provide the basis on which the intervention will be made. Periodic reassessment will determine whether alterations in the nutrition intervention are required.

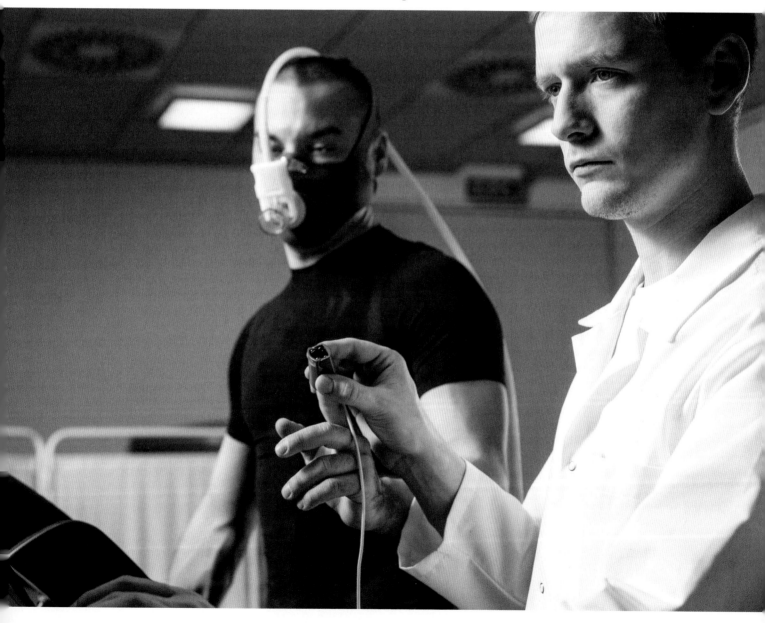

Categories included in the nutrition assessment are food and nutrition-related history, anthropometric measurements, biochemical data, medical tests and procedures, nutrition-focused physical findings, client history, and comparative standards.

A complete history includes not only intake but also eating patterns, diet quality, and variety of foods consumed, as well as any consumption of alcohol, caffeine, and dietary supplements.

In the absence of instruments validated for the athletic population, those developed for the general population are typically used, including a 24-hour recall, a 3- to 7-day food record, and a food frequency questionnaire.

Challenges specific to the assessment of the athlete include periodized training cycles, temporary manipulation of the diet, diets specific to training vs competition days, the use of dietary supplements, sports foods and products, and adequacy of preexercise and postexercise fueling.

Biochemical assessments of particular concern in the athlete's assessment are the oxygen-carrying nutrients (iron, folic acid, vitamin B-12), bone-building nutrients (vitamin D and calcium), hormones, and markers of hydration status.

Collected data must be compared with evidence-based standards.

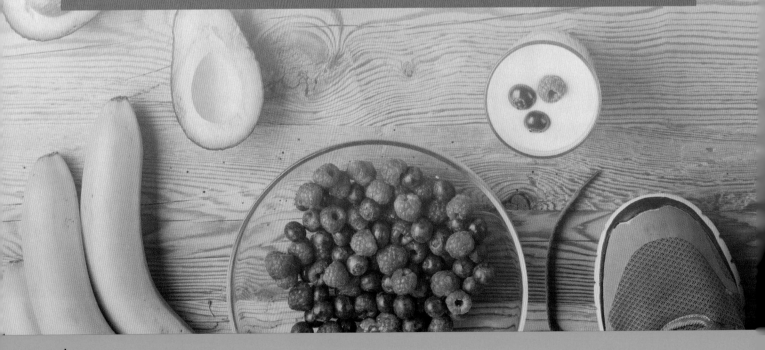

1. Myers EF. Nutrition Care Process and Model and the International Dietetics and Nutrition Terminology: what do they have to do with public policy? *Nutr Today.* 2014;49(1):26-31. doi:10.1097/NT.0000000000000015.

2. Academy of Nutrition and Dietetics. Sports Nutrition Care Manual. http://nutritioncaremanual.org/. 2016. Accessed June 16, 2016.

3. Riebe D, Franklin BA, Thompson PD, et al. Updating ACSM's recommendations for exercise preparticipation health screening. *Med Sci Sports Exerc.* 2015;47(11)2473-2479. doi:10.1249/MSS.0000000000000664.

4. American College of Sports Medicine. *ACSM's Guidelines for Exercise Testing and Prescription;* V 37. 8th ed. Philadelphia, PA: Wolters Kluwer. Lippencott Williams & Wilkins; 2010.

5. Prochaska J, Velicer W. The transtheoretical model of health behavior change. *Am J Health Promot.* 1997;12(1):38-48.

6. Thomas DT, Erdman KA, Burke LM. Position of the Academy of Nutrition and Dietetics, Dietitians of Canada, and the American College of Sports Medicine: Nutrition and Athletic Performance. *J Acad Nutr Diet.* 2016;116(3):501-528. doi:10.1016/j.jand.2015.12.006.

7. Maughan RJ, Shirreffs SM. IOC Consensus Conference on Nutrition in Sport, 25-27 October 2010, International Olympic Committee, Lausanne, Switzerland. *J Sports Sci.* 2011;29(suppl 1):1S. doi:10.1080/02640414.2011.619339.

8. Steinmuller PL, Kruskall LJ, Karpinski CA, Manore MM, Macedonio MA, Meyer NL. Academy of Nutrition and Dietetics: Revised 2014 standards of practice and standards of professional performance for registered dietitian nutritionists (competent, proficient, and expert) in sports nutrition and dietetics. *J Acad Nutr Diet.* 2014;114(4):631-641. doi:10.1016/j.jand.2013.12.021.

9. Knuiman P, Kramer IF. Contributions to the understanding of the anabolic properties of different dietary proteins. *J Physiol.* 2012;590(12):2839-2840. doi:10.1113/jphysiol.2012.233684.

10. Pi-Sunyer FX, Becker DM, Bouchard C, et al, for the NHLBI Obesity Education Initiative Expert Panel on the Identification, Evaluation, and Treatment of Overweight in Adults. Clinical guidelines on the identification, evaluation, and treatment of overweight and obesity in adults: executive summary. *Arch Intern Med.* 1998;68(4):1855-1867.

11. Ode JJ, Pivarnik JM, Reeves MJ, Knous JL. Body mass index as a predictor of percent fat in college athletes and nonathletes. *Med Sci Sports Exerc.* 2007;39(3):403-409. doi:10.1249/01.mss.0000247008.19127.3e.

12. Kruschitz R, Wallner-Liebmann SJ, Hamlin MJ, et al. Detecting body fat—a weighty problem BMI versus subcutaneous fat patterns in athletes and non-athletes. *PLoS One.* 2013;8(8):1-9. doi:10.1371/journal.pone.0072002.

13. Gallagher D, Heymsfield SB, Heo M, Jebb SA, Murgatroyd PR, Sakamoto Y. Healthy percentage body fat ranges: an approach for developing guidelines based on body mass index. *Am J Clin Nutr.* 2000;72(3):694-701.

14. BMI percentile calculator for child and teen metric version. Centers for Disease Control and Prevention website. http://nccd.cdc.gov/dnpabmi/Calculator.aspx?CalculatorType=Metric. Accessed September 28, 2015.

15. Barlow SE. Expert committee recommendations regarding the prevention, assessment, and treatment of child and adolescent overweight and obesity: summary report. *Pediatrics.* 2007;120(suppl 4):164S-192S. doi:10.1542/peds.2007-2329C.

16. Flegal KM. Waist circumference of healthy men and women in the United States. *Int J Obes (Lond).* 2007;31(7):1134-1139. doi:10.1038/sj.ijo.0803566.

17. Deakin V. Measuring nutritional status of athletes: clinical and research perspectives. In: Burke L, Deakin V, eds. *Clinical Sports Nutrition.* 4th ed. North Ryde, Australia: McGraw-Hill; 2010:20-43.

18. Heaney S, O'Connor H, Gifford J, Naughton G. Comparison of strategies for assessing nutritional adequacy in elite female athletes' dietary intake. *Int J Sport Nutr Exerc Metab.* 2010;20(3):245-256.

19. Moffatt RJ, Tomatis VB, Harris DA, Deetz AM. Estimation of food and nutrient intake of athletes. In: Driskell J, Wolinsky I, eds. *Nutritional Assessment of Athletes.* 2nd ed. Boca Raton, FL: CRC Press; 2010:3-50.

20. Koehler K, Braun H, De Marees M, et al. Parallel assessment of nutrition and activity in athletes: validation against doubly labelled water, 24-h urea excretion, and indirect calorimetry. *J Sports Sci.* 2010;28(13):1435-1449. doi:10.1080/02640414.2010.513482.

21. Thompson FE, Subar AF, Loria CM, Reedy JL, Baranowski T. Need for technological innovation in dietary assessment. *J Am Diet Assoc.* 2010;110(1):48-51. doi:10.1016/j.jada.2009.10.008.

22. Freedman LS, Commins JM, Moler JE, et al. Pooled results from 5 validation studies of dietary self-report instruments using recovery biomarkers for energy and protein intake. *Am J Epidemiol.* 2014;180(2):172-188. doi:10.1093/aje/kwu116.

23. Improved measures of diet and physical activity program Genes, Environment, and Health Initiative (GEI). National Heart, Lung, and Blood Institute Obesity Research, National Institutes of Health. www.nhlbi.nih.gov/research/resources/obesity/completed/geis.htm. Updated July 2014. Accessed November 20, 2015.

24. Jospe MR, Fairbairn KA, Green P, Perry TL. Diet app use by sports dietitians: a survey in five countries. *JMIR Mhealth Uhealth.* 2015;3(1):e7. doi:10.2196/mhealth.3345.

25. Ptomey LT, Willis EA, Honas JJ, et al. Validity of energy intake estimated by digital photography plus recall in overweight and obese young adults. *J Acad Nutr Diet*. 2015;115(9):1392-1399. doi:10.1016/j.jand.2015.05.006.

26. Maughan RJ. Water and electrolyte loss and replacement in training and competition. In: Maughan RJ, ed. *Sports Nutrition: The Encyclopaedia of Sports Medicine*. Vol XIX. 2nd ed. Chichester, UK: John Wiley & Sons; 2013:174-184.

27. Maughan RJ. Quality assurance issues in the use of dietary supplements, with special reference to protein supplements. *J Nutr*. 2013;143(11):1843S-1847S. doi:10.3945/jn.113.176651.

28. Wiens K, Erdman KA, Stadnyk M, Parnell JA. Dietary supplement usage, motivation, and education in young, Canadian athletes. *Int J Sport Nutr Exerc Metab*. 2014;24(6):613-622. doi:10.1123/ijsnem.2013-0087.

29. Arensberg ME, Costello R, Deuster PA, Jones D, Twillman G. Summit on human performance and dietary supplements summary report. *Nutr Today*. 2014;49(1):7-17. doi:10.1097/NT.0000000000000013.

30. Diehl K, Thiel A, Zipfel S, Mayer J, Schnell A, Schneider S. Elite adolescent athletes' use of dietary supplements: characteristics, opinions, and sources of supply and information. *Int J Sport Nutr Exerc Metab*. 2012;22(3):165-174.

31. Torres-McGehee TM, Pritchett KL, Zippel D, Minton DM, Cellamare A, Sibilia M. Sports nutrition knowledge among collegiate athletes, coaches, athletic trainers, and strength and conditioning specialists. *J Athl Train*. 2012;47(2):205-211.

32. Hornstrom GR. Nutrition knowledge, practices, attitudes, and information sources of Mid-American Conference college softball players. *Food Nutr Sci*. 2011;02(02):109-117. doi:10.4236/fns.2011.22015.

33. Contento IR. Nutrition education: linking research, theory, and practice. *Asia Pac J Clin Nutr*. 2008;17(1):176-179.

34. Di Noia J, Prochaska JO. Dietary stages of change and decisional balance: a meta-analytic review. *Am J Health Behav*. 2010;34(5):618-632. doi:10.5993/AJHB.34.5.11.

35. Prochaska and DiClemente's Stages of Change Model. UCLA Center for Human Nutrition website. www.cellinteractive.com/ucla/physcian_ed/stages_change.html. Accessed October 2, 2015.

36. Stuntz CP, Edwards JC, Kaye M. Individual and social predictors of performance-enhancing and dietary supplement use among male NCAA Division III athletes. *J Issues Intercoll Athl*. 2014;7:187-206.

37. Aronson D. Ask the expert. Today's Dietitian magazine website. www.todaysdietitian.com/news/enews_0909_03.shtml. Accessed October 17, 2015.

38. Burke L, Deakin V, eds. *Clinical Sports Nutrition*. 4th ed. North Ryde, Australia: McGraw-Hill; 2010:100

39. Ainsworth BE. How to assess the energy costs of exercise and sport. In: Maughan RJ, ed. *Sports Nutrition: The Encyclopaedia of Sports Medicine*. Vol XIX. 2nd ed. Chichester, UK: John Wiley & Sons; 2013:61-71.

40. McArdle WD, Katch FI, Katch VI, eds. *Exercise Physiology: Nutrition, Energy, and Human Performance*. 8th ed. Baltimore, MD: Walter Kluwer Health, Lippincott Williams & Wilkins; 2015.

41. MedGem overview. Microlife Medical Home Solutions website. www.mimhs.com/medgem/solutions/intermediate0/med/overview/. Accessed October 17, 2015.

42. Zhao D, Xian X, Terrera M, et al. A pocket-sized metabolic analyzer for assessment of resting energy expenditure. *Clin Nutr*. 2014;33(2):341-347. doi:10.1016/j.clnu.2013.06.001.

43. Thompson J, Manore MM. Predicted and measured resting metabolic rate of male and female endurance athletes. *J Am Diet Assoc*. 1996;96(1):30-34. doi:10.1016/S0002-8223(96)00010-7.

44. Gerrior S, Juan W, Basiotis P. An easy approach to calculating estimated energy requirements. *Prev Chronic Dis*. 2006;3(4):A129.

45. Loucks AB, Kiens B, Wright HH. Energy availability in athletes. *J Sports Sci*. 2011;29(suppl 1):7S-15S. doi:10.1080/02640414.2011.588958.

46. Diagnosis of diabetes and prediabetes. National Diabetes Information Clearinghouse, National Institute of Diabetes and Digestive and Kidney Diseases. NIH Publication No 12–4642. http://diabetes.niddk.nih.gov/dm/pubs/diagnosis/. Published June 2014. Accessed August 1, 2016.

47. Stone NJ, Robinson J, Lichtenstein AH, et al. 2013 ACC/AHA guideline on the treatment of blood cholesterol to reduce atherosclerotic cardiovascular risk in adults: a report of the American College of Cardiology/American Heart Association Task Force on Practice Guidelines. *J Am Coll Cardiol*. 2014;63(25):2890-2932. doi:10.1161/01.cir.0000437741.48606.98.

48. Sawka MN, Burke LM, Eichner ER, Maughan RJ, Montain SJ, Stachenfeld NS. Exercise and fluid replacement. *Med Sci Sports Exerc*. 2007;39(2):377-390. doi:10.1249/mss.0b013e31802ca597.

49. American College of Sports Medicine. *ACSM's Guidelines for Exercise Testing and Prescription*. 9th ed. Philadelphia, PA: Wolters Kluwer, Lippincott Williams & Wilkins; 2013.

50. Cheuvront SN, Kenefick RW, Zambraski EJ. Spot urine concentrations should not be used for hydration assessment: a methodology review. *Int J Sport Nutr Exerc Metab*. 2014;25(3):293-297. doi:10.1123/ijsnem.2014-0138.

51. Kenefick RW, Cheuvront SN. Hydration for recreational sport and physical activity. *Nutr Rev*. 2012;70(suppl 2):137S-142S. doi:10.1111/j.1753-4887.2012.00523.x.

52. Hew-Butler T, Rosner MH, Fowkes-Godek S, et al. Statement of the Third International Exercise-Associated Hyponatremia Consensus Development Conference, Carlsbad, California, 2015. *Clin J Sport Med*. 2015;25(4):303-320.

53. Woolf K, Manore M. B-vitamins and exercise: does exercise alter requirements? *Int J Sport Nutr Exerc Metab*. 2006;16(5):453-484.

54. Grimaldi AS, Parker BA, Capizzi JA, et al. 25(OH) vitamin D is associated with greater muscle strength in healthy men and women. *Med Sci Sports Exerc*. 2013;45(1):157-162. doi:10.1249/MSS.0b013e31826c9a78.

55. von Hurst PR, Beck KL. Vitamin D and skeletal muscle function in athletes. *Curr Opin Clin Nutr Metab Care*. 2014;17(6):539-545. doi:10.1097/MCO.0000000000000105.

56. Wortsman J, Matsuoka LY, Chen TC, Lu Z, Holick MF. Decreased bioavailability of vitamin D in obesity. *Am J Clin Nutr*. 2000;72(3):690-693.

57. Larson-Meyer DE, Willis KS. Vitamin D and athletes. *Curr Sport Med Rep*. 2010;9(4):220-226. doi:10.1249/JSR.0b013e3181e7dd45.

58. Haub M, Loest H, Hubach K. Assessment of vitamin status of athletes. In: Driskell J, Wolinsky I, eds. *Nutritional Assessment of Athletes*. 2nd ed. Boca Raton, FL: CRC Press; 2010:289-310

59. Pasricha S, Low M, Thompson J, Farrell A, De-Regil LM. Iron supplementation benefits physical performance in women of reproductive age: a systematic review and meta-analysis. *J Nutr*. 2014;144(6):906-914. doi:10.3945/jn.113.189589.

60. Rowland T. Iron deficiency in athletes: an update. *Am J Lifestyle Med*. 2012;6(4):319-327. doi:10.1177/1559827611431541.

61. Akabas SR, Dolins KR. Micronutrient requirements of physically active women: what can we learn from iron? *Am J Clin Nutr*. 2005;81(5):1246S-1251S.

62. US Olympic Committee. *Iron Status in Athletes*. 2014. www.researchgate.net/publication/270215096_Iron_Requirements_and_Iron_Status_of_Athletes. Accessed September 5, 2016.

63. Longo DL, Camaschella C. Iron-deficiency anemia. *N Engl J Med*. 2015;372(19):1832-1843. doi:10.1056/NEJMra1401038.

64. Thomas DT, Erdman KA, Burke LM. American College of Sports Medicine Joint Position Statement. Nutrition and athletic performance. *Med Sci Sports Exerc*. 2016;48(3):543-568.

65. Nattiv A, Loucks AB, Manore MM, Sanborn CF, Sundgot-Borgen J, Warren MP, for the American College of Sports Medicine. American College of Sports Medicine position stand. The female athlete triad. *Med Sci Sports Exerc*. 2007;39(10):1867-1882. doi:10.1249/mss.0b013e318149f111.

66. Donnelly JE, Blair SN, Jakicic JM, Manore MM, Rankin JW, Smith BK. Appropriate physical activity intervention strategies for weight loss and prevention of weight regain for adults. *Med Sci Sports Exerc*. 2009;41(2):459-471. doi:10.1249/MSS.0b013e3181949333.

67. Mountjoy M, Sundgot-Borgen J, Burke L, et al. The IOC consensus statement: beyond the female athlete triad—relative energy deficiency in sport (RED-S). *Br J Sports Med*. 2014;48(7):491-497. doi:10.1136/bjsports-2014-093502.

68. Professional resources. American Academy of Pediatrics. www.aap.org/en-us/professional-resources/Pages/Professional-Resources.aspx. Accessed October 17, 2015.

69. Turocy PS, DePalma BF, Horswill CA, et al. National Athletic Trainers' Association position statement: safe weight loss and maintenance practices in sport and exercise. *J Athl Train*. 2011;46(3):322-336.

70. Buell JL, Franks R, Ransone J, Powers ME, Laquale KM, Carlson-Phillips A. National Athletic Trainers' Association position statement: evaluation of dietary supplements for performance nutrition. *J Athl Train*. 2013;48(1):124-136. doi:10.4085/1062-6050-48.1.16.

71. Granger LR, Johnson CL, Malina RM, et al. National Athletic Trainers' Association position statement: preventing, detecting, and managing disordered eating in athletes. *J Athl Train*. 2008;43(1):80-108. doi: 10.4085/1062-6050-43.1.80.

CHAPTER 9

ANTHROPOMETRIC MEASUREMENTS AND BODY COMPOSITION

Carrie Hamady, MS, RD, LD, and Amy Morgan, PhD, FACSM

INTRODUCTION

Anthropometric measurements, such as body weight, height, and waist circumference, along with body composition, are key components for assessing an athlete. Monitoring changes in weight and height helps to evaluate the growth of a young athlete and can serve as a predictor of health and wellness in adulthood. Assessment of body composition can also be an indicator of energy balance, effects of training, and overall disease risk. Therefore, the purpose of this chapter is to define body weight and body composition, describe body composition measurement techniques, and illustrate how diet can assist an athlete in achieving body composition goals.

Anthropometric Measurements

Weight and height are the most common anthropometric measurements taken during an assessment of athletes. To ensure accuracy, weight should be taken with a calibrated scale and not as a self-reported measurement from the athlete. Depending on the purpose of the visit (eg, weekly diet reviews, quarterly assessments, or seasonal physicals), weights should be taken on the same scale at every visit for consistency. Height should be taken with a stadiometer, which can be attached to the scale or affixed to the wall for reliability. For young athletes who are still growing, measurement of height should be performed at every visit to assess changes. A height can then be taken at the yearly physical once it has been determined that the athlete is through growing, which can vary from person to person.

Weight and height can be used to determine body mass index (BMI). BMI is often thought of as a measure of body composition; however, it does not provide any values related to body fat or muscle content. BMI, calculated as weight (kg) divided by height (m^2), is described by the Centers for Disease Control and Prevention as a potential "indicator of high body fatness." Because there is no way to determine percent fat from this method, BMI is a tool used to "screen for weight categories that may lead to health problems."[1] See Table 9.1 for examples of BMI classifications. In athletes, the use of BMI is limited, primarily because muscularity may lead to a high BMI without high body fatness. In many cases, athletes may be characterized as obese when utilizing standard ranges for BMI when, in fact, they are not overly fat. Thus, while BMI is universally available, is affordable, and requires minimal time to assess, it is only a screening tool and not a measure of body composition. See Table 9.1 for classifications of BMI.

Waist circumference can also be used to identify distribution of fat and therefore is a marker of disease risk. Individuals who carry excess visceral fat in their abdominal region can experience metabolic changes leading to insulin resistance, hypercholesterolemia, hormonal imbalances, and hypertension. As a result, they are at higher risk for many chronic diseases, such as cardiovascular disease, diabetes, stroke, and certain cancers.[2,3] According to the National Institutes of Health (NIH), a healthy waist measurement is less than 35 in for a woman and less than 40 in for a man.[4]

Waist circumference can be measured at the natural waist or at the umbilicus. To be consistent with NIH recommendations, an umbilicus measurement is taken as follows [5]:

Locate the upper hip bone and the top of the right iliac crest. Place a measuring tape in a horizontal place around the abdomen at the level of the iliac crest. Before reading the tape measure, ensure that the tape is snug, but does not compress the skin, and is parallel to the floor. The measurement is made at the end of a normal expiration.

Table 9.1 Body Mass Index Classifications[1]

Classification	Value
Underweight	<18.5
Normal	18.5–24.9
Overweight	25.0–29.9
Obesity (class I)	30.0–34.9
Obesity (class II)	35.0–39.9
Extreme obesity (class III)	≥40.0

DEFINITION OF BODY COMPOSITION

In the context of sport, body composition can contribute to performance, injury risk, and effective goal setting and interventions. Often, when individuals hear the term body composition, his or her immediate reaction is to think about body fat and not about the other components that contribute to the overall makeup of the body (eg, muscle, water, bone, minerals). Body composition can be described in terms of a two-compartment, three-compartment, or four-compartment model. For the purposes of this chapter, the two-compartment model—(1) lean body mass, which includes muscle, bone, and organs, and (2) fat mass—will be utilized. While they are not exactly synonymous, it is important to note that for many purposes the terms *lean body mass* (LBM) and *fat-free mass* are used interchangeably.

In the sport or athletic setting, body composition assessment is inclusive of bone, fat, and muscle, although there is often a focus on body weight or amount of fat. While it may be important to measure fat or body weight to gauge or track the health of an athlete, there are many events in which individuals of various sizes and body compositions can be successful, such as baseball, softball, football, soccer, basketball, and tennis. For other events, body weight and composition may significantly affect an athlete's performance, perhaps because there are weight classes (eg, boxing, wrestling) or because the athlete needs to propel his or her body through space (eg, diving, gymnastics) in an efficient, athletic, and artistic manner. In any case, it is important to work on an individual basis to help an athlete maintain a healthy level of body weight, fat mass, and LBM. See Box 9.1 for a discussion on measuring body composition in athletes.

Box 9.1 Why Measure Body Composition in Athletes?

In the assessment of many sport medicine professionals, there are three reasons why one may choose to measure weight or body composition in athletes. These are: (1) to address concerns about the health of an athlete, (2) to determine contributions to performance, and (3) to best prepare an individual for a sport-specific performance. These reasons are not independent, and in most cases, body composition is measured for some combination of these factors.

BODY COMPOSITION TO GAUGE HEALTH

It is important to determine if an individual has too little or too much body fat: Both situations are a cause for concern for long-term health of an athlete. Body fat is typically reported as a percentage of total body weight (percent body fat). The reference values for percent fat are determined in large part by gender, age, and activity level.[6] In general, men will have a lower percent fat than women, and fat content tends to increase with age, particularly for those over age 40. As one might suspect, athletes and highly active individuals are leaner and have a lower percent fat than those who are less active.

However, all individuals have a certain amount of body fat that is imperative to overall health and, therefore, is referred to as essential body fat. Essential fat is found in vital organs, such as the heart, lungs, liver, spleen, kidneys, intestines, muscles, and the central nervous system. In women, essential fat is also necessary for the production of sex-specific hormones. Typically, women require about 10% to 13% essential fat and men 2% to 5%.[7]

In general, high levels of fat are associated with a multitude of health concerns, including cardiovascular disease, type 2 diabetes, metabolic disease, and some cancers.[2,3] Other secondary issues, such as joint problems (eg, osteoarthritis), limited functional movement, and compromised independence, can result from long-term obesity.[8] Conversely, low levels of fat are also problematic, primarily in women. In general, women who have too little fat may be at risk for reduced or no menstrual cycle, decreasing estrogen levels, and impaired development of bone.[9-11] This can increase the risk of developing osteopenia and osteoporosis later in life, despite participation in activities that are associated with bone health in other women of a similar age.[9-11]

BODY COMPOSITION AS A CONTRIBUTOR TO PERFORMANCE

Perhaps one of the best uses of body composition measures in healthy individuals is to assess muscle (lean mass) in athletes, particularly over time. If an individual is underperforming, either in practice or competition, low levels of muscle mass may be a contributing factor because the athlete does not have adequate muscle to perform at a level necessary to compete.

A second way to use muscle or lean tissue as an indicator of performance is to complete periodic assessments to identify trends. For example, measuring body composition at pre-, mid-, and postseason will provide longitudinal evidence of gains or losses of muscle and fat across the season. If a coach has noted a drop in an athlete's performance, it may be due to a loss of muscle. In this case, it becomes necessary for the athlete to work with strength and conditioning coaches who can provide appropriate exercises to maintain muscle and with registered dietitian nutritionists (RDNs) for guidance on the most appropriate dietary intake so the athlete can maintain performance across a season.

BODY COMPOSITION TO BEST PREPARE AN ATHLETE FOR PERFORMANCE

The assessment of body composition should not be a one-time measure during the season. It can be helpful for planning training regimens during the off-season as well. As discussed previously, an athlete should work with the strength and conditioning coach, along with the RDN, to develop a plan to regain any LBM lost during a season and to determine how to prevent this from happening the next season. Conversely, if an athlete gained weight or fat mass after the season, the athlete should work with the trainers and RDNs to achieve an optimal body composition before the next season. Trying to make significant changes to body composition during the season is not advised due to the potential for adverse effects on performance or endurance. The overall goal is to begin the preseason in peak shape to maximize the benefits of the training sessions. See the Changing Body Composition section of this chapter for more details.

BODY COMPOSITION TECHNIQUES

There are a variety of methods to estimate body composition. Until recently, all techniques for living humans were compared with underwater weighing (UWW), also referred to as hydrodensitometry. While

UWW is often described as the gold standard and has traditionally been considered the criterion method, it is time intensive and less comfortable than numerous other techniques[13] (for an excellent overview of techniques, see *ACSM's Resource Manual for Guidelines for Exercise Testing and Prescription*.[12] In addition, UWW is mainly available only within an exercise physiology laboratory and thus less accessible than other methods. Newer techniques, such as dual energy x-ray absorptiometry (DXA), are more precise and technologically advanced than UWW. When determining which technique is best for your program or athletes, there are a variety of factors to consider, including cost, precision, comfort level, and time required per test (for both the athlete and the technician). Generally, skinfold thickness or air displacement plethysmography (ADP) can provide the relevant information while being cost-effective and efficient. See Table 9.2 for an outline of these factors. The following section will provide a short description of the most common techniques, as well as a discussion of the considerations for each. For the purposes of this chapter, the techniques will be divided into two categories: (1) traditional clinical techniques and (2) advanced techniques.

Table 9.2 Factors to Consider When Choosing a Body Composition Technique

Method	Availability	Accuracy	Time	Cost
Bioelectrical impedance analysis	Limited	Moderate–high[a]	1–3 min	Low–medium
Skinfold thickness	High	Moderate–high[a]	~5 min	Low
Underwater weighing	Limited	Historical gold atandard	5–15 min	Medium
Air displacement plethysmography	Limited	High	≤10 min	High
Dual-energy x-ray absorptiometry	Limited	Modern standard	≤10 min	High

[a] Accuracy dependent on external factors, such as participants following pretest precautions and availability of a trained technician.

Traditional Clinical Techniques

Two methods have been identified in this category: (1) bioelectrical impedance analysis (BIA) and (2) measures of skinfold thickness.

BIOELECTRICAL IMPEDANCE ANALYSIS

BIA involves asking an athlete to use a device that allows a minimal, undetectable, electrical current to pass through the body. This device measures the resistance to the flow of the electrical current; in general, there is more resistance to flow in an individual with less water-containing tissue. As fat contains little water and muscle is well fortified with water, more resistance is indicative of an individual with a higher percent fat and vice versa.

One of the benefits of BIA is that it is a fairly quick measure (1 to 3 minutes per person), so many athletes can be tested in a short time. It is also a fairly accurate measure of percent fat (ie, standard error of the estimate between 2.7% and 6.3% compared with UWW) when high-quality equipment is utilized *and* when stringent pretest criteria are maintained (see Box 9.2 on page 180 for pretest criteria).[14] However, it is important to note that in athletes, BIA tends to underestimate percent fat compared with UWW.[15]

There is large variability in the quality of BIA devices; within reason, more expensive devices tend to be more accurate. The cost of BIA machines ranges from very inexpensive models that test using two points of contact (about $50 for a home model) to more costly, research-grade machines with up to eight points of contact through direct skin contact or via electrodes affixed to the skin ($4,000 or more). Local availability of a quality device may be limited. Adherence to pretest criteria (see Box 9.2) is vital for accuracy. Because results are determined by body fluid, testing in anything but a normally hydrated state (euhydration) will negatively affect the results. If suggested pretest criteria are not followed, results will not be accurate.

> **Box 9.2** Bioelectrical Impedance Analysis Pretest Criteria
>
> - No food or drink for 2 hours
> - No caffeine use or heavy exercise for 4 hours
> - No alcohol consumption for 12 hours
> - Maintenance of test position for 5 minutes

SKINFOLD THICKNESS

The other measure in this category is the method that uses skinfold thickness to estimate percent fat. Within the traditional clinical techniques category, skinfold thickness measurement is readily available, fairly accurate, low cost, and requires only about 5 minutes per athlete. See Figures 9.1 through 9.7 for images of these measurements. There are, however, certain standards that must be met to ensure accuracy.

Three factors can affect the accuracy of an estimate of percent fat by skinfold thickness. First, measures need to be taken at the correct anatomical location. Each standardized site is clearly demarcated by bony landmarks.[6,16] These locations need to be identified and the skinfold thickness measured when the athlete is in the correct body position. In general, this is an anatomical position without twisting or bending to make the site more available to the tester. Twisting and bending may affect the skin and thus the size of the subsequent fold. A second contributor to accuracy is equipment. While there are a variety of calipers available, inexpensive ones with thin spring mechanisms may stretch or lose recoil over time, changing the force of the caliper on the fold. This may have a small impact on the measured size of the folds over time. For high-quality folds and research purposes, either Lange or Harpenden calipers are recommended because these tools provide a constant pressure of approximately 10 g/mm^2. Most importantly, skinfold thickness is most accurately measured when taken by a trained technician. Training includes learning from an expert and practicing until repeated measures at the same, properly identified site are consistently within 1 to 3 mm. This is a learned skill. When all of the aforementioned criteria are met and the proper equations are utilized for the specific population that is being tested, estimates of percent fat from skinfold thickness are within about 3.5% of UWW.[17]

As indicated earlier, the cost of skinfold thickness is fairly low. It includes the cost of calipers, which range from about $20 to $500, and any fees charged by the technician. The time per athlete depends mainly on the number of skinfold thickness sites measured. For best results, three measures should be taken at each site, and the median value used. While measuring more sites results in higher accuracy, there may be a reasonable trade-off because measuring more sites takes more time, and "good enough" values may be achieved with fewer sites. The number of sites should be determined by the purpose of the data. For health and across-season data, fewer sites (minimum of three) can be used. If the data are to be used for research, more sites (eg, five to seven, depending on the equation) are appropriate. In terms of availability, it is easy to purchase or gain access to calipers, while the availability of a trained technician may be more difficult. Because of the need to measure each site three times, the skinfold thickness method is a bit more time intensive than BIA, requiring about 5 minutes per athlete. However, skinfold thickness can be measured with limited pretest considerations, improving accessibility. Caution should be exercised if those being tested are sweaty or have used lotion at the test sites, which makes the skin slippery and more difficult to pinch, reducing accuracy. Finally, keep in mind that if measures will be repeated at the end of the season, athletes should report in the same state, and skinfold thickness should be taken by the same trained technician as in previous sessions to ensure consistency. See Box 9.3 (page 182) for skinfold analysis equations.

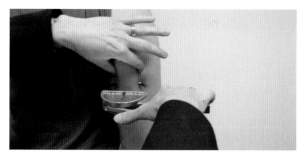

FIGURE 9.1 Demonstration of the triceps skinfold measure. A vertical pinch is made on the midline of the posterior (back) surface of the arm (over the triceps muscle) midway between the acromion process (bony tip of the shoulder) and olecranon process (approximately the elbow joint).

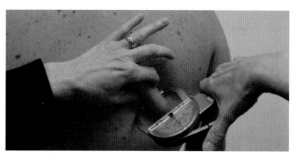

FIGURE 9.5 Demonstration of the subscapular skinfold measure. The diagonal pinch (at about 45°) is made following the natural fold of the skin 1 to 2 cm below the inferior angle of the scapula on a line running laterally (away from the body).

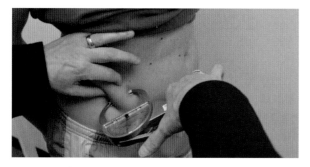

FIGURE 9.2 Demonstration of the iliac crest (suprailiac) skinfold measure. A diagonal pinch downward and medially (approximately 45°) is made immediately above the iliac crest on a vertical line from the front of the axilla (armpit).

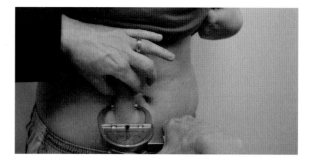

FIGURE 9.6 Demonstration of the abdominal skinfold measure. A vertical pinch is made 1 to 2 cm to the right of the umbilicus.

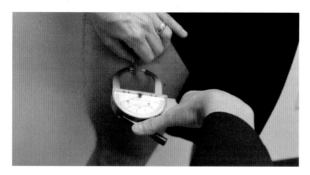

FIGURE 9.3 Demonstration of thigh skinfold measure. A vertical pinch is made at the midpoint of the anterior (front) surface of the thigh, midway between patella (knee cap) and inguinal fold (crease at top of thigh).

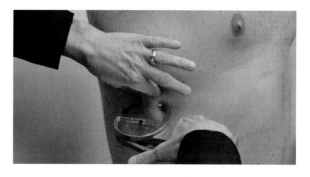

FIGURE 9.7 Demonstration of the midaxillary skinfold measure. A vertical pinch is made with the athlete's arm held at chest height, then follow a horizontal line from the bottom of the xiphoid process (breastbone) to the side of the torso until below the axilla (armpit).

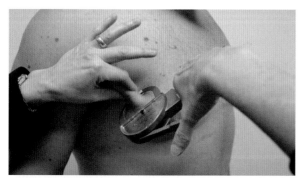

FIGURE 9.4 Demonstration of the (pectoral) chest skinfold measure usually taken in men only. A diagonal pinch (about 45°) is taken on a line midway between the axilla and the nipple.

Generalized skinfold equations for three sites:

Men (chest, abdomen, thigh):

Body density = 1.10938 − 0.0008267 (sum of three skinfolds) + 0.0000016 (sum of three skinfolds)^2 − 0.0002574 (age)

Women (triceps, suprailiac, thigh):

Body density = 1.099421 − 0.0009929 (sum of thre skinfolds) + 0.0000023 (sum of three skinfolds)^2 − 0.0001392 (age)

Calculation of % fat from body density:

Body fat (%) = (495/body density) − 450

Advanced Techniques

This section provides very brief descriptions of the three most common advanced methods of measuring body composition. These methods are UWW, ADP, and DXA. While all three are considered highly accurate measures of body composition, all three require specialized, costly equipment. Therefore, accessibility to such options is usually limited to hospitals or large universities that may have this equipment available, often through an exercise physiology laboratory. Because of the equipment cost and specialized nature of the test, it is not unusual for charges to range from $20 to $200 per athlete and sometimes higher for DXA testing. See Table 9.3 for a breakdown of equipment and maintenance costs. Of these three techniques, ADP (measured through a device marketed under the brand name Bod Pod) and DXA are the best options in terms of athlete comfort during the test. The last factor to be considered for these three techniques is the time required to complete the assessment. Generally, ADP and DXA can be completed in 10 minutes or less. The time required for UWW varies for each individual; it is important to note that it requires three to five tests per session. The first time someone experiences UWW, there is a learning curve that requires extra time, and participant comfort plays a large role in how long each person will take. With repeated measures, time per test will diminish.

Table 9.3 Equipment and Maintenance Costs for Advancd Body Composition Techniques

Technique	Initial Cost	Estimated Yearly Maintenance
Underwater weighing	$2,000–$15,000 Depends on use of pool, newly built, or commercially available tank	Minimal; water for filling and electrical costs for pump
Air displacement plethysmography (Bod Pod)	$20,000–$40,000 new Dependent on testing options	$4,000–$5,000 under maintenance contract
Dual energy x-ray absorptiometry	$90,000–$200,000 dependent on model and options	$5,000–$10,000 under maintenance contract

AIR DISPLACEMENT PLETHYSMOGRAPHY

ADP requires an individual to sit in an egg-shaped chamber wearing tight-fitting clothing. This technique measures body volume by measuring the amount of air displaced when the athlete is seated in the chamber. The only people who should not be tested in this device are individuals over 500 lbs (equipment scale limit) and those with diagnosed claustrophobia. With some assistance, accessibility is available to those who use wheelchairs. Results from ADP are comparable to UWW in most populations (ie, within 2% to 3%), although it has been shown to overestimate percent fat in some populations (eg, collegiate female athletes[20]) and underestimate percent fat in others (eg, collegiate football players[21]). To improve accuracy, there is a need for more population-specific options built into the software. See Figures 9.8 and 9.9.

DUAL ENERGY X-RAY ABSORPTIOMETRY

DXA is a tool that has been used mainly to determine bone density in medical or research settings. However, because this technology can measure the three compartments of bone, muscle, and fat, use of specialized software with DXA can also provide both muscle mass and body-fat measurements. Further, total body and regional values (eg, trunk, limbs) can be ascertained. Participant comfort is not a concern because athletes can be tested in any light clothing without zippers or jewelry. One challenge in testing athletes may be body size; an extremely large or tall individuals may extend beyond the range of the scanner or have to lie in a more cramped position, distorting regional measures. While exposure to x-rays may be an initial concern, a whole-body measurement is comparable to background radiation levels.[12] For athletes with spinal cord injuries, DXA is the most accurate because segmental or regional measurements can be taken. For example, if an athlete is paralyzed from the waist down, the athlete may have muscle atrophy in the lower half of the body, thus resulting in higher percent body fat in that area. As a result, the athlete's upper body may be highly muscular, so the assessment of the upper body will provide the relevant information for this individual.

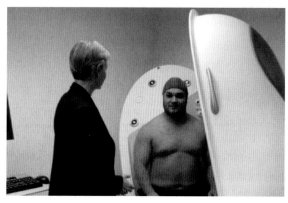

FIGURE 9.8 View of a participant seated in the Bod Pod.

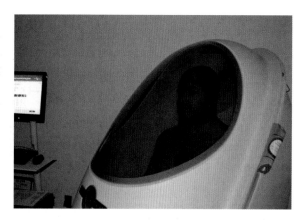

FIGURE 9.9 View of a participant being tested in the Bod Pod.

UNDERWATER WEIGHING

UWW has been considered the gold standard in body composition assessment and has been used in exercise physiology labs for more than 50 years. This test requires an individual to be submerged underwater while suspended from a calibrated weighing scale and expire as much air as possible from the lungs. Weight is measured in the water after all of the air has been expired and the person is motionless.

Limits to this technique include the discomfort experienced with the maximal expiration, the difficulty testing those not comfortable in the water, and the challenges of accessibility for those who use wheelchairs because ladders are often required to get in or out. Because this is the method involved in much of the classic body composition research, many regression equations are derived using UWW as the standard.

SPECIALIZED POPULATIONS

For athletes with amputations or spinal cord injuries, there may be a need to adjust caloric intake recommendations due to changes in overall body mass and muscle mass. Athletes who have had an amputation will need to have their calorie needs and weight goals adjusted according to which limb was removed. To determine ideal body weight, start with the Hamwi equation and then subtract the percentage of body weight that has been amputated.[22] See Box 9.4 for a sample of this equation. See Table 9.4 for more information on calculating ideal body weight for missing limbs.

Sample equation for below-the-knee amputation in a 5-ft 10-in man:

Ideal body weight (IBW) = 166 lb x 5.9% (weight of amputated area) = 9.8 lb

Adjusted IBW = 166 lb − 9.8 lbs. = 156.2 lb ± 10%

The new adjusted ideal body weight can be used when determining calorie and weight goals for this athlete. Assessment of body composition should be accurate using the techniques described previously, unless the athlete does not have a limb needed for the essential measurements for skinfold thickness. In that case, one of the advanced body-fat testing techniques could be used.

Table 9.4 Percent Weight by Body Part

Body Part	Percent Weight of Body Part
Arm	5.0%
Foot	1.5%
Portion of leg below knee	5.9%
Portion of leg above knee	8.1%
Whole leg	16.0%

For athletes with paraplegia or quadriplegia, adjustments should be made for caloric needs, ideal body weight, and body-fat testing. An athlete with paraplegia will typically see a loss of 5% to 10% of body weight due to muscle atrophy, and an athlete with quadriplegia will see a decrease of 10% to 15%. This loss in muscle should be taken into account when calculating desired body weight or energy needs. See Box 9.5 for an example of calculating ideal body weight for a female with paraplegia.

Box 9.5 Sample Equation

Sample equation for a 5-ft 6-in woman with paraplegia:

Ideal body weight (IBW) = 130 lb x [5% up to 10% (difference in needs with paraplegia)]

Calculations: 130 lb − [6.5 lb up to 13 lb]

Adjusted IBW = 123.5 to 117 lb ±10%

As stated previously, DXA is the preferred method for assessing body composition because it allows for segmental measurements.[23] For example, if the athlete is paralyzed from the waist down, the body fat in the lower half of the body would be significantly higher than that in the upper half. Because the upper torso is used for the sport, it is more important to know the percent fat for that section of the body as opposed to overall fat mass.

OTHER CONSIDERATIONS

Once an athlete, and possibly the coach, is informed of the percent fat result, it may be determined that the athlete should make changes in LBM or fat mass or a combination of the two. If a change is desired, the athlete would benefit from the assistance of a strength coach as well as an RDN. It is essential to note that diet alone cannot alter body composition—a combination of exercise and diet is needed. This section reviews some practical nutritional implications for changing body composition, including the appropriate time to change body composition, how to monitor changes, potential effects on performance, and limitations in assessing body composition. See Chapter 11 for more on diet strategies for weight loss or weight gain.

Changing Body Composition

Goals for changing body composition should be established on an annual training cycle to promote realistic and timely approaches to changes in behavior or training schedules. Otherwise, some athletes may feel pressure to engage in unhealthy practices that could result in negative outcomes on performance. Some athletes, such as offensive or defensive linemen, shot putters, and powerlifters, may want to gain weight in the off-season to start the season stronger than the year before. During this training period, the clinician should assess weight weekly to determine if weight gain is occurring too rapidly or too slowly. Target weight gain should be 0.25 to 0.5 kg/wk to avoid negative side effects.[24] Rapid weight gains can cause adverse metabolic reactions, such as changes in hormone levels, increases in triglyceride production, and decreases in mitochondria efficiency.[25] Calorie levels should be adjusted based on the amount of weight gained until the final weight goal is achieved.

After determining body composition, some athletes may choose to focus on decreasing fat mass after their season is over while trying to either maintain or gain LBM. To achieve this, the athlete should work with an RDN to establish a calorie goal and macronutrient distribution tailored to individual needs based on training schedules and body weight or composition goals. To decrease fat mass, diet will need to have a calorie deficit, yet provide adequate protein to promote the maintenance or growth of LBM during high-intensity training with a range of 1.2 to 2.0 g/kg/d.[26,27] To minimize the use of protein for energy so that it will be available for synthesis, adequate energy, mainly in the form of carbohydrate, should be provided to meet caloric needs.[28] Weight loss should occur slowly. Athletes may be able to maintain fat-free mass and performance at a greater level when weight loss is limited to less than 1% per week.[22] The goal is to establish the smallest deficit in calories that produces desired results to avoid metabolic adaptations.[25] When weight loss occurs too quickly, the athlete loses more LBM and is at risk for negative effects once the weight-loss phase ends.[22,25] Potential side effects can include rapid weight gain, increased hunger, and alterations to energy expenditure.

Focus must be placed on both diet and exercise when the athlete desires to change fat mass and maintain or gain LBM over a period of more than 2 weeks. In fact, diet alone can lead to more loss of LBM when trying to lose weight.[29] Therefore, exercise—namely, resistance training—needs to accompany the changes in diet; aerobic exercise could potentially contribute to the loss of LBM.[30] It is the combination of exercise and proper nutrition that will bring the desired changes to body composition to achieve personal goals and maximize performance. See Chapters 10 and 11 for a more complete discussion of energy balance and weight management.

Timing of Body Composition Changes

Another consideration is the timing of weight-loss or weight-gain interventions. Starting an aggressive plan to alter body composition during the active season is not recommended. Instead, the athlete should address body composition goals in the off-season to begin preseason in peak shape. The macronutrient distribution recommended for changing body composition is often not high enough in carbohydrate to meet the needs for optimal performance.[29] Given that all athletes have different needs and training goals, there will be some exceptions to the rule. However, when attempting to lose weight or fat mass, there is always the potential to lose LBM as well, which could negatively affect an athlete during the competitive season. Additionally, there are nutritional barriers to the management of body composition. These include limited access to healthy foods, limited time or skills for food preparation, lack of daily routine, and exposure to catering with unlimited portion sizes and energy-dense foods.[31] Therefore, the role of the clinician during the off-season is not only to help with body composition goals but also to help find creative solutions to these barriers.

Frequency and Error of Measurements

As a general rule, the minimum time between measures of body composition is 3 months. This is because changes in body composition are not usually measurable in shorter periods due, in large part, to the variability of measurement for most methods. For example, suppose the first time an athlete is assessed, his or her percent fat measurement is 17%. If the assumption is that the measurement error is within 3%, the percent fat is actually 17% ± 3% If a subsequent measure indicates a value of 15% and the same error is assumed, the individual's percent fat is then between 12% and 18%. In this example, it is not definitive that there is truly a change in the individual's body composition due to the overlap in percent body fat from the two measurements. Therefore, measurements taken too frequently may give a false sense of change when it is possible that no relevant changes have occurred.

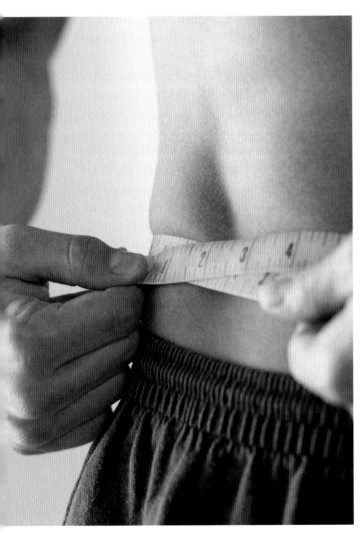

Another concern regarding frequent assessments is the potential for negative alterations in dietary or activity behavior in response to findings. If the previous example is considered and an individual is not made aware of the error inherent in the measure, he or she may unnecessarily change behaviors to alter body composition. These changes could have negative long-term consequences. These examples highlight the caution that is necessary when interpreting and communicating results of body composition testing.

Girth Measurement

Although not an ideal tool to assess body composition, many individuals rely on girth measures at certain sites as a short-term assessment (ie, usually in periods of less than 3 months) to determine if an athlete is progressing in adding muscle or losing fat. While this may seem like a solution, there are several drawbacks. If an increase is noted at a specific site, girth size does not indicate whether the increase in size is from an increase in muscle (a preferred improvement) or an increase in fat (not preferred). Conversely, a decrease in size at a specific site may indicate a loss from muscle or fat. Because girth encompasses both of these components, there is no way to identify which interpretation is accurate. Coupling skinfold thickness measures with girth does not solve this dilemma, as discussed in the previous section, because appreciable changes in fat in less than 3 months cannot be accurately measured. This is an example of when reliance on other performance measures (eg, strength) is more appropriate to determine if muscle quality has improved.

Limitations of Body Composition Data in Relation to Performance

While body composition is a useful tool for the assessment of athletes, it is important to exercise caution in the use and interpretation of these measures. There are many other variables that contribute much more significantly to athletic performance, such as muscular strength and endurance, cardiovascular endurance, and skill level within the sport. These variables can be improved and maximized through an appropriate training regimen; daily performance (in training or competition) can be maximized through appropriate nutritional fueling and hydration status.

There are published values that depict common body composition ranges for a variety of sports.[32-35] What is clear from these numbers is that there is quite a range between sexes and across sports. Keep in mind that these are averages; they do not dictate guidelines that need to be enforced within a sport. Encouraging an athlete to meet a specific level of percent fat that is not realistic for the athlete's physiological makeup is counterproductive, particularly if performance has been good.

As discussed previously, the use of body composition is quite helpful for tracking both fat and muscle composition within an athlete and for identifying someone who may be at risk for health or performance concerns. The use of body composition measurements is best used to assist athletes in maximizing performance across a season.

ANTHROPOMETRIC SKILLS

Historically, didactic programs in dietetics have included very little, if any, hands-on anthropometric training. As a result, many current practicing RDNs lack these skills. More recently, many of these programs have created nutrition assessment courses that go beyond discussing anthropometrics to include hands-on training. Several options are available for RDNs who were never trained in anthropometrics. Many of the manufacturers of body composition equipment offer training by a representative. If an RDN works with a degreed exercise physiologist, the physiologist who has received training in anthropometrics may be willing to train the RDN. Nutrition and dietetics practitioners can also complete certification programs that include anthropometrics, such as those offered by the American College of Sports Medicine and the National Strength and Conditioning Association. Lastly, the highly regarded International Society for the Advancement of Kinanthropometry trains and accredits people throughout the world in anthropometry. There are four levels of training, and they require reaccreditation every 4 years. (See the society's website for more information: www.isakonline.com/home.)

KEY TAKEAWAYS

Measures of percent fat in athletes should be used when there are concerns about health, performance, or injury, or to help determine levels of muscle or lean tissue.

Use body composition measures as a tool to track muscle and LBM across a season.

Choose the technique that will meet needs while minimizing time and discomfort.

RDNs and strength and conditioning professionals can work together to help athletes adjust LBM and percent fat, ideally during the off-season.

Suggest a combination of exercise and proper nutrition to help the athlete bring about the desired body composition changes to maximize performance and begin preseason in peak shape.

Keep in mind that other variables, such as muscular strength and endurance, cardiovascular endurance, and skill level within the sport, should be used in conjunction with body composition measures.

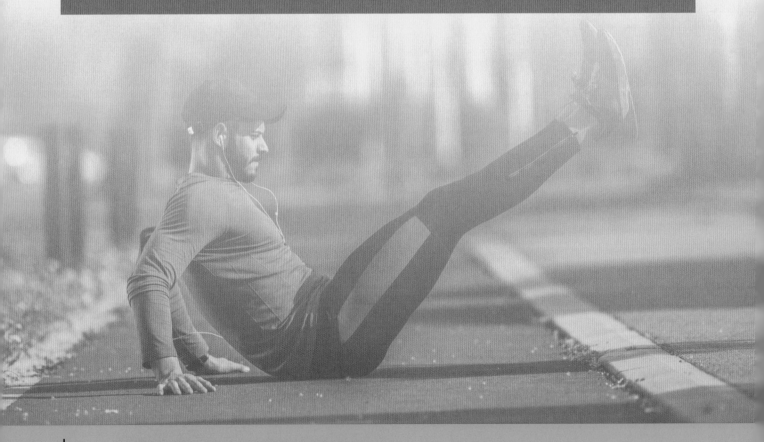

REFERENCES

1. About adult BMI. Centers for Disease Control and Prevention website. www.cdc.gov/healthyweight/assessing/bmi/adult_bmi/. Updated May 15, 2015. Accessed September 26, 2016.

2. Eckel RH. Obesity and heart disease: a statement for healthcare professionals from the Nutrition Committee, American Heart Association. *Circulation*. 1997;96(9):3248-3250.

3. How is metabolic syndrome diagnosed? National Heart, Lung and Blood Institute, National Institutes of Health website. www.nhlbi.nih.gov/health/health-topics/topics/ms/diagnosis. Updated November 6, 2015. Accessed September 27, 2016.

4. What are the health risks of overweight and obesity? National Heart, Lung and Blood Institute, National Institutes of Health website. www.nhlbi.nih.gov/health/health-topics/topics/obe/risks. Updated July 6, 2012. Accessed September 27, 2016.

5. National Heart, Lung, and Blood Institute Obesity Education Initiative. The practical guide: identification, evaluation, and treatment of overweight and obesity in adults. www.nhlbi.nih.gov/files/docs/guidelines/prctgd_c.pdf. Published October 2000. Accessed September 27, 2016.

6. Pescatello LS. *ACSM's Guidelines for Exercise Testing and Prescription*. 9th ed. Philadelphia, PA: Wolters Kluwer/Lippincott Williams & Wilkins; 2014.

7. American College of Sports Medicine. *ACSM's Health-Related Physical Fitness Assessment Manual*. 2nd ed. Philadelphia, PA: Wolters Kluwer/Lippincott Williams & Wilkins; 2008.

8. Marsh AP, Rejeski WJ, Espeland MA, et al. Muscle strength and BMI as predictors of major mobility disability in the Lifestyle Interventions and Independence for Elders pilot (LIFE-P). *J Gerontol A Biol Sci Med Sci*. 2011;66(12):1376-1383.

9. Gordon CM, Nelson LM. Amenorrhea and bone health in adolescents and young women. *Curr Opin Obstet Gynecol*. 2003;15(5):377-384.

10. Nattiv A, Loucks AB, Manore MM, Sanborn CF, Sundgot-Borgen J, Warren MP, American College of Sports Medicine. American College of Sports Medicine Position Stand. The female athlete triad. *Med Sci Sports Exerc*. 2007;39(10):1867-1882.

11. Maimoun L, Georgopoulos NA, Sultan C. Endocrine disorders in adolescent and young female athletes: impact on growth, menstrual cycles and bone mass acquisition. *J Clin Endocrinol Metab*. 2014;99(11):4037-4050.

12. American College of Sports Medicine. *ACSM's Resource Manual for Guidelines for Exercise Testing and Prescription*. 7th ed. Philadelphia, PA: Wolters Kluwer/Lippincott Williams & Wilkins; 2013.

13. Ackland TR, Lohman TG, Sundgot-Borgen J, et al. Current status of body composition assessment in sport: review and position statement on behalf of the ad hoc research working group on body composition, health and performance, under the auspices of the IOC Medical Commission. *Sports Med*. 2012;42(3);227-249.

14. Graves JE, Kanaley JA, Garzarella L, Pollock ML. Anthropometry and body composition assessment. In: Maud PJ, Foster C, eds. *Physiological Assessment of Human Fitness*. 2nd ed. Champaign, IL: Human Kinetics; 2006:185-225.

15. Dixon CB, Deitrick RW, Pierce JR, Cutrufello PT, Drapeau LL. Evaluation of the BOD POD and leg-to-leg bioelectrical impedance analysis for estimating percent body fat in National Collegiate Athletic Association Division III collegiate wrestlers. *J Strength Cond Res*. 2005;19(1):85-91.

16. Lohman TG, Roche AF, Martorell R. *Anthropometric Standardization Reference Manual*. Champaign, IL: Human Kinetics; 1988.

17. Heyward VH, Wagner, DR. *Applied Body Composition Assessment*. 2nd ed. Champaign, IL: Human Kinetics; 2004.

18. Jackson AS, Pollock ML. Practical assessment of body composition. *Phys Sportsmed*. May 1985;13(5):76-90.

19. Brozek J, Henschel A. *Techniques for Measuring Body Composition*. Washington, DC: National Academy of Science; 1961:223-244.

20. Vescovi JD, Hildebrandt L, Miller W, Hammer R, Spiller A. Evaluation of the BOD POD for estimating percent fat in female college athletes. *J Strength Cond Res*. 2002;16(4):599-605.

21. Collins MA, Millard-Stafford ML, Sparling PB, et al. Evaluation of the BOD POD for assessing body fat in collegiate football players. *Med Sci Sports Exerc*. 1999;31(9):1350-1356.

22. Garthe I, Raastad T, Refsnes PE, Koivisto A, Sundgot-Borgen J. Effects of two different weight-loss rates on body composition and strength and power-related performance in elite athletes. *Int J Sport Nutr Exerc Metab*. 2011;21(2);97-104.

23. Jones LM, Goulding A, Gerrard DF. DEXA: a practical and accurate tool to demonstrate total and regional bone loss, lean tissue loss, and fat mass gain in paraplegia. *Spinal Cord*. 1998;36(9):637-640.

24. American College of Sports Medicine. American College of Sports Medicine position stand. Progression models in resistance training for healthy adults. *Med Sci Sports Exerc*. 2009;41(3):687-708.

25. Trexler ET, Smith-Ryan AE, Norton LE. Metabolic adaptations to weight loss: implications for the athlete. *J Int Soc Sports Nutr*. 2014;11(7):1-7.

26. Burke LM. New guidelines for carbohydrate intakes in sport from the International Olympic Committee. *SCAN Pulse*. 2012;31(3):7-11.

27. Mettler S, Mitchell N, Tipton KD. Increased protein intake reduces lean body mass during weight loss in athletes. *Med Sci Sports Exerc Metab*. 2010;42(2):326-337.

28. Rodriguez NR, Vislocky LM, Gaine PC. Dietary protein, endurance exercise, and human skeletal-muscle protein turnover. *Curr Opin Clin Nutr Metab Care*. 2007;10(1):40-45.

29. Phillips S. Dietary protein for athletes: from requirements to metabolic advantage. *Appl Physiol Nutr Metab*. 2006;31(6):647-654.

30. Phillips SM, Van Loon LJ. Dietary protein for athletes: from requirement to optimum adaptation. *J Sports Sci*. 2011;29(suppl 1):29S-38S.

31. Thomas DT, Erdman KA, Burke LM. American College of Sports Medicine joint position statement. Nutrition and athletic performance. *Med Sci Sports Exerc*. 2016;48(3):543-568.

32. Jeukendrup A, Gleeson M. *Sport Nutrition*. 2nd ed. Champaign, IL: Human Kinetics; 2010

33. Bentzur KM, Kravitz L, Lockner DW. Evaluation of the BOD POD for estimating percent body fat in collegiate track and field female athletes: a comparison of four methods. *J Strength Cond Res*. 2008;22(6):1985-1991.

34. Glodt Baker AJ. *Evaluation of the Body Composition of Female Collegiate Athletes Using the BOD POD* [master's thesis]. Lexington: University of Kentucky; 2012.

35. Ode JJ, Pivarnik JM, Reeves MJ, Knous JL. Body mass index as a predictor of percent body fat in college athletes and nonathletes. *Med Sci Sports Exerc*. 2007;39(3)403-409.

CHAPTER 10

ENERGY BALANCE

Christopher Melby, DrPH, Hunter L Paris, MS, and Rebecca Foright, MS

INTRODUCTION

Rapid increase in obesity throughout the United States and many other countries has spawned a weight-loss industry fraught with quick-fix approaches, diet gimmicks, misinformation, and confusion for the public. Athletes and other active individuals attempting to achieve a desired body weight and composition for reasons of health, metabolic fitness, and sports performance are not immune to marketing and uncertainty. A foundational understanding of the factors that affect energy balance will enable health practitioners to provide their clients with the most accurate scientific approaches possible and can help practitioners and clients sort through vast amounts of misinformation clamoring for their attention.

Energy balance is a function of energy input to the body consumed as carbohydrates, proteins, fats, and alcohol and the energy expenditure of the body at rest, during physical activity, and while processing ingested food.

The magnitude and direction (positive or negative) of energy balance are reflected by changes in energy stores based on the equation:

$$\Delta ES = EA - EEx$$

where ΔES is the change in bodily energy stores, EA is the energy ingested and available to the human body, and EEx is total body energy expenditure.[1] If food energy availability (input) and bodily energy expenditure (output) are equal, the energy stores in the body (glycogen, proteins, and fats) remain fairly constant over time, and the individual is said to be in energy balance or at zero energy balance.

A state of positive energy balance is characterized by greater energy input than expenditure, resulting in an increase in body energy stores. A state of negative energy balance is characterized by greater energy expenditure than energy intake, which causes a decrease in bodily energy stores. In this chapter, the fundamental principles of energy balance will be examined, setting the stage for Chapter 11, which discusses dietary approaches to body weight regulation. The concepts presented in this chapter have relevance to competitive and recreational athletes attempting to alter body weight and composition, as well as to non-athletes initiating diet and exercise changes. A central theme of the chapter is the dynamic nature of energy balance, wherein changes in energy intake can result in changes in energy expenditure and vice versa, which can have substantial effects on energy storage and body weight regulation. Box 10.1 (page 192) defines some of the terms that will be used throughout this chapter.

FOUNDATIONAL PRINCIPLES OF BIOENERGETICS

The key principles that underlie body weight regulation come from the field of bioenergetics. Energy is defined as the capacity to do work, and, in the case of the human body, this work is a biological and physical function that includes a variety of cellular processes such as transport of ions against their concentration gradients, the synthesis of various compounds such as glycogen and proteins and skeletal muscle contraction for physical activity.

ATP: adenosine triphosphate

BAT: brown adipose tissue

ETS: electron transport system

ExEE: exercise energy expenditure

NAD: nicotinamide adenine dinucleotide

NEAT: nonexercise activity thermogenesis

PA: physical activity

PAEE: physical activity energy expenditure

PAL: physical activity level

RMR: resting metabolic rate

TCA cycle: tricarboxylic acid cycle (Kreb's cycle)

TDEE: total daily energy expenditure

TEF: thermic effect of food

Figures 10.1 and 10.2 provide schematic overviews of several fundamental aspects of energy metabolism in the human body. The energy available to athletes in food comes from macronutrients synthesized by plants and other animals (eg, proteins) and is used to synthesize the primary energy (the "currency") of the body: adenosine triphosphate (ATP). This energy contained in the chemical bonds of the ATP molecule is used for biologic work. Upon hydrolysis of ATP to adenosine diphosphate (ADP) and inorganic phosphate (P_i), energy is released (exergonic process), which is used for vital cellular functions. The daily ATP requirement is met not by tapping into a large reservoir of stored ATP but primarily by rapidly resynthesizing ATP from ADP and P_i in the mitochondria. If the ATP-resynthesizing processes were somehow impaired, the amount of stored, available ATP would be sufficient to provide only several seconds worth of energy to contracting skeletal muscle, thus highlighting the need and ability of the body to recycle ADP into ATP.[2] This process of creating the high-energy phosphoanhydride bond of ATP from ADP and P_i is highly endergonic, with the necessary energy input coupled to the highly exergonic process of the oxidation of macronutrients, including carbohydrates, fatty acids, and deaminated amino acids. In oxidation reactions catalyzed by dehydrogenase enzymes, hydrogen atoms are removed from macronutrient intermediates by the coenzymes nicotinamide adenine dinucleotide (NAD+) and flavin adenine dinucleotide (FAD), resulting in the reduction of these molecules to NADH and $FADH_2$. These reduced coenzymes, in turn, undergo oxidation in the electron transport system, where electrons are passed between conjugate redox pairs in the respiratory chain to ultimately reduce oxygen to form water. These oxidation/reduction reactions result in protons being pumped from the mitochondrial matrix across the inner mitochondrial membrane, resulting in the generation of a membrane potential and a pH gradient. This potential energy is then used to drive the endergonic process of ATP synthesis from ADP and P_i as the hydrogen ions (protons) move back across the inner mitochondrial membrane by way of a specific conductance pathway associated with ATP synthase.

In this way, oxidation reactions are coupled to phosphorylation of ADP, hence the term oxidative phosphorylation to describe the synthesis of ATP inside the mitochondria. Given the importance of oxygen as the final oxidizing agent in the electron transport chain and the liberation of carbon dioxide by decarboxylation of macronutrient substrates, determining the rate of oxygen consumption and carbon dioxide production via indirect calorimetry provides an accurate measure of whole-body energy expenditure, except when substantial amounts of ATP are produced anaerobically. The latter can occur when exercise intensity approaches maximal capacity and the demand for ATP exceeds the capacity of skeletal muscle fibers to generate the ATP entirely by mitochondrial oxidative phosphorylation.

FIGURE 10.1 Plant Photosynthesis and Human Glucose Metabolism Synthesis of glucose in plants occurs in photosynthesis. Plants require radiant energy from the sun to synthesize glucose from carbon dioxide and water. After ingestion of glucose from plants, the human body will use the energy contained within the chemical bonds of glucose molecules to provide what is necessary to synthesize adenosine triphosphate (ATP) from adenosine diphosphate (ADP) and inorganic phosphate (P_i). ATP is the primary energy currency used by cells to perform biological work such as skeletal muscle contraction. The diagram shows how the exergonic process of glucose metabolism (oxidation) in cellular respiration provides the energy required for ATP synthesis. Lipids and proteins (amino acids) also undergo oxidation to provide the necessary energy for ATP synthesis.

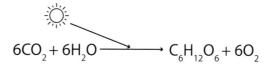

Photosynthesis in plants:

$$6CO_2 + 6H_2O \longrightarrow C_6H_{12}O_6 + 6O_2$$

Cellular metabolism:

$$C_6H_{12}O_6 + 6O_2 \longrightarrow 6CO_2 + 6H_2O$$

Energy

ADP + P_i → ATP

Energy for biologic work

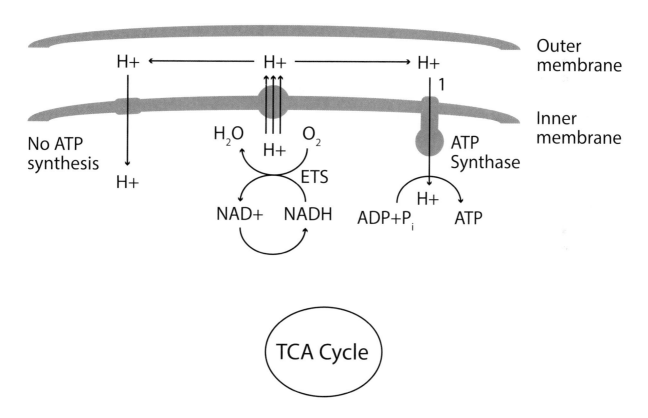

FIGURE 10.2 Simplified Mitochondrial Bioenergetics. In the tricarboxylic acid cycle (TCA) (also called the Kreb's cycle), oxidation reactions catalyzed by dehydrogenase enzymes result in the removal of hydrogen atoms from substrates by the coenzymes nicotinamide adenine dinucleotide (NAD+) and flavin adenine dinucleotide (FAD; not shown in diagram) resulting in the reduction of these molecules to NADH and $FADH_2$. These reduced coenzymes, in turn, undergo oxidation in the electron transport system; electrons are passed between conjugate redox pairs in the respiratory chain to ultimately reduce oxygen to form water. These oxidation/reduction reactions cause protons to move from the mitochondrial matrix across the inner mitochondrial membrane, resulting in the generation of a membrane potential and a pH gradient. As shown in scenario A, this energy is then used to drive the endergonic process of adenosine triphosphate (ATP) synthesis from adenosine diphosphate and inorganic phosphate as the hydrogen ions (protons) move back across the inner mitochondrial membrane by way of a specific conductance pathway associated with ATP synthase. If protons "leak" back into the matrix (inner portion of the mitochondrion) by conduction pathways not linked to ATP synthase shown by scenario B (eg, by uncoupling proteins found in highly thermogenic brown adipose tissue [BAT]), the coupling efficiency of oxidation and phosphorylation is reduced, and more heat and fewer ATP molecules are synthesized relative to the amount of oxygen consumed.

THE ENERGY BALANCE EQUATION: A SIMPLE CONCEPT WITH LAYERS OF COMPLEXITY

The first law of thermodynamics states that energy is neither created nor destroyed, but it is transformed from one form to another. In humans, the energy balance equation is based on this law because we must account for the energy we ingest (macronutrients) and the energy we expend in carrying out the processes vital to life. The energy balance equation dictates that energy available from foods and beverages in excess of expenditure—that is, a positive energy balance—will result in increased energy stores. Conversely, when energy expenditure is greater than what is metabolically available from our ingested food, negative energy balance will result in depletion of the body's energy stores.

Owing to episodic food intake via meals and snacks consumed during the day and episodic levels of daily physical activity and exercise, athletes are almost always in a state of acute energy imbalance. For example, during a meal, acute excess energy is available without a substantial increase in energy expenditure, making mealtimes a brief period characterized by an acute state of positive energy balance and storage of macronutrients. On the other hand, exercise during practice for a sport and other forms of physical activity during the day are characterized by an acute state of energy deficit as energy expenditure is substantially greater than energy intake. Thus, while energy intake and energy expenditure can be quantified for brief periods, determination of chronic energy balance requires averaging acute energy balance over days, weeks, and months.[3]

During times of positive energy balance, adipocytes (fat cells) are the major storage depot for excess energy, with triacylglycerol molecules within adipocytes being the primary means of storing this energy. Clearly, an excessive expansion of adipose tissue mass can jeopardize athletic performance and is associated with increased risk for a host of chronic inflammatory diseases such as type 2 diabetes and coronary heart disease.[4] The sequelae of excessive adiposity could lead one to assume that a lower fat mass means better health. However, adipose tissue plays an important functional role in ensuring that adequate energy is available during times of short-term (fasting) and long-term (hypocaloric diets) energy deprivation, as well as long-distance endurance exercise. Adipose tissue also has an important endocrine role, secreting regulatory signaling molecules such as leptin (discussed later in this chapter), which influences both energy intake and energy expenditure.[5] Thus, an excessively low degree of adiposity can detrimentally affect human health, and potentially performance, depending on the sport.

Despite the perceptions that some individuals are seemingly susceptible to weight gain and excessive fat storage, it is impossible to increase body energy stores without energy intake exceeding energy expenditure. We simply cannot defy the first law of thermodynamics in an attempt to explain why some individuals are more prone to weight gain than others. An understanding of the various determinants of both sides of the balance—energy expenditure and intake—demonstrates the many nuances and complexities of this equation (see Figure 10.3). Chapter 11 provides information regarding achievement of weight management goals for sport-specific athletes.

Metabolic Efficiency

The second law of thermodynamics dictates that the cellular reactions that generate ATP are less than perfectly efficient—that is, at least a portion of energy released from oxidation of macronutrients will be lost as heat rather than all of the available energy being conserved in the phosphoanhydride bonds of ATP molecules. Note that even under normal conditions, cellular oxidation of glucose results in greater heat production than energy conserved as ATP. Metabolic efficiency maximizes ATP production relative to heat loss, while metabolic inefficiency is characterized by increased heat production and lessened synthesis of ATP molecules relative to the potential energy in a macronutrient.[5]

The foundational principles of mitochondrial bioenergetics reveal that oxidation reactions in the mitochondria result in protons being pumped from the matrix, creating a proton gradient. If these protons "leak" back into the matrix by conduction pathways not linked to ATP synthase (eg, by uncoupling proteins

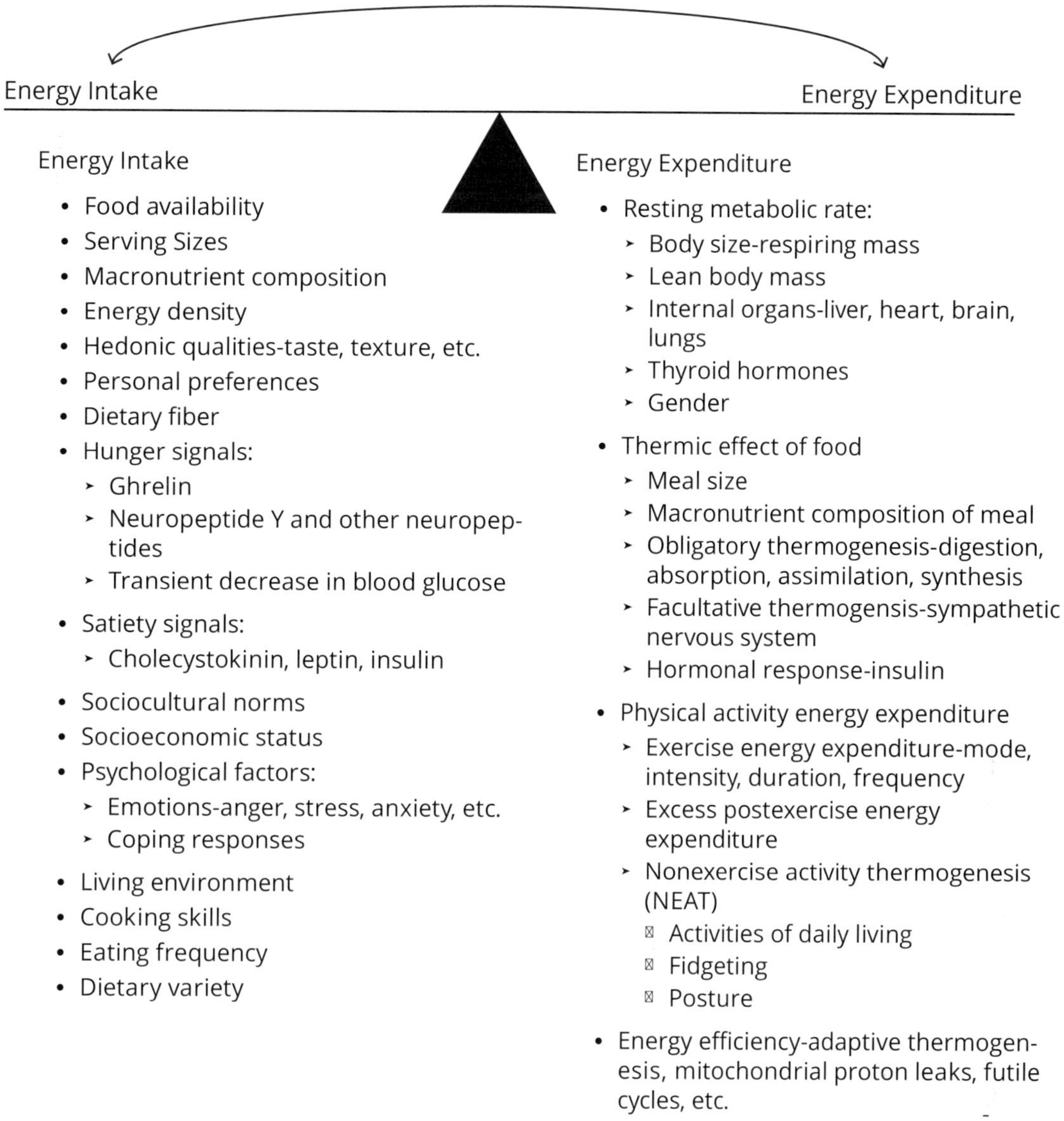

Energy Intake ⟷ Energy Expenditure

Energy Intake

- Food availability
- Serving Sizes
- Macronutrient composition
- Energy density
- Hedonic qualities-taste, texture, etc.
- Personal preferences
- Dietary fiber
- Hunger signals:
  - Ghrelin
  - Neuropeptide Y and other neuropeptides
  - Transient decrease in blood glucose
- Satiety signals:
  - Cholecystokinin, leptin, insulin
- Sociocultural norms
- Socioeconomic status
- Psychological factors:
  - Emotions-anger, stress, anxiety, etc.
  - Coping responses
- Living environment
- Cooking skills
- Eating frequency
- Dietary variety

Energy Expenditure

- Resting metabolic rate:
  - Body size-respiring mass
  - Lean body mass
  - Internal organs-liver, heart, brain, lungs
  - Thyroid hormones
  - Gender
- Thermic effect of food
  - Meal size
  - Macronutrient composition of meal
  - Obligatory thermogenesis-digestion, absorption, assimilation, synthesis
  - Facultative thermogensis-sympathetic nervous system
  - Hormonal response-insulin
- Physical activity energy expenditure
  - Exercise energy expenditure-mode, intensity, duration, frequency
  - Excess postexercise energy expenditure
  - Nonexercise activity thermogenesis (NEAT)
    - Activities of daily living
    - Fidgeting
    - Posture
- Energy efficiency-adaptive thermogenesis, mitochondrial proton leaks, futile cycles, etc.

FIGURE 10.3 Interactive Energy Balance The dynamic or interactive energy balance equation predicts that body energy stores are a function of energy intake and energy expenditure, both influenced by a multitude of factors. Sizable changes in energy intake usually evoke compensatory behavioral and metabolic changes in energy expenditure that defend the initial body weight. Conversely, sizable changes in energy expenditure may evoke changes in energy intake. These compensatory changes vary substantially between individuals and are related to neuroendocrine adjustments and cognitive factors.

found in highly thermogenic brown adipose tissue [BAT]), the coupling efficiency of oxidation and phosphorylation is reduced, and more heat and fewer ATP molecules are synthesized relative to the amount of oxygen consumed. A person who produces more heat and less ATP per mole of substrate would thus be less energy efficient compared with an individual who produces more ATP relative to the amount of substrate oxidized. It follows, then, that energy inefficiency is characterized by an increased quantity of substrate required to synthesize a given amount of ATP, which, in turn, will require more oxygen consumption (reducing oxygen to water) in the cellular mitochondria.

There is considerable interest in variable efficiency rates of cellular energy transduction, which could theoretically help explain differences in susceptibility and resistance to obesity among humans living in the same obesigenic environment.[2] The commonly observed phenomenon that individuals subjected to the same magnitude of energy deficit or surplus do not lose or gain the same amount of weight, respectively, can be at least partly due to individual differences in energy efficiency in response to dieting or overeating.[6] Different types of fat cells can impact energy efficiency. There are two distinct types of adipose tissue: white and brown. White adipose tissue is the primary site of energy storage and is responsible for the secretion of various hormones, including leptin. BAT is responsible for the dissipation of energy in the form of heat, by way of less efficient coupling of oxidation and phosphorylation. BAT was once thought to only exist in human infants; however, human adults have variable amounts of brown fat depots.[7] Published observations of variation in the ability of brown fat to increase energy expenditure via uncoupling mitochondrial oxidation from ATP synthesis and the observation that the amount of brown fat in adults is inversely correlated with body mass index provide credible evidence for human differences in metabolic efficiency.[8] Interestingly, there is accumulating evidence that white adipocytes can undergo some degree of "browning," (also referred to as "beiging") resulting in beige-colored adipocytes with increased mitochondria that, upon stimulation, also exhibit greater uncoupled oxidative phosphorylation and thus more heat production.[9] There is considerable interest in the possibility that exercise could cause the browning of white adipose tissue by way of a newly discovered myokine called irisin. Researchers first reported that skeletal muscle of exercising mice secreted irisin, which stimulated mitochondrial biogenesis and the browning of white adipocytes. These changes were associated with increased energy expenditure and reduced energetic efficiency.[10] However, a number of recently published studies tempered the initial excitement about the possible role of exercise. In one study, investigators found that while messenger RNA translated into the irisin protein was increased in men following a 12-week endurance exercise training program, circulating irisin was actually reduced after the 12 weeks of exercise, and there was little evidence for exercise-induced browning of white adipose tissue.[11] Along these lines, in a cross-sectional comparison of endurance-trained athletes with lean sedentary counterparts, endurance training was actually associated with lower cold-stimulated BAT activity.[12] Furthermore, in a population-based sample of over 700 men and women, circulating irisin concentrations were inversely associated with exercise capacity in men, although there was a trend toward a positive association of irisin with exercise capacity in women.[13] These findings have suggested that in humans there is little to no effect of chronic exercise on circulating irisin-induced beiging of white adipose tissue. However, research strongly suggests that some of the incongruities in study results stem from the inability to accurately measure the irisin peptide. When using a better detection method, irisin increases with aerobic exercise.[14] If this controversy is adequately resolved by more accurate measures of irisin, and exercise is found to stimulate beiging of adipocytes via myokine, this would be yet another benefit of exercise to body weight regulation. More research is required to adequately determine the effect of exercise on irisin and beiging of white adipocytes.

Important Energy Balance Concepts

Four specific principles are important for understanding the energy balance equation: (1) the laws of thermodynamics are inviolable; (2) the large variation in human responses to controlled diet and exercise changes likely results, at least in part, from differences in energetic efficiency that may be linked to genetic and epigenetic variation;[15] (3) changing one side of the energy balance equation will usually result in involuntary metabolic or behavioral changes on the other side; and (4) human responses to diet and exercise that seem contrary to our understanding of bioenergetics (eg, as individuals losing far less weight than predicted based on their purported decreases in energy intake and increases in exercise) are not violations of the laws of thermodynamics. These apparent violations are due, instead, to substantial limitations in our ability to accurately measure energy intake and availability and total energy expenditure and its individual components, as well as our limited ability to measure changes in energetic efficiency in response to external perturbations, such as changes in diet and exercise.

NEUROENDOCRINE REGULATION OF ENERGY BALANCE

Both energy intake and expenditure can be readily modified by voluntary behavior—after all, the amount and types of food we eat and our level of physical activity are choices we make. However, over the past several decades, considerable evidence has emerged showing that energy balance is regulated by a host of neuroendocrine factors. This notion is summarized by Jeffrey Friedman, MD, PhD, an internationally recognized scientist known for his work in molecular genetics, energy regulation, and obesity. He states, "The simplistic notion that weight can be controlled by 'deciding' to eat less and exercise more is at odds with substantial scientific evidence illuminating a precise and powerful biologic system that maintains body weight within a relatively narrow range."[16] Although this view of the magnitude of genetic control over body weight is not shared by all scientists, it does highlight the fact that physiological regulatory controls of body weight do exist.

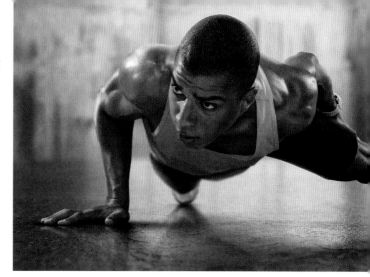

The hypothalamus, a portion of the central nervous system located just above the brainstem, integrates a host of signals from the liver, gut, and adipose tissue to regulate energy expenditure and the initiation, termination, and frequency of eating. The arcuate nucleus (ARC) is one of several important nuclei in the hypothalamus involved in the regulation of energy expenditure and intake. The ARC is composed of two neuronal populations with reciprocal functions. Neurons coexpressing neuropeptide Y (NPY) and agouti-related protein (AgRP) work in concert to increase food intake and decrease energy expenditure when stimulated.[17] Weight loss and the associated changes in various hormone concentrations activate these neurons to counter the weight loss by promoting positive energy balance and weight regain. Alternatively, the stimulation of neurons expressing proopiomelanocortin (POMC) induces decreases in food intake and increases in energy expenditure. These neurons are activated by homeostatic adjustments in response to weight gain to drive a negative energy balance and weight loss.[18]

Adiposity-Related Signals

Two circulating hormones have been identified as adiposity-related signals—insulin and leptin. As adiposity increases, so do circulating insulin and leptin concentrations.[19,20] The former results from the well-characterized compensatory hyperinsulinemia in response to insulin resistance. Elevation of leptin occurs as a direct consequence of increased fat mass, the primary site of leptin synthesis and secretion.[21] Effects on energy intake and expenditure are two of the many functions of these two major adiposity-related signals, as shown in Figure 10.4 (see page 198). These two hormones communicate to the brain the magnitude of the body's adiposity. Leptin receptors are located throughout the brain,[22] including both populations of ARC neurons. Binding to the leptin receptor in the ARC leads to a signaling cascade that ultimately inhibits NPY/AgRP neurons and excites POMC neurons to exert an antiadiposity effect.[23] In this way, increasing leptin concentrations due to increasing fat mass will promote weight loss. Like leptin, insulin interacts with the ARC of the hypothalamus to exert its anorexigenic effects. Insulin binds to the insulin receptor to inhibit NPY/AgRP neurons and reduce food intake.[24] Provided an individual does not develop insulin or leptin resistance, as body weight fluctuates, changes in circulating concentrations of leptin and insulin will activate/inhibit these neuronal circuits to return body weight to its preestablished level.

Powerful homeostatic regulation of food intake occurs such that severe energy restriction leading to weight loss typically results in a strong internal drive to eat, whereas an overabundance of food intake and weight gain is often followed by a reduction in food intake. These homeostatic compensatory responses, observed in both animals and humans, support the notion that body weight and composition are regulated within a usual range for a given individual. There are many factors that determine this range, including genetic, environmental, and socioeconomic factors.[25] Substantial deviations from this range are met with metabolic and feeding changes that alter energy expenditure and intake in an effort to return body weight to its preestablished level.[26] For example, as adipose tissue expands, adiposity-related signals, insulin and

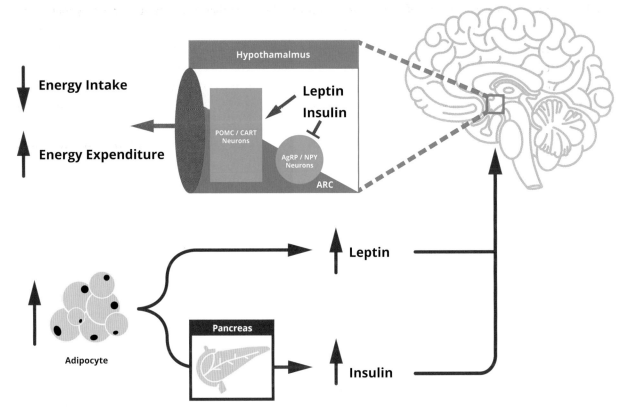

FIGURE 10.4 Effects of Leptin and Insulin on Energy Intake and Expenditure Leptin and insulin are considered adiposity-related signals—that is, they alert the brain to the amount of body fat stores present. As body fat increases, synthesis and release of leptin into circulation also increases. Insulin is secreted from the pancreas, not from adipocytes, but the amount circulating is proportional to the amount of body fat. Therefore, increased storage of fat is associated with increased blood concentrations of both leptin and insulin. These hormones travel to the brain where they bind to their respective receptors located on neurons throughout the hypothalamus, including specific neurons in the arcuate nucleus. They inhibit the expression of two orexigenic (hunger-stimulating) neuropeptides—agouti-related peptide and neuropeptide Y. These same hormones stimulate neurons that express the anorexigenic (hunger-suppressing) neuropeptides—proopiomelanocortin and cocaine- and amphetamine-regulated transcript. These latter neuropeptides also stimulate an increase in energy expenditure. Thus, as adipose tissue expands, the increased circulation of these hormones results in homeostatic adjustments to limit this expansion by decreasing energy intake and increasing energy expenditure.

leptin, increase in circulation.[27-29] Through their effect on specific hypothalamic neurons, the signals stimulate increased energy expenditure and encourage a greater sense of satiety leading to decreased food intake. Loss of body fat reduces these signals, leading to decreased energy expenditure and increased food intake.[28,29] This communication between adipose tissue and the brain suggests that the control of body weight extends beyond volitional behavior. There are also a number of peptides released by the digestive tract that interact with the hypothalamus to regulate short-term hunger and satiety. These will be briefly discussed in a later section.

The rapid increase in human obesity may seem to be at odds with the set-point theory because it would appear that corrective internal actions must be lacking in a substantial portion of the population in the face of our current obesigenic environment. However, it is likely that the obesity-prone person regulates body weight, but at a higher set point than the obesity-resistant individual,[28] akin to an individual with hypertension regulating his or her blood pressure via endocrine and neural inputs, but at a higher level than normal. It is also possible that impairments in regulation occur such that the brain becomes resistant to peripheral signals such as leptin and insulin. The possibility also exists that most humans exhibit a stronger, more powerful defense against weight loss than against weight gain.[30] Regardless, it is evident that compensatory changes in energy intake occur in both obese and nonobese individuals (including athletes) in response to energy excesses or deficiencies.[31,32] The magnitude of these compensatory responses is probably under both genetic control and environmental influences.

It seems logical that the dramatic increase in overweight and obesity over the past 30 to 40 years would be primarily due to environmental changes, given that any significant shifts in the human genetic constitution would not occur during such a brief time. Note, however, that in earlier years, an underlying genetic predisposition might have been masked by an environment in which hard manual labor and lack of palatable food were the norms. However, such a genetic predisposition, coupled with our current obesigenic environment, could readily result in an obese phenotype today.[33] The individual contributions of genes and voluntary behavior in ultimately determining a person's body weight are unknown. The "either/or" debate (genetic/biological determinism vs voluntary choices) is not particularly helpful in dealing with individuals. What is important is to seek understanding of the behavioral and metabolic features of the individual, with the aim of developing the most effective personalized approach to achieving a healthy and competitive body weight and composition.

ENERGY EXPENDITURE

There are four components of total daily energy expenditure (TDEE) that make up one side of the energy balance scale: resting metabolic rate (RMR), the thermic effect of food (TEF), NEAT, and exercise energy expenditure (ExEE). Physical activity energy expenditure (PAEE) would include both NEAT and ExEE (see Figure 10.3). A brief discussion of each of the four components follows.

Resting Metabolic Rate

RMR is the energy expended by an individual for cellular processes necessary to maintain life while lying supine in a postabsorptive, awakened state.[34] For sedentary individuals, the RMR accounts for approximately 70% to 75% of daily energy expenditure.[35] For an athlete who engages in hours of exercise training each day, RMR may account for up to half of total daily energy expenditure.[36] There are many factors that influence RMR, the most pronounced being body size (especially lean body mass), with greater respiring tissue mass accounting for greater energy expenditure. Among adults, RMR is generally lower in women than men, mostly due to differences in lean body mass. Resting metabolism decreases with advancing age, primarily resulting from age-related declines in lean mass. RMR decreases approximately 2% per decade in healthy adult women and approximately 3% per decade in healthy adult men.[37] Although skeletal muscle accounts for a sizable portion of lean tissue, the internal organs, including the liver, heart, brain, kidneys, and lungs, together expend far more energy *at rest* than skeletal muscle. Numerous hormones affect RMR as well, especially the thyroid hormone triiodothyronine. Individuals with a hypoactive thyroid gland have lower metabolic rates than their body size would predict, and they tend to readily gain weight and experience profound fatigue until the condition is corrected. On the other hand, a hyperactive thyroid gland leads to decreased energy efficiency characterized by increased RMR and weight loss.

MEASUREMENT OF RESTING METABOLIC RATE

Typically RMR is measured for 30 to 60 minutes in the early morning, approximately 10 to 12 hours after the previous evening's meal while lying quietly in a recumbent position in a thermoneutral environment.[34] Most often, RMR is measured via indirect calorimetry, a process involving the measurement of respiratory gases. Because oxygen (O_2) utilization in the mitochondria is directly tied to ATP synthesis and heat production, the measurement of oxygen consumption (and often carbon dioxide [CO_2] production as well) is used to accurately quantify energy expenditure. A ventilatory mask, mouthpiece, or canopy is used in conjunction with a metabolic cart equipped with a flow meter and CO_2 and O_2 analyzers. The energy equivalent per liter of O_2 ranges between 4.6 and 5.0 kcal, depending on the relative proportion of fats, carbohydrates, and deaminated amino acids oxidized. Based on the oxygen consumption per minute and the energy equivalent per liter of oxygen, energy expenditure per minute is determined, which is then extrapolated to a 24-hour period. Some handheld measurement devices are also available. These devices are less expensive and can provide reasonably accurate measurements of RMR, but they are generally not capable of measuring the energy costs of exercise when ventilation rates are much higher than during rest.[38]

ESTIMATION OF RMR BY PREDICTION EQUATIONS

Because indirect calorimetry is not accessible by all athletes, many RMR prediction equations have been developed. These typically include such variables as body size, age, and sex, with more sophisticated equations including some measure of lean and fat mass. Some commonly used equations are provided in Box 10.2. Unfortunately, the development of RMR equations for athletes has lagged behind those established for the general population, and it is possible that the accuracy of the common equations overestimate RMR values in obese individuals, owing to their lower lean to fat mass ratio, while these same equations may underestimate RMR in athletes, who typically exhibit a higher lean to fat mass ratio than characteristic of the general population. Given that the Cunningham equation for RMR estimation is based on fat-free mass, this equation would appear to work fairly well for athletes.[39]

Box 10.2 Equations for Estimating Resting Metabolic Rate[40-44]

There is likely not a single best equation for all athletes because there is substantial diversity in body composition among athletes competing in different sports. If fat-free mass (FFM) can be accurately determined, the Cunningham equation often works well, but as the amount of body fat increases in athletes, its contribution to resting metabolic rate (RMR) will increase, which is not accounted for in this particular equation. For female athletes, the Owen equation is often used, as it was derived specifically from the study of elite female athletes. However, the number of female athletes studied to derive this equation was quite small (n = 8). The example in this box uses the Mifflin-St Jeor equation, but the reader is encouraged to use each of the equations for the sample athlete to identify the range of predicted RMR values.

Harris-Benedict Equation[40]

Men: RMR (kcal/d) = 66.4730 + 13.7516W + 5.0033H − 6.7750A

Women: RMR (kcal/d) = 665.0955 + 9.5634W + 1.8496H − 4.6756A

Where W = weight (kg); H = height (cm); A = age (y).

Cunningham Equation[41]

Men: RMR (kcal/d) = 370 + 21.6FFM

Women: RMR (kcal/d) = 370 + 21.6FFM

Where FFM = kg fat-free mass

Owen Equation[42,43]

Men: RMR (kcal/d) = 879 + 10.2W

Women: RMR (kcal/d) = 795 + 7.18W

Female athletes: RMR (kcal/d) = 50.4 + 21.1W

Where W = weight (kg)

Mifflin-St Jeor Equation[44]

Men: RMR (kcal/d) = 10W + 6.25H − 5A + 5

Women: RMR (kcal/d) = 10W + 6.25H − 5A − 161

Where W = weight (kg); H = height (cm); A = age (y)

Example

A 30-year-old male endurance athlete (very active) who is 1.75 m tall (5 ft 9 in) and weighs 73 kg (160.6 lb). Using the Mifflin-St Jeor equation:

RMR = (10 × 73) + (6.25 × 175) − (5 × 30) + 5 = 1,679 kcal/d

EFFECT OF EXERCISE ON RMR

In a number of studies, endurance-trained athletes exhibited higher RMR values than nonathletes. However, this phenomenon does not seem to result from any adaptations to exercise training. It is more likely that the combination of high ExEE and high energy intake (high flux) in these athletes can temporarily, but not permanently, increase their RMR when measured the morning after exercise.[45] However, there is little evidence that the amount of physical activity for health maintenance and weight control used by recreational exercisers will produce any permanent increases in RMR, with the possible exception of such exercise in older individuals.[46]

Some fitness enthusiasts have promoted the idea that because regular weight lifting can increase skeletal muscle mass, such exercise will substantially increase RMR. Although this may be an attractive notion, a sizable increase in muscle mass is likely to occur only for the individual who becomes a serious weight lifter. The contribution of each pound of muscle mass to *resting* energy expenditure is far less than that of a similar mass of such internal organs as the liver and heart, so one would have to substantially increase muscle mass to increase RMR. Most people who lift weights for health rather than for bodybuilding or sports competition will not increase their muscle mass enough to produce more than a small increase in RMR. For the serious weight trainer, a single prolonged strenuous bout of weight lifting may increase RMR when measured the following morning.[47] Nevertheless, it is clear that for both athletes and nonathletes, young and old, the major impact of both endurance and resistance exercise on total daily energy expenditure occurs during the activity itself and not from any substantial increases in RMR.

Thermic Effect of Food

TEF is defined as the increase in energy expenditure above RMR in response to ingestion of food. This increase in energy expenditure is attributable to obligatory components that include digestion, absorption, transport, and assimilation of the food we eat, as well as a facultative component. The latter is the portion of TEF resulting from the increase in sympathetic nervous system activity that accompanies food consumption.

MEASUREMENT OF THERMIC EFFECT OF FOOD

TEF is usually measured in the same way as RMR, via indirect calorimetry. A meal of known macronutrient and calorie content is provided, and increase in energy expenditure above RMR is measured over 3 to 6 hours, with more accurate determinations made over at least 5 to 6 hours.[35] The average TEF for a mixed meal accounts for approximately 10% of energy ingested. The thermic effect of the individual macronutrients varies considerably, with fat having the lowest at approximately 3% of ingested fat calories, followed by carbohydrates at 5% to 10% of ingested carbohydrate energy, and proteins having the highest thermic effect at 20% to 30% of protein calories.[48]

Physical Activity Energy Expenditure

PAEE is the energy expenditure above resting values that results from skeletal muscle contraction, including that required for movement, balance, and maintenance of posture. This component can be further divided into the ExEE and NEAT.

EXERCISE ENERGY EXPENDITURE

Exercise is defined as volitional movement done to improve or maintain one or more features of either health- or performance-related physical fitness.[49] Exercise is typically the most variable component of daily energy expenditure, and for the athlete attempting to modify body weight and composition, it is obviously the component under the most volitional control. The energetic cost of daily exercise is based on the frequency, duration, intensity, and mode of exercise. On a given day, it can range from zero calories for the nonexerciser to several thousand calories for an individual who participates in a long-distance endurance event, such as a marathon. Athletes who participate in regular strenuous and prolonged exercise training have very high TDEE values, which may require conscientious efforts to obtain adequate energy intake. For example, a study estimated the energy requirements in competitive cyclists to be approximately 4,300 kcal/d while in training and less than 2,400 kcal/d on very sedentary days.[45]

The energy expended for a given exercise bout is usually determined by indirect calorimetry done in a laboratory and then extrapolated to a free-living situation with adjustments made for body size. A compendium of the energy expenditure values for many modes, durations, and intensities of exercise has been published by the American College of Sports Medicine. These values are useful in helping determine the contribution of PAEE to TDEE and energy balance.[50] Often the energetic cost of exercise is expressed in metabolic equivalents, or METs, which are multiples of RMR. For example, if an athlete expends 1.0 kcal/min at rest, and during a given training session has an ExEE of 13 kcal/min, his or her exercise intensity is:

$$13 \text{ kcal/min} \div 1.0 \text{ kcal/min} = 13 \text{ METs}$$

Energy expenditure is elevated for a period following exercise, with greater energy expenditure during this recovery period occurring with higher-intensity exercise. This phenomenon is a function of numerous factors, including elevated body temperature and elevated circulating catecholamines (epinephrine and norepinephrine). This excess postexercise energy expenditure should be considered part of the total ExEE.

NONEXERCISE ACTIVITY THERMOGENESIS

NEAT is the energy expenditure resulting from physical activity not considered exercise, such as activities of daily living and fidgeting. Maintaining body posture is also part of NEAT. This component of TDEE is difficult to measure and is often determined by default after measuring the other three components and subtracting them from TDEE or by using lightweight sensors to detect posture and motion. Primarily owing to the work of James Levine at the Mayo Clinic, NEAT is now widely recognized as an important and highly variable component of TDEE.[51,52] People who are obese spend more time sitting during the day than those who are not obese individuals.[53] Sitting energy expenditure is lower than standing, as the latter requires muscle contractions necessary to maintain balance.[54] Therefore, altering daily activities, such as taking the flight of stairs instead of the elevator, can contribute to TDEE.

Determining Total Daily Energy Expenditure

Determining TDEE to identify a person's energy requirements, while difficult to measure accurately, can be undertaken by a variety of methods. Whole-room calorimeters are used by some scientists but are not available for most people. Even when used by scientists, their use typically underestimates TDEE because ambulation is limited within the small chamber. The use of stable isotopes of hydrogen and oxygen (ie, doubly labeled water) provides accurate measures of TDEE in a free-living environment, but use of this approach is very expensive and impractical apart from access to a major research institution. The factorial method involves measuring individual components of TDEE and then summing these to determine TDEE. However, this approach is very labor intensive and impractical.

Pedometers, accelerometers, and heart rate monitors can be useful in quantifying physical activity, especially when accompanied by activity diaries. Technological advances have made accelerometer-based activity monitors such as watches and fitness bands available to individuals. While the features and capabilities of these devices vary, they all attempt to provide the user with information on TDEE. These monitors estimate RMR using anthropometric data entered by the user—height, weight, gender, and age—and then base TDEE on estimates of calories expended above this RMR value. Some devices attempt to calculate calories for specific activities, while others use additional measurements, such as the temperature of the skin or barometric pressure, to more accurately consider intensity and activity. Initial research on the efficacy of some of these devices has shown promising results for increasing physical activity and weight loss.[55] When evaluated more directly and compared with research-grade instruments, these monitors showed strong validity for measuring step count but only moderate validity for measuring TDEE, with some devices differing in energy expenditure estimates by up to 900 kcal. Between different devices and activities, validity of the monitors varied widely.[56,57] Additionally, wearable global positioning system (GPS) tracking devices, such as GPS watches, are more frequently being used to quantify workload, describe intensity, and estimate energy expenditure. GPS is a satellite-based system that continuously monitors location and then computes caloric expenditure based on anthropometric data and distance traveled. When energy expenditure estimates from multiple GPS devices were compared against a validated accelerometer-based measure while walking at varying speeds, GPS watches showed lower reliability than the accelerometer, especially at increased speeds. The researchers concluded that GPS watches may be limited in their ability to provide accurate values for energy expenditure: Caution is advised when using these devices for such purposes.[58] Taken together, activity monitors may prove useful for keeping track of steps and physical activity but should be used reservedly when attempting to closely track caloric expenditure, especially over a wide range of activities.

Conversion of data from steps walked, accelerometer counts, or changes in heart rate to precise energy expenditure values can be problematic. In light of these issues, TDEE is commonly estimated by multiplying either estimated or measured RMR by a specified physical activity level (PAL), which is a factor based on estimated PAEE. For a sedentary person, the estimates are likely to be more accurate, owing to a small contribution of physical activity to TDEE. However, for athletes, there is substantial room for error based on the significant contribution of ExEE to TDEE. The PAL values have been derived from a variety of methods, including the factorial approach and the use of doubly labeled water. Table 10.1 provides the PAL values established by the Institute of Medicine (IOM) based on a compilation of doubly labeled water values in free-living individuals.[36] The PALs range from 1.25 for an extremely sedentary person with limited opportunity for ambulation to more than 2.5 for an athlete who spends hours per day in exercise training. For example, in the study mentioned earlier, the competitive cyclists had resting metabolic rates of approximately 1,800 kcal/d and estimated TDEE values of 4,300 kcal/d, with a calculated PAL of 4,300 kcal/1,800 kcal = approximately 2.4. Interestingly, on sedentary days, these same athletes exhibited TDEE reflective of a PAL of approximately 1.42.[45]

Table 10.1 Institute of Medicine Physical Activity Levels[9]

Physical Activity Level (PAL) Category	Mean PAL Value (Range)	Example
Sedentary	1.25 (1.1–1.39)	A person with a sedentary occupation who spends his or her entire day sitting
Low level of physical activity	1.50 (1.40–1.59)	An office worker who sits most of the day other than the walking necessary to perform tasks of daily living
Active	1.75 (1.60–1.89)	An athlete who exercises approximately 1 h/d or a person with an active vocation equivalent to walking 6–8 mile/d
Very active	2.20 (1.90–2.50)	A competitive athlete engaging in several hours of vigorous exercise training

Another means of estimating TDEE has been provided by the IOM. The US Department of Health and Human Services contracted with an expert panel of scientists to develop estimates of daily energy intake commensurate with good nutrition.[36] Based on studies using doubly labeled water to quantify TDEE in free-living individuals, the panel established mathematically derived equations that use age, height, body weight, and physical activity factors to estimate TDEE. These male- and female-specific equations are provided in Table 10.2 (page 204).[36] Note that the physical activity (PA) coefficients used in these equations are not the same as PALs. Box 10.3 (page 205) provides a comparison of two estimations of an athlete's energy requirements, one using the Mifflin-St Jeor formula and the other using the IOM equation. TDEE for this person varied by several hundred kilocalories, demonstrating the difficulty in accurately determining TDEE.

Sex	Estimated Energy Requirement, kcal/d	Physical Activity Coefficients
Male	$662 - 9.53A^a + [PA^b \times (15.9W^c + 540H^d)]$	1.00: Sedentary 1.11: Low active 1.25: Active 1.48: Very active
Female	$354 - 6.91A + [PA \times (9.36W + 726H)]$	1.00: Sedentary 1.12: Low active 1.27: Active 1.45: Very active

[a] A = age in years
[b] PA = physical activity
[c] W = weight in kilograms
[d] H = height in meters

ENERGY INTAKE

There are many factors that affect energy intake among active individuals, including the availability and palatability of food, macronutrient composition, social norms, peer pressure, economics, and psychological and emotional factors, to name a few (see Figure 10.3, page 195). Hall and colleagues have described energy intake as a function of the dynamic interplay between homeostatic feedback (hormonal signals from the periphery to the brain), hedonic feedback (stimulation of brain reward centers by foods and even food images), and cognitive feedback (self-regulation and feedback from the environment, including such things as measured body weight, social norms, etc).[59] While a thorough discussion of this dynamic interplay is beyond the scope of this chapter, some important aspects of neuroendocrine regulation are described later. Insulin and leptin are adiposity-related signals secreted from the periphery with effects on food intake mediated through the central nervous system. However, in humans, appetite and food intake are also regulated by a host of hunger and satiety signals originating from the gastrointestinal tract. Ghrelin, the only known orexigenic hormone, is produced primarily by the stomach.[60] This peptide is the endogenous ligand for the growth hormone secretagogue receptor type 1a, which is located throughout the body. Ghrelin binds to its receptor on vagal afferent neurons to mediate effects on appetite regulation.[61] These vagal afferents terminate on the nucleus tractus solitarius, which is connected to the ARC through noradrenergic neurons. Outside of the ARC, ghrelin has an additional effect in driving food intake through the stimulation of the reward centers of the brain. Fasting and weight loss lead to increases in circulating ghrelin concentrations to promote food intake. These concentrations drop rapidly with meal ingestion, proportional to meal calorie content.[62]

There are numerous peptide hormones released by the gastrointestinal tract that are anorexigenic—that is, they decrease hunger and increase satiety. Cholecystokinin (CCK) is secreted by the intestines upon food ingestion. Its role in digestion includes stimulating enzyme release from the pancreas and bile duct, slowing gastric emptying, and enhancing intestinal motility. CCK decreases hunger and increases satiety by way of its interactions with the vagus nerve.[63] Additionally, circulating CCK can cross the blood-brain barrier and directly affect the central nervous system. Weight loss decreases circulating CCK concentrations, a phenomenon shown to persist for at least 1 year and possibly much longer after initial weight loss.[2] Glucagon-like peptide 1 (GLP-1) is another anorexigenic hormone secreted by the gastrointestinal tract in response to food intake. GLP-1 increases stimulate the vagus nerve to decrease hunger and increase satiety. Peptide YY (PYY) is cosecreted with GLP-1, mediating its effects through binding to the Y family of G-protein–coupled receptors. PYY also acts to decrease hunger and increase satiety. Concentrations are lowest during fasting and peak about an hour after eating. Calorie content consumed and dietary composition of ameal will affect secretion of these gastrointestinal peptides.[64] These gut peptides, along with still other neuroendocrine signals not discussed in this chapter, coalesce to form the complicated web of signals that must be integrated to determine all aspects of food intake. While the hypothalamus controls the homeostatic regulation of food intake, vast brain circuits beyond the hypothalamus are involved in the initiation and duration of food intake and feeding behavior based on cognitive and hedonic feedback. When activated, these feedback pathways are capable of overriding the homeostatic control mechanisms designed to maintain energy balance.

It is unclear how exercise affects the secretion of these neuroendocrine factors, manipulating hunger and food intake. Studies have demonstrated how exercise is able to increase, decrease, or not affect ratings of hunger, and these changes in hunger often fail to result in predictable changes in actual food intake.[65-70] The same ambiguous conclusions have been drawn when measuring the effects of exercise on the concentrations of the hormones and peptides involved in regulating food intake.[70] The discrepancy in the results of these studies may be due to differences in exercise intensity, duration, and mode; participant characteristics such as sex, adiposity, and fitness level; whether or not exercise was performed in a fed or fasted state; or even differences in the test meal composition and the amount of time during which intake was monitored after the exercise bout.

Effect of Dietary Composition on Energy Intake

There is evidence that habitual intake of high-fat, mixed meals promotes higher energy intake than lower-fat meals.[71] It seems that the higher energy content of the former is less well noticed, a phenomenon termed passive overconsumption. Given the higher energy intake and the fact that of the three macronutrients, dietary fat is the weakest at promoting its own oxidation, one can envision why overfeeding and fat deposition can so readily occur when dietary composition is high in fat. Note, however, that individuals who consume high-fat, low-carbohydrate diets to lose weight are ingesting more than their usual intake of calories and still lose weight. In reality, such diets are typically hypocaloric because the reduction in carbohydrate calories is greater than the increase in fat and protein calories.

Measurement of Energy Intake

Just like the measurement of energy expenditure, the accurate determination of one's energy intake is also fraught with difficulties. Self-reported energy intake can be derived from diet recalls, diet records, and food frequency questionnaires using computer software with the US Department of Agriculture database for nutrient composition of foods. However, self-reported intake often substantially underestimates actual energy intake.[72-75] Inaccuracies in dietary self-reports severely limit their usefulness in attempting to accurately quantify energy intake. Accurately measuring energy intake is difficult enough in itself, but energy intake is not always synonymous with metabolizabled energy in the form of macronutrients absorbed into circulation and available for energy use by cells in the body. The efficiency of absorption is not readily measured. It can be affected by a variety of factors including the composition of microbiota in the gut. For a brief discussion of this topic see Box 10.4.

Box 10.4 Emerging Research on Gut Microbiome

One area of emerging research on energy intake and availability is that of the gut microbiome. Humans host trillions of bacteria in the gut, and because this microbiome is involved with such processes as amino acid synthesis, degradation of otherwise indigestible foods, and glucose and lipid metabolism, it may have important implications for whole-body energy balance.

Firmicutes and *Bacteroidetes* are the most common bacterial divisions in the gut, and the activity and relative abundance of these organisms has been implicated in health and disease. A comparison of obese vs lean individuals showed that obesity is associated with changes in these two bacterial divisions and that weight loss correlates with a change in the gut biota. Furthermore, when germ-free mice were colonized with the gut bacteria from an obese donor, these mice showed a significantly greater increase in body fat compared with germ-free mice colonized with a lean microbiota *despite there being no difference in food intake*. This would indicate that energy expenditure or the amount of metabolizabled energy from the food is altered by these changes, although it is unclear how.[74]

Energy harvesting describes an elevated ability to absorb energy from the diet, thus decreasing energy losses in the stool. The ability of certain intestinal bacteria to convert portions of nondigestible carbohydrates, such as nondigestible starch and certain dietary fibers, to short-chain fatty acids that are readily absorbed from the gut may be one explanation linking gut microbiota to energy balance and body weight and composition. While there is still lack of clarity on whether or not individuals more prone to weight gain have increased energy harvest efficiency due to the type of microbial colonization, even small daily adjustments in energy availability could have effects on body weight over the long term. Bacteria in the gastrointestinal tract could also affect energy harvest by directly influencing intestinal microvasculature, glucose metabolism through the absorption of monosaccharides, and lipid metabolism and storage.[75] Future research will determine the extent to which gut micriobiota influence energy intake and expenditure and whether or not altering the composition of microbiota by dietary changes can have relevant effects on body weight and composition.

If an individual's body weight and body composition are stable, energy availability and energy expenditure will be similar over time. Estimating energy expenditure by using an appropriate PAL or equation in Table 10.2 and then balancing that with caloric consumption in a weight-stable individual is more likely to provide an accurate estimate of energy intake than self-reported dietary intake. However, self-reported levels of physical activity used to establish an appropriate PAL (Table 10.1) or PA coefficient (Table 10.2) are often overestimated, and one must consider this possibility when there is a large mismatch between self-reported dietary intake and estimated energy requirements.[76]

COMPLEXITIES OF THE ENERGY BALANCE EQUATION

An overly simplistic view of the energy balance equation may lead to projections or even promises of the magnitude of weight loss or weight gain an athlete should achieve based on his or her diet or exercise changes. However, these projections often assume that all other factors that affect the energy balance equation remain the same. Such a static equation fails to account for homeostatic behavioral and metabolic adjustments in response to perturbations in energy intake and expenditure that render the static energy balance equation inadequate to accurately depict the reality of the human experience. Less than predicted changes in body weight and composition can lead to both athlete and counselor discouragement and frustration. Kevin Hall, PhD, at the National Institutes of Health, has written extensively about the dynamic aspects of energy balance, and the interested reader is referred to one of his reviews.[77]

Dietary-Induced Changes in Energy Balance

In the same manner that acute and chronic exercise can influence energy balance by affecting TDEE and energy intake, so, too, can dietary changes affect energy balance leading to increases or decreases in body energy stores.

ENERGY DEFICIT LEADING TO WEIGHT LOSS

Many studies show that during the dynamic phase of weight loss (active weight loss), a hypoenergetic diet results in a decrease in RMR and TDEE. Decreases in energy expenditure with active weight loss can be attributed to a loss of respiring body mass as well as a decrease in energy expenditure per unit of body mass, the latter reflecting an increase in energy efficiency. However, there is considerable controversy about whether this increased energy efficiency persists when the individual has maintained this lost weight for a considerable time. Increased energy efficiency persists in the reduced weight state could help explain the inability of so many individuals to maintain weight loss and the reported high levels of exercise and calorie-counting required of many individuals to maintain long-term weight loss.[78] A well-controlled inpatient study sheds some important light on this controversy. Not surprisingly, the investigators found that individuals who lost 10% or more of their body weights over a 5- to 8-week period had a reduced TDEE greater than what could be accounted for by loss of body mass when measured within a few weeks of the weight loss. In the same study, another cohort of individuals who had maintained 10% or more weight loss for a minimum of 1 year was examined. The TDEE of this group was also significantly lower than predicted by their metabolic body size. The authors concluded that weight loss produces increased energy efficiency (lower energy requirements) that persists long term in individuals able to maintain the weight loss.[79] In an attempt to explain their findings, the same research group found in a separate study that weight loss was associated with an increased skeletal muscle work efficiency at very low exercise intensities (eg, pedaling a bicycle at 10 to 25 Wof power).[80] As individuals lose weight, their TDEE decreases due to the loss of metabolically active tissue. However, TDEE actually decreases *beyond* what would be predicted by this loss in tissue, thus leading to a reduced caloric expenditure in the rested state and making sustained weight loss more difficult.

Given the aforementioned issues, the following scenario describes inappropriate use of the energy balance equation to determine the amount of weight to be lost by a dieting client. Suppose the health practitioner and client agree that a 17-lb weight loss would improve the athlete's sports performance. They set a goal of reducing energy intake by 500 kcal/d, with specific daily food reductions identified after a comprehensive dietary assessment. Given that a pound of fat is equivalent to approximately 3,500 kcal, they might conclude that the dietary change would lead to a loss of 1 lb of fat per week (500 kcal/d × 7 days = 3,500 kcal), which, over a 4-month period (17 weeks), would result in a 17-lb decrease in body fat. However, the eventual weight loss is far less than predicted, and both client and professional are disappointed and frustrated. In reality, a static equation is not useful because changes in food intake can result in metabolic and behavioral changes in factors that influence energy expenditure. Owing to the hypocaloric state, RMR will decrease to an extent greater than explained by loss of respiring tissue mass (ie, metabolic efficiency increases). Also, compared with the prediet state, the energy cost of any particular weight-bearing movement decreases as body mass is lost, and TEF is reduced as less food is consumed. Thus, an initial 500-kcal deficit shrinks over time with subsequent reduction in the velocity of weight loss. Additionally, not all weight loss is body fat (typically about 75% fat loss, 25% lean), and the energy content of fat and lean tissue are not the same.[81] One can see that given the dynamics induced by an energy deficit, the specific amount of weight lost in a given period is not readily predictable. Adding to this complexity are the difficulties in accurately reducing energy intake by 500 kcal, the possible changes in ExEE that can occur when dieting, and the considerable interindividual variation in changes in RMR and PAEE that can occur in response to a reduction in energy intake over a number of months.

Not only does diet-induced weight loss lead to decreases in energy expenditure as described previously, but it is also associated with increases in hunger and decreases in satiety. The term energy gap has been coined to identify the decrease in energy expenditure and the increase in hunger that accompanies diet-induced weight loss. Animal studies performed by Paul MacLean, PhD, have shown that while weight loss produces many favorable changes in cardiometabolic features, numerous metabolic changes almost inevitably lead these animals to regain their lost weight.[82] This anabolic profile following weight loss in humans is characterized by reduced RMR; reduced TEF; increased metabolic efficiency; reduced circulating leptin and insulin; increased orexigenic peptides, such as ghrelin; and reduced anorexigenic peptides, such as PYY. These physiological changes result in the energy gap, in which the animal desires more calories than it requires. These metabolic changes induced by caloric restriction can readily alter energy balance following weight loss and appear to be major contributors to lack of successful long-term weight loss in many dieters. Registered dietitian nutritionists should be cognizant of the energy-gap phenomenon and seek ways to help their clients attenuate the decline in energy expenditure and the increase in hunger after weight loss. A high ExEE can help attenuate the drop in TDEE and allows for greater calorie intake without resulting in positive energy balance. Following diet-induced weight loss, individuals maintaining a relatively high TDEE via exercise with adequate calorie intake (a high flux state) can attenuate the energy gap by increasing subjective feelings of fullness and increasing RMR compared with a sedentary low flux state.[83] Chapter 11 provides information on possible ways to attenuate the increase in hunger, including the use of preload liquids such as water and water-based soups and higher protein intakes.

ENERGY EXCESS LEADING TO WEIGHT GAIN

For the active individual attempting to gain weight (including athletes wanting to increase lean body mass), increase in energy intake is crucial. However, increased energy consumption may be offset by compensatory changes in metabolism, such that TDEE will increase and thus attenuate increases in lean body mass. These compensatory changes in energy expenditure are highly variable, as are the magnitude of weight gain and increases in lean mass and body fat. For example, in several studies in which individuals were overfed an additional 1,000 kcal/d for several months, there were three- to fivefold differences in the magnitude of weight gain between the highest and lowest gainers.[84,85] In a study from the Mayo Clinic, there was a 10-fold difference in the amount of body fat deposition between the highest and lowest gainers, despite the same magnitude of overfeeding between study participants (1,000 kcal in excess of maintenance requirements).[84] Overfeeding increases RMR in most individuals beyond what would be expected by their changes in body size; that is, overfeeding results in decreased energy efficiency. Also, increases in TEF and the energy cost of movement contribute to an increase in TDEE. Adding to the complexity are the dramatic changes in NEAT that can occur in some individuals. In the Mayo Clinic study, an increase in NEAT was a much stronger predictor of attenuated weight gain than were increases in RMR and TEF.[84]

Exercise-Induced Changes in Energy Balance

Just as a change in energy intake can influence energy expenditure, an increase in PAEE can also influence energy intake. Although physical activity is obviously the best means of increasing energy expenditure, the effects on weight loss of exercise alone typically reveal modest results[86] unless substantial increases in ExEE occur without compensatory increases in energy intake.[87] The reasons why an exercise-only approach to weight loss produces such small losses of body weight for many individuals is worthy of discussion (see Box 10.5).

The magnitude of an exercise-induced energy deficit and weight loss can be affected by more than just the energy cost of the exercise, as compensatory changes in both NEAT and energy intake may occur. Just as with dieting and overfeeding, there is substantial individual variability in the amount of weight loss due to exercise, as highlighted in a study by King and colleagues. In this experimental investigation, people who are overweight or obese underwent prescribed and supervised exercise (500 kcal/session) for 5 days per week for 12 weeks. The average weight loss was 3.7 kg (8.1 lb), similar to that predicted using the static energy balance equation, suggesting no metabolic or compensatory changes. However, there was a very large individual response, with 4 of the 30 study participants actually gaining weight, and in the remaining 26 subjects the weight loss ranged from 1 kg (2.2 lb) to 14.7 kg (32.3 lb). This occurred despite rigorous

Suppose that a sedentary individual attempting to lose some weight decides to do so by starting an exercise program. He establishes a goal of walking for 40 minutes a day, 5 days per week. Based on our understanding of energy balance issues, how much weight might this individual expect to lose over the course of several weeks and months if he tenaciously sticks to his new exercise regimen? The following information provided about this individual will be helpful to our discussion:

- Resting energy expenditure = 1.25 kcal/min = 1,800 kcal/d
- Sitting/standing energy expenditure = 1.5 kcal/min
- Exercise characteristics:
  - Duration: 40 min/exercise session
  - Frequency: 5 times/wk
  - Intensity: 5 metabolic equivalents = 6.25 kcal/min
- Gross daily energy cost of 40 minutes exercise: 6.25 kcal/min × 40 min = 250 kcal/d
- Net energy cost of exercise: 250 kcal – (40 min × 1.5) = 190 kcal/d
- Net energy cost of exercise per week: 190 kcal × 5 d/wk = 950 kcal/wk

These data show that while the gross energy cost of the walking exercise is 250 kcal for 40 minutes, the net energy cost is 60 kcal less, owing to the fact that even if the person had not exercised, he would have expended at least 60 kcal during the 40 minutes while sitting or standing. Without any compensatory changes in dietary intake or other components of energy expenditure, the projected energy deficit over the course of a single month would be less than 4,000 kcal, equivalent to a monthly weight loss of slightly more than 1 lb, assuming no other metabolic or behavioral compensations, which is highly unlikely. This weight loss is far less than one might expect from a month-long diet. A head-to-head comparison of the amount of weight loss achieved by exercise only vs diet only is somewhat unfair, as the magnitude of energy deficit created by a hypocaloric diet is usually far greater than that created by starting an exercise program.

control and supervision of the exercise program so that all individuals were achieving the same energy cost of exercise. The major predictor of the magnitude of weight change was the change in energy intake that accompanied the exercise.[88] These findings suggest that in response to initiating sizable weekly energy expenditure in exercise, some individuals increase their energy intakes, whereas other individuals actually reduce them. Why there is a difference in response is not understood, but it is clear that there are very large differences in body weight and composition changes in response to the same amount of exercise.[89]

It is also possible that in response to an increase in ExEE, compensatory decreases in NEAT could offset the impact on energy balance. In a study at the University of Vermont, elderly individuals who initiated an endurance exercise training program failed to significantly increase their TDEE, presumably because of a compensatory decline in NEAT during the nonexercise portion of the day.[90] However, there remains the possibility that the reverse could be true in some individuals—that is, their NEAT may increase with improved physical fitness (see Figure 10.5 on page 210).

On the other end of the spectrum, a sudden cessation of ExEE can also have implications for body-weight regulation. This might occur, for example, when an athlete experiences a debilitating injury or when a collegiate athlete, accustomed to a life of daily, regimented physical activity, graduates and no longer has the regular mandates of training and team practice. These scenarios exemplify a transition from a high flux state—wherein a high TDEE must be matched with a high energy intake—to a low energy flux state where energy intake must be substantially decreased to match the new state of low TDEE. Failure to lower energy intake in response to reduced energy expenditure, either mandated by injury or by personal choice, will necessarily lead to a positive energy balance and an increase in adiposity. Unfortunately, owing to reduced exercise, atrophy of skeletal muscle often occurs as well.

While little is known regarding the specific physiological phenomena in the initial hours and days of reduced physical activity, these circumstances can result in substantial metabolic changes over time. One study found that with just 2 days of no exercise in endurance-trained individuals, insulin sensitivity dropped to those of sedentary levels.[91] Additionally, increasing adiposity often accompanies retirement from sports participation. An estimated 30% of retired American football players have metabolic syndrome,[92] with a 60% prevalence in retired linemen specifically.[93] In another study, competitive cyclists exercised at a moderate-heavy intensity for 3 consecutive days, and then abstained from exercise for the 2

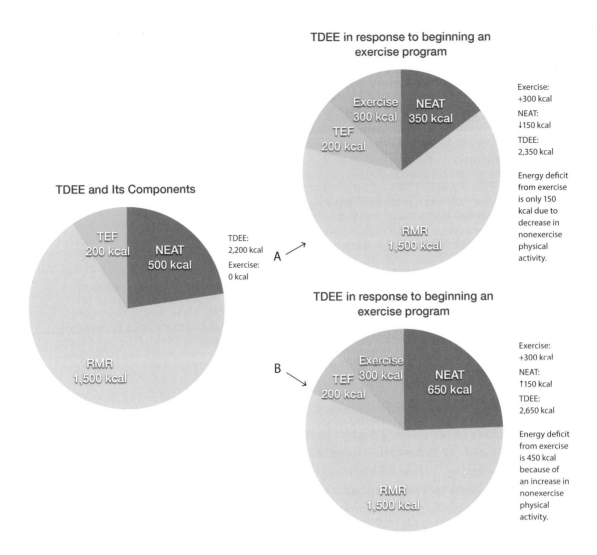

FIGURE 10.5 Illustration of Change in Energy Balance in a Sedentary Person This figure illustrates two possible scenarios depicting the change in energy balance of a sedentary individual who begins an exercise program to create an energy deficit. Initially the person is in energy balance with a total daily energy expenditure (TDEE) of 2,200 kcal (physical activity level = 1.47), based on a resting metabolic rate of 1,500 kcal, a thermic effect of food of 200 kcal, and nonexercise activity thermogenesis (NEAT) of 500 kcal. The person begins an exercise program and adds a net 300 kcal to the energy expenditure side of the energy balance equation. However, as can be seen in scenario A, the person compensates by reducing the activities of daily living, so the net change in energy expenditure is 300 kcal, not 150 kcal.[41,42] In scenario B, in addition to the increase in exercise energy expenditure, the person actually increases NEAT by 150 kcal, and the net increase in TDEE is 450 kcal. Note that any change in energy intake as a result of a change in exercise must also be considered when looking at the overall impact on energy balance of beginning an exercise program.

days following, while maintaining a high-energy intake. In just these 2 days, individuals displayed an RMR that was reduced from a high flux state and regained weight that had been lost in the previous 3 days of exercise.[45] Taken together, these data show potential implications for reductions in energy expenditure on body weight and markers for metabolic health and warrant modifications in intake during these periods. Though specific recommendations pertaining to alterations in total calories and macronutrient ratios are yet to be firmly established, changes in insulin sensitivity and resting metabolism lend support to the necessity of reevaluating nutrition strategies when transitioning out of a high flux condition.

EFFECT OF ACUTE EXERCISE ON POSTEXERCISE ENERGY EXPENDITURE

There was a common belief that upon completion of an exercise bout, individuals would continue to expend energy at an excess rate for a prolonged time, possibly up to 24 hours based on studies done almost 50 years ago. This excess postexercise energy expenditure was thought to be a substantial contributor to TDEE in those who exercised. However, based on more carefully controlled studies, this is usually not the case. Although research has clearly shown that energy expenditure remains increased at higher than preexercise resting baseline levels immediately after exercise, the magnitude of this postexercise elevation of energy expenditure is almost always quite small unless the exercise bout is of high intensity and prolonged duration. Endurance exercise of the intensity and duration commonly done by recreational exercisers (for example, walking for 30 to 60 minutes or jogging at a pace of 8 to 10 minutes per mile for 30 minutes) typically results in a return to baseline of energy expenditure well within the first hour of recovery.[94] The postexercise energy bonus for this type of exercise probably accounts for only about 10 to 30 additional kilocalories expended beyond the exercise bout itself.[95] In athletes performing high-intensity, long-duration exercise, postexercise energy expenditure may remain elevated longer and could contribute a bit more to TDEE.[45,94] Endurance athletes who are in a state of high energy flux (high energy intake and expenditure) may have postexercise elevations detectable the morning after exercise,[45] but it is the rare individual who can regularly achieve this state of high flux. The average person who does considerably less strenuous exercise will likely experience little meaningful contribution of this postexercise bonus to his or her TDEE.

Several studies suggest that vigorous weight-lifting exercise may increase energy expenditure to more than usual resting values for several hours and possibly even until the morning of the following day.[47,96] However, the average person at the gym who spends more time socializing than exercising will not experience prolonged elevation of postexercise energy expenditure after a bout of resistance exercise. The possibility remains that, for both endurance and resistance exercise, accumulation of even modest excess postexercise energy expenditure over the course of months and years can substantially impact energy expenditure. Yet, it is clear that the vast majority of energy expenditure occurs during the exercise itself rather than after.

EFFECT OF ACUTE EXERCISE ON ENERGY INTAKE

Numerous studies have examined the effects of acute and chronic exercise on energy intake. Many experimental studies indicate that following acute strenuous exercise, the energy cost of the exercise is not completely compensated for by increased energy intake during the next 24 hours.[65,97] Donnelly and colleagues conducted a systematic review of published studies and concluded that there is no consistent evidence that is increased exercise affects energy intake or dietary macronutrient intake.[98] These conclusions suggest that in athletes who exhibit their desired body composition and increase exercise training to maximize performance may need to intentionally increase their energy intake accordingly.

SUMMARY

Individual behavioral and metabolic characteristics affect acute and chronic energy balance and fundamentally explain the various body shapes and sizes present within the human population, including athletes. Energy balance is, at the core, a simple concept: if energy intake exceeds expenditure, the excess energy will be stored in the body, primarily as fat, unless concomitant exercise or physical maturation favors greater storage as lean body mass; if energy expenditure exceeds intake, body energy stores will be lost. However, energy balance is best understood as a dynamic equation rather than a static one, wherein changes to one side of the scale can produce unintentional compensatory metabolic and behavioral changes in the other side of the scale. Because body weight is regulated by a host of neuroendocrine factors, because adaptive changes to energy intake and expenditure can modify energy balance and energy efficiency, and because there are considerable difficulties in accurately quantifying both intake and expenditure, the simplicity of this concept gives way to considerable complexity. Even with intact regulatory systems, it seems that in the face of our current obesigenic environment, the regulatory systems of many humans are poorly equipped to adequately protect against excess body weight and fat gain. Maintaining relatively high daily energy expenditure via

ExEE and NEAT can help protect against unhealthy weight gain in the face of our current abundance of highly palatable food. Although body fat stores can be reduced by creating an energy deficit, severe energy restriction by dieting can result in metabolic adaptations that sabotage maintenance of lost weight. Increases in physical activity can contribute to increased energy expenditure, but the magnitude of this increase is often quite small for the beginning exerciser. Realistic expectations regarding energy intake and expenditure and their effects on body weight and composition must replace the often mythical promises marketed to hopeful consumers by advertisements, gimmickry, and fad diets. Understanding the behavioral and metabolic features of the elite or recreational athlete is important in developing the most effective individualized approaches to facilitate their achievement of a healthy and competitive body weight and composition.

KEY TAKEAWAYS

Energy balance is, at the core, a simple concept—if energy availability from food and beverage intake exceeds expenditure, the excess energy will be stored in the body, primarily as fat, unless concomitant exercise or physical maturation favors greater storage as lean body mass; if energy expenditure exceeds intake, body energy stores will be lost.

Energy balance is best understood as a dynamic equation rather than a static one, wherein changes in energy expenditure often evoke compensatory voluntary or involuntary changes in energy intake. Conversely, changes in energy intake evoke compensatory changes in energy expenditure.

Total daily energy expenditure is the sum of the RMR, the TEF, and PAEE, including exercise and nonexercise activity thermogenesis.

Energy intake is influenced by neuroendocrine factors that regulate hunger and satiety. However, personal, social, and environmental factors, including the availability of high-energy–dense foods and low levels of physical activity, can override the homeostatic regulation of body weight and contribute to increased body fat.

Weight loss is usually associated with an increase in hunger and a reduction in energy expenditure—called the energy gap—which is a major contributor to the common occurrence of weight regain. Regular exercise may help attenuate the energy gap by contributing to increased energy expenditure and enabling higher energy intake without accompanying weight gain.

Understanding the behavioral and metabolic features of the elite or recreational athlete is important in developing the most effective individualized approaches to facilitate his or her achievement of a healthy and competitive body weight and composition.

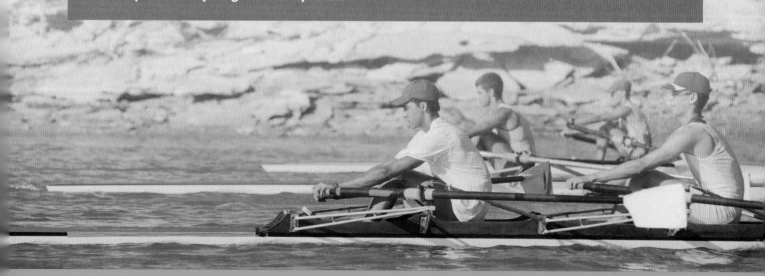

1. Schutz Y. Dietary fat, lipogenesis and energy balance. *Physiol Behav.* 2004;83(4):557-564.

2. Harper ME, Green K, Brand MD. The efficiency of cellular energy transduction and its implications for obesity. *Annu Rev Nutr.* 2008;28:13-33.

3. Chow CC, Hall KD. Short and long-term energy intake patterns and their implications for human body weight regulation. *Physiol Behav.* 2014;134:60-65.

4. Emanuela F, Grazia M, Marco de R, Maria Paola L, Giorgio F, Marco B. Inflammation as a link between obesity and metabolic syndrome. *J Nutr Metab.* 2012;2012:476380. Published online March 1, 2012. doi: 10.1155/2012/476380.

5. Wells JC. The evolution of human adiposity and obesity: where did it all go wrong? *Dis Model Mech.* 2012;5(5):595-607.

6. Leibel RL, Rosenbaum M, Hirsch J. Changes in energy expenditure resulting from altered body weight. *N Engl J Med.* 1995;332(10):621 628.

7. Virtanen KA, Lidell ME, Orava J, et al. Functional brown adipose tissue in healthy adults. *N Engl J Med.* 2009;360(15):1518-1525.

8. Cypess AM, Lehman S, Williams G, et al. Identification and importance of brown adipose tissue in adult humans. *N Engl J Med.* 2009;360(15):1509-1517.

9. Petrovic N, Walden TB, Shabalina IG, Timmons JA, Cannon B, Nedergaard J. Chronic peroxisome proliferator-activated receptor gamma (PPARgamma) activation of epididymally derived white adipocyte cultures reveals a population of thermogenically competent, UCP1-containing adipocytes molecularly distinct from classic brown adipocytes. *J Biol Chem.* 2010;285(10):7153-7164.

10. Bostrom P, Wu J, Jedrychowski MP, et al. A PGC1-alpha-dependent myokine that drives brown-fat-like development of white fat and thermogenesis. *Nature.* 2012;481(7382):463-468.

11. Norheim F, Langleite TM, Hjorth M, et al. The effects of acute and chronic exercise on PGC-1alpha, irisin and browning of subcutaneous adipose tissue in humans. *FEBS J.* 2014;28(3)1:739-749.

12. Vosselman MJ, Hoeks J, Brans B, et al. Low brown adipose tissue activity in endurance-trained compared with lean sedentary men. *Int J Obes (Lond).* 2015;39(12):1696-1702.

13. Kersholt N, Ewert R, Nauck M, et al. Association of circulating irisin and cardiopulmonary exercise capacity in healthy volunteers: results of the Study of Health in Pomerania. *BMC Pulm Med.* 2015;15:41.

14. Jedrychowski MP, Wrann CD, Paulo JA, et al. Detection and quantitation of circulating human irisin by tandem mass spectrometry. *Cell Metab.* 2015;22(4):734-740.

15. Albuquerque D, Stice E, Rodriguez-Lopez R, Manco L, Nobrega C. Current review of genetics of human obesity: from molecular mechanisms to an evolutionary perspective. *Mol Genet Genomics.* 2015;290(4):1191-1221.

16. Friedman JM. Modern science versus the stigma of obesity. *Nat Med.* 2004;10(6):563-569.

17. Morton GJ, Schwartz MW. The NPY/AgRP neuron and energy homeostasis. *Int J Obes Relat Metab Disord.* 2001;25(suppl 5):56S-62S.

18. Hagan MM, Rushing PA, Schwartz MW, et al. Role of the CNS melanocortin system in the response to overfeeding. *J Neurosci.* 1999;19(6):2362-2367.

19. Considine RV, Sinha MK, Heiman ML, et al. Serum immunoreactive-leptin concentrations in normal-weight and obese humans. *N Engl J Med.* 1996;334(5):292-295.

20. Polonsky KS, Given BD, Van Cauter E. Twenty-four-hour profiles and pulsatile patterns of insulin secretion in normal and obese subjects. *J Clin Invest.* 1988;81(2):442-448.

21. Friedman JM. A tale of two hormones. *Nat Med.* 2010;16(10):1100-1106.

22. Funahashi H, Yada T, Suzuki R, Shioda S. Distribution, function, and properties of leptin receptors in the brain. *Int Rev Cytol.* 2003;224:1-27.

23. Elias CF, Aschkenasi C, Lee C, et al. Leptin differentially regulates NPY and POMC neurons projecting to the lateral hypothalamic area. *Neuron.* 1999;23(4):775-786.

24. Schwartz MW, Marks JL, Sipols AJ, et al. Central insulin administration reduces neuropeptide Y mRNA expression in the arcuate nucleus of food-deprived lean (Fa/Fa) but not obese (fa/fa) Zucker rats. *Endocrinology.* 1991;128(5):2645-2647.

25. Keijer J, Hoevenaars FP, Nieuwenhuizen A, van Schothorst EM. Nutrigenomics of body weight regulation: a rationale for careful dissection of individual contributors. *Nutrients.* 2014;6(10):4531-4551.

26. Keesey RE, Powley TL. Body energy homeostasis. *Appetite.* 2008;51(3):442-445.

27. Schwartz MW, Baskin DG, Kaiyala KJ, Woods SC. Model for the regulation of energy balance and adiposity by the central nervous system. *Am J Clin Nutr.* 1999;69(4):584-596.

28. Schwartz MW, Niswender KD. Adiposity signaling and biological defense against weight gain: absence of protection or central hormone resistance? *J Clin Endocrinol Metab.* 2004;89(12):5889-5897.

29. Niswender KD, Baskin DG, Schwartz MW. Insulin and its evolving partnership with leptin in the hypothalamic control of energy homeostasis. *Trends Endocrinol Metab.* 2004;15(8):362-369.

30. Schwartz MW, Woods SC, Seeley RJ, Barsh GS, Baskin DG, Leibel RL. Is the energy homeostasis system inherently biased toward weight gain? *Diabetes.* 2003;52(2):232-238.

31. Major GC, Doucet E, Trayhurn P, Astrup A, Tremblay A. Clinical significance of adaptive thermogenesis. *Int J Obes (Lond).* 2007;31(2):204-212.

32. Melby CL, Schmidt WD, Corrigan D. Resting metabolic rate in weight-cycling collegiate wrestlers compared with physically active, noncycling control subjects. *Am J Clin Nutr.* 1990;52(3):409-414.

33. Ravussin E, Bogardus C. Energy balance and weight regulation: genetics versus environment. *Br J Nutr.* 2000;83(suppl 1):17S-20S.

34. Bullough RC, Melby CL. Effect of inpatient versus outpatient measurement protocol on resting metabolic rate and respiratory exchange ratio. *Ann Nutr Metab.* 1993;37(1):24-32.

35. Levine JA. Measurement of energy expenditure. *Public Health Nutr.* 2005;8(7A):1123-1132.

36. Brooks GA, Butte NF, Rand WM, Flatt JP, Caballero B. Chronicle of the Institute of Medicine physical activity recommendation: how a physical activity recommendation came to be among dietary recommendations. *Am J Clin Nutr.* 2004;79(5):921S-930S.

37. Roberts SB, Dallal GE. Energy requirements and aging. *Public Health Nutr.* 2005;8(7A):1028-1036.

38. Nieman DC, Trone GA, Austin MD. A new handheld device for measuring resting metabolic rate and oxygen consumption. *J Am Diet Assoc.* 2003;103(5):588-592.

39. Thompson J, Manore MM. Predicted and measured resting metabolic rate of male and female endurance athletes. *J Am Diet Assoc.* 1996;96(1):30-34.

40. Harris JA, Benedict FG. A biometric study of human basal metabolism. *Proc Natl Acad Sci U S A.* 1918;4(12):370-373.

41. Cunningham JJ. Body composition as a determinant of energy expenditure: a synthetic review and a proposed general prediction equation. *Am J Clin Nutr.* 1991;54(6):963-969.

42. Owen OE, Holup JL, D'Alessio DA, et al. A reappraisal of the caloric requirements of men. *Am J Clin Nutr.* 1987;46(6):875-885.

43. Owen OE, Kavle E, Owen RS, et al. A reappraisal of caloric requirements in healthy women. *Am J Clin Nutr.* 1986;44(1):1-19.

44. Mifflin MD, St Jeor ST, Hill LA, Scott BJ, Daugherty SA, Koh YO. A new predictive equation for resting energy expenditure in healthy individuals. *Am J Clin Nutr.* 1990;51(2):241-247.

45. Bullough RC, Gillette CA, Harris MA, Melby CL. Interaction of acute changes in exercise energy expenditure and energy intake on resting metabolic rate. *Am J Clin Nutr.* 1995;61(3):473-481.

46. Bell C, Day DS, Jones PP, et al. High energy flux mediates the tonically augmented beta-adrenergic support of resting metabolic rate in habitually exercising older adults. *J Clin Endocrinol Metab.* 2004;89(7):3573-3578.

47. Melby C, Scholl C, Edwards G, Bullough R. Effect of acute resistance exercise on postexercise energy expenditure and resting metabolic rate. *J Appl Physiol (1985).* 1993;75(4):1847-1853.

48. van Baak MA. Meal-induced activation of the sympathetic nervous system and its cardiovascular and thermogenic effects in man. *Physiol Behav.* 2008;94(2):178-186.

49. Caspersen CJ, Powell KE, Christenson GM. Physical activity, exercise, and physical fitness: definitions and distinctions for health-related research. *Public Health Rep.* 1985;100(2):126-131.

50. Ainsworth BE, Haskell WL, Whitt MC, et al. Compendium of physical activities: an update of activity codes and MET intensities. *Med Sci Sports Exerc.* 2000;32(suppl 9):498S-504S.

51. Levine JA, Vander Weg MW, Hill JO, Klesges RC. Non-exercise activity thermogenesis: the crouching tiger hidden dragon of societal weight gain. *Arterioscler Thromb Vasc Biol.* 2006;26(4):729-736.

52. Levine JA. Nonexercise activity thermogenesis—liberating the life-force. *J Intern Med.* 2007;262(3):273-287.

53. Levine JA, Lanningham-Foster LM, McCrady SK, et al. Interindividual variation in posture allocation: possible role in human obesity. *Science.* 2005;307(5709):584-586.

54. Levine JA, Schleusner SJ, Jensen MD. Energy expenditure of nonexercise activity. *Am J Clin Nutr.* 2000;72(6):1451-1454.

55. Lewis ZH, Lyons EJ, Jarvis JM, Baillargeon J. Using an electronic activity monitor system as an intervention modality: a systematic review. *BMC Public Health.* 2015;15:585.

56. Lee JM, Kim Y, Welk GJ. Validity of consumer-based physical activity monitors. *Med Sci Sports Exerc.* 2014;46:1840-1848.

57. Ferguson T, Rowlands AV, Olds T, Maher C. The validity of consumer-level, activity monitors in healthy adults worn in free-living conditions: a cross-sectional study. *Int J Behav Nutr Phys Act.* 2015;12:42.

58. Hongu N, Orr BJ, Roe DJ, Reed RG, Going SB. Global positioning system watches for estimating energy expenditure. *J Strength Cond Res.* 2013;27(11):3216-3220.

59. Hall KD, Hammond RA, Rahmandad H. Dynamic interplay among homeostatic, hedonic, and cognitive feedback circuits regulating body weight. *Am J Public Health*. 2014;104(7):1169-1175.

60. Kojima M, Hosoda H, Date Y, Nakazato M, Matsuo H, Kangawa K. Ghrelin is a growth-hormone-releasing acylated peptide from stomach. *Nature*. 1999;402(6762):656-660.

61. le Roux CW, Neary NM, Halsey TJ, et al. Ghrelin does not stimulate food intake in patients with surgical procedures involving vagotomy. *J Clin Endocrinol Metab*. 2005;90(8):4521-4524.

62. le Roux CW, Patterson M, Vincent RP, Hunt C, Ghatei MA, Bloom SR. Postprandial plasma ghrelin is suppressed proportional to meal calorie content in normal-weight but not obese subjects. *J Clin Endocrinol Metab*. 2005;90(2):1068-1071.

63. Rogers RC, Hermann GE. Mechanisms of action of CCK to activate central vagal afferent terminals. *Peptides*. 2008;29(10):1716 1725.

64. Moran TH. Gut peptides in the control of food intake. *Int J Obes (Lond)*. 2009;33(suppl 1):7S-10S.

65. King NA, Lluch A, Stubbs RJ, Blundell JE. High dose exercise does not increase hunger or energy intake in free living males. *Eur J Clin Nutr*. 1997;51(7):478-483.

66. Thompson DA, Wolfe LA, Eikelboom R. Acute effects of exercise intensity on appetite in young men. *Med Sci Sports Exerc*. 1988;20(3):222-227.

67. Pomerleau M, Imbeault P, Parker T, Doucet E. Effects of exercise intensity on food intake and appetite in women. *Am J Clin Nutr*. 2004;80(5):1230-1236.

68. King NA, Snell L, Smith RD, Blundell JE. Effects of short-term exercise on appetite responses in unrestrained females. *Eur J Clin Nutr*. 1996;50(10):663-667.

69. Imbeault P, Saint-Pierre S, Almeras N, Tremblay A. Acute effects of exercise on energy intake and feeding behaviour. *Br J Nutr*. 1997;77:511-521.

70. Bilski J, Manko G, Brzozowski T, et al. Effects of exercise of different intensity on gut peptides, energy intake and appetite in young males. *Ann Agric Environ Med*. 2013;20(4):787-793.

71. Stubbs RJ, Harbron CG, Murgatroyd PR, Prentice AM. Covert manipulation of dietary fat and energy density: effect on substrate flux and food intake in men eating ad libitum. *Am J Clin Nutr*. 1995;62(2):316-329.

72. Goldberg GR, Black AE, Jebb SA, et al. Critical evaluation of energy intake data using fundamental principles of energy physiology: 1. Derivation of cut-off limits to identify under-recording. *Eur J Clin Nutr*. 1991;45(12):569-581.

73. Melby CL, Ho RC, Jeckel K, Beal L, Goran M, Donahoo WT. Comparison of risk factors for obesity in young, nonobese African-American and Caucasian women. *Int J Obes Relat Metab Disord*. 2000;24(11):1514-1522.

74. Turnbaugh PJ, Ley RE, Mahowald MA, Magrini V, Mardis ER, Gordon JI. An obesity-associated gut microbiome with increased capacity for energy harvest. *Nature*. 2006;444(7122):1027-1031.

75. Lau E, Carvalho D, Pina-Vaz C, Barbosa JA, Freitas P. Beyond gut microbiota: understanding obesity and type 2 diabetes. *Hormones (Athens)*. 2015;14(3):358-369.

76. Prince SA, Adamo KB, Hamel ME, Hardt J, Connor Gorber S, Tremblay M. A comparison of direct versus self-report measures for assessing physical activity in adults: a systematic review. *Int J Behav Nutr Phys Act*. 2008;5:56.

77. Hall KD, Sacks G, Chandramohan D, et al. Quantification of the effect of energy imbalance on bodyweight. *Lancet*. 2011;378(9793):826-837.

78. Wing RR, Hill JO. Successful weight loss maintenance. *Annu Rev Nutr*. 2001;21:323-341.

79. Rosenbaum M, Hirsch J, Gallagher DA, Leibel RL. Long-term persistence of adaptive thermogenesis in subjects who have maintained a reduced body weight. *Am J Clin Nutr*. 2008;88(4):906-912.

80. Goldsmith R, Joanisse DR, Gallagher D, et al. Effects of experimental weight perturbation on skeletal muscle work efficiency, fuel utilization, and biochemistry in human subjects. *Am J Physiol Regul Integr Comp Physiol*. 2010;298(1):79R-88R.

81. Jequier E. Energy metabolism in obese patients before and after weight loss, and in patients who have relapsed. *Int J Obes*. 1990;14(suppl 1):59-64; discussion 64-57.

82. Maclean PS, Bergouignan A, Cornier MA, Jackman MR. Biology's response to dieting: the impetus for weight regain. *Am J Physiol Regul Integr Comp Physiol*. 2011;301(3):581R-600R.

83. Paris HL, Foright RM, Werth KA, et al. Increasing energy flux to decrease the biological drive toward weight regain after weight loss - A proof-of-concept pilot study. *Clinical Nutrition ESPEN*. 2016;11:12e-20e.

84. Levine JA, Eberhardt NL, Jensen MD. Role of nonexercise activity thermogenesis in resistance to fat gain in humans. *Science*. 1999;283(5399):212-214.

85. Bouchard C, Tremblay A, Despres JP, et al. The response to long-term overfeeding in identical twins. *N Engl J Med*. 1990;322(2):1477-1482.

86. Christiansen T, Paulsen SK, Bruun JM, Ploug T, Pedersen SB, Richelsen B. Diet-induced weight loss and exercise alone and in combination enhance the expression of adiponectin receptors in adipose tissue and skeletal muscle, but only diet-induced weight loss enhanced circulating adiponectin. *J Clin Endocrinol Metab*. 2010;95(2):911-919.

87. Bouchard C, Tremblay A, Nadeau A, et al. Long-term exercise training with constant energy intake. 1: effect on body composition and selected metabolic variables. *Int J Obes.* 1990;14(1):57-73.

88. King NA, Hopkins M, Caudwell P, Stubbs RJ, Blundell JE. Individual variability following 12 weeks of supervised exercise: identification and characterization of compensation for exercise-induced weight loss. *Int J Obes (Lond).* 2008;32(1):177-184.

89. Donnelly JE, Hill JO, Jacobsen DJ, et al. Effects of a 16-month randomized controlled exercise trial on body weight and composition in young, overweight men and women: the Midwest Exercise Trial. *Arch Intern Med.* 2003;163(11):1343-1350.

90. Goran MI, Poehlman ET. Endurance training does not enhance total energy expenditure in healthy elderly persons. *Am J Physiol.* 1992;263(5 pt 1):950e-957e.

91. Oshida Y, Yamanouchi K, Hayamizu S, Nagasawa J, Ohsawa I, Sato Y. Effects of training and training cessation on insulin action. *Int J Sports Med.* 1991;12(5):484-486.

92. Miller MA, Croft LB, Belanger AR, et al. Prevalence of metabolic syndrome in retired National Football League players. *Am J Cardiol.* 2008;101(9):1281-1284.

93. Booth FW, Roberts CK. Linking performance and chronic disease risk: indices of physical performance are surrogates for health. *Br J Sports Med.* 2008;42(12):950-952.

94. Phelain JF, Reinke E, Harris MA, Melby CL. Postexercise energy expenditure and substrate oxidation in young women resulting from exercise bouts of different intensity. *J Am Coll Nutr.* 1997;16(2):140-146.

95. Sedlock DA, Fissinger JA, Melby CL. Effect of exercise intensity and duration on postexercise energy expenditure. *Med Sci Sports Exerc.* 1989;21(6):662-666.

96. Osterberg KL, Melby CL. Effect of acute resistance exercise on postexercise oxygen consumption and resting metabolic rate in young women. *Int J Sport Nutr Exerc Metab.* 2000;10(1):71-81.

97. Melby CL, Osterberg KL, Resch A, Davy B, Johnson S, Davy K. Effect of carbohydrate ingestion during exercise on post-exercise substrate oxidation and energy intake. *Int J Sport Nutr Exerc Metab.* 2002;12(3):294-309.

98. Donnelly JE, Herrmann SD, Lambourne K, Szabo AN, Honas JJ, Washburn RA. Does increased exercise or physical activity alter ad-libitum daily energy intake or macronutrient composition in healthy adults? A systematic review. *PLoS One.* 2014;9(1):e83498.

CHAPTER 11

WEIGHT MANAGEMENT

Marie Dunford, PhD, RD, and Michele A. Macedonio, MS, RDN, CSSD

INTRODUCTION

Many athletes look for a performance edge by changing their weight and body composition. Changing the amount of weight, skeletal muscle, or body fat has potential performance advantages if goals are set appropriately. Unfortunately, athletes may set inappropriate weight and body composition goals or try to achieve their goals too quickly or during the wrong part of the competitive season. Such changes may be detrimental to performance and negatively impact health.[1]

A sports registered dietitian nutritionist (RDN) can help an athlete assess his or her weight and body composition and compare the measures to those of successful athletes in their sport who often have similar, but not identical, body composition, shape, and size. This assessment allows the athlete to set weight range and body composition goals that support performance without negatively affecting training, recovery, and health. Once appropriate goals are established, the sports RDN also helps the athlete develop an eating plan well matched to his or her sport, training schedule, and food preferences. This chapter reviews the factors that need to be considered when establishing weight and body composition goals and a case study that illustrates how to practically apply this information.

WEIGHT MANAGEMENT GOALS OF ATHLETES

Depending on his or her individual characteristicsand the demands of the sport, an athlete may want to (1) increase skeletal muscle mass, (2) increase skeletal muscle mass and slightly increase body fat, (3) increase skeletal muscle mass and decrease body fat simultaneously, (4) decrease body fat, or (5) increase body fat. As shown in Table 11.1, these changes may result in increased or decreased size and improved strength, power, speed, or cardiovascular endurance, which may enhance performance.[2-7]

Table 11.1 Weight Goals and Expected Performance Outcomes[2-7]

Goal	Expected Performance Outcomes	Examples
Increase skeletal muscle mass	Increase strength and power	Sprinters, bodybuilders
Increase skeletal muscle mass and slightly increase body fat	Increase size and strength; be better matched physically to opponents	Athletes in contact sports, especially as they progress to elite levels
Increase skeletal muscle mass and decrease body fat simultaneously	Increase strength and power; increase power-to-weight ratio	Athletes in "ball" sports, cyclists, rowers, wrestlers
Decrease body fat	Increase speed; improve vertical or horizontal distance	Long-distance runners, gymnasts, figure skaters, high jumpers
Increase body fat	Increase size (mass)	Power lifters, sumo wrestlers

Most athletes engage in some form of resistance training to maintain or increase muscular strength, power, and endurance. It is often beneficial for novice athletes or those moving to more demanding levels of competition (eg, high school to college, college to professional) to substantially increase skeletal muscle size, which often coincides with increased strength and muscle endurance. However, for many athletes, muscular strength and endurance are more important than increased size because too much muscle can result in decreased speed or perceived decreases in flexibility or agility. For example, a distance runner who gains too much skeletal muscle mass may find that speed is actually decreased because more effort must be made to transport the extra body weight associated with the extra muscle. In addition, excess weight from skeletal muscle can damage joints and ligaments.[5]

Changes in body fat can also substantially influence performance. Excess body fat is detrimental for many athletes because it reduces speed.[2] Excess body fat represents dead weight because the excess weight must be carried but does not contribute to muscle power. Decreasing excess body fat may have a positive effect on performance. However, trying to achieve an ever-lower percentage of body fat is a performance disadvantage because lean body mass and strength may be lost and health problems can develop, such as disrupted hormonal balance or disordered eating behaviors.[5] Although not mentioned as frequently as fat loss, some athletes may need to increase body mass by gaining body fat. Physical size alone can be a performance advantage, especially in contact sports. In these cases, additional body fat may aid the athlete's performance.

DETERMINING OPTIMAL PERFORMANCE WEIGHT AND BODY COMPOSITION RANGES

Optimal performance weight and body composition are unique to each individual, so genetic predisposition is associated with success in the sport, and the individual's current physical characteristics must be compared. Factors to consider when determining an optimal performance weight range are listed in Box 11.1 and discussed in this chapter, but not all may apply to a particular athlete.[1,5]

Box 11.1 Factors to Consider in Setting Weight-Management Goals[1-5]

Sport-Related Characteristics
- Sport
- Position
- Relative need for power and endurance
- Power-to-weight ratio
- Relative need for speed, flexibility, agility, and mobility

Physique-Related Characteristics
- Body weight
- Body composition
- Body size
- Body build
- Metabolic syndrome phenotype
- Body appearance

Sport-Related Characteristics

Certain physical characteristics are associated with success in particular sports. For example, all competitive bodybuilders have a high percentage of skeletal muscle mass and a low percentage of body fat. Conversely, sumo wrestlers are large-bodied, with a considerable amount of body fat. Elite distance runners tend to be lightweight and light-boned, and they have a relatively low percentage of body fat because these characteristics are associated with efficiently moving the body a long distance as quickly as possible. Appearance may be a factor in scoring, such as in women's gymnastics and figure skating. Thus, some sports have greater physical uniformity among competitors, especially at the elite levels of competition (see Box 11.2). Successful athletes in individual, noncontact sports, such as tennis and golf, are of many body weights, sizes, and shapes.[1,5]

Box 11.2 Weight and Body Composition Uniformity Among Athletes[1-5]

More Body Composition Uniformity
- Baseball catchers
- Basketball centers, point guards
- Bodybuilders
- Figure skaters
- Football linemen
- Gymnasts
- Long-distance cyclists
- Long-distance runners
- Powerlifters
- Rhythmic gymnasts

Less Body Composition Uniformity
- Baseball pitchers
- Divers
- Golfers
- Recreational triathletes
- Tennis players

In contact sports, such as football, basketball, rugby, mixed martial arts, and ice hockey, being physically well matched to one's opponents is often a key to success, but physical size alone is not the determining factor in most sports. The relative need for power, speed, or endurance and the need to be agile, flexible, or mobile may be particularly important, a key to the individual's success. The physical characteristics of successful athletes in the sport should be considered as a guideline, but in many sports, there is room for tremendous individual variability.[1,2,5]

POSITION PLAYED

Physical uniformity may be associated with position. For example, a football lineman tends to be physically similar to other linemen but different in weight and body composition compared with running backs, linebackers, and receivers. Linemen tend to have a greater percentage of body fat than the other players on the team so that they are less easily pushed around by other linemen. In contrast, wide receivers have less body fat than lineman because of their need for superior running speed.[8] Linebackers benefit from quick running speed and the agility to change direction quickly but also need enough mass to stop a run. Particularly in contact sports, position may dictate the need for an athlete of particular size, weight, or body composition.

In many team sports, there is a range of weights and body compositions for a given position. For example, in soccer, some defenders are more muscular and weigh more than others who are lighter weight and have comparatively less muscle, yet each can succeed as a defender. Weight and body composition vary in baseball outfielders, in part because of their offensive skills. Some hit for power while others hit to get on base, steal bases, and score on base hits. Power hitters benefit from greater body weight, whereas fast base runners are likely to have a body composition associated with speed (eg, relatively low percentage of body fat). Sports in which position plays a major role include baseball, basketball, football, ice and field hockey, lacrosse, rugby, soccer, and softball.[1]

RELATIVE NEED FOR POWER AND ENDURANCE

Athletes are often characterized as strength and power or endurance athletes (see Figure 11.1). For example, short-distance runners, such as 100-m and 200-m runners, depend primarily on explosive power.

They have substantial upper- and lower-body skeletal muscle mass and a relatively heavy body weight. As the distance increases to the middle distances (eg, 1,500 ms), body composition begins to change as the race favors endurance rather than power. The 1,500-m runner is less muscular and lighter weight than the 100-m runner. Long-distance runners, such as marathon runners, tend to be light in weight and have a relatively low percentage of body fat because these characteristics are associated with efficiently moving the body quickly over a long distance. Cycling and swimming are other sports in which the distance covered influences the relative need for power and endurance, and, therefore, weight and body composition.[1,2,5]

Those who rely only on strength or explosive power include bodybuilders, powerlifters, and certain field athletes, such as shot-putters and discus, hammer, and javelin throwers. Powerlifters and throwers benefit from being large-bodied and strong. Body fat adds to total body weight, which can be a performance advantage because it adds mass. However, too high a percentage of body fat can be a health disadvantage, particularly if the excess fat is abdominal fat.[9]

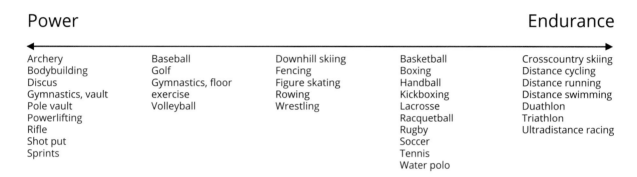

Power   Endurance

Archery	Baseball	Downhill skiing	Basketball	Crosscountry skiing
Bodybuilding	Golf	Fencing	Boxing	Distance cycling
Discus	Gymnastics, floor	Figure skating	Handball	Distance running
Gymnastics, vault	exercise	Rowing	Kickboxing	Distance swimming
Pole vault	Volleyball	Wrestling	Lacrosse	Duathlon
Powerlifting			Racquetball	Triathlon
Rifle			Rugby	Ultradistance racing
Shot put			Soccer	
Sprints			Tennis	
			Water polo	

FIGURE 11.1 The Power-Endurance Continuum Some sports depend predominantly on power, as shown on the left side of the continuum, whereas others depend to a large degree on endurance capacity, as shown on the right. Many sports require a blend of power and endurance. It may be helpful to determine the relative position of the athlete's sport or position on the continuum so that realistic weight and body composition goals can be established.[1,2,4]

Most sports require a combination of power and endurance. For example, basketball and soccer require intermittent short bursts of power (eg, fast break, breakaway play) as well as cardiovascular endurance. Body weight and composition must be fine-tuned for the athlete to be able to do both well. Particularly challenging are those sports that require several power and endurance events, such as decathlon. Decathletes must have a body composition that is not too muscular (a disadvantage when running the 1,500-m race) or too low in weight (a disadvantage when shot-putting).

Body composition is also a factor in cardiovascular conditioning. Reducing excess body fat may improve cardiovascular endurance and allow athletes to continue to perform well near the end of the game. This is especially important in sports with overtime periods, such as basketball, soccer, and lacrosse.[10] Although conditioning is important for all athletes, improved cardiovascular endurance may be the primary goal for performance-focused recreational athletes and older players who are competing for playing time with younger players. Such players often try to reduce excess body fat as a way to improve endurance and performance.[11]

POWER-TO-WEIGHT RATIO

Power-to-weight ratio refers to the amount of power (ie, explosive skeletal muscle strength) that can be generated per pound or kilogram of body weight. A high power-to-weight ratio is a performance advantage in many sports, the result of a relatively low percentage of body fat and a relatively high percentage of skeletal muscle for the total amount of body weight. For example, male professional distance cyclists tend to have approximately 7% to 10% body fat. Excess body fat is dead weight because it must be moved but does not contribute to muscle power.[1,5]

Examples of sports that benefit from a high power-to-weight ratio include boxing, wrestling, martial arts, rowing (crew), high jumping, pole vaulting, distance running, gymnastics, swimming, diving, and cycling. A high power-to-weight ratio is also advantageous for athletes in positions that cover a large area of the field, rink, or court and depend on speed, such as many basketball, ice hockey, lacrosse, rugby, figure skating, and soccer positions.

Power-to-weight ratio can be changed by increasing skeletal muscle mass to increase power or decreasing body fat to decrease body weight. Unless an athlete has a large amount of excess body fat, maximizing power by increasing muscle mass is more likely to benefit performance than minimizing body fat. Athletes need to be aware that extreme changes in either direction can be detrimental to performance. For example, too great an increase in skeletal muscle mass can increase body weight too much, which can reduce speed. Conversely, decreasing body fat too much can hurt performance because there is not enough body fat to support rigorous training and competition. There can also be health-related problems brought on by these changes, such as joint problems or changes in hormone concentrations as a result of an eating disorder.[5]

RELATIVE NEED FOR SPEED, MOBILITY, FLEXIBILITY, AND AGILITY

The need for speed and mobility influences goals for body weight and composition. Some athletes may benefit from an increase in lower-body muscle mass and a decrease in body fat to increase sprint speed. Others may benefit from maintenance of muscle mass but a decrease in excess body fat. Because speed is easily measured, the impact of weight and body composition changes on speed can be easily assessed. Some athletes say that too much muscle reduces their flexibility and agility.[5]

WEIGHT CERTIFICATION REQUIREMENTS

Boxing, wrestling, some of the martial arts, and lightweight crew (rowing) are examples of sports with weight categories. Weight-regulated sports put considerable emphasis on scale weight because the athlete cannot compete until weight is certified. There is a theoretical performance advantage to being at the top rather than the bottom of the weight category, and this may influence the athlete to choose to compete in a weight category that is below a biologically comfortable weight.[1,5]

The need to have weight certified cannot be overlooked as a significant factor in the athlete's preparation for competition. Unfortunately, the fastest way to manipulate scale weight is to reduce body water. To do so, athletes restrict water intake, lose excessive amounts through sweating, and take diuretics. These are dangerous practices, especially when they are combined because body temperature can be elevated to a medically unsafe and sometimes fatal level.[1,5]

In the past, wrestling was the poster child for hazardous practices used to "make weight" or "cut weight," terms used to describe large and rapid losses in scale weight through extraordinary measures (eg, starvation, severe dehydration, excessive exercise). Some wrestlers died from these practices, and wrestling now has rules that require the establishment of a minimum weight category before the beginning of the season based on body composition and proper hydration. However, not all weight-regulated sports have adopted such rule changes, and athletes in those sports remain at risk for potential medical problems and detrimental performance outcomes (eg, fainting, lack of concentration).[5] For additional information on wrestling, see the Wrestling At a Glance section located on page 576-577.

Physique-Related Characteristics

The challenge for both athletes and the professionals who work with them is to determine ranges for weight and body composition compatible with excellent performance, good health, *and* the individual's genetic potential and unique characteristics.

BODY WEIGHT

Weight is usually expressed as a single number, although it should be stated as a weight range. Using a weight range helps to account for the error inherent in any form of measurement and helps prevent misinterpretations due to natural day-to-day fluctuations in body weight, especially in water weight. A baseline weight is one of the first assessment measures taken, but an appropriate weight range cannot be established until information is known about the individual athlete's height, body build, and body composition, as well as the sport and position played.[1,5]

BODY COMPOSITION

Body composition assessment is necessary to set an appropriate weight range and to monitor changes in lean body mass and storage fat. An accurate assessment is critical, as explained in Chapter 9. However, the most accurate measures are not readily accessible or affordable to most athletes. Many have access to only one method, which will need to be repeated over time to track any changes.

Body composition cannot predict success in any sport, but it can affect optimal performance.[3] Table 11.2 lists the body composition of competitive athletes in some sports as reported in the scientific literature.[1,5] These figures are only guidelines and should be used cautiously.

Table 11.2 Estimated Body Composition of Selected Well-Trained Athletes[5]		
Sport	**Position or Distance**	**% Body Fat**
Men		
Baseball, collegiate	All positions	11.0–17.0
Baseball, professional	All positions	8.5–12.0
Basketball, professional	Centers	9.0–20.0
	Forwards	7.0–14.0
	Guards	7.0–13.0
Cycling, road, professional	Long distance	7.0–10.0
Football (American), college (NCAA Division I)	Defensive backs	7.0–14.5
	Receivers	9.0–16.5
	Quarterbacks	14.0–22.0
	Linebackers	12.5–23.5
	Defensive linemen	14.5–25.0
	Offensive linemen	18.5–28.5
Ice hockey, elite	Forwards and defensemen	10.0–11.5
Judo, national team	All weight classes	8.5–19.0
Rugby, professional	All positions	9.0–20.0
Running, elite	Middle distance	8.0–16.5
	Long distance	12.0–18.0

Continued on next page

Sport	Position or Distance	% Body Fat
Table 11.2 Estimated Body Composition of Selected Well-Trained Athletes[5] (Continued)		
Soccer, college	All positions	13.0–19.0
Soccer, professional or college	All positions	7.5–18.0
Swimming or diving, college	Middle distance or diving	17.0–30.0
	Long distance	20.0–34.0
Tennis, elite		8.0–18.0
Water polo, national team		6.5.0–17.5
Wrestling, college		6.5–16.0
Women		
Ice hockey, elite	All positions	14.0–18.0
Running, elite	Middle distance	8.0–16.5
	Long distance	12.0–18.0
Soccer, collegiate	All positions	13.0–19.0
Swimming or diving, college	Middle distance or diving	17.0–30.0
Swimming or diving, masters	Long distance	20.0–34.0
Tennis, elite		15.0–25.0

BODY SIZE

Body size refers to height, weight, and body build. Body size has increased in many high school, collegiate, and professional sports over the past 50 years, including football, basketball, ice hockey, baseball, and tennis.[12-16] A dramatic increase has been seen in the weight of football linemen at every level, from professional to youth. Some of this weight has been an increase in abdominal fat, a known health risk and a likely performance disadvantage due to a lack of fitness and speed.[16,17]

Although there are exceptions, many athletes need to increase body size as they move to the next level of competition (eg, high school to college, college to professional). In many cases, this means an increase in skeletal muscle mass and body weight. It may also mean a small increase in body fat; in some positions, such as football linemen, it can mean a substantial increase in fat. Although body size can be manipulated, it is ultimately determined by genetics. It is important to note that in the United States, puberty occurs between the ages of 11 and 19, so there is wide variability in when an athlete achieves full physical maturity.[1,5]

BODY BUILD

Body build, also referred to as somatotype, may be useful when discussing the influence of genetic predisposition on body composition. Classification is based on three categories: endomorphic, mesomorphic, or ectomorphic. Endomorphs tend to be stocky with wide hips and are at risk for easily gaining body fat, particularly in the abdominal area. Mesomorphs tend to gain skeletal muscle mass relatively easily and generally do not gain excessive amounts of body fat. Ectomorphs appear to be thin. Some individuals clearly fall into one of the three categories, but many reflect more than one somatotype.[1,5]

Body build is associated with certain sports. For example, shot-putters tend to be endomorphs, body-builders tend to be mesomorphs, and distance runners tend to be ectomorphs.[5] Visual appraisal does not quantify body dimensions, but it is a way to draw general observations about successful performance related to physique. Until an individual reaches full physical maturity, it may be difficult to accurately assess physique.

METABOLIC SYNDROME PHENOTYPE

Metabolic syndrome is characterized by a clustering of metabolic disorders and risk factors: abdominal obesity; hypertension; dyslipidemia, including elevated triglycerides and low high-density lipoprotein cholesterol; glucose intolerance; and insulin resistance (see Table 11.3).

These features are associated with a higher risk for cardiovascular disease and type 2 diabetes. The prevalence of metabolic syndrome in the US adult population is approximately 25%, but the percentage increases with age.[18] Small studies of high school, collegiate, and professional football linemen have found a high incidence of metabolic syndrome, perhaps as high as 50% of linemen. Early screening is recommended, particularly for large-bodied, heavyweight athletes prone to increased abdominal fat.[19,20] In one study of collegiate football players, 62% had prehypertension and 20% were diagnosed with hypertension.[21]

There is emerging evidence that some female athletes in sports emphasizing strength may have hyperandrogenism, resulting in menstrual dysfunction, such as amenorrhea, and a tendency to abdominal obesity with accompanying insulin resistance and dyslipidemia. Some of these individuals meet the criteria for polycystic ovary syndrome. Menstrual dysfunction in female athletes as a result of a long-term energy deficit has been well studied as part of the female athlete triad. In contrast to those athletes, female athletes with hyperandrogenism typically do not suffer from an energy deficit or reduced bone mineral density. Early screening for any type of menstrual dysfunction is recommended, and intervention will be based on the individual's reproductive hormone profile.[22]

Table 11.3 Diagnostic Criteria for Metabolic Syndrome[18]

Measure	Criteria[a]
Waist circumference	>102 cm (>40 in) in men >88 cm (>35 in) in women
Triglycerides	>150 mg/dL (1.7 mmol/L) or drug treatment for elevated triglycerides
High-density lipoprotein cholesterol (HDL-C)	<40 mg/dL (0.9 mmol/L) in men <50 mg/dL (1.1 mmol/L) in women or drug treatment for reduced HDL-C
Blood pressure	>130 mm Hg systolic blood pressure or >85 mm Hg diastolic blood pressure or drug treatment for hypertension
Fasting blood glucose	>100 mg/dL (5.6 mmol/L) or drug treatment for elevated glucose

[a] Any three of the five criteria constitute a diagnosis of metabolic syndrome.

BODY APPEARANCE

Body appearance cannot be overlooked when setting weight and body composition goals. An obvious example is the sport of bodybuilding, where competitors are scored on body appearance. Weight and body composition are part of the subjective scoring of other aesthetic sports, such as women's gymnastics and figure skating. Dissatisfaction with weight, body shape, or body image can lead to disordered eating and eating disorders in both men and women.[23-25]

For most athletes, body appearance is not part of the scoring. However, popular athletes featured in visual media may feel pressure to attain and maintain an athletic physique. Some sports, such as women's high jump, pole vaulting, and beach volleyball, feature tight-fitting clothing that reveals the body's contour. In general, female athletes are more concerned than male athletes with physical appearance, particularly perceived fatness, and are more likely to restrict energy intake and use weight-loss supplements.[26] Appearance is one reason that athletes of both sexes may use anabolic steroids. Interestingly, an athletic appearance is so socially powerful that some high school nonathletes use anabolic steroids to achieve a body composition associated with rigorous athletic training.[27]

FOUR-STEP PROCESS FOR ACHIEVING WEIGHT AND BODY COMPOSITION GOALS

The goal for an athlete is an optimal performance weight range that reflects a healthy body composition. Although the specific goals will depend on the individual, the process used to achieve the goals is universal. Four steps are critical:

1. Assessment

2. Goal Setting

3. Action Plan

4. Evaluation And Reassessment

Assessment

No two athletes are the same. Assessment is the starting point for any successful plan designed to achieve body weight and body composition goals. A proper assessment creates a picture of an individual athlete's current status, providing baseline information that is used for setting realistic and achievable goals for where an athlete wants to be. This baseline information also becomes the basis for individual action plans designed to reach desired weight and body composition ranges and serves as a point of comparison. The more information an assessment provides, the better able an athlete is to create a successful action plan and to gauge progress. Box 11.3 summarizes the assessment measurements used to create an individualized and targeted nutrition plan geared to help athletes set target goals, design effective action plans, and evaluate and reassess progress.[1]

PHYSICAL ASSESSMENT

Height and weight measurements are easy to do and necessary to determine optimal performance weight. Athletes in some sports and positions are similar in height and weight. Height measurements are necessary when assessing weight because many formulas include height as a factor. Stadiometers provide the most accurate height measurement and make measuring quick and simple. However, in the absence of a stadiometer, height can be measured by having the athlete stand barefoot on a hard surface and against a wall, looking straight ahead with head, shoulders, buttocks, and heels touching the wall. The athlete should stand as tall and straight as possible. With a ruler or other flat straightedge placed on the head of the athlete, the wall is marked at the underside of the 90° angle where the ruler meets the wall. Then, the distance from the ground to the marking on the wall is measured.[1,5]

Optimal weight is relative to height. Weight-class sports specify weight categories with specific weight ranges, so weight is a key issue for these athletes. To some degree, body weight is an important factor for all athletes. Weight measurements should be taken in the morning after urinating and before eating or drinking, using the same properly calibrated scale, with the athlete wearing minimal clothing. Note that one weight measurement does not tell the whole story. To most accurately assess progress toward one's goal, serial weights should be taken regularly and uniformly. Regular weight checks also help an athlete keep tabs on hydration status and provide athletes with a basis for rehydration strategies.[1,5]

Body mass index (BMI) is not used with athletes to determine overweight or obesity status. However, for those athletes who strive for a low body weight and a low body fat, BMI may be a necessary assessment measure as an indication of health status. The World Health Organization defines underweight in adults as a BMI of less than 18.5, which may indicate malnutrition, presence of an eating disorder, or other health problems. In those younger than 20 years of age, underweight is defined as a BMI below the 5th percentile.[1,5]

Girth measurements provide a tool for measuring body size and proportion and for screening for excessive abdominal fat accumulation. Although not a direct measure of body composition, measuring the girth, or circumference, at six sites is helpful in tracking change in body composition over time.[1,5] Girth measurements are inexpensive and easy to take. For the most accuracy, a flexible but inelastic tape measure is used to measure circumference, typically at the waist, hips, thighs, calves, arms, and chest. Changes in girth measurements can indicate that the current plan is working. Waist circumference is one diagnostic criterion for metabolic syndrome (see Table 11.3 on page 225).[18]

Body composition is an important factor in determining optimal performance weight. Accurate body composition measurement is necessary for a comprehensive nutrition assessment because body weight is only part of the picture. The composition of that weight is often the more important part. For practical purposes, the body is divided into two major compartments: fat and lean. Body fat is either essential fat or storage fat. Essential fat, present in the heart, lungs, liver, spleen, and lipid-rich tissues of the central nervous system, is necessary for normal physiological functioning. In women, there is additional sex-specific essential fat that has biological functions for reproduction and other hormonal functions. Essential fat in women is approximately four times that of men. Storage fat is primarily in adipose tissue, including visceral fat that protects organs from trauma and fat beneath the skin. To maintain health and normal body function, lower limits for body fat percentage are set at 3% for men and 12% for women. These lower limits are for reference only, and even the leanest athletes typically exceed these percentages of body fat.[1,5]

Fat-free mass (FFM) and lean body mass (LBM), although often used interchangeably, are not the same. Lean body mass contains a small percentage of non–sex-specific essential fat (approximately 3% of body mass), whereas fat-free mass contains no fat (FFM = body mass – fat mass). In fully hydrated, healthy adults, the main difference between FFM and LBM is essential fat. LBM is generally the term used in body composition measurement. The percentage of LBM is often part of equations used to determine energy needs.[1,5]

Obtaining an accurate body composition measure is not as easy as measuring body weight, height, and girth. For a detailed explanation of body composition methods and their strengths and weaknesses, refer to Chapter 9.

PHYSIOLOGICAL ASSESSMENT

Physiological measurements that provide valuable baseline information about the athlete include those obtained at a physical exam, such as biochemical assays and clinical examination, and measurements of metabolic rate, nutrient intake, and exercise expenditure. For a detailed explanation of how to conduct a comprehensive sports nutrition assessment, refer to Chapter 8.

When available, laboratory tests allow the sports RDN to evaluate the nutritional status of the athlete by ascertaining whether biochemical parameters are within healthful ranges. Once collected, this information can be used as a target for dietary modifications and as a measure of progress. A clinical examination includes past and present medical history, family history, signs of disease or illness, and habits that may affect health, such as sleep patterns.[1]

An understanding of an athlete's usual dietary intake is an indispensable part of a comprehensive assessment. The more complete and accurate the diet record, the more likely that the prescribed meal plan will be precisely tailored to the athlete's energy and nutrient needs. A detailed 3- to 5-day diet record and nutrient analysis is the preferable method of collecting dietary information, if time allows and the athlete is willing to record all foods and beverages consumed. This method of diet assessment not only provides a view of the athlete's usual eating patterns but also a measure of the quantity and the quality of the food intake. The information provides the basis for a nutrition plan designed to help the athlete reach body weight and body composition goals. Dietary intake studies reveal that people routinely underestimate portions when recording food intake.[28] Therefore, it is crucial to instruct athletes to eat as they usually do and to record portions as accurately and completely as possible so that the information reflects usual food intake and meal patterns. Nutrient analysis software can be used to analyze the nutrient content of a food record, but it is only as good as the database on which the program is based. For the most complete information, the US Department of Agriculture National Nutrient Database for Standard Reference (https://ndb.nal.usda.gov) should form the foundation for the nutrient analysis program.[29] When time or unwillingness prohibits the collection of a 3- to 5-day diet record, other methods of collecting dietary intake information can be employed, including 24-hour recall, food frequency questionnaire, or a usual diet intake pattern. In any case, it is important to explain how this information will be used in designing a personalized and precise meal plan. The more complete and accurate the information collected, the more effective the meal plan and menu pattern will be.

Knowledge of metabolic rate provides an energy baseline that forms the foundation for a targeted, realistic, and effective weight-management plan. Resting metabolic rate (RMR) refers to the energy requirement needed for all metabolic processes of the active cell mass required to maintain normal regulatory balance and body functions at rest.[5] As explained in Chapter 10, RMR can be estimated by measuring oxygen consumption via indirect calorimetry or by using prediction equations (see Box 10.2 on page 200 in Chapter 10).

Physical activity, also referred to as exercise energy expenditure, has a profound effect on total daily energy expenditure (TDEE). For athletes, the energy needed for training, conditioning, and performance represents a substantial proportion of total daily energy needs. World-class athletes, for instance, can almost double their TDEE with 3 to 4 hours of intense training.[5] It is important that athletes record daily exercise and note both the intensity and duration of the exercise. An accurate determination of TDEE is difficult because of the variability of the contribution of physical exercise. Refer to Chapter 10 for information on how best to estimate TDEE.

Performance measurements, such as running speed or relative peak power, allow athletes to determine a baseline and track improvements in performance. Running speed is easy to measure. Relative peak power measures power-to-weight ratio. The 30-second Wingate test measures both average and peak power of the lower body. Upper-body power can be measured by using a modified Wingate test or an arm ergometer.[2]

Goal Setting

Careful interpretation of the assessment measures will determine if the athlete's current weight and body composition are appropriate. Begin by determining whether body composition is well matched to the sport (see Table 11.2, pages 223–223) and the athlete's genetic predisposition for leanness.

Although the athlete may want to focus only on weight or body composition goals, it is important that athletes set at least three related goals. A minimum of one goal should be set in each area—performance, weight and body composition, and health. Performance-based goals may range from simply finishing an event, such as a marathon or triathlon, to very specific goals, such as decreasing performance time by 10 seconds. A weight range should be set to reflect an appropriate body composition range. As shown in Box 11.4, a formula can be used to help set the weight range.[29] For many athletes, the health goal may be continued good health, but some may need to set specific goals, such as continuing to menstruate, decreasing abdominal fat, or bringing a biochemical parameter into a healthful range. In each case, goals need to be SMART. SMART, an acronym that athletes can easily remember, signifies the essential qualities of effective goals: specific, measurable, achievable, realistic, and time driven.

Box 11.4 Calculating Target Weight

The following formula, calculated using both a lower and higher percentage body fat, is used to establish a weight range. To use this formula, an assessment of body composition must be done because fat-free mass must be known. This formula assumes that the athlete is adequately hydrated.[28]

Target body weight = Current fat-free mass ÷ (1 − % Desired body fat)

Example

A long-distance cyclist currently weighs 187 lb. His body composition is 87% fat-free mass (163 lb) and 13% body fat. His goal is 8% to 10% body fat with no change in lean mass. An appropriate weight range to reflect this body composition goal is 177 to 181 lb (assuming all weight is lost from adipose tissue).

Target body weight = 163 lb ÷ (1 − 0.08) = 163 lb ÷ 0.92 = 177 lb

Target body weight = 163 lb ÷ (1 − 0.1) = 163 lb ÷ 0.9 = 181 lb

This same formula may be used no matter how the athlete wants to change body composition. For example, if this cyclist wanted to increase muscle mass by 5 lb to 168 lb and decrease body fat at the same time, his estimated weight range would be 183 to 187 lbs (168 lb ÷ 0.92 and 168 lb ÷ 0.9).

Action Plan

The fundamental features of an effective action plan include the following:
- appropriate energy intake;
- adequate amounts of protein, carbohydrate, and fat;
- proper macronutrient proportions;
- a variety of foods to ensure adequate amounts of vitamins, minerals, fiber, and water;
- proper timing of nutrient intake to aid in recovery;
- appropriate training plan and daily physical activity; and
- personal food preferences, cost, and convenience.

ENERGY INTAKE: The number of calories needed daily cannot be predicted with precision, but an assessment of RMR and usual physical activity can help establish an estimate. For those who want to gain weight by increasing skeletal muscle mass, a rule of thumb for men is baseline calorie intake plus 400 to 500 kcal daily. For women, adding 300 to 400 kcal more than baseline is recommended. However, individuals vary to a great degree, and recommended daily energy intake must be individualized.[1]

To reduce weight by reducing body fat, a guideline is baseline intake minus 300 to 500 kcal/d for men and minus 200 to 300 kcal/d for women. Greater reductions in daily energy intake may leave the athlete unable to maintain or increase energy output from physical activity and exercise.[1] A reasonable weight-loss goal for athletes is approximately 0.7% loss of body weight per week.[3]

To gain skeletal muscle mass and lose body fat simultaneously, energy intake and nutrient timing must be as precise as possible. A starting point for daily intake is baseline requirements plus 300 kcal/d for men and plus 200 kcal/d for women. However, close monitoring is needed, and total energy intake may need to be adjusted by 50- to 100-kcal increments daily until the desired outcome is reached. For those who wish to increase body fat, energy intake more than baseline is necessary.[1]

PROTEIN INTAKE: In general, the amount of protein recommended for athletes daily is 1.4 to 2.0 g/kg.[3,5] The recommended protein intake to increase skeletal muscle mass in strength athletes is typically approximately 1.7 to 2.0 g/kg/d, assuming caloric intake is adequate. A common question asked by health professionals is whether athletes should use a high-protein diet when attempting weight loss. It is well known that low-calorie diets in humans can lead to negative nitrogen balance and a significant loss of lean body mass.[3,5] Several studies in overweight and women who are obese have shown that the loss of LBM can be reduced (but not prevented entirely) with higher protein diets.[30]

Unfortunately, the amount of protein in a high-protein diet is often not clearly defined. A common recommendation for athletes consuming a moderately caloric restricted diet (~0.7% loss of body weight per week) is a protein intake of approximately 1.5 g/kg/d, in an effort to protect against the loss of lean body mass. A study by Mettler and colleagues found that a diet containing protein at a high level (~2.3 g/kg or ~35% of total caloric intake) helped to preserve LBM, but this diet was consumed for a very short time (2 weeks), and it is not known if other levels of protein or other time frames are equally effective.[31] A position paper on nutrition and athletic performance from the Academy of Nutrition and Dietetics, Dietitians of Canada, and the American College of Sports Medicine states that during energy restriction, protein needs can be higher than 2.0 g/kg, but at this time a definitive amount is not known.[3] More research is needed.

The major concern with high-protein, calorie-reduced diets is carbohydrate content, which may not be sufficient to restore muscle glycogen and support training and performance over many weeks or months. It is prudent for athletes to work with a sports RDN when they are attempting to lose weight, protect against the loss of LBM, maintain their level of training, or maintain or improve their performance. Determining the amount of protein needed to achieve all of these goals is likely to require some trial and error. The other macronutrients— carbohydrate and fat—will also need to be fine-tuned.

Another issue is the amount of leucine consumed. Leucine is a branched-chain amino acid that activates a key signaling pathway needed to build and maintain skeletal muscle mass. Leucine, along with resistance exercise, is necessary for optimal muscle protein synthesis. Both the amount and timing of leucine impact the maximal synthesis of skeletal muscle protein. Recommendations for adult athletes include 20 to 25 g (0.25 g/kg) of high-quality protein per meal with at least 2.2 g of leucine per meal. Whey protein and cow's milk are examples of excellent sources of protein and leucine. Older athletes may be anabolically resistant to optimal skeletal muscle protein synthesis and may benefit from 30 to 40 g (0.4 g/kg) of high-quality protein per meal, which should also provide sufficient leucine.[32] For more information on aging athletes, see Chapter 14.

CARBOHYDRATE AND FAT INTAKE: Regardless of the athlete's weight management goals, carbohydrate should be sufficient to resynthesize muscle glycogen stores daily (~3 to 12 g/kg). Fat restriction should be moderate. A rule-of-thumb calculation for moderate fat intake is approximately 1 g/kg/d or about 25% to 30% of total energy intake. Restricting fat intake to less than 20% of total energy intake is not recommended.[3] Current body weight is typically used to make calculations about the necessary grams per kilograms per day. As body weight decreases, especially to a large degree, recalculations are necessary to reflect the athlete's current (now lower) body weight.[5]

ACTION PLAN SUMMARY: Generally, athletes are encouraged to distribute food and beverage intake throughout the day by eating three meals and two or three snacks, assuring energy and nutrient availability when most needed.[33] This distribution of calories and nutrients helps athletes be adequately fueled before exercise and fully recover after exercise. Some postexercise carbohydrate and high-quality protein are necessary for the adequate resynthesis of muscle glycogen and the repair and synthesis of skeletal muscle, respectively. Consuming high-quality protein throughout the day may be beneficial for athletes restricting caloric intake because protein is associated with increased satiety as well as providing some protection against loss of skeletal muscle mass due to energy restriction.[3,5] Food intake and training must be coordinated. Each diet plan must be individualized, incorporating personal food preferences, religious beliefs, convenience, and cost.

Evaluation and Reassessment

Even a plan that seems perfect on paper needs evaluation. Evaluation allows the athlete to determine if goals are being met. If progress is too slow or too fast, adjustments can be made before training, performance, or health is impacted. Reassessment of many of the original assessment measures is invaluable for tracking progress and, at times, adjusting the original goals. A case study illustrating a comprehensive plan of a linebacker in the National Football League appears in Box 11.5.

Box 11.5 Case Study of a National Football League Linebacker

An outside linebacker who is 6 feet 1 inch (1.85 m) and weighs 226 lb (7 kg), with 19% body fat (43 lb [19.5 kg]) and 183 lb (83.2 kg) of lean mass, wants to be "ripped" by training camp. During his first 2 years in the National Football League (NFL), this athlete struggled to maintain his weight during the season. He lives alone and prepares his own meals. During the season, the team provides breakfast and lunch, but he often finds he is too tired after a day of intense training to prepare a full dinner, and he is concerned that his nutrition may be lacking.

The athlete's goal is to earn a starting linebacker position in the upcoming season. To do this, he needs to gain strength and increase speed and agility. Wanting to be in peak condition when he reports to the team for conditioning, this athlete is engaged in an intense 6-hour workout 4 days a week at a high-level training facility during the break between the end of the season and off-season workouts.

Together, the athlete and the sports registered dietitian nutritionist (RDN) collected the necessary nutrition assessment data, set realistic achievable goals, planned an effective nutrition strategy to support his training regimen, and set benchmarks for evaluation and reassessment.

Step 1: Assessment

In the assessment, the sports RDN collected the following data:

- Height: 6 ft 1 in (1.85 m)
- Weight: 226 lb (102.7 kg)
- Somatotype: Mesomorph/ectomorph
- Body composition (BOD POD):
  - ~19% body fat
  - ~43 lb (19.5 kg) body fat
  - ~183 lb (83.2 kg) lean mass
- Metabolic rate: 2,510 kcal
- Dietary intake: 2,805 kcal
- Average daily physical activity: 1,828 kcal

The assessment of height and weight indicates that the athlete's current size is sufficient to play in the NFL, but his weight and percentage of lean body mass are lower than those of many of his competitors. His mesomorphic/ectomorphic body build suggests that he can gain skeletal mass, but perhaps not as easily as a true mesomorph. A detailed 3-day record of dietary intake reveals that his average daily energy intake is 2,805 kcal.

Due to his large body size and large amount of skeletal muscle mass, the energy needed to support his resting metabolic rate are substantial, approximately 2,500 kcal/d. In addition, he expends more than 1,800 kcal/d, due in large part to his rigorous workouts. It is quickly apparent that his current intake does not meet the predicted amount of calories he needs daily to maintain current weight and body composition. This is predominantly due to his fatigue after hours of working out and his lack of cooking skills. However, he likes to eat and enjoys a wide variety of foods. He will need to consume substantially more calories if he wishes to increase skeletal muscle mass.

Step 2: Goal Setting

When asked, the athlete could quickly list his goal: earn a starting position by being stronger and quicker than the other linebackers on the team. But he was not able to translate this goal into measurable objectives. For example, when the sports dietitian asked him how much he thought he should weigh or how quickly he expected to gain skeletal muscle mass, his answers suggested weight and body composition goals that were unrealistic. The sports RDN helped him establish some realistic goals and an appropriate time frame in which to meet them (see the chart below). For example, he wanted to increase body mass as well as lean mass for greater bulk and strength. A goal weight of 230 to 233 lb was established by calculating a realistic gain of lean mass (0.5 to 0.75 lb gain over 8 weeks) and adding it to his current weight. In working with the sports RDN, he was able to establish goals that were SMART—specific, measurable, achievable, realistic, and time driven.

Continued on next page

Goal	Objective
Earn a starting position.	Gain 0.75 lb/wk. After 8 weeks, reach goal weight range of 230–233 lb.
Gain strength to become the strongest linebacker on the team by camp.	Gain 0.5–0.75 lb lean mass per week. After 8 weeks, increase lean mass by 6 lb.
Gain speed and agility to become the quickest linebacker on the team by camp.	After 8 weeks, achieve a body fat of 18%–19%.

Step 3: Action Plan

The athlete's action plan had four basic objectives:

- Increase calorie intake.
- Consume a high-carbohydrate, moderate-protein, moderate-fat diet.
- Distribute food intake over the course of the day to fuel activity and reduce fatigue.
- Consume a recovery snack immediately after exercise.

The athlete's initial meal plan of 4,800 kcal/d was based on his total energy expenditure of approximately 4,338 kcal plus an additional 500 kcal to cover the metabolic cost of building additional skeletal muscle tissue. Macronutrient distribution was based on 1.7 g protein per kiolgram body weight and 8 g carbohydrate per kiolgram body weight. The 4,800 kcal were distributed in a meal pattern of three meals plus two snacks. Preexercise meals and postexercise snacks were designed to ensure adequate fuel, sufficient high-quality protein, and proper rehydration and to support maximum muscle growth.

Using the 3-day food records, the sports RDN made suggestions for increasing portion sizes of certain foods and incorporating ready-to-eat or easy-to-prepare foods into meals and snacks. A supermarket tour proved helpful, as did a few basic cooking classes, a list of suggested dinner meals, preworkout and postworkout snack options, and several easy recipes.

Step 4: Evaluation and Reassessment

The evaluation and reassessment step involved the following tasks:

- Keep a food intake record and evaluate for energy intake, macronutrient balance, and nutrient adequacy.
- Record weight weekly.
- Measure body composition after 4 and 8 weeks; compare strength, power, and performance before and after the 8-week program.

The effectiveness of the initial meal plan was determined by monitoring weight. After 2 weeks it was decided that an additional 200 kcal/d might be needed to achieve the target weekly weight gain. When the additional calories were added, weekly weight gain stayed on target. At the end of 8 weeks, this athlete had reached his body weight goal of 232 lb (105.5 kg). A reassessment of his body composition indicated 18% body fat and a gain of 6 lbs (2.7 kg) in lean body mass. Having reached his preseason goals, this athlete followed a modified plan during the season, and, for the first time in his NFL career, he was able to maintain his target weight throughout the season. In addition, this was an injury-free season in which he started 16 games at weak-side linebacker and was ranked first on the team with a career-high 143 tackles. He moved from weak-side to middle linebacker, where he started the final eight games of the season.

Follow-up

Two years later, the linebacker suffered a severe knee sprain midway through the season and was placed on injured reserve. He was committed to arriving at off-season workouts in peak condition. At the end of the season, he once again engaged in a rigorous strength and conditioning program, 6 hours a day, 4 days a week, at the same training facility where he had trained 2 years prior. During the time he was on injured reserve, his weight dropped to 229 lb (104.1 kg). A body composition assessment determined that he was 19% body fat and 185.5 lbs (84.3 kg) of lean body mass. During the 8-week conditioning program, his goal was to increase total weight to 232 lb (105.5 kg) with 18% body fat. With his starting weight of 229 lb (104.1 kg), this meant a gain of 3.5 lb (1.6 kg) lean mass and a loss of 0.5 lb (0.23 kg) of body fat. Because he needed to slightly trim body fat and slowly gain muscle, his meal plan was modified to a 4,800-kcal meal plan with 1.9 g protein per kilogram body weight and 8 g carbohydrate per kilogram body weight. Weekly monitoring of weight indicated just less than a ½ lb gain per week. By the end of the conditioning program, this athlete had reached his goals.

SUMMARY

Weight management goals and plans must be highly individualized. Factors that determine optimal weight and body composition ranges include sports-related characteristics, such as position played, relative need for power and endurance, and need for speed, mobility, flexibility, and agility. Physique-related characteristics, such as body size, build, weight, composition, and appearance, must also be considered. Achieving optimal weight and body composition goals requires assessment, goal setting, an action plan, and evaluation and reassessment.

KEY TAKEAWAYS

Make a checklist of sport- and physique-related factors to review and prioritize when counseling an athlete.

Use the checklist as a teaching tool to help athletes understand the many factors to be considered when setting weight and composition goals.

Conduct a comprehensive nutrition assessment.

Help the athlete set reasonable, realistic, and achievable weight and body composition goals periodized to the performance season and the physical demands on the athlete.

Create a nutrition plan with the athlete that is tailored to the athlete's preferences and personal circumstances.

Routinely monitor and assess progress and adjust the nutrition plan as needed.

REFERENCES

1. Macedonio M, Dunford M. *The Athlete's Guide to Making Weight*. Champaign, IL: Human Kinetics; 2009.

2. Kinney WL, Wilmore JH, Costill DL. *Physiology of Sport and Exercise*. 6th ed. Champaign, IL: Human Kinetics; 2015.

3. Thomas DT, Erdman KA, Burke LM. Position of the Academy of Nutrition and Dietetics, Dietitians of Canada, and the American College of Sports Medicine: nutrition and athletic performance. *J Acad Nutr Diet*. 2016;116(3):501-528.

4. Manore MM. Weight management for athletes and active individuals: a brief review. *Sports Med*. 2015;45(suppl 1):83-92.

5. Dunford M, Doyle JA. *Nutrition for Sport and Exercise*. 3rd ed. Belmont, CA: Cengage Learning; 2015.

6. Pasiakos SM, McLellan TM, Lieberman HR. The effects of protein supplements on muscle mass, strength, and aerobic and anaerobic power in healthy adults: a systematic review. *Sports Med*. 2015;45(1):111-131.

7. Zillmann T, Knechtle B, Rüst CA, Knechtle P, Rosemann T, Lepers R. Comparison of training and anthropometric characteristics between recreational male half-marathoners and marathoners [Erratum in *Chin J Physiol*. 2013;56(4):243]. *Chin J Physiol*. 2013;56(3):138-146.

8. Melvin MN, Smith-Ryan AE, Wingfield HL, Ryan ED, Trexler ET, Roelofs EJ. Muscle characteristics and body composition of NCAA Division I football players. *J Strength Cond Res*. 2014;28(12):3320-3329.

9. Bosch TA, Burruss TP, Weir NL, et al. Abdominal body composition differences in NFL football players. *J Strength Cond Res*. 2014;28(12):3313-3319.

10. Collins SM, Silberlicht M, Perzinski C, Smith SP, Davidson PW. The relationship between body composition and preseason performance tests of collegiate male lacrosse players. *J Strength Cond Res*. 2014;28(9):2673-2679.

11. Rüst CA, Knechtle B, Knechtle P, Rosemann T. Similarities and differences in anthropometry and training between recreational male 100-km ultra-marathoners and marathoners. *J Sports Sci*. 2012;30(12):1249-1257.

12. Yamamoto JB, Yamamoto BE, Yamamoto PP, Yamamoto LG. Epidemiology of college athlete sizes, 1950s to current. *Res Sports Med*. 2008;16(2):111-127.

13. Montgomery DL. Physiological profile of professional hockey players—a longitudinal comparison. *Appl Physiol Nutr Metab*. 2006;31(3):181-185.

14. Crotin RL, Forsythe CM, Bhan S, Karakolis T. Changes in physical size among major league baseball players and its attribution to elite offensive performance. *J Strength Cond Res*. 2014;28(10):2705-2708.

15. Anzell AR, Potteiger JA, Kraemer WJ, Otieno S. Changes in height, body weight, and body composition in American football players from 1942 to 2011. *J Strength Cond Res*. 2013;27(2):277-284.

16. Skinner AC, Hasty SE, Turner RW II, Dreibelbis M, Lohr JA. Is bigger really better? Obesity among high school football players, player position, and team success. *Clin Pediatr (Phila)*. 2013;52(10):922-928.

17. Grundy SM, Cleeman JI, Daniels SR, et al; American Heart Association; National Heart, Lung, and Blood Institute. Diagnosis and management of the metabolic syndrome: an American Heart Association/National Heart, Lung, and Blood Institute Scientific Statement [Errata in *Circulation*. 2005;112(17):e297,e298]. *Circulation*. 2005;112(17):2735-2752.

18. Steffes GD, Megura AE, Adams J, et al. Prevalence of metabolic syndrome risk factors in high school and NCAA division I football players. *J Strength Cond Res*. 2013;27(7):1749-1757.

19. Helzberg JH, Camilo J, Waeckerle JF, O'Keefe JH. Review of cardiometabolic risk factors among current professional football and professional baseball players. *Phys Sportsmed*. 2010;38(3):77-83.

20. Buell JL, Calland D, Hanks F, et al. Presence of metabolic syndrome in football linemen. *J Athl Train*. 2008;43(6):608-616.

21. Karpinos AR, Roumie CL, Nian H, Diamond AB, Rothman RL. High prevalence of hypertension among collegiate football athletes. *Circ Cardiovasc Qual Outcomes*. 2013;6(6):716-723.

22. Javed A, Kashyap R, Lteif AN. Hyperandrogenism in female athletes with functional hypothalamic amenorrhea: a distinct phenotype. *Int J Womens Health*. 2015;7:103-111.

23. Goltz FR, Stenzel LM, Schneider CD. Disordered eating behaviors and body image in male athletes. *Rev Bras Psiquiatr*. 2013;35(3):237-242.

24. Kong P, Harris LM. The sporting body: body image and eating disorder symptomatology among female athletes from leanness focused and nonleanness focused sports. *J Psychol*. 2015;149(1-2):141-160.

25. Muller SM, Gorrow TR, Schneider SR. Enhancing appearance and sports performance: are female collegiate athletes behaving more like males? *J Am Coll Health*. 2009;57(5):513-520.

26. Calfee R, Fadale P. Popular ergogenic drugs and supplements in young athletes. *Pediatrics*. 2006;117(3):e577-e589.

27. Poslusna K, Ruprich J, de Vries JH, Jakubikova M, van't Veer P. Misreporting of energy and micronutrient intake estimated by food records and 24 hour recalls, control and adjustment methods in practice. *Br J Nutr*. 2009;101(suppl 2):73S-85S.

28. Ahuja JK, Moshfegh AJ, Holden JM, Harris E. USDA food and nutrient databases provide the infrastructure for food and nutrition research, policy, and practice. *J Nutr.* 2013;143(2):241S-2419S.

29. Rankin JW. Weight loss and gain in athletes. *Curr Sports Med Rep.* 2002;1(4):208-213.

30. Carbone JW, McClung JP, Pasiakos SM. Skeletal muscle responses to negative energy balance: effects of dietary protein. *Adv Nutr.* 2012;3(2):119-126.

31. Mettler S, Mitchell N, Tipton KD. Increased protein intake reduces lean body mass loss during weight loss in athletes. *Med Sci Sports Exerc.* 2010;42(2):326-337.

32. Doering TM, Reaburn PR, Phillips SM, Jenkins DG. Post-exercise dietary protein strategies to maximize skeletal muscle repair and remodeling in masters endurance athletes: a review. *Int J Sport Nutr Exerc Metab.* 2016;26(2):168-178. doi: 10.1123/ijsnem.2015-0102. Epub September 24, 2015.

33. Ivy J, Ferguson-Stegall LM. Nutrient timing: the means to improving exercise performance, recovery, and training adaptation. *Am J Lifestyle Med.* 2014;8(4):246-259.

SECTION 3

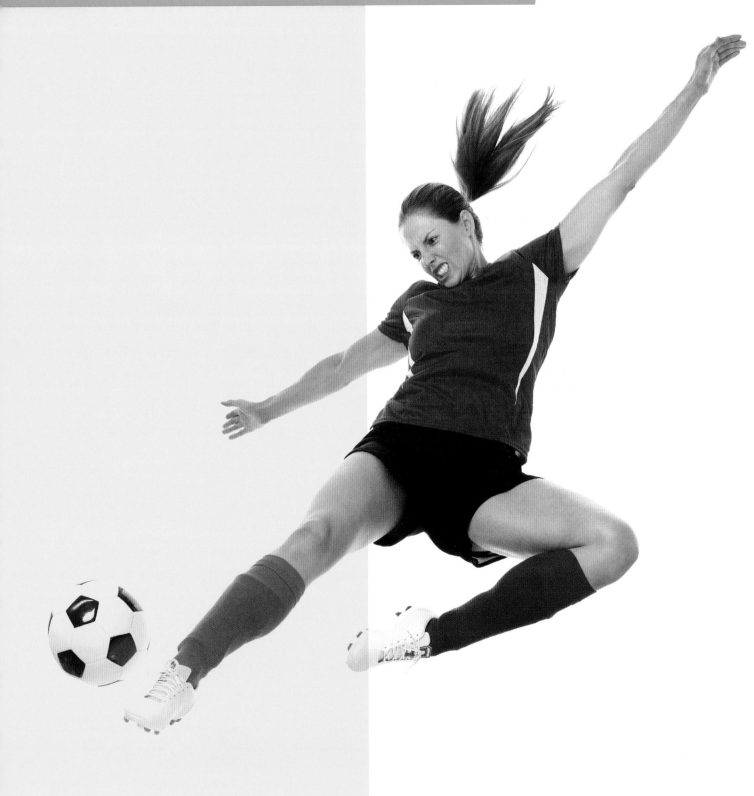

PRINCIPLES IN PRACTICE

Athletics is not restricted to the young elite or the professional athlete. Today, children participate in competitive sports, as do older adults. This section provides the sports dietitian with insight into the physiological and health-related issues of diverse populations. Understanding the unique needs of these populations will help the sports dietitian develop plans to meet the needs of each athlete, whether it is a collegiate athlete who is challenged by lack of cooking skills or an athlete with diabetes who needs medical nutrition therapy. In this section, life cycle issues are discussed in chapters dealing with youth, college-age, and older athletes (Chapters 12, 13, and 14, respectively). A chapter on elite athletes (Chapter 15) is included to highlight the opportunities and challenges faced by the sports dietitian when planning nutrition strategies for high-performing athletes. The unique nutritional needs of vegetarian athletes, pregnant athletes, athletes with disordered eating, and those with type 1 and type 2 diabetes are also included in this section (Chapters 16 through 20).

CHAPTER 12

CHILD AND ADOLESCENT ATHLETES

Roberta Anding, MS, RD, LD, CDE, CSSD, FAND

INTRODUCTION

The popularity of youth sports in the United States is at an all-time high. Data from the 2000 Census estimated that the total youth sports participation was greater than 50 million children and adolescents.[1] The National Federation of State High School Associations (NFHS) reports that in the 2013 to 2014 school year, high school sports participation was approximately 7.7 million (58% male and 42% female adolescents). Throughout the United States, football has nearly twice as many participants (1,093,234) as other sports. Other top sports for boys include outdoor track and field (580,321), basketball (541,054), baseball (482,629), and soccer (417,419). The most popular sports programs for girls include outdoor track and field (478,885), basketball (433,344), volleyball (429,634), soccer (374,564), and fast-pitch softball (364,297). The number of high school participants has increased every year for the past 20 years. Absent from this data set are statistics regarding cheerleading, which has experienced a surge in popularity over the past decade. A survey by NFHS estimates that more than 400,000 young women are participating in cheerleading in the United States, making it as popular as other traditional sports for girls.[2] Parents and volunteer coaches are often responsible for guidance on hydration, nutrition, and training in younger athletes. In high school, the coaches often assume more than one role, and their expertise in nutrition varies. Given the prevalence of youth sports, the expertise of a sports dietitian is needed to promote evidenced-based principles for performance and proper nutrition for growth and development.

BENEFITS OF YOUTH SPORTS

The benefits of youth sports are numerous and are both physical and psychosocial. Physical activity should be considered an essential component of normal growth and development and should be routinely assessed as a vital sign in the electronic medical record. Sports can provide an outlet for youth to begin and maintain physical activity. Regular physical activity in the formative years has been shown to be a predictor of a healthier body weight and regular exercise patterns in adulthood.[3,4] Not surprisingly, children who

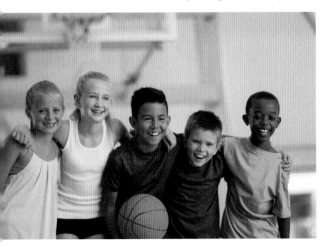

participate in sports have greater levels of cardiovascular fitness, lower abdominal fat, and reduced arterial stiffness.[5] In addition to improving cardiorespiratory fitness, regular physical activity has been shown to improve lipid profiles in youth, most notably triglyceride and high-density lipoprotein cholesterol levels, although the improvement is often modest.[6] The dose of exercise to improve lipids is consistent with the duration and frequency of a minimum of 40 minutes per day 5 days per week over a 4-month period.[7] This level of exercise is consistent with a sports season for children and teens. The psychological benefits of regular exercise for children and teens include improved self-esteem, increased social interaction, and a decrease in depressive symptoms.[8]

Bone Density

Regular physical activity is also essential for the development and maintenance of bone mineral density. The osteogenic force of physical activity is related to the local and specific mechanical loading of the bone. The tensile and compressive forces of specific resistance or strength-producing programs can promote bone development. According to the National Strength and Conditioning Association position paper, when properly performed and supervised, a comprehensive strength and conditioning program is safe to initiate in children as young as 5 to 6 years old, although more typically a strength program begins at age 12.[9]

Additionally, numerous sport-specific studies have demonstrated targeted areas of bone development based on the loading forces. Studies with gymnasts show improved bone density in wrists and the proximal portion of the femur given the nature of the sport.[10,11] Although research results vary, consistent load-bearing exercise in the prepubertal phase of adolescence can promote an increase in bone accrual of 0.6% to 1.7% per year.[12] In a review article by Hind, prepubertal children who exercised regularly experienced mean percent increases of 0.9% to 4.9% in bone parameters over 6 months in early pubertal development.[13] Less bone accrual was realized in late adolescence or young adulthood, indicating the role of exercise in bone accrual during childhood and early puberty.[8] A longitudinal study of soccer players demonstrated that the osteogenic benefits of exercise in adolescents can have a positive impact on bone health after they complete their competitive years. Thirty years after they stopped playing, former soccer players had a higher bone mineral density and larger bone mass compared with sedentary counterparts, indicating that playing sports during adolescence may have long-lasting health benefits.[14] In a review article by Tenforde and Fredericson, the loading of bone in sports can be characterized by high impact (gymnastics, hurdling), loading impact (soccer, basketball), and nonimpact (swimming, cycling) sports.[15] Higher impact loading sports result in a favorable improvement in bone geometry, whereas nonimpact sports are either neutral or detrimental to bone accrual. Optimal bone development during childhood and adolescence is predicated on energy availability and a normal hormonal milieu.

Physical Activity and Obesity

Multiple studies have highlighted the known benefits of physical fitness and nutrition on health, including lower body fat, improved lipids, lower blood pressure, and improved insulin sensitivity in youth.[7] Over the past 25 years, the rate of obesity in US youth has doubled, and the rate in adolescents is even more alarming. The incidence of type 2 diabetes is increasing faster in the adolescent population than in adults, with an increase of 30.5% from 2001 to 2009.[16] Sports and physical activity are an integral component of obesity and type 2 diabetes prevention. Type 2 diabetes is often characterized by peripheral insulin resistance and the inability of the pancreatic β cells to maintain euglycemia in the fasted and postprandial state. Approximately 90% of the glucose uptake is in skeletal muscle in a healthy individual. However, a consequence of obesity is the reduction of this peripheral uptake of glucose to approximately 50% of baseline with a further reduction in those with type 2 diabetes.[17] Increased visceral fat distribution and hepatic steatosis have been shown to be directly related to insulin resistance in the pediatric population.[18] The prevailing mechanism for the development of type 2 diabetes has historically centered on peripheral insulin resistance. Newer models have highlighted the role of mitochondrial dysfunction as an additional mechanism. Mitochondrial dysfunction is characterized by alterations in oxidative phosphorylation, enzymatic defects, and lipid metabolism. Cardiorespiratory fitness is an indirect measure of oxidative phosphorylation, and exercise also plays a unique role in the improvement of mitochondrial function and quality. In mitochondrial dysfunction, lipid oxidation is impaired, and fatty acid metabolites accumulate, contributing to insulin resistance. Although the exact pathophysiology of type 2 diabetes in youth is yet to be completely elucidated, it is clear that consistent, vigorous exercise (>80% maximal heart rate[19]) can improve the markers of insulin sensitivity, irrespective of changes in body composition. The Diabetes Prevention Program has demonstrated that increased activity (150 minutes per week) and weight loss (5% to 7% of initial weight) in adults can reduce the development of diabetes in high-risk individuals, but less is known about children and teens. In children, increased adiposity, including increased visceral fat, has been linked with the development of metabolic syndrome. A Finnish pediatric prospective study showed higher baseline fasting insulin levels in children who later developed metabolic syndrome.[20] The results of this study suggest that insulin resistance in obese children precedes the metabolic and atherogenic complications.

Adolescents who are overweight and who participated in a structured exercise program for 3 to 5 days per week for 3 to 8 months improved insulin sensitivity up to 50%.[21,22] In this context, organized sport can be considered a public health strategy for preventing diabetes in youth. With increasing pressure to have larger linemen in football, prepubertal boys or boys in early puberty may seek to gain weight but lack the androgen to add significant lean mass. Therefore, increasing body weight is likely to be adipose tissue and not lean body mass, thus increasing the likelihood of insulin resistance. The progressive assessment of abdominal girth among adolescents and screening for acanthosis nigricans in athletes is critical for preventing type 2 diabetes in this vulnerable population. Waist circumference cutoffs for the diagnosis of metabolic syndrome have been established based on age, gender, and ethnicity, which can be useful for the practicing sports dietitian (see Table 12.1).[23] Given the magnitude of the pediatric obesity epidemic, sports dietitians will regularly encounter young athletes with metabolic syndrome.

Table 12.1 Optimal Waist Circumference Thresholds (cm) for Predicting Cardiovascular Risk Clustering in Adolescents Based on Ethnicity[24]

Age, y	Hispanic Boys	Hispanic Girls	Non-Hispanic White Boys	Non-Hispanic White Girls	Non-Hispanic Black Boys	Non-Hispanic Black Girls
12	76.5	77.1	73.1	71.5	66.8	74.6
13	81.6	79.1	74.2	78.0	72.6	75.6
14	80.3	79.6	76.1	74.8	75.0	80.0
15	83.5	79.8	77.2	77.6	76.5	82.7
16	83.7	81.2	82.1	78.5	74.7	84.6
17	85.0	82.4	85.1	77.6	77.9	86.8
18	87.1	82.5	83.5	78.0	79.0	86.9
19	87.5	86.4	86.3	85.0	78.6	87.2

The lifelong costs of obesity are staggering. The direct financial cost of pediatric obesity is $14.1 billion per year.[24] In addition to the increased risk of type 2 diabetes, a teen who is obese is more likely to become an adult who is overweight or obese and has an increased risk of heart disease, hypertension, cancer, and osteoarthritis. Other significant health concerns include nonalcoholic fatty liver disease, sleep apnea, and asthma.[25] Physical activity and dietary regulation can be seen as the cornerstone of obesity prevention and management. In obesity prevention and management, it is difficult to separate the distinct roles of exercise and diet. Although the causes of obesity are multifactorial, the factors driving this epidemic remain the steady increase in calories coupled with decreases in physical activity.[26] Reduced intake of sugar-sweetened beverages has been highlighted as a specific dietary intervention to reduce pediatric obesity. The most recent clinical report of the American Academy of Pediatrics recommends reducing intake of all sugar-sweetened beverages as a strategy to prevent pediatric obesity.[27] Recent data indicate that children and adolescents have reduced their intake of sugar-sweetened sodas and fruit drinks with added sugar. However, as the intake of these beverages decreases, consumption of sweetened coffees, teas, and sports drinks increases.[28]

It is important for sports dietitians to keep abreast of the changing beverage consumption patterns of children and teens to provide guidance for athletes. Although genetics and inherited predispositions to body morphology ultimately influence body size, musculature, and body fatness, positive energy balance is the major contributor to excess body fatness.[29] It is critical for the sports dietitian to play a role in weight management in this vulnerable population. Nutritional recommendations must be altered to lower body fat and maintain adequate calories for activity. In practical terms, registered dietitian nutritionists can use a sedentary to low-active cofactor as a starting point. Tables 12.2 and 12.3 provide guidance on calorie calculations for children and adolescents.

Table 12.2 Equations to Calculate Estimated Energy Requirements[a]

Energy Requirement	Sex	Calculation (EER), kcal/d
Estimated Energy Requirements (EER) for 9- to 19-year olds[b]	Boys	$EER = 88.5 - (61.9 \times age\ [y]) + PA^c \times (26.7 \times wt\ [kg] + 903 \times ht\ [m]) + 25$
	Girls	$EER = 135.3 - (30.8 \times age\ [y]) + PA \times (10 \times wt\ [kg] + 934 \times ht\ [m]) + 25$
EER for persons aged ≥19 years[d]	Men	$EER = 662 - 9.53 \times age\ (y) + PA \times [(15.91 \times wt\ [kg] + 539.6 \times ht\ [m])]$
	Women	$EER = 354 - 6.91 \times age\ (y) + PA \times [(9.36 \times wt\ [kg] + 726 \times ht\ [m])]$

[a] EER is the average dietary energy intake that is predicted to maintain energy balance in healthy-weight individuals of a defined age, sex, weight, height, and level of physical activity consistent with good health. In children and pregnant and lactating women, the EER includes the needs associated with growth at rates consistent with good health.

[b] EER = Total energy expenditure + Energy deposition

[c] PA = physical activity

[d] For each year below 30, add to the EER 7 kcal/d for women and 10 kcal/day for men. For each year above 30, subtract from the EER 7 kcal/d for women and 10 kcal/d for men.

Adapted from *Dietary Reference Intakes: The Essential Guide to Nutrient Requirements.* 2006 by the National Academy of Sciences, Courtesy of the National Academies Press, Washington, DC.

Table 12.3 Physical Activity Coefficients[a] for Use in Estimated Energy Requirement Equations for Adolescents or Adult Women

	Sedentary[b] (PAL[c] 1.0–1.39)	Low Active[d] (PAL 1.4–1.59)	Active[e] (PAL 1.6–1.89)	Very Active[f] (PAL 1.9–2.5)
Adolescents aged 14–18 years old	1.0	1.16	1.31	1.56
Women aged 19 years and older	1.0	1.12	1.27	1.45

[a] Physical activity coefficients are used in the estimated enerdy requirements (EER) equations and are based on ranges of physical activity levels.

[b] Sedentary refers to typical daily living activities (eg, household tasks, walking to the bus).

[c] PAL = physical activity level. PAL is the ratio of the total energy expenditure to the basal energy expenditure.

[d] Low active refers to typical daily living activities PLUS 30 to 60 minutes of daily moderate activity (eg, walking at 5 to 7 km/h).

[e] Adtive refers to typical daily living activities PLUS at least 60 minutes of daily moderate activity.

[f] Very active refers to typical daily living activities PLUS at least 60 minutes of daily moderate activity PLUS an additional 60 minutes of vigorous activity or 120 minutes of moderate activity.

Adapted from *Dietary Reference Intakes: The Essential Guide to Nutrient Requirements.* 2006 by the National Academy of Sciences, Courtesy of the National Academies Press, Washington, DC.

Psychosocial Stigma of Obesity

Psychosocial stigma for children or adolescents who are overweight or obese can be significant. Weight teasing and bullying are pervasive in today's society. In a study by Neumark-Sztainer and colleagues, the prevalence of weight teasing was reported in a sample of over 4,700 youths who were overweight orobese.[30] Of the sample, 63% of the girls and 58% of the boys who were obese (body mass index [BMI] > 95 percentile) reported weight teasing. These subjects also reported weight teasing within their families. Weight teasing was associated with an increase in binge eating and placed the youth at greater risk of further obesity. Subsequent research indicates that body dissatisfaction in youth who are overweight is an additional risk factor for eating disorders and disordered eating behaviors.[31] Although the exact prevalence of weight teasing in youth sports is unknown, 42% of those reported being bullied by adult perpetrators including coaches.[32]

Psychological Benefits of Sports

Youth sports can promote healthy psychosocial development and positive attributes. Physical activity in children and adolescents is thought to be a key determinant of cognitive development. Cognitive development is broadly defined as the ability to acquire knowledge through a variety of mechanisms, including experiences and sensory input. High cognitive function is an important determinant of health, and, conversely, poor cognitive functioning is linked to increased morbidity and mortality.[33,34] Literature suggests that active children and teens have higher levels of cognitive function, reported as improved memory and concentration and better classroom behavior, leading to better academic performance.[35-39] Well-structured sports participation has been specifically linked to learning values, skills, self-control, persistence, and responsibility.[36] Sports can also promote resilience and the ability to rebound from disappointment.[37] Sports participation in high school has been associated with improved mental health and reduced depression. Proposed mechanisms are complex but include neurobiological factors and improved social factors, such as a sense of connectedness and belonging.[38-39] High school girls who are active in sports are more likely to graduate high school, have fewer pregnancies as adolescents, and demonstrate greater self-esteem than those who do not participate in sports.[40]

Despite the noted benefits, sports participation can also have negative consequences. Most children and teens report having fun as a primary reason for participation. Conversely, when a sport is no longer enjoyable, children and teens report becoming less active or finding something else that is more fun. A recent comprehensive review by the International Olympic Committee cautions against early specialization, which is a contributor to increased injury rates and burnout.[41,42] Sports dietitians should be attuned to the signs and symptoms of depression and burnout as part of an initial assessment. Children and adolescents are vulnerable to inappropriate coaching and instructions. Children and adolescents who live at the coaching facility, such as those in world class ballet, gymnastics, and figure skating, are at particular risk given their young age and potential social isolation from family and friends.

PHYSICAL GROWTH AND DEVELOPMENT

Prepubertal Stage

In the prepubertal phase or sexual maturity rating 1, boys and girls share many physical attributes. Body composition analyses are similar between girls and boys, with a percent body fat of 16% to 17% fat and relatively similar amounts of lean weight.[43] Height, weight, injury risks, hemoglobin levels, and physical attributes of strength and endurance are similar between boys and girls.[44-45] During the prepubertal phase, rate of growth is about 5 cm/y in boys and girls. The activation of the pituitary-gonadal axis signals the onset of puberty, and the physiological changes become gender specific. During early puberty, linear growth increases markedly in both sexes from approximately 5 cm/y in prepubertal boys and girls to 8.3 cm/year in pubertal girls and 9.5 cm/y in pubertal boy. Weight velocity increases from 3 kg/y in prepubertal boys to 9 kg/y during puberty; less is known about pubertal girls. The changes in biological landmarks are sex specific.

Pubertal Development

Puberty is the process of physical and psychological maturation from childhood to adulthood. It is characterized by physical and psychological changes that influence nutritional needs and food choices. The biological changes include increases in height and weight, body composition changes, increases in calorie and protein needs, sexual development, and increases in skeletal mass and density. Although the biological changes during puberty are consistent, the timing and tempo of these landmarks can vary and are influenced by genetics, sex, and nutritional status (eg, malnutrition and obesity). The impact of genetics in determining the cascade of pubertal events is estimated to be 41% to 71%.[46] Therefore, pubertal development is the interaction of genetic traits with components of the environment. The age of menarche has declined steadily in the United States over the past 50 years. Overweight and obesity are part of the etiology of this decline, but other variables are emerging as well. Researchers have found that brominated flame retardants, phytoestrogens, phenols, and phthalates have the potential to affect the timing of puberty.[47,48] The alteration of normal pubertal development has the potential to impact body composition and nutritional needs. Girls who experience early menarche (age < 11 years) are more likely to become overweight and are less sensitive to insulin than girls who experience menarche later in adolescence (age > 14 years).[49,50]

Given the variability in timing and tempo of pubertal events, chronological age is not a reliable marker for predicting growth and nutritional requirements. Tanner stages (also known as sexual maturity ratings) are the best gauge of the current stage of growth and development. In females, the sexual maturity rating is based on appearance and development of breasts and pubic hair. In males, Tanner stages are characterized by testicular and penile development, along with the development and patterning of pubic hair. Although it is not in the scope of the sports registered dietitian nutritionist (RDN) to conduct this level of physical exam, these biological landmarks can be done as an adolescent self-assessment. Self-assessment of sexual maturity ratings does not replace a physical exam by a trained pediatrician but can be useful in distinguishing the prepubertal and pubertal phase.[51] Because calorie and protein needs are determined by Tanner stages, this assessment can guide the dietitian in the development of an appropriate nutrition plan. Table 12.4 illustrates the Tanner staging process and the nutritional implications.

Table 12.4 Sexual Maturity Rating and Nutritional Implications

Girls

Stage	Development	Nutritional Implications
Stage 1	No pubic hair or maturation of genitalia	Calories based on Dietary Reference Intake
Stage 2	Sparse pubic hair Small breast buds Increased sweat gland activity Initiation of peak height velocity (PHV); growth spurt of 3–5 in Average age: 10.6 y	Calories increase to their highest levels in adolescence Girls experience an increase peak in weight velocity ~6–9 mo before PHV; they "grow out, then up"
Stage 3	Pubic hair increases and is darker and curly Breasts are larger Acne may occur End of PHV	Nutritional guidance needed to improve nutrient density
Stage 4	Menarche begins at average age of 12.5 y 98% of adult height achieved	May occur earlier in girls who are obese May be delayed with malnutrition or decreased energy availability
Stage 5	Adult breasts and pubic hair Increase in fat and muscle mass	

Continued on next page

Boys

Stage	Development	Nutritional Implications
Stage 1	No pubic hair or maturation of genitalia	Calories based on Dietary Reference Intake
Stage 2	Penile enlargement Scrotum reddens and changes texture Increased activity of sweat glands	Lack of androgen limits lean mass accrual Strength training can improve neuromuscular control and strength without increase in mass
Stage 3	Faint noticeable mustache Voice begins to change Acne may occur Beginning of PHV; growth spurt of 6–8 in	Peak weight velocity and peak height velocity coincide Calories and protein increase to their highest levels
Stage 4	Voice deepens Acne may be severe	Muscle mass increases
Stage 5	Able to grow full beard Linear growth ceases between age 18–21 y	Muscle mass increases Calorie and protein needs equal to an adult male

Adapted from *Dietary Reference Intakes: The Essential Guide to Nutrient Requirements.* 2006 by the National Academy of Sciences, Courtesy of the National Academies Press, Washington, DC.

PUBERTAL DEVELOPMENT IN GIRLS

The first hallmark of puberty in girls is the development of breast buds at an average age of 10.6 years, signaling the onset of Tanner stage 2. Peak weight velocity occurs in girls before the peak height velocity. In practical terms, girls "grow out" and then "grow up." Peak height velocity follows early in the pubertal process for girls during Tanner stage 2 and slows during Tanner stage 3. Menarche occurs during Tanner stage 4, which, on average, occurs at age 12.5 years in the United States. About 98% of adult height is achieved by Tanner stage 4. As part of a nutrition assessment, all sports dietitians should assess age of menarche to gauge the phase of growth and development because this ultimately influences caloric need. However, there are ethnic and racial differences in pubertal timing. Research indicates that African American girls may enter puberty earlier than their white and Hispanic peers.[52] In a large practice-based study, 48% of African American girls had reached Tanner stage 2 by age 8, contrasting with the average age of onset of 10.6 years. In addition, obesity during the prepubescent phase can hasten the onset of puberty. In a study of Chinese girls, the girls who were obese entered Tanner stage 2 at age 8.8 years of age whereas the girls who were lean entered this phase of growth and development at age 9.3 years.[53] Childhood obesity hastens the onset of puberty via increased estradiol. Girls who experience early puberty will have a slightly extended period of growth compared with girls who experience a more typical pattern. Just as overnutrition can hasten the onset of puberty in girls, undernutrition may delay the onset and tempo of the pubertal cascade.

Evidence from developing countries shows that menarche occurs at an older age in malnourished teens, suggesting that food insecurity or caloric restriction may delay menarche through nutritional mechanisms.[54] Although there is controversy in the literature, data on underfueled young athletes indicate that intensive training may delay the onset of puberty, suggestive of low energy availability. In response to this growing concern over gymnasts, the Scientific Commission of the International Gymnastics Federation convened a committee to review the literature on the effects of intensive training on the growth and development of female gymnasts. The short stature and later maturation of female gymnasts have often been attributed to the demands of training and the emphasis on leanness; however, after extensive review, these characteristics are considered within the normal range of variability for the population.[41,55]

Less information is available about other sports. Sports dietitians should take a detailed menstrual history to assess for the possibility of low energy availability.

After puberty, young women develop less strength than their male counterparts. Strength-trained female athletes can achieve approximately 70% of the total strength of their male counterparts and 30% to 50% of the upper body strength secondary to a relative decrease in lean mass compared with their male counterparts. Estrogen and progesterone promote the deposition of more body fat than muscle, possibly limiting strength gains. Females increase body fat levels from approximately 16% during the prepubertal phase to about 23% in adulthood.[43,44,48,56,57] Muscle fiber types are not gender specific; however, females have an overall smaller muscle fiber size. Therefore, many of the physiological changes during puberty affecting sports performance can be attributed to hormonal and body composition changes. Pubertal changes and performance changes in females are summarized in Box 12.1.

Box 12.1 Pubertal Changes Affecting Sports Performance in Females[58]

Increase in percent body fat
Reduced hemoglobin levels
Lung volume and aerobic capacity reduced
Early maturers have increased levels of adiposity
Improved balance and flexibility

PUBERTAL DEVELOPMENT IN BOYS

In boys, the first physical signs of maturation include testicular enlargement and a change in scrotal color. The average age of onset of Tanner stage 2 in boys is 11.6 years old. Peak height velocity in boys occurs in Tanner stage 3, about the same time as peak weight velocity, with the coinciding increase in caloric requirements. Height velocity accelerates from approximately 5 cm/y to 9.5 cm/y. Compared with girls, boys have a prolonged period of growth, resulting in about a 13 cm greater height. As androgen levels increase, there is a significant increase in lean body mass. Weight velocity increases from 3 kg/year in prepubertal boys to 9 kg/y during puberty. Lean mass doubles from about the age of 10 through 17, further increasing calorie requirements.[59] The increase in androgen not only increases lean weight but also allows for muscular hypertrophy with strength training. Increasing calories and protein in the absence of adequate androgen increases the likelihood of weight gain, which can lead to significant obesity. The sports RDN should assess stage of growth and development and provide education on normal growth and development. During adolescence, boys often struggle with gaining weight secondary to the needs of growth and development and fueling their sport. A late-maturing boy is more likely to use or abuse performance-enhancing supplements to improve body composition.[60]

Obesity has an impact on growth parameters, although there in not universal agreement on the effect. Puberal boys who are obese have lower serum sex hormone–binding globulin and consequently lower total testosterone levels compared with healthy-weight peers. In addition, obesity can cause an increase in the aromatization of testosterone to estradiol, which can increase the rate of skeletal maturation and increase the risk of gynecomastia.[61] Although the role of obesity and sexual maturation is established in girls, there is not universal agreement on the role of obesity and sexual maturation in boys. Unlike in girls, Biro and colleagues found that in a population-based cohort of 346 boys, the boys who had a greater fat mass as measured by the sum of skinfolds had less advanced sexual maturation by age 12 years.[47] Boys who had a higher BMI and greater adiposity reached a maturation stage at an older age. In a longitudinal, population-based study, Lee and colleagues reported that a higher BMI z-score trajectory during early to middle childhood may be associated with later onset of puberty among boys.[62] These findings suggest that greater body fat mass is *not* linked to an earlier onset of puberty among boys. In a conflicting study, De Leonibus and colleagues suggest that obesity in males results in an earlier onset and completion of puberty in boys as well as girls.[63] More research is needed to determine the role of obesity and excess fatness on pubertal timing in males.

Normal Psychological Development

The transition from childhood to adolescence also marks a period of psychosocial development. This chapter will not examine this development in depth, but the sports dietitian should recognize the hallmarks of this transition because they can impact the nutrition care process. The three major areas of psychological development for the adolescent are cognition, psychosocial relationships, and emotional development.

Transition from concrete to abstract thinking is a normal developmental task of adolescence. Younger children often think in a concrete manner. Concrete thinkers rely on what they see or objects that are physically present and struggle with the extrapolation from a known item to an unknown. The world exists as good or bad or right or wrong; concrete thinkers struggle with shades of gray. As a simple example, consider a sports dietitian's counsel reducing intake of sugar-sweetened beverages for improvement of nutritional status for many children and teens. If you counsel a concrete thinker on reducing lemonade consumption, you may see the concrete thinker only reduce intake of this specific beverage. Reducing consumption of a single beverage is what was heard, and the inability to think abstractly may limit how the child comprehends the recommendation. Often the perceived noncompliance is a failure of the provider to use developmentally appropriate language. Nutrition education for the concrete thinker needs to be precise and succinct, with clear instructions. Nutrition concepts should be prescriptive and have limited choices. Youths who remain concrete thinkers in high school may be frustrated with higher-functioning abstract concepts, such as advanced mathematics or too many choices in meal planning.

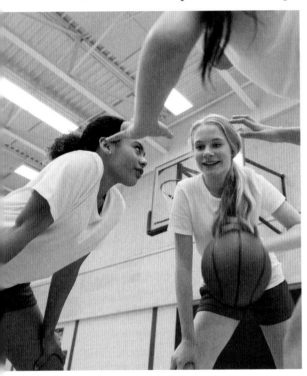

Abstract thinking implies the ability to imagine things not yet experienced. Adolescents who are able to think abstractly can speculate about all possibilities, not just the known. Abstract thinkers may want to understand the "why" and may require more time and effort in a counseling session.[64] The emergence of abstract thinking allows the adolescent to develop more comprehensive thought, possibly through the development of the personal fable or the imaginary audience. This concept is based on the belief that an imaginary group, often peers, are always watching or thinking about the individual. Also viewed as adolescent egocentricism, the concept of the personal fable may contribute to the belief that they are invincible. This belief can predispose the adolescent to increased risk-taking behavior because consequences only happen to others, not to them.[65] Among athletes, this can translate into anabolic steroid use, diet pills for weight loss, and drinking and driving. Additionally, the adolescent brain appears more sensitive to reward, including sweet substances, during early adolescence. This enhanced reward sensitivity in adolescence may increase the likelihood of the rewarding properties of abuse of drugs and alcohol.[66]

Psychosocial development of normal adolescence includes identity formation and autonomy. Erickson postulated that identity formation is an essential developmental task of adolescence.[67] Identity is defined as who the adolescent is, separate and apart from the family of origin. Some risk taking is central to the formation of an identity. During this critical stage of development, teens may experiment with dietary trends, lifestyles, and mannerisms. An identity related to sports is often formed during this phase. Jessor suggested that appropriate risk taking can serve as a key social and personal determinant of self-confidence.[68] This developmental task progresses through adolescence and in early adolescence is characterized (ages 12 to 14) by forming same-sex peer groups with less interest in family activities and parental guidance. During middle adolescence (ages 15 to 17), the peer group becomes mixed and becomes the primary social group for the teen; family conflict can escalate. Sports dietitians may be valuable educators at this time as the adolescent still seeks guidance from responsible adults other than his or her parents. In late adolescence (ages 18 to 21), separation from the family of origin has developed. Conflict with family may decline.

Additionally, during this phase of adolescence, the sports dietitian should consider interviewing the older teen separate from their parents.

EXERCISE PHYSIOLOGY IN CHILDREN AND TEENS

Nutritional requirements for athletes are determined based on the type, intensity, and duration of the sport. Most nutrition guidelines set for adults use well-established concepts of exercise physiology. However, growth, development, and pubertal status can influence muscular function and fuel utilization. The surge in the hormones associated with puberty (growth hormone, insulin-like growth factor, catecholamines, and sex steroid hormones) may indeed affect nutritional requirements. For ethical reasons, limited studies exist outlining the physiological differences among children, adolescents, and adults. Sports dietitians should use adult guidelines for calculating nutrient needs when the athlete reaches Tanner 5.

Children and young adolescents have limited endogenous carbohydrate stores. Glycogen storage capacity and the response to diets of different macronutrient distributions have not been studied extensively in children and adolescents due to the invasive nature of intervention studies. In an animal model, researchers suggested that puberty may be related to a lower glycogen storage capability.[69] The regulation of glucose metabolism is mediated in part through insulin metabolism. Puberty is considered an insulin-resistant state secondary to a rise in growth hormone and sex steroid hormones. Prepubertal children have insulin responses similar to those of adults. However, during Tanner stages 2 through 4, insulin sensitivity can be reduced by 30%.[70]

As such, fatty acid oxidation is higher in boys and girls than in adults.[71] Therefore, children are biologically equipped for sustained aerobic activity vs anaerobic sports based on maturation landmarks. Although conflicting reports about substrate metabolism between children and adults exist, the majority of research indicates adult and child differences in substrate metabolism, with children exhibiting a higher fat oxidation than adults.[71] One study of five 11-year-old boys found that phosphofructokinase (glycolytic) activity was approximately 40% of reported adult values.[72] In an additional study, Kaczor and colleagues reported that lactate dehydrogenase activity in skeletal muscle of 3- to 11-year-old children was only about 28% of the value determined in adulthood.[73] Given the predominance of fat oxidation and the limited ability to store carbohydrate in childhood, as well as enzymatic immaturity, carbohydrate recommendations during exercise may be less than that of adults, although practical guidelines are lacking.[74]

It is unclear exactly when during adolescence the shift occurs favoring an adult metabolic pattern. This may contribute to conflicting study results in teens. In addition, less is known regarding the metabolic differences between girls and boys. Given the increase in lean mass, particularly in boys, it may be prudent to evaluate enzymatic activity based on fat-free mass (FFM).[75] A study by Stephens and colleagues suggests that the enhanced metabolism of fat appears to be dominant through midpuberty.[76] In a conflicting recent study by Couto and colleagues, a higher-carbohydrate diet (70%) given to boys aged 13 through 18 years indicated an improved overall performance vs a low-carbohydrate diet (25%); the performance included a 400-m end-of-race sprint.[77] This may be due to maturational changes or the impact of training on glucose disposal. There may also be a study difference in training and overall diet. Although there appears to be some difference between adolescents and adults, international experts have suggested that the carbohydrate needs of teens can be calculated using adult guidelines given the intensity and duration of sport.[78]

THERMOREGULATION AND FLUID REQUIREMENTS

The long-standing belief that children and adolescents are physiologically impaired in regulating temperature compared with adults has been challenged by more recent science. Children have higher levels of relative evaporative cooling and sweating efficiency, thus yielding lower mass-dependent heat storage.[79] Therefore, the current perspective is that adequately hydrated youth athletes are not at a thermoregulatory disadvantage compared with similarly fit, hydrated, and acclimatized adults during exercise in the heat.[80]

Although children and teens can tolerate thermal loads in a similar fashion as adults, there are pubertal-related differences in the dissipation of heat loads. Children and teens rely less on sweating to promote thermal equilibrium and more on blood flow redistribution, with heat dissipation through radiative and conductive cooling.[78] Children rely more on dry heat dissipation by their larger relative skin surface area than on evaporative heat loss, which controls thermoregulation in adults. With training, children and teens become more efficient at peripheral vasodilation vs alterations in sweat rate.[81] In essence, this means a lower sweat rate and accompanying lower sodium losses. The link between dehydration and athletic performance in children is limited. It is well established that dehydration levels of 2% to 7% can cause a decrement of performance in distance events lasting over an hour in adults. One study has examined the link between dehydration and performance in children. Wilk and colleagues found that dehydration levels of 1% negatively affected endurance performance in 10- to 12-year-old boys.[82] As with other maturational landmarks, the transition from radiant cooling to evaporative cooling is driven by puberty, and this transition appears to be complete by the end of puberty, at about Tanner stage 5.[83]

Fluid replacement guidelines for children can be calculated as an hourly fluid intake of 13 mL/kg (6 mL/lb) body weight. Postexercise rehydration requirements have been estimated at 4 mL/kg (2 mL/lb) for each hour of exercise to avoid initiating subsequent exercise in a dehydrated state.[84] Alternatively, the policy statement from the American Academy of Pediatrics on climatic heat stress and exercising children and adolescents suggests 100 to 250 mL every 20 minutes for 9- to 12-year-olds and 1 to 1.5 L/h for 13- to 18-year-olds, assuming adequate hydration status prior to activity.[85]

Preexisting illness, along with fitness level, may predispose children and adolescents to heat-related illnesses. Chronic illnesses such as diabetes insipidus, poorly controlled type 1 and type 2 diabetes, obesity, cystic fibrosis, febrile illnesses, and Graves disease are examples of illnesses that may alter fluid balance.[86,87] The cause of heat-related illness in children and adolescents may not be due to impaired thermoregulatory response but rather due to compromised preactivity hydration status.[88] Children may have less access to fluid during a school day than a teen who can drink during change of classes. Additionally, a recent bout of a gastrointestinal illness is a risk factor for dehydration if fluid balance is not corrected before initiation of activity. Alcohol and some dietary supplements may also increase this risk and should be included in the assessment. The sports dietitian should assess for preexisting chronic illness and medication use as risk factors for dehydration.

In practical terms, although children and teens are not at a unique metabolic disadvantage, the level of coaching and training in the pediatric population may increase the risk of a heat-related illness. Additionally, many youth sports are supervised by parents, and there is no certified athletic trainer providing on-field guidance on fluid intake and supervision. Sports RDNs can educate teams, parent groups, booster clubs, and inexperienced coaches in the middle school and high school levels on evidenced-based guidelines for proper hydration.[89]

As with adults, consideration of the type of beverage consumed is important. Using American College of Sports Medicine (ACSM) guidelines, as well as the policy statement from the American Academy of Pediatrics, the use of a sports drink for exercise greater than 1 hour to promote adequate fluid consumption and rehydration may be indicated.[85,90] If the exercise is greater than an hour in the heat, a sports drink provides the necessary electrolytes, carbohydrates, and fluid. Water is recommended for exercise lasting less than an hour. Children and teens should be educated on the proper use of sports drinks and avoid consumption during meals when either low-fat milk or water is the preferable.

NUTRITION ASSESSMENT AND NUTRIENT NEEDS

As with adults, a nutrition assessment for the pediatric athlete should be comprehensive and age specific. The determination of energy needs is well established in children, and the estimation of those needs can be found in Table 12.2 and 12.3 (page 241).

During adolescence, energy needs are increased to promote normal growth and development, as well as to meet the energy demands of sport participation. In middle school and high school, athletes may compete for their school and participate in club sports outside of school. Given the inherent challenges with Tanner staging, any calorie calculation for an adolescent athlete should be considered an estimate. During midpuberty, the increase in sex steroids increases the ability to add lean mass. For young athletes, the accrual of lean mass through puberty and strength and conditioning increases the overall calorie need. The prediction equations developed by Cunningham and Harris-Benedict are recommended by the ACSM and the Academy of Nutrition and Dietetics position paper for estimation of the resting metabolic rate in athletes.[91,92] The Cunningham prediction model incorporates FFM and differences in body composition between athletes and nonathletes. In contrast, the prediction equations by Harris-Benedict do not include FFM but instead include total body weight and sex. Given the higher percent of lean weight of most athletes, an equation that includes FFM may be advantageous but not readily available. Research has suggested that the recently developed De Lorenzo weight-based equation may be easier to use in clinical practice. Early research by Thompson and colleagues suggests that the Cunningham equation is highly accurate for endurance athletes.[93] The Cunningham equation has also been validated in recreational athletes.[94] However, in heavily muscled athletes, it may underestimate calorie needs.[95] If FFM is available, the Cunningham equation for calculating resting metabolic rate is: $500 + (22 \times \text{FFM (kg)})$.

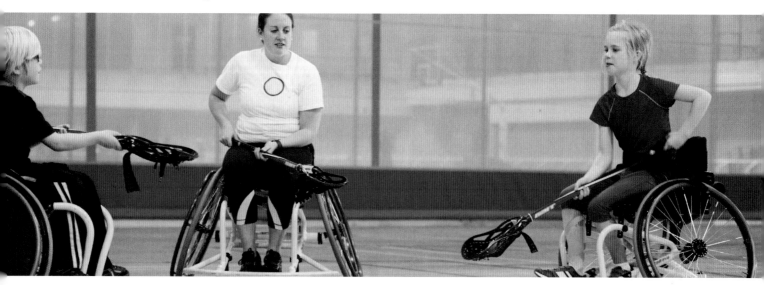

Research using these prediction equations with developing adolescents has not been validated. However, the estimates for additional needs for growth and development have been estimated. Through his research, Torun has estimated the caloric burden for synthesizing new tissue in well-nourished children and teens at 2 kcal/g of daily weight gain, although this cannot be practically assessed. The calorie burden for growth and development is small but not irrelevant. However, the energy needs of training and competition have the greatest impact on calorie needs beyond resting energy expenditure (REE).[96]

More recently, the concept of energy availability has emerged as a strategy to estimate energy needs. Energy availability is defined as dietary intake minus exercise energy expenditure using kilograms of FFM and is the amount of energy available to the body to perform all other functions after the cost of exercise is subtracted. The concept was first studied in females as part of the female athlete triad, where an energy availability of 45 kcal/kg FFM per day was found to be associated with energy intake for optimal health and performance. Inadequate energy availability is considered chronic reduction in energy availability below 30 kcal/kg FFM per day and is associated with a loss or impairment of physiological function. Chronic energy deficiency is often not reliably indicated by low body weight, and energy balance cannot be assumed by stable body weight.[97] The Harris-Benedict equation has been used to predict REE in many published reports of REE in women who are underweight.[98,99] A reduced ratio of measured REE to predicted REE by the Harris-Benedict equation is often in the range of 60% to 80% in clinical models of starvation, such as anorexia nervosa. Less is known about the impact of the underfueled child athlete. The use of energy availability has limited validity in childhood and, as such, clear guidelines on the use of this calculation in pediatric practice are lacking.

Physiological alterations at the metabolic level in the underfueled athletes include decreased REE; suppressed triiodothyronine (T_3), insulin-like growth factor-1, and leptin concentrations; and elevated reverse T_3, ghrelin, peptide YY, and cortisol concentrations.[100-102] The underfueled athlete will often experience a downregulation of metabolic rate to compensate for chronic reduction in calories. In a clinical setting, the downregulation of metabolic rate can be manifested by bradycardia, hypothermia, and postural orthostatic tachycardia syndrome (POTS). Sports RDNs should regularly assess body temperature (< 97°), heart rate (< 50 bpm), and orthostatic dizziness as part of the assessment. Gastroparesis is also common and can alter normal hunger and satiety cues. Therefore, the concept of intuitive eating may be flawed in athletes. Sports dietitians can use these surrogate measures of body temperature, heart rate, and POTS to objectively assess or augment the determination of energy availability when FFM data are not available. Box 12.2 outlines considerations included in the assessment of an adolescent athlete.

Box 12.2 Nutrition Assessment Checklist: Adolescent Athlete

Concrete vs abstract thinker
☐ Dictates education style

Body composition
☐ Changes dependent on Tanner stage
☐ Percent body fat

Acanthosis nigricans
☐ Indicative of insulin resistance
☐ Assess menstrual status as amenorrhea may be present

Sugar-sweetened beverages (including sports drinks)
☐ Coffee drinks
☐ Energy drinks
☐ Inappropriate use of sports drinks

Daily eating pattern
☐ Is breakfast consumed daily?
☐ Snacks—frequency, what type of items?
☐ Fast-food consumption

Enjoyment of sports
☐ Overtraining
☐ Monopolizes all free time

Age of menarche
☐ Mother's age of menarche
☐ Delayed

Alcohol use
☐ Consider interviewing adolescent alone

Supplement use
☐ Late-developing male at higher risk
☐ Team sports indicate higher risk

Dietary Assessment

Dietary assessment of an athlete's energy intake can be derived from weighed or measured food records (typically measuring intake for 3 to 7 days), 24-hour recall, or from food frequency questionnaires. An inherent challenge in the pediatric population is the poor historical recalls of children and adolescents. Parents should be part of the interview process with children. Children may need six to nine 24-hour recalls to establish recall reliability. Teens may require three to six recalls.[103] Given the limited amount of time in a clinical sports nutrition practice, dietary recalls may provide insight on food patterning but not necessarily energy intake. Athletes often consume sports nutrition foods and sports drinks during practice, and the amount consumed is difficult to estimate. It is not surprising that adolescent athletes report intakes lower than the suggested calculations.[104] Digital dietary histories may prove particularly useful in a younger athlete population.[105]

As with all populations, the pediatric population has unique vitamin and mineral needs. RDNs are well equipped to assess and screen for nutrient deficiencies. Vulnerable nutrients identified in the pediatric population, include vitamin D, calcium, iron, potassium, and dietary fiber. Inadequate intakes of calcium, potassium, and dietary fiber can be alleviated by including dairy foods, vegetables, fruits, and whole grains.[106] However, given the limited food sources of vitamin D, this can be an especially vulnerable nutrient.

Alcohol may also be a source of calories for children and adolescents and is rarely assessed in an underage population. Among young people who consume alcohol, the proportion who drink heavily is higher than among adult drinkers, rising from approximately 50% in those 12 to 14 years old to 72% among those 18 to 20 years old.[107] Not surprisingly, high school is a time when drinking rates increase drastically, given the propensity of risk-taking behaviors. Between 36% and 50% of high school students currently drink alcohol, and up to 60% of them report binge drinking (drinking five or more drinks on one occasion for men or four or more drinks on one occasion for women).[108] Alcohol consumption is more common in boys than girls and more common in whites than other ethnicities.[109] In studies of adolescent athletes, approximately 24% report binge drinking.[110] Adolescents who use alcohol are also at risk for abusing anabolic steroids.[111] Athletes involved in team sports are more likely to abuse alcohol than those in individual sports.[112] Nutritional status, particularly related to B vitamins, magnesium, and other trace minerals, can be compromised by excessive alcohol intake.

PROTEIN NEEDS IN THE CHILD AND ADOLESCENT ATHLETE

A key component in the evaluation of protein needs in adolescents is the assumption of caloric adequacy. Often the lack of calories allows for the production of energy from noncarbohydrate precursors, such as protein, via gluconeogenesis. All estimates of protein requirements are predicated on adequate energy balance. In addition to determining how to meet the demands of often intensive training regimens, estimates of protein needs in the athletic adolescent population must account for increased needs for growth and development.[113] Nitrogen balance studies have been conducted in select adolescent athletes and indicate that positive nitrogen balance is achieved with a protein intake ranging between 1.35 and 1.6 g of protein per kilogram per day.[114,115] Dietary intake patterns have shown that protein intake of adolescent male athletes is about 1.5 g/kg/day. Among all adolescents, protein intake as a percent of calories has increased in all ethnic groups with the exception of African American adolescents. From 1999 to 2000 and 2009 to 2010, protein intake as a percent of calories increased from 13.5% to 14.7% in boys and from 13.4% to 14.3% in girls.[116] Less is known on the protein needs of female adolescent athletes. Given the research restrictions in the pediatric population, the physiology of protein metabolism and synthesis comes from data on the adult population. Participation in sports, particularly team sports, may improve nutritional status, eating patterns, and nutrient intakes in teens, including overall protein intake.[117] This is further supported byRDN-observed fueling before, during, and after sports. Male dietary patterns often closely mimic the dietary recommendations, whereas girls are less likely to meet the recommendations. Both boys and girls often fall short of carbohydrate needs.[118]

Protein status may be compromised in adolescents following restrictive diets, dietary fads, or inappropriately planned vegetarian diets. Sports dietitians are crucial in planning diets adequate in calories to ensure that protein is spared from being used as an energy source, protein consumption is spaced throughout the day, and fad diets are avoided by this vulnerable population. Lean sources of protein should be stressed in an effort to limit animal-based saturated fat.

DIETARY FAT IN THE CHILD AND ADOLESCENT ATHLETE

Quality sources of dietary fat can serve as valuable calorie sources in children and adolescents struggling with caloric adequacy. Often an athlete who is underweight is encouraged to consume high-fat, fried foods or foods of poor nutrient density to gain weight. Dietary habits are formed, and preferences are developed in childhood and adolescence; therefore, it is imperative to provide guidance on the appropriate food sources of dietary fat. High-fat diets, ketogenic diets, and low carbohydrate availability are concepts not studied in the healthy pediatric population. Data from the HELENA study suggest that as dietary fat increases, there is an increase in truncal fat, regardless of the level of physical activity in adolescents.[119] However, there is conflicting research on the role of dietary fat and adiposity in children. Ambrosini and colleagues demonstrated a relationship between increasing dietary fat and total body fatness.[120] However, a large study of Australian children suggested no relationship between macronutrient percentages and BMI.[121] The role of fat and adiposity in adolescent athletes is unclear, but RDNs should be careful not to promote high-fat diets. It is also unclear if all fatty acids stimulate the same physiological response.

Although fats can be a valuable source of calories, promoting the optimal type and amount of fat is important. In a study by Bachman and colleagues, sources of dietary fats included oils from potato chips, salad dressing, and nuts and seeds.[122] Major contributors of solid fats were grain-based desserts, cheese, and sausages for all Americans. Among children and adolescents, major contributors of solid fats included pizza, grain-based desserts, and whole milk.[123]

Dietary fat has a protein-sparing effect, provided adequate calories are consumed. Additions of unsaturated oils in a variety of foods, such as nuts, nut butters, avocados, salad dressings, and mayonnaise, can add valuable calories. RDNs are in a position to provide valuable guidance for increasing dietary fats. Controlling the ratio of n-6 to n-3 fatty acids is also a central issue for optimal brain development. The National Health and Nutrition Examination Survey (NHANES) 2009–2010 provided information on dietary intake of n-3 and n-6 fatty acids among adults.[124] NHANES reported that mean daily intake of α-linolenic acid was 1.77 g among men and 1.38 g among women. Mean daily intake of eicosapentaenoic acid (EPA) was 40 mg among men and 30 mg among women. Mean daily intake of docosahexaenoic acid (DHA) was 80 mg for men and 60 mg for women. There is little difference between mean intakes by sex, race and ethnicity, or income. In an international review of fatty acid intake in children and adolescents, most children and teens worldwide exceeded the recommended limits for saturated fat and fell short of the recommended intake of polyunsaturated fatty acids (PUFAs).[125] The mean consumption of intakes of total EPA and DHA varied between 45 mg and 150 mg in children and between 40 mg and 160 mg in adolescents. The brain continues to grow postnatally, and myelinogenesis remains incomplete until early adulthood. The role of DHA in brain development and cognitive function is well established. The composition of the brain is about 60% fat, making it one of the highest fat organs in the body. The majority of the fats are polyunsaturated: EPA, DHA, and arachidonic acid.[126] DHA is the dominant long-chain omega-3 PUFA in the brain and has been shown to accumulate in areas of the brain associated with learning and memory, such as the cerebral cortex and hippocampus.[127,128] The fatty acid content of the brain is dietary dependent; the phospholipids in the brain can be modified by diet.[129] Given the central role of long-chain fats, n-3 fatty acids deserve special attention in pediatrics. DHA has been shown to improve cognition, learning, memory, and school performance.[130] Given the limited food sources of DHA, children and teens who do not consume cold-water fish will most likely not meet target guidelines.[131] A survey of adolescents' knowledge regarding omega-3 fatty acids demonstrated that teens can recognize the role of n-3 fatty acids in heart health but lack knowledge on the roles of these long-chain PUFAs in brain or cognitive function. Additionally, most teens (79%) were not educated by their health care providers on the roles of n-3 fatty acids.[132] RDNs, as the food and nutrition experts, can provide valuable education on this important dietary fat and should plan diets with optimal health in mind. Supplementation with n-3 fatty acids (EPA and DHA) should be considered to optimize brain function. Box 12.3 lists the age-specific recommended adequate intake of n-3 fatty acids.

VITAMIN D

Attention has turned to vitamin D deficiency in the pediatric population, as it has in the adult population. Using the Institute of Medicine (IOM) criteria with the end point of fracture, approximately 10.3% of US children age 6 to 18 years (population estimate 5.5 million) have 25-hydroxyvitamin D (25[OH]D) levels less than 16 ng/mL, based on NHANES data.[133] Although there may be controversy in the literature on optimum levels, the IOM, the American Academy of Pediatrics, and the Pediatric Endocrine Society define the parameters for vitamin 25(OH)D adequacy as follows:

- Sufficient: > 20 ng/mL
- Insufficient: 15 to 20 ng/mL
- Deficient: < 15 ng/mL[134,135]

However, other studies, most notably from the orthopedic literature on adults, suggest the following parameters for vitamin 25 (OH)D:

- Sufficient: ≥ 32 ng/mL
- Insufficient: 20 to 32 ng/mL
- Deficient:< 20 ng/mL[136,137]

These values are based on cutoffs believed to optimize intestinal calcium absorption and prevent hyperparathyroidism. The role of vitamin D and bone mineral accrual is well established and beyond the scope of this chapter. Bone formation peaks during puberty, and the establishment of adequate bone density in childhood is critical for long-term bone health throughout adulthood. Pubertal girls with hypovitaminosis D seem to be at risk of not reaching maximum peak bone mass, particularly at the lumbar spine.[139] Maintaining vitamin D blood levels at or above 20 ng/mL throughout the year may be needed to improve the bone markers in adolescents.[140]

Research investigating the relationship of vitamin D deficiency and muscular status in the pediatric population is sparse. Ward and colleagues assessed serum 25(OH)D in girls age 12 to 14 years and measured muscle power. Vitamin D levels were significantly associated with muscle power and force in adolescent girls. Vitamin D myopathy is associated with fatigue and lack of participation in physical education.[141] Inadequate vitamin D status may result in fatigue and diminished muscle oxygenation, consequently negatively affecting muscle strength and causing weakness.[142] Sport performance criteria, such as higher jump velocities and jump heights, are significantly improved with adequate levels of vitamin D.[143] Muscle biopsies from adult athletes with low vitamin D levels have demonstrated atrophic changes in fast-twitch type II muscle fibers, which are crucial to most athletes.[144] However, the supplementation of adolescents with vitamin D in a randomized controlled trial indicated that despite improvements in 25(OH)D status, treatment with vitamin D was not shown to increase bone mineral accretion, bone geometry or strength, muscle force, or power. Improvements were found in jump velocity in girls with the lowest baseline 25(OH)D concentrations.[141] Research showing the lack of effect of vitamin D intervention after the period of peak mineral and muscle mass accretion suggests that supplementation with vitamin D earlier in pediatrics may be required.

Accumulating data suggests that a deficiency of vitamin D may also contribute to iron deficiency anemia. Research by Sim and colleagues has established the link between vitamin D deficiency and increased prevalence of anemia in adults, likely due to the role of vitamin D in erythropoiesis.[145] Atkinson and colleagues demonstrated among white children that 25(OH)D levels in the upper quartiles (≥ 20 ng/mL) were associated with a nearly 0.2 g/dL higher hemoglobin compared with those less than 20 ng/mL.[146]

In African American children, hemoglobin was higher among those with 25(OH)D levels above 11 ng/mL, highlighting ethnic differences. It is clear that sports dietitians should consider vitamin D status when working with child and adolescent athletes.

CALCIUM

Calcium requirements are 1,000 mg/day for children (4 to 8 years) and 1,300 mg/day for preadolescents and adolescents. Although it is possible to meet these requirements through diet alone, calcium intake of children and adults in the United States is generally lower than daily recommendations, especially for children age 9 to 18 years and those who are Hispanic or African American.[147] Adequate calcium is important for the development of peak bone mass in children and adolescents, especially during puberty. Inadequate calcium intake in adolescence may also increase the likelihood of bone disease in adults.[148] Approximately half of total body calcium is laid down during puberty in girls and up to two-thirds in boys by the end of puberty.[149,150] Although calcium-fortified foods are available, milk and milk products provide about 50% of total calcium intake within the United States and are the leading sources of dietary calcium for children age 2 years and older.

During pubertal growth, bone growth outpaces bone mineralization, which, in essence, decreases bone mineral deposition. A research study by Faulkner and colleagues demonstrated the nadir of bone mineral density coincides with peak height velocity in both boys and girls.[151] This coincides with an increase in distal radius fractures during periods of rapid growth and development, suggesting that the relative lack of bone mineral density is clinically significant. As opposed to other biological processes where recovery is possible, the lack of calcium and poor bone mineralization during puberty may permanently impact bone development and increase the risk of osteoporosis in adulthood.[152] Sources of dietary calcium are shown in Table 12.5. RDNs should plan diets with a focus on adequate dietary sources of calcium.

Table 12.5 Calcium Content of Selected Foods[153]

Food	Serving Size	Milligrams per Serving
Almond milk, vanilla, sweetened	8 oz	451
Yogurt, plain, low fat	8 oz	415
Mozzarella, part skim	1.5 oz	333
Sardines, canned in oil, with bones	3 oz	325
Yogurt, fruit, low-fat	8 oz	313–384
Cheddar cheese	1.5 oz	307
Milk, nonfat	8 oz	299
Soy milk, calcium-fortified	8 oz	299
Milk, reduced fat (2% milk fat)	8 oz	293
Milk, buttermilk, low fat	8 oz	284
Milk, whole (3.25% milk fat)	8 oz	276
Orange juice, calcium fortified	6 oz	261
Tofu, firm, made with calcium sulfate	½ cup	253
Salmon, pink, canned, solids with bone	3 oz	181
Cottage cheese, 1% milk fat	1 cup	138

Continued on next page

Table 12.5 Calcium Content of Selected Foods[153] (Continued)

Food	Serving Size	Milligrams per Serving
Tofu, soft, made with calcium sulfate	½ cup	138
Ready-to-eat cereal, calcium fortified	1 cup	100–1,000
Frozen yogurt, vanilla, soft serve	½ cup	103
Turnip greens, fresh, boiled	½ cup	99
Kale, raw, chopped	1 cup	100
Ice cream, vanilla	½ cup	84
Chinese cabbage, bok choy, raw, shredded	1 slice	74
Bread, white	1 slice	73
Pudding, chocolate, ready to eat, refrigerated	4 oz	55
Tortilla, corn, ready to bake/fry	one, 6-in diameter	46
Tortilla, flour, ready to bake/fry	one, 6-in diameter	32
Sour cream, reduced fat, cultured	2 Tbsp	31
Bread, whole wheat	1 slice	30
Broccoli, raw	½ cup	21
Cream cheese, regular	1 Tbsp	14

IRON

Iron needs during adolescence are increased primarily due to the rapid expansion of blood volume in male and female adolescents. Menarche also significantly impacts iron needs. Iron deficiency is the most prevalent mineral deficiency in the United States, affecting 9% to 16% of female adolescents.[154] The causes of iron deficiency and subsequent anemia in the young athlete are multifactorial and include increased needs, lack of dietary iron, coexistence of vitamin D deficiency, and such chronic illnesses as undiagnosed celiac disease or *Helicobacter pylori* infection. Among athletes, overuse of nonsteroidal anti-inflammatory drugs and footstrike hemolysis can also contribute to low iron status.

In the US diet, the richest sources of heme iron, the most bioavailable form, include lean red meats and seafood. Dietary sources of nonheme iron include some vegetables, nuts, beans, and fortified grain products, including sports bars. Approximately half of the dietary iron comes from fortified cereals, bread, and grain products. Poorly planned vegetarian or vegan diets can increase the risk of iron deficiency. Diets that eliminate breads, fortified grains, or cereals can also reduce the intake of nonheme iron.

Undiagnosed chronic illnesses can contribute to iron deficiency. In cases of iron-deficiency anemia that are refractory to treatment, celiac disease is diagnosed in 1.8% to 14.6% of patients.[155] *H pylori* is often an undiagnosed cause of iron deficiency. *H pylori* is more common in females. In a study of female high school athletes, the prevalence of *H pylori* immunoglobulin G antibodies was 14% and iron deficiency was about 50%.[156]

The assessment of iron deficiency and iron-deficiency anemia in a pediatric practice are routinely done by measuring hematocrit and hemoglobin, and neither of these methods is sensitive or specific. The use of ferritin levels is not routine in general pediatrics. Female athletes may experience an elevated risk of iron deficiency and iron-deficiency anemia and show declines in physical and cognitive performance. In response to intense training, hepcidin, a peptide hormone that inhibits intestinal iron absorption and sequesters iron in the macrophage, increases. The inflammatory response and the synthesis of proinflammatory cytokines, such as interleukin-6, act to stimulate hepcidin expression, in turn reducing iron absorption and sequestering iron in the macrophage. Ferritin levels may be reduced.[157] Hepcidin release may also be a marker of overreaching and overtraining.[158] Table 12.6 illustrates dietary sources of iron.

Table 12.6 Food Sources of Iron[153]		
Food	**Serving Size**	**Milligrams per Serving**
Breakfast cereals, fortified with 100% of the daily value for iron	1 serving	18
Oysters, eastern, cooked with moist heat	3 oz	8
White beans, canned	1 c	8
Chocolate, dark, 45%–69% cacao solids	3 oz	7
Beef liver, pan fried	3 oz	5
Lentils, boiled and drained	½ c	3
Spinach, boiled and drained	½ c	3
Tofu, firm	½ c	3
Kidney beans, canned	½ c	2
Sardines, Atlantic, canned in oil, drained solids with bones	3 oz	2
Chickpeas, boiled and drained	½ c	2
Tomatoes, canned, stewed	½ c	2
Beef, braised bottom round, trimmed to 1/8″ fat	3 oz	2
Potato, baked, flesh and skin	1 medium	2
Cashew nuts, oil roasted	1 oz (18 nuts)	2
Green peas, boiled	½ c	1
Chicken, roasted, meat and skin	3 ounces	1
Rice, white, long grain, enriched, parboiled, drained	½ c	1
Bread, whole wheat	1 slice	1
Bread, white	1 slice	1
Raisins, seedless	¼ c	1
Spaghetti, whole wheat, cooked	1 c	1

Continued on next page

Table 12.6 Food Sources of Iron[153] (Continued)		
Food	Serving Size	Milligrams per Serving
Tuna, bluefin, fresh	3 oz	1
Turkey, roasted, breast meat and skin	3 oz	1
Nuts, pistachio, dry roasted	1 oz (49 nuts)	1
Broccoli, boiled and drained	½ c	1
Egg, hard boiled	1 large	1
Rice, brown, long or medium grain, cooked	1 c	1

ERGOGENIC AIDS IN THE ADOLESCENT ATHLETE

Rates of ergogenic aids usage to enhance body composition have been reported as high as 58% among high school athletes.[159] In the transition from adolescence to adulthood, young adult males who played a sport in high school were 15.6% more likely to use performance-enhancing supplements than their nonathletic peers.[160] High school athletes are more likely to try to increase muscle mass by changing their diets, increasing exercise, or using protein supplements than students who do not participate in sports.[161] This provides an excellent opportunity for sports dietitians to educate cleints on appropriate fueling strategies to achieve those goals within the limits of Tanner staging.

Research in the adult population has illustrated the effectiveness of dietary supplements to augment sports performance (for further discussion, see Chapter 7). In the pediatric population, due to ethical constraints, less research is available on the safety of these products. Despite the lack of strong clinical support in pediatrics, a study in 2012 showed that 1.2 million athletes younger than 18 years in the United States reported using a supplement specifically to enhance sport performance in the previous 30 days. In this study, a multivitamin mineral product accounted for 90% of the purchases for sports enhancement.[162]

Creatine is one of the most popular supplements used by teenagers. The ACSM and the American Academy of Pediatrics state that the evidence on potential side effects of creatine supplementation in people younger than 18 years is inadequate to formulate valid conclusions as to the risk-to-benefit ratio of creatine supplementation. Therefore, creatine supplementation is not advised for the pediatric population.[163,164] Sports dietitians should exercise caution in recommending sports-enhancing supplements in a pediatric population. Sports dietitians also play a critical role in educating student athletes, coaches, and parents on the potential for supplements to be contaminated with unknown and potentially banned substances.

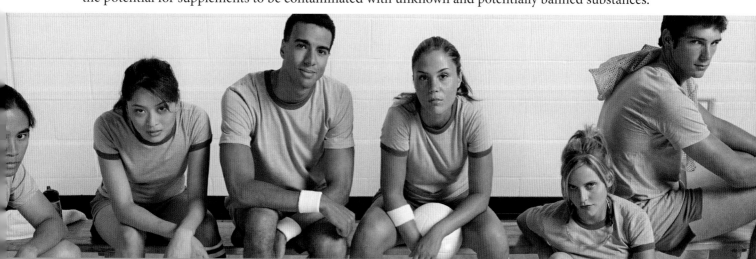

KEY TAKEAWAYS

The nutritional needs of the child and adolescent athlete are based on gender and stages of growth and development.

Tanner staging, or sexual maturity ratings, should guide the sports dietitian in planning appropriate nutrition education.

Sports dietitians should assess developmental learning styles.

Include key recommendations for carbohydrate, protein, fat, vitamin/mineral intake, and hydration goals.

Relative energy deficiency and/or the female athlete triad should be assessed in high-risk athletes.

Vitamin D, calcium, and iron are nutrients of concern in a growing population.

Sports dietitians should exercise caution in recommending performance-enhancing supplements to children and adolescent athletes.

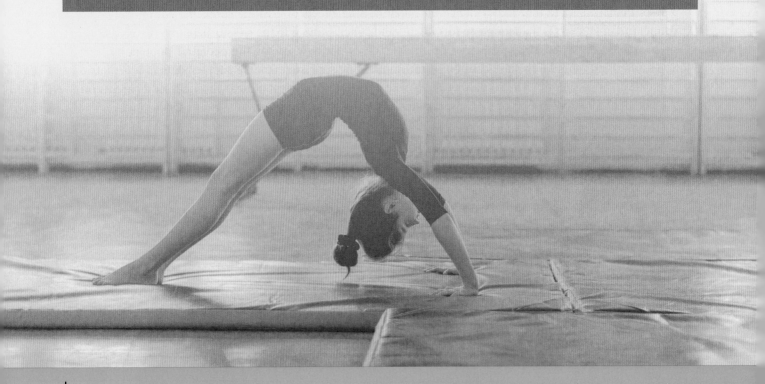

REFERENCES

1. Census 2000 Gateway. US Census Bureau website. www.census.gov/main/www/cen2000.html. Updated July 19, 2003. Accessed July 21, 2017.

2. National Federation of State High School Associations. 2013-2014 High School Athletics Participation Survey. 2015; www.nfhs.org/ParticipationStatistics/PDF/2013-14_Participation_Survey_PDF.pdf. Accessed June 27, 2017.

3. Singh AS, Mulder C, Twisk JW, van Mechelen W, Chinapaw MJ. Tracking of childhood overweight into adulthood: a systematic review of the literature. *Obes Rev.* 2008;9(5):474-488.

4. Mamun AA, Hayatbakhsh MR, O'Callaghan M, Williams G, Najman J. Early overweight and pubertal maturation—pathways of association with young adults' overweight: a longitudinal study. *Ibt J Obes.* 2009;33(1):14-20.

5. Stigman S, Rintala P, Kukkonen-Harjula K, Kujala U, Rinne M, Fogelholm M. Eight-year-old children with high cardiorespiratory fitness have lower overall and abdominal fatness. *Int J Pediatr Obes.* 2009;4(2):98-105.

6. Thackray AE, Barrett LA, Tolfrey K. Acute high-intensity interval running reduces postprandial lipemia in boys. *Med Sci Sports Exerc.* 2013;45(7):1277-1284.

7. Strong WB, Malina RM, Blimkie CJ, et al. Evidence based physical activity for school-age youth. *The J Pediatr .* 2005;146(6):732-737.

8. Eime RM, Young JA, Harvey JT, Charity MJ, Payne WR. A systematic review of the psychological and social benefits of participation in sport for adults: informing development of a conceptual model of health through sport. *Int J Behav Nutr Phys Act.* 2013;10:135.

9. Faigenbaum AD, Kraemer WJ, Blimkie CJ, et al. Youth resistance training: updated position statement paper from the National Strength and Conditioning Association. *J Strength Cond Res.* 2009;23(5 suppl):S60-S79.

10. MacKelvie KJ, Petit MA, Khan KM, Beck TJ, McKay HA. Bone mass and structure are enhanced following a 2-year randomized controlled trial of exercise in prepubertal boys. *Bone.* 2004;34(4):755-764.

11. Morris FL, Naughton GA, Gibbs JL, Carlson JS, Wark JD. Prospective ten-month exercise intervention in premenarcheal girls: positive effects on bone and lean mass. *J Bone Miner Res.* 1997;12(9):1453-1462.

12. Specker B, Thiex NW, Sudhagoni RG. Does exercise influence pediatric bone? A systematic review. *Clin Orthop Relat Res.* 2016;473(11)3658-1672.

13. Hind K, Burrows M. Weight-bearing exercise and bone mineral accrual in children and adolescents: a review of controlled trials. *Bone.* 2007;40(1):14-27.

14. Tveit M, Rosengren BE, Nilsson JA, Karlsson MK. Exercise in youth: high bone mass, large bone size, and low fracture risk in old age. *Scand J Med Sci Sports.* Aug 2015;25(4):453-461.

15. Tenforde AS, Fredericson M. Influence of sports participation on bone health in the young athlete: a review of the literature. *PM R.* 2011;3(9):861-867.

16. Dabelea D, Mayer-Davis EJ, Saydah S, et al. Prevalence of type 1 and type 2 diabetes among children and adolescents from 2001 to 2009. *JAMA.* 2014;311(17):1778-1786.

17. Wittmeier KD, Wicklow BA, MacIntosh AC, et al. Hepatic steatosis and low cardiorespiratory fitness in youth with type 2 diabetes. *Obesity.* 2012;20(5):1034-1040.

18. Fabbrini E, Sullivan S, Klein S. Obesity and nonalcoholic fatty liver disease: biochemical, metabolic, and clinical implications. *Hepatology.* 2010;51(2):679-689.

19. Garber CE, Blissmer B, Deschenes MR, et al. American College of Sports Medicine position stand. Quantity and quality of exercise for developing and maintaining cardiorespiratory, musculoskeletal, and neuromotor fitness in apparently healthy adults: guidance for prescribing exercise. *Med Sci Sports Exerc.* 2011;43(7):1334-1359.

20. Magnussen CG, Koskinen J, Chen W, et al. Pediatric metabolic syndrome predicts adulthood metabolic syndrome, subclinical atherosclerosis, and type 2 diabetes mellitus but is no better than body mass index alone: the Bogalusa Heart Study and the Cardiovascular Risk in Young Finns Study. *Circulation.* 2010;122(16):1604-1611.

21. Kang HS, Gutin B, Barbeau P, et al. Physical training improves insulin resistance syndrome markers in obese adolescents. *Med Sci Sports Exerc.* 2002;34(12):1920-1927.

22. Gutin B, Barbeau P, Owens S, et al. Effects of exercise intensity on cardiovascular fitness, total body composition, and visceral adiposity of obese adolescents. *Am J Clin Nutr.* 2002;75(5):818-826.

23. Messiah SE, Arheart KL, Lipshultz SE, Miller TL. Body mass index, waist circumference, and cardiovascular risk factors in adolescents. *J Pediatr.* 2008;153(6):845-850.

24. Trasande L, Chatterjee S. The impact of obesity on health service utilization and costs in childhood. *Obesity.* 2009;17(9):1749-1754.

25. Andersen LB, Sardinha LB, Froberg K, Riddoch CJ, Page AS, Anderssen SA. Fitness, fatness and clustering of cardiovascular risk factors in children from Denmark, Estonia and Portugal: the European Youth Heart Study. *Int J Pediatr Obes.* 2008;3 (suppl 1):58-66.

26. Abbott RA, Davies PS. Habitual physical activity and physical activity intensity: their relation to body composition in 5.0-10.5-y-old children. *Eur J Clin Nutr.* 2004;58(2):285-291.

27. Daniels SR, Hassink SG, Committee on the role of the pediatrician in primary prevention of obesity. *Pediatrics.* 2015;136(1):e275-e292.

28. Mesirow MS, Welsh JA. Changing beverage consumption patterns have resulted in fewer liquid calories in the diets of US Children: National Health and Nutrition Examination Survey 2001-2010. *J Acad Nutr Pediatr.* 2015;115(4):559-566,e4.

29. Woodruff SJ, Hanning RM, Barr SI. Energy recommendations for normal weight, overweight and obese children and adolescents: are different equations necessary? *Obe Rev.* 2009;10(1):103-108.

30. Neumark-Sztainer D, Falkner N, Story M, Perry C, Hannan PJ, Mulert S. Weight-teasing among adolescents: correlations with weight status and disordered eating behaviors. *Int J Obes Relat Metab Disord.* 2002;26(1):123-131.

31. Goldschmidt AB, Wall MM, Loth KA, Neumark-Sztainer D. Risk factors for disordered eating in overweight adolescents and young adults. *J Pediatr Psychol.* 2015;40(10):1048-1055.

32. Puhl RM, Peterson JL, Luedicke J. Weight-based victimization: bullying experiences of weight loss treatment-seeking youth. *Pediatrics.* Jan 2013;131(1):e1-e9.

33. Gale CR, Batty GD, Tynelius P, Deary IJ, Rasmussen F. Intelligence in early adulthood and subsequent hospitalization for mental disorders. *Epidemiology.* 2010;21(1):70-77.

34. Gale CR, Cooper R, Craig L, et al. Cognitive function in childhood and lifetime cognitive change in relation to mental wellbeing in four cohorts of older people. *PLoS One.* 2012;7(9):e44860.

35. Gottfredson LS, Deary IJ. Intelligence predicts health and longevity, but why? *Curr dir Psychol Sci.* 2004;13(1):1-4.

36. Zarrett N, Fay K, Li Y, Carrano J, Phelps E, Lerner RM. More than child's play: variable- and pattern-centered approaches for examining effects of sports participation on youth development. *Dev Psychol.* 2009;45(2):368.

37. Eccles JS, Barber BL, Stone M, Hunt J. Extracurricular activities and adolescent development. *J Soc Issues.* 2003;59(4):865-889.

38. Jewett R, Sabiston CM, Brunet J, O'Loughlin EK, Scarapicchia T, O'Loughlin J. School sport participation during adolescence and mental health in early adulthood. *J Adolesc Health.* 2014;55(5):640-644.

39. Dishman RK, Hales DP, Pfeiffer KA, et al. Physical self-concept and self-esteem mediate cross-sectional relations of physical activity and sport participation with depression symptoms among adolescent girls. *Health Psychol.* 2006;25(3):396-407.

40. Agostini R, Titus S. *Medical and Orthopedic Issues of Active and Athletic Women.* Hanley & Belfus; 1994.

41. Bergeron MF, Mountjoy M, Armstrong N, et al. International Olympic Committee consensus statement on youth athletic development. *BR J Sports Med.* 2015;49(13):843-851.

42. DiFiori JP, Benjamin HJ, Brenner J, et al. Overuse injuries and burnout in youth sports: a position statement from the American Medical Society for Sports Medicine. *Clin J Sport Med.* 2014;24(1):3-20.

43. Spear BA. Adolescent growth and development. *J Am Diet Assoc.* 2002;102(3 suppl):S23-S29.

44. Wilmore JH. The application of science to sport: physiological profiles of male and female athletes. *Can J Sport Scie.* 1979;4(2):103-115.

45. Patel DR, Nelson TL. Sports injuries in adolescents. *Med Clin North Am.* 2000;84(4):983-1007.

46. Tanner JM. *Fetus into Man: Physical Growth from Conception to Maturity.* Harvard University Press; 1990.

47. Biro FM, Khoury P, Morrison JA. Influence of obesity on timing of puberty. *Int J Androl.* 2006;29(1):272-277; discussion 286-290.

48. Wolff MS, Teitelbaum SL, Pinney SM, et al. Investigation of relationships between urinary biomarkers of phytoestrogens, phthalates, and phenols and pubertal stages in girls. *Environ Health Perspect.* 2010;118(7):1039-1046.

49. Wilson DA, Derraik JG, Rowe DL, Hofman PL, Cutfield WS. Earlier menarche is associated with lower insulin sensitivity and increased adiposity in young adult women. *PLoS One.* 2015;10(6):e0128427.

50. Elks CE, Ong KK, Scott RA, et al. Age at menarche and type 2 diabetes risk: the EPIC-InterAct study. *Diabetes Care.* 2013;36(11):3526-3534.

51. Rasmussen AR, Wohlfahrt-Veje C, Tefre de Renzy-Martin K, et al. Validity of self-assessment of pubertal maturation. *Pediatrics.* 2015;135(1):86-93.

52. Ramnitz MS, Lodish MB. Racial disparities in pubertal development. *Semin Reprod Med.* 2013;31(5):333-339.

53. Zhai L, Liu J, Zhao J, et al. Association of obesity with onset of puberty and sex hormones in Chinese girls: a 4-year longitudinal study. *PLoS One.* 2015;10(8):e0134656.

54. Belachew T, Hadley C, Lindstrom D, Getachew Y, Duchateau L, Kolsteren P. Food insecurity and age at menarche among adolescent girls in Jimma Zone Southwest Ethiopia: a longitudinal study. *Reprod Biol Endocrinol.* 2011;9:125.

55. Malina RM, Baxter-Jones AD, Armstrong N, et al. Role of intensive training in the growth and maturation of artistic gymnasts. *Sports Med.* 2013;43(9):783-802.

56. Malina R. Effects of physical activities on growth in stature and adolescent growth spurt. *Med Sci Sports Exerc.* 1994;26:759.

57. Komi PV, ed. *Strength and Power in Sport.* Oxford, UK: Blackwell Scientific Publications; 1993.

58. Greydanus DE, Omar H, Pratt HD. The adolescent female athlete: current concepts and conundrums. *Pediatr Clin North Am.* 2010;57(3):697-718.

59. Gong EJ, Spear BA. Adolescent growth and development: Implications for nutritional needs. *J Nutr Educ.* 1988;20(6):273-279.

60. Yager Z, O'Dea JA. Relationships between body image, nutritional supplement use, and attitudes towards doping in sport among adolescent boys: implications for prevention programs. *J Int Soc Sports Nutr.* 2014;11(1):13.

61. Vandewalle S, De Schepper J, Kaufman JM. Androgens and obesity in male adolescents. *Curr Opin Encocrinol Diabetes Obes.* 2015;22(3):230-237.

62. Lee JM, Kaciroti N, Appugliese D, Corwyn RF, Bradley RH, Lumeng JC. Body mass index and timing of pubertal initiation in boys. *Arch Pediatr Adolesc Med.* 2010;164(2):139-144.

63. DeLeonibus C, Marcovecchio M, Chiavaroli V, Chiarelli F, Mohn A. Timing of puberty and physical growth in obese children. *Pediatr Obes.* 2014;9(4):292-299.

64. Sturdevant MS, Spear BA. Adolescent psychosocial development. *J Am Diet Assoc.* 2002;102(3 suppl):S30-S31.

65. Vartanian L. Revisting the imaginary audience and personal fable constructs of adolescent egocentricism: a conceptual review. *Adolescence.* 2000;35(140):639-661.

66. Spear LP. Adolescent neurodevelopment. *J Adolesc Health.* 2013;52(2 suppl 2):S7-S13.

67. Erickson E. *Identity, Youth and Crisis.* New York, NY: Wiley Online Library; 1969.

68. Jessor R. Successful adolescent development among youth in high-risk settings. *Amer Psychol.* 1993;48(2):117.

69. Baneree S, Saenger P, Hu M. Fat accretion and the regulation of insulin mediated glycogen synthesis after puberty in the rat. *Am J Physiol* 1997;2734(pt 2):R1534-1539.

70. Bloch CA, Clemons P, Sperling MA. Puberty decreases insulin sensitivity. *J Pediatr.* 1987;110(3):481-487.

71. Riddell MC. The endocrine response and substrate utilization during exercise in children and adolescents. *J Appl Physiol.* 2008;105(2):725-733.

72. Eriksson B. Muscle metabolism in children—a review. *Acta Paediatr Scand.* 1980;283:20-28.

73. Kaczor JJ, Ziolkowski W, Popinigis J, Tarnopolsky MA. Anaerobic and aerobic enzyme activities in human skeletal muscle from children and adults. *Pediatr Res.* 2005;57(3):331-335.

74. Foricher JM, Ville N, Gratas-Delamarche A, Delamarche P. Effects of submaximal intensity cycle ergometry for one hour on substrate utilisation in trained prepubertal boys versus trained adults. *J Sports Med Phys Fitness.* 2003;43(1):36-43.

75. Brandou F, Savy-Pacaux AM, Marie J, Brun JF, Mercier J. Comparison of the type of substrate oxidation during exercise between pre and post pubertal markedly obese boys. *Int J Sports Med.* 2006;27(5):407-414.

76. Stephens B, Cole A, Mahon A. The influence of biological maturation on fat and carbohydrate metabolism during exercise. *Int J Sport Nutr Exerc Metab* 2006;16(2):166-179.

77. Couto PG, Bertuzzi R, de Souza CC, et al. High carbohydrate diet induces faster final sprint and overall 10,000-m times of young runners. *Pediatr Exerc Sci.* 2015;27(3):355-363.

78. Desbrow B, McCormack J, Burke LM, et al. Sports Dietitians Australia position statement: sports nutrition for the adolescent athlete. *Int J Sport Nutr Exerc Metab.* 2014;24(5):570-584.

79. Inbar O, Morris N, Epstein Y, Gass G. Comparison of thermoregulatory responses to exercise in dry heat among prepubertal boys, young adults and older males. *Exp Physiol.* 2004;89(6):691-700.

80. Bergeron MF. Youth sports in the heat: recovery and scheduling considerations for tournament play. *Sports Med.* 2009;39(7):513-522.

81. Falk B. Effects of thermal stress during rest and exercise in the paediatric population. *Sports Med.* 1998;25(4):221-240.

82. Wilk B, Yuxiu H, Bar-Or O. Effect of hypohydration on aerobic performance of boys who exercise in the heat. *Med Sci Sports Exerc.* 01/2002;34(5):S48.

83. Falk B, Dotan R. Children's thermoregulation during exercise in the heat: a revisit. *Appl Physiol Nutr Metab.* 2008;33(2):420-427.

84. Rowland T. Fluid replacement requirements for child athletes. *Sports Med.* 2011;41(4):279-288.

85. Council on Sports,Medicine and Fitness, Council on School Health, Bergeron MF, Devore C, Rice SG. Policy statement—climatic heat stress and exercising children and adolescents. *Pediatrics.* 2011;128(3):e741-e747.

86. Karet FE. Disorders of water and acid-base homeostasis. *Nephron Physiol.* 2011;118(1):28-34.

87. Bar-Or O, Blimkie CJ, Hay JA, MacDougall JD, Ward DS, Wilson WM. Voluntary dehydration and heat intolerance in cystic fibrosis. *Lancet.* Mar 21 1992;339(8795):696-699.

88. Yardley JE, Stapleton JM, Carter MR, Sigal RJ, Kenny GP. Is whole-body thermoregulatory function impaired in type 1 diabetes mellitus? *Curr Diabetes Rev.* 1 2013;9(2):126-136.

89. Bass SL, Inge K. Thermoregulation in young athletes exercising in hot environments. *Int Sports Med J.* 2001;2(5):1-6.

90. American College of Sports Medicine, Sawka MN, Burke LM, et al. American College of Sports Medicine position stand. Exercise and fluid replacement. *Med Sci Sports Exerc.* 2007;39(2):377-390.

91. Mifflin MD, St Jeor ST, Hill LA, Scott BJ, Daugherty SA, Koh YO. A new predictive equation for resting energy expenditure in healthy individuals. *Am J Clin Nutr.* 1990;51(2):241-247.

92. Owen OE, Kavle E, Owen RS, et al. A reappraisal of caloric requirements in healthy women. *Am J Clin Nutr..* 1986;44(1):1-19.

93. Thompson J, Manore MM. Predicted and measured resting metabolic rate of male and female endurance athletes. *J Am Diet Assoc.* 1996;96(1):30-34.

94. ten Haaf T, Weijs PJ. Resting energy expenditure prediction in recreational athletes of 18-35 years: confirmation of Cunningham equation and an improved weight-based alternative. *PLoS One.* 2014;9(9):e108460.

95. Carlsohn A, Scharhag-Rosenberger F, Cassel M, Mayer F. Resting metabolic rate in elite rowers and canoeists: difference between indirect calorimetry and prediction. *Ann Nutr Metab.* 2011;58(3):239-244.

96. Torun B. Energy requirements of children and adolescents. *Public Health Nutr.* 2005;8(7A):968-993.

97. Leibel RL, Rosenbaum M, Hirsch J. Changes in energy expenditure resulting from altered body weight. *N Engl J Med.*1995;332(10):621-628.

98. Marra M, Polito A, De Filippo E, et al. Are the general equations to predict BMR applicable to patients with anorexia nervosa? *Eat Weight Disorder.* 2002;7(1):53-59.

99. Polito A, Fabbri A, Ferro-Luzzi A, et al. Basal metabolic rate in anorexia nervosa: relation to body composition and leptin concentrations. *Am J Clin Nutr.* 2000;71(6):1495-1502.

100. Danforth E Jr, Burger AG. The impact of nutrition on thyroid hormone physiology and action. *Annu Rev Nutr.* 1989;9:201-227.

101. De Souza MJ, Lee DK, VanHeest JL, Scheid JL, West SL, Williams NI. Severity of energy-related menstrual disturbances increases in proportion to indices of energy conservation in exercising women. *Fertil Steril.* 2007;88(4):971-975.

102. Laughlin GA, Yen SS. Nutritional and endocrine-metabolic aberrations in amenorrheic athletes. *J Clin Endocrinol Metab.* 1996;81(12):4301-4309.

103. Ollberding NJ, Couch SC, Woo JG, Kalkwarf HJ. Within- and between-individual variation in nutrient intake in children and adolescents. *J Acad Nutr Diet.* 2014;114(11):1749-1758,e5

104. Aerenhouts D, Deriemaeker P, Hebbelinck M, Clarys P. Energy and macronutrient intake in adolescent sprint athletes: a follow-up study. *J Sports Sci.* Jan 2011;29(1):73-82.

105. Baker LB, Heaton LE, Stein KW, Nuccio RP, Jeukendrup AE. Validity and relative validity of a novel digital approach for 24-h dietary recall in athletes. *Nutr J.* 2014;13:41.

106. McGuire S. US Department of Agriculture and US Department of Health and Human Services, Dietary Guidelines for Americans, 2010. 7th ed. Washington, DC: US Government Printing Office. *Adv Nutr.* 2011;2(3):293-294.

107. Office of Juvenile Justice and Dellinquency Prevention. Drinking in America: Myths, Realities, And Prevention Policy. Washington, DC: US Department of Justice; 2005.

108. Alcohol and Public Health. Centers for Disease Control and Prevention website. 2016; www.cdc.gov/alcohol/. Accessed July 17, 2016.

109. Siqueira L, Smith VC, Committee on substance abuse. binge drinking. *Pediatrics.* 2015;135(3):e718-e726.

110. Diehl K, Thiel A, Zipfel S, Mayer J, Schneider S. Substance use among elite adolescent athletes: findings from the GOAL Study. *Scand J Med Sci Sports.* 2014;24(1):250-258.

111. Bahrke MS, Yesalis CE, Kopstein AN, Stephens JA. Risk factors associated with anabolic-androgenic steroid use among adolescents. *Sports Med.* 2000;29(6):397-405.

112. Kulesza M, Grossbard JR, Kilmer J, Copeland AL, Larimer ME. Take one for the team? Influence of team and individual sport participation on high school athlete substance use patterns. *J Child Adoles Subst Abuse*. 2014;23(4):217-223.

113. Aerenhouts D, Zinzen E, Clarys P. Energy expenditure and habitual physical activities in adolescent sprint athletes.*J Sports Sci Med*. 2011;10(2):362-368.

114. Aerenhouts D, Van Cauwenberg J, Poortmans JR, Hauspie R, Clarys P. Influence of growth rate on nitrogen balance in adolescent sprint athletes. *Int J Sport Nutr Exerc Metab*. 2013;23(4):409-417.

115. Boisseau N, Vermorel M, Rance M, Duche P, Patureau-Mirand P. Protein requirements in male adolescent soccer players. *Eur J Applied Physiol*. 2007;100(1):27-33.

116. Ervin RB, Ogden CL. Trends in intake of energy and macronutrients in children and adolescents from 1999-2000 through 2009-2010. *NCHS Data Brief*. 2013(113):1-8.

117. Croll JK, Neumark-Sztainer D, Story M, Wall M, Perry C, Harnack L. Adolescents involved in weight-related and power team sports have better eating patterns and nutrient intakes than non-sport-involved adolescents. *J Am Diet Assoc*. 2006;106(5):709-717.

118. Baker LB, Heaton LE, Nuccio RP, Stein KW. Dietitian-observed macronutrient intakes of young skill and team-sport athletes: adequacy of pre, during, and postexercise nutrition. *Int J Sport Nutr Exerc Metab*. 2014;24(2):166-176.

119. Labayen I, Ruiz JR, Ortega FB, et al. High fat diets are associated with higher abdominal adiposity regardless of physical activity in adolescents; the HELENA study. *Clin Nutr*. 2014;33(5):859-866.

120. Ambrosini GL, Emmett PM, Northstone K, Howe LD, Tilling K, Jebb SA. Identification of a dietary pattern prospectively associated with increased adiposity during childhood and adolescence. *Int J Obes*. 2012;36(10):1299-1305.

121. Elliott SA, Truby H, Lee A, Harper C, Abbott RA, Davies PS. Associations of body mass index and waist circumference with: energy intake and percentage energy from macronutrients, in a cohort of Australian children. *Nutr J*. 2011;10:58.

122. Bachman JL, Reedy J, Subar AF, Krebs-Smith SM. Sources of food group intakes among the US population, 2001-2002. *J Am Diet Assoc*. 2008;108(5):804-814.

123. Reedy J, Krebs-Smith SM. Dietary sources of energy, solid fats, and added sugars among children and adolescents in the United States. *J Am Diet Assoc*. 2010;110(10):1477-1484.

124. US Department of Agriculture, Agricultural Research Service. Total Nutrient Intakes: Percent Reporting and Mean Amounts of Selected Vitamins and Minerals from Food and Dietary Supplements, by Gender and Age, What We Eat in America, NHANES 2009-2010. www.ars.usda.gov/ba/bhnrc/fsrg. Published 2012. Accessed July 3, 2017.

125. Harika RK, Cosgrove MC, Osendarp SJ, Verhoef P, Zock PL. Fatty acid intakes of children and adolescents are not in line with the dietary intake recommendations for future cardiovascular health: a systematic review of dietary intake data from thirty countries. *BR J Nutr*. 2011;106(3):307-316.

126. Gharami K, Das M, Das S. Essential role of docosahexaenoic acid towards development of a smarter brain. *Neurochem Int*. 2015;89:51-62.

127. Chung WL, Chen JJ, Su HM. Fish oil supplementation of control and (n-3) fatty acid-deficient male rats enhances reference and working memory performance and increases brain regional docosahexaenoic acid levels. *J of Nutr* 2008;138(6):1165-1171.

128. Gamoh S, Hashimoto M, Sugioka K, et al. Chronic administration of docosahexaenoic acid improves reference memory-related learning ability in young rats. *Neuroscience*. 1999;93(1):237-241.

129. Anding RH, Hwang DH. Effects of dietary linolenate on the fatty acid composition of brain lipids in rats. *Lipids*. 1986;21(11):697-701.

130. Richardson AJ, Burton JR, Sewell RP, Spreckelsen TF, Montgomery P. Docosahexaenoic acid for reading, cognition and behavior in children aged 7-9 years: a randomized, controlled trial (the DOLAB Study). *PLoS One*. 2012;7(9):e43909.

131. Rahmawaty S, Charlton K, Lyons-Wall P, Meyer BJ. Dietary intake and food sources of EPA, DPA and DHA in Australian children. *Lipids*. 2013;48(9):869-877.

132. Harel Z, Riggs S, Vaz R, White L, Menzies G. Omega-3 polyunsaturated fatty acids in adolescents: knowledge and consumption. *J Adolesc Health*. 2001;28(1):10-15.

133. Karalius VP, Zinn D, Wu J, et al. Prevalence of risk of deficiency and inadequacy of 25-hydroxyvitamin D in US children: NHANES 2003-2006. *J Pediatr Endocrinol Metab*. 2014;27(5-6):461-466.

134. Misra M, Pacaud D, Petryk A, et al. Vitamin D deficiency in children and its management: review of current knowledge and recommendations. *Pediatrics*. 2008;122(2):398-417.

135. Wagner CL, Greer FR, American Academy of Pediatrics Section on B, American Academy of Pediatrics Committee on N. Prevention of rickets and vitamin D deficiency in infants, children, and adolescents. *Pediatrics*. 2008;122(5):1142-1152.

136. Mitchell DM, Henao MP, Finkelstein JS, Burnett-Bowie SA. Prevalence and predictors of vitamin D deficiency in healthy adults. *Endocr Pract.* 2012;18(6):914-923.

137. Bischoff-Ferrari HA, Giovannucci E, Willett WC, Dietrich T, Dawson-Hughes B. Estimation of optimal serum concentrations of 25-hydroxyvitamin D for multiple health outcomes. *Am J Clin Nutr.* 2006;84(1):18-28.

138. Institute of Medicine. *Dietary Reference Intakes for Energy, Carbohydrate, Fiber, Fat, Fatty Acids, Cholesterol, Protein, and Amino Acids.* Washington, DC: National Academies Press; 2002.

139. Saggese G, Baroncelli GI, Bertelloni S. Puberty and bone development. *Best Pract Res Clin Endocrinol Metab.* 2002;16(1):53-64.

140. Cashman KD, Hill TR, Cotter AA, et al. Low vitamin D status adversely affects bone health parameters in adolescents. *Am J Clin Nutr.* 2008;87(4):1039-1044.

141. Ward KA, Das G, Berry JL, et al. Vitamin D status and muscle function in post-menarchal adolescent girls. *J Clin Endocrinol Metab.* 2009;94(2):559-563.

142. Boland R. Role of vitamin D in skeletal muscle function. *Endocr Rev.* 1986;7(4):434-448.

143. Close G, Russell J, Cobley J, et al. Assessment of vitamin D concentration in non-supplemented professional athletes and healthy adults during the winter months in the UK: implications for skeletal muscle function. *J Sports Sci.* 2013;31(4):344-353.

144. Bartoszewska M, Kamboj M, Patel DR. Vitamin D, muscle function, and exercise performance. *Pediatr Clin North Am.* 2010;57(3):849-861.

145. Sim JJ, Lac PT, Liu IL, et al. Vitamin D deficiency and anemia: a cross-sectional study. *Ann Hematol.* 2010;89(5):447-452.

146. Atkinson MA, Melamed ML, Kumar J, et al. Vitamin D, race, and risk for anemia in children. *J Pediatr.* 2014;164(1):153-158 e151.

147. Bailey RL, Dodd KW, Goldman JA, et al. Estimation of total usual calcium and vitamin D intakes in the United States. *J Nutr.* 2010;140(4):817-822.

148. Abrams SA. Calcium and vitamin D requirements for optimal bone mass during adolescence. *Curr Opin Clin Nutr Metab Care.* 2011;14(6):605-609.

149. Golden NH, Abrams SA, Committee on N. Optimizing bone health in children and adolescents. *Pediatrics.* 2014;134(4):e1229-1243.

150. Lloyd T, Rollings N, Andon MB, et al. Determinants of bone density in young women. I. Relationships among pubertal development, total body bone mass, and total body bone density in premenarchal females. *J Clin Endocrinol Metab.* 1992;75(2):383-387.

151. Faulkner RA, Davison KS, Bailey DA, Mirwald RL, Baxter-Jones AD. Size-corrected BMD decreases during peak linear growth: implications for fracture incidence during adolescence. *J Bone Miner Res.* 2006;21(12):1864-1870.

152. Sandler RB, Slemenda CW, LaPorte RE, et al. Postmenopausal bone density and milk consumption in childhood and adolescence. *Am J Clin Nutr.* 1985;42(2):270-274.

153. US Department of Agriculture, Agricultural Research Service, Nutrient Data Laboratory. USDA National Nutrient Database for Standard Reference, Release 28. September 2015. www.ars.usda.gov/northeast-area/beltsville-md/beltsville-human-nutrition-research-center/nutrient-data-laboratory/docs/usda-national-nutrient-database-for-standard-reference/. Accessed July 3, 2017.

154. Sekhar DL, Murray-Kolb LE, Kunselman AR, Paul IM. Identifying factors predicting iron deficiency in United States adolescent females using the ferritin and the body iron models. *Clin Nutr.* Jun 1 2015;10(3):e118-e123.

155. Fernandez-Banares F, Monzon H, Forne M. A short review of malabsorption and anemia. *World J Gastroenterol.* 2009;15(37):4644-4652.

156. Sandstrom G, Rodjer S, Kaijser B, Borjesson M. *Helicobacter pylori* antibodies and iron deficiency in female adolescents. *PLoS One.* 2014;9(11):e113059.

157. McClung JP, Karl JP. Iron deficiency and obesity: the contribution of inflammation and diminished iron absorption. *Nutr Rev.* 2009;67(2):100-104.

158. Ziemann E, Kasprowicz K, Kasperska A, Zembron-Lacny A, Antosiewicz J, Laskowski R. Do high blood hepcidin concentrations contribute to low ferritin levels in young tennis players at the end of tournament season? *J Sports Sci Med.* 2013;12(2):249-258.

159. Kayton S, Cullen RW, Memken JA, Rutter R. Supplement and ergogenic aid use by competitive male and female high school athletes. *Med Sci Sports Exerc.* 2002;34(5):S193.

160. Dodge TL, Jaccard JJ. The effect of high school sports participation on the use of performance-enhancing substances in young adulthood. *J Adolesc Health.* 2006;39(3):367-373.

161. Eisenberg ME, Wall M, Neumark-Sztainer D. Muscle-enhancing behaviors among adolescent girls and boys. *Pediatrics.* 2012;130(6):1019-1026.

162. Evans MW Jr, Ndetan H, Perko M, Williams R, Walker C. Dietary supplement use by children and adolescents in the United States to enhance sport performance: results of the National Health Interview Survey. *J Prim Prev.* 2012;33(1):3-12.

163. Gomez J, American Academy of Pediatrics Committee on Sports Medicine and Fitness. Use of performance-enhancing substances. *Pediatrics*. 2005;115(4):1103-1106.

164. Terjung RL, Clarkson P, Eichner ER, et al. American College of Sports Medicine roundtable. The physiological and health effects of oral creatine supplementation. *Med Sci Sports Exerc*. 2000;32(3):706-717.

CHAPTER 13

COLLEGE ATHLETES

Jennifer Ketterly, MS, RDN, CSSD, and Caroline Mandel, MS, RD, CSSD

INTRODUCTION

Today there are nearly 500,000 student-athletes participating in 43 sports at more than 1,000 National Collegiate Athletic Association (NCAA) member institutions (see Table 13.1).[1] Because of the rigorous demands of athletic participation, academic pressures, and the realities of college life, student-athletes are at nutritional risk. College athletes may be predisposed to poor nutrition, poor recovery, fatigue, and injury due to poor eating habits, lack of resources, or rigid training diets. Over the past 25 years, interest and investment in sports dietetics at university athletic departments has increased dramatically, starting with the United States' first collegiate sports dietitian, Kristine Clark PhD, RD, FACSM, at Penn State in 1991. What followed was a surge in the recognition of the role that sports nutrition plays in the health and success of the student-athlete. In 1994, Clark wrote an article detailing the scope of her practice, re-marking that, "Athletic departments in colleges and universities are beginning to recognize the role a sports nutrition professional plays in providing both clinical nutrition services to athletes and nutrition education programs to teams, coaches, and trainers."[2] As of this writing, there were nearly 80 full-time registered dietitian nutritionists (RDNs) providing nutrition services to Division I athletic departments in the United States.

Table 13.1 Division I, II, and III National Collegiate Athletic Associate Member Institutions[1]

	Division I		Division II		Division III		National Collegiate Athletic Association TOTAL	
Total Members	345		306		438		1,089	
	Teams	Athletes	Teams	Athletes	Teams	Athletes	Teams	Athletes
Men	3,005	96,154	2,208	65,853	3,779	109,048	9,012	271,055
Women	3,614	83,080	2,557	46,781	4,151	77,953	10,322	207,814
Total	6,619	179,234	4,765	112,634	7,930	187,001	19,334	478,869

COLLEGIATE SPORTS DIETITIANS

Being a modern collegiate sports dietitian demands expert-level skills and proficiencies in clinical nutrition, counseling, medical nutrition therapy (MNT), exercise physiology, and administration to successfully establish and manage the programming, operations, and management needs of sports nutrition departments. Box 13.1 defines the skills, responsibilities, and characteristics of competent, proficient, and expert-level practitioners in sports dietetics.[3]

These positions require a food and nutrition professional with experience working as part of a multi-disciplinary team, counseling athletes on a variety of nutrition concerns ranging from everyday eating to performance nutrition and facilitating nutrition education seminars to diverse athletic groups.

What makes this position unique is that the collegiate sports dietitian's role goes beyond clinical responsibilities and includes the administration and coordination of nutrition services compliant with NCAA guidelines. Understanding training schedules, physiological demands of training and competing, common injuries, body composition goals, and team culture and beliefs of multiple sports teams is another unique aspect of the collegiate sports dietitian position. An advanced degree, with additional coursework in the exercise sciences, is helpful. Many collegiate sports dietitians working with student-athletes have achieved the certified specialist in sports dietetics credential offered by the Commission on Dietetic Registration.

Box 13.1 Definitions of Competent, Proficient, and Expert Practitioner[3]

Competent Practitioner: A registered dietitian nutritionist (RDN) who is either just starting practice after having obtained RDN registration by the Commission on Dietetic Registration or an experienced RDN who has recently assumed responsibility to provide nutrition services in a new focus area. This individual acquires additional on-the-job skills and engages in tailored continuing education to further enhance knowledge and skills obtained in formal education.

Proficient Practitioner: An RDN who is generally 3 or more years beyond entry into the profession, has obtained operational job performance skills, and is successful in the focus area. These RDNs demonstrate additional knowledge, skills, and experience. They may acquire specialist credentials to demonstrate proficiency in the focus area.

Expert Practitioner: An RDN who is recognized within the profession and has mastered the highest degree of skill and knowledge in a focus area of dietetics through additional knowledge, formal academic preparation, experience, or training. These RDNs exhibit characteristics that include leadership and vision and demonstrate effectiveness in planning, achieving, evaluating, and communicating targeted outcomes. They may have an expanded or specialist role, or both, and may possess an advanced credential. The practice is more complex, and the practitioner has a high degree of autonomy and responsibility.

Collegiate sports dietitians provide nutrition counseling and education to student-athletes in 43 sports. This nutrition counseling and education enhances adaptation to training and can have the following benefits:

- improved health and exercise performance,
- improved recovery from strenuous training,
- optimization of hydration status,
- reduced risk of injury and illness,
- achievement and maintenance of appropriate body weight and body composition, and
- responsible use of dietary supplements and reduced risk of using contaminated or banned substances.

The collegiate sports dietitian needs to be knowledgeable about the energy systems used to train and compete in each sport and have an understanding of the sport's terminology and team culture. While emphasizing sports nutrition strategies to enhance athletic performance, the sports dietitian is also a jack-of-all-trades in that he or she counsels athletes about making good choices in the dining hall, at training-table meals, and at the grocery store. The sports dietitian also teaches cooking skills for off-campus living. The collegiate sports dietitian provides MNT for diagnoses such as type 1 diabetes, celiac disease, gluten sensitivity, food allergies and intolerances, gastrointestinal complaints, and eating disorders. In addition to educating student-athletes, the collegiate sports dietitian educates coaches, athletic trainers, and other department personnel on the use of sports foods, drinks, and dietary supplements that are in compliance with the rules and bylaws of the NCAA, as well as the International Olympic Committee (IOC) for athletes involved in Olympic sports.[4,5]

The collegiate sports dietitian typically wears many hats, including administrator, foodservice coordinator, clinician, educator, and academician. However, each athletic department is unique, and the primary support role of the collegiate sports dietitian can therefore vary. Depending on the athletic department's priority needs, financial abilities, and administrative and staff awareness or readiness, collegiate sports dietitians can exist in a variety of service models. A sports nutrition department or staff of full-time RDNs undoubtedly allows for the greatest impact and provision of a wider scope of services covering administrative, clinical, educational, and academic responsibilities and can even include foodservice projects such as work with the dining hall or training table and development of fueling stations. The collegiate sports dietitian who works independently for a multisport athletic department either in a full-time or part-time capacity may narrow his or her focus to meeting the clinical and educational needs of the student-athlete population while serving only in a consultative manner on other administrative and foodservice projects. Some college and university athletic departments may choose or may only be able to commit to a consultant arrangement for collegiate sports dietitian services, in which case the collegiate sports dietitian most likely takes direction from the department's identified priority needs. The department's key stakeholders often help define these high needs. In sum, collegiate sports dietitian services can be offered and delivered via a variety of arrangements based on the athletic resources and needs. The demand for high performers in these environments will likely continue to expand as student wellness and athlete welfare reemerge as significant needs of modern times and new generations.

Administrative Responsibilities

Given the advancement of the collegiate athletics nutrition environment, full-time collegiate sports dietitians have assumed a great deal of administrative responsibilities, in addition to carrying out the expected clinical and educational roles. Because the collegiate sports dietitian is often working without the benefit of other nutrition coworkers or preexisting nutrition infrastructure, these administrative skills are critical to build an effective nutrition service model for the athletic department's multisport program. For example, a valuable role for the collegiate sports dietitian is in negotiating, managing, or contributing to nutrition-related contracts to facilitate decision making for optimal nutrition outcomes. This could mean that the collegiate sports dietitian develops a relationship with a local pharmacy and negotiates a purchasing procedure for vitamin and mineral supplements at contracted bid or discounted costs. There may be potential for similar relationships and negotiations with lab services to test for iron deficiency, with grocery stores to become a primary vendor for preworkout and postworkout foods, and with distributors or nutritional supplement companies to provide practice and game-time hydration and recovery products. Being able to negotiate cost-effective purchases and contribute to sports marketing contract discussions allows the collegiate sports dietitian to offer added value to the athletic department and ultimately affect the delivery of high-quality, cost-effective nutrition to the student-athletes.

Collegiate sports dietitians may also develop and administer policies, procedures, and protocols; create and facilitate multidisciplinary treatment teams; work with foodservice staff; and function as an athletic department representative. Policies, procedures, and protocols for the following situations are often necessary in a collegiate athletic setting:

- referrals to the collegiate sports dietitian,
- eating disorders prevention, care, and treatment,
- nutritional supplement purchasing, evaluation, and distribution,
- weight and body composition analysis,
- iron-deficiency screening,
- female athlete triad screening and monitoring, and
- other nutrition-related sports medicine protocols (eg, cramping and stress fracture prevention and postsurgical rehabilitation support).

Use of multidisciplinary treatment and performance teams can enhance communication among providers and other support personnel to facilitate care for the student-athlete. Eating disorder treatment teams are crucial to managing the integrative nature of these diseases. Creating performance teams with members of the athletic training and strength and conditioning staff can be an effective way to communicate about an athlete's goals and progress while fostering respect for each discipline involved in the athlete's care. A body composition team may also be useful in some situations and with select teams.

In addition to the development and negotiation of contracts and participation in treatment and performance teams, the collegiate sports dietitian has to consider how to deliver individual outpatient services to student-athletes. To manage this practice, one typically needs to develop efficient appointment procedures, determine initial and follow-up consultations, develop forms, implement appropriate documentation, and ensure that standards of practice and confidentiality are followed. Individual consultations can take place in a variety of university and athletic department facilities. For example, campus health sports medicine clinics and athletic training rooms are two common sports nutrition service locations, in addition to specified nutrition office space. In any setting, it is important to market nutrition services to student-athletes and other support personnel because many will likely have had little experience working with a collegiate sports dietitian. Services are used more often when athletes know where and how to find the collegiate sports dietitian and when services are offered at convenient times. It is important to consider class schedule variances throughout the week, typical treatment and practice times, and the athlete's path through campus when drafting an appointment schedule. For efficient scheduling, use an appointment service, online calendar and scheduling, and assistance from administrative support personnel and sports medicine clinics.

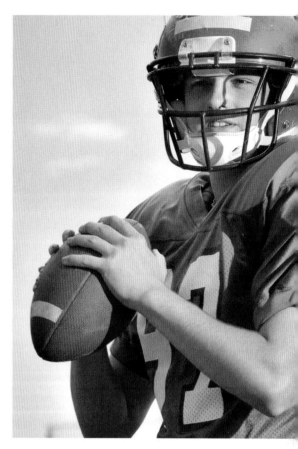

Clinical Responsibilities

In the clinical role, the sports dietitian provides individualized nutrition education and counseling to the student-athlete. This may be done by self-referral or referral by another member of the athletic department. The reasons that a student-athlete may be referred to the sports dietitian include fatigue, poor eating habits, hydration concerns, weight management, body composition testing, iron deficiency, disordered eating, supplement questions, history of chronic dieting, food allergies, vegan or vegetarian meal planning, gastrointestinal complaints, or medical diagnoses such as diabetes, high cholesterol, or hypertension. Also, the collegiate sports dietitian can refer student-athletes to the appropriate member of the athletic medicine team, campus resources, or off-campus resources, such as an eating disorder support group, as necessary. The collegiate sports dietitian assesses the student-athletes dietary intake patterns and then educates and counsels the athlete on an appropriate performance diet to help him or her reach desired health and performance goals. The collegiate sports dietitian works to develop rapport with the student-athlete and uses various counseling strategies, such as goal-setting, behavior modification, relapse prevention, cognitive-behavioral therapy, and motivational interviewing. The collegiate sports dietitian has an arsenal of tools at his or her disposal, including evidence-based sports nutrition guidelines, MNT protocols for nutrition diagnoses, and best practice as determined by extensive practical experience in sports dietetics.

The collegiate sports dietitian participates in student-athlete preparticipation physicals in a variety of ways. Many sports dietitians have developed nutritional needs assessment tools to identify athletes at risk for poor eating habits and those who need individualized nutrition counseling. Screening questions cover weight and dieting history, meal patterns, shopping habits and cooking skills, restaurant frequency, frequently consumed foods, and use of supplements or vitamins. The sports dietitian works closely with the athletic medicine staff to screen for nutrition-related issues such as iron-deficiency anemia, inappropriate supplement use, weight-management concerns, disordered eating, and the female athlete triad. Quatramoni describes collegiate athletes' vulnerability to nutritional risks due to demands of sport and college life and

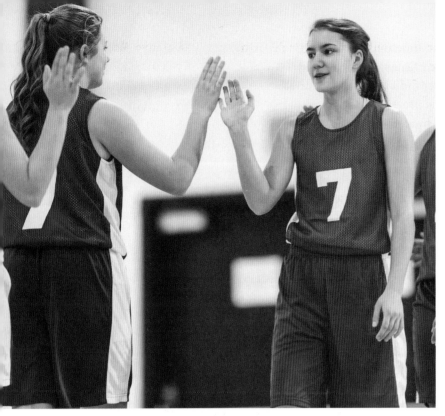

recommends the Female Athlete Screening Tool as useful for identifying eating pathology for referral and intervention.[6,7] In 2014, the Female Athlete Triad Coalition published a consensus statement on screening, diagnosis, treatment, and return to play for athletes dealing with the female athlete triad.[8] Also in 2014, the IOC published its consensus statement introducing a more comprehensive term of relative energy deficiency in sport (RED-S) to propose a replacement for the term "female athlete triad".[9] More information about athletes and eating disorders is found in Chapter 18.

Foodservice Responsibilities

The foodservice opportunities for collegiate sports dietitians have increased dramatically due to changes in NCAA regulations as to what types of foods and beverages athletic departments are permitted to provide to student athletes and when they may provide them. Working within the foodservice industry is now a significant and logical part of working in a collegiate environment. The training table, a phrase referring to meals served only to student-athletes in a closed setting, can be provided in an on-site athletic dining facility or residence dining hall or catered to a locker room, team lounge, or other athletic space. In addition, athletic departments can now offer additional meals and unlimited snacks as part of athletic participation. Many schools offer these additional foods and snacks at locations called fueling stations. Fueling stations can be set up as temporary or mobile food and supplement distribution points in locker rooms, weight rooms, concession stands, or other convenient locations, or they may be built into a fixed space to serve as a centralized location for all teams. Training tables and fueling stations are both ideal places for the sports dietitian to deliver nutrition education messages and help athletes select performance foods. Both are important examples of the planning, budgeting, and staffing responsibilities of the collegiate sports RDN. Other examples of roles that a sports dietitian can have in the foodservice environment include the following:

- Help negotiate fair and appropriate meal costs for the training table.
- Help outline food-quality standards.
- Advocate for adequate staff and staffing patterns at the training table to allow for optimal service.
- Encourage food-related data collection and forecasting models to achieve cost-effective operations.
- Develop or review cycle menus and suggest alternative preparation methods or items to meet sports nutritional needs and requirements.
- Provide nutrition analysis of menu items and develop a format for posting nutrient information at point-of-sale or online.
- Arrange adequate ordering, receiving, and delivery processes to manage the supply chain.
- Help plan and coordinate foodservice needs for team travel and hotel stays. Teams will often stay in hotels with foodservice availability (for both home and travel games). The sports dietitian is the perfect liaison between the team and hotel and can effectively plan the meals and communicate with the hotel staff on food-quality standards, preparation method, buffet arrangements, special dietary needs, and budgetary limitations to ensure that the meal is appropriate, convenient, time efficient, and conducive to the travel itinerary.

Lastly, the collegiate sports dietitian often functions as an athletic department representative. Recruiting events, campus committees, and community-sponsored functions are examples of situations in which the sports dietitian may be asked to participate and represent the athletic department. Serving as an ambassador for the department in a professional and collegial manner provides an opportunity to develop relationships inside and outside the department while building awareness and furthering the respect for the sports dietitian's services.

Nutrition Education Responsibilities

As an educator, the collegiate sports dietitian develops and conducts sports nutrition seminars for sports teams, coaches, and athletic medicine staff, including athletic trainers, team physicians, physical therapists, and sports counselors. Providing sports nutrition education for coaches and athletic medicine staff helps to make sure everyone is on the same page and provides a consistent nutrition message to the student-athlete. Nutrition knowledge has been shown to play an important role in adapting optimal nutrition practices, thus positively affecting athletic performance. Several studies have demonstrated that knowledge of correct performance nutrition and recovery principles among high school athletes, coaches, and incoming collegiate freshman student-athletes is limited or lacking.[10-13] Rockwell and colleagues assessed nutrition knowledge, opinions, and practices of coaches and athletic trainers from 21 sports at an NCAA Division I institution. Participants responded correctly to 67% of nutrition knowledge questions. Coaches and athletic trainers from women's sports gave more correct responses than those from men's sports. Coaches and athletic trainers who had 15 or more years of experience gave more correct responses than those with fewer years of experience.[14] Torres-McGehee and colleagues reported that of 579 Division I, II, and III participants surveyed, 77.8% of athletic trainers and 81.6% of strength and conditioning specialists had adequate sports nutrition knowledge, whereas 35.9% of coaches and 9% of student-athletes had adequate knowledge.[15] Table 13.2 suggests sports nutrition topics relevant for student-athletes.

Other educational approaches range from low tech to high tech and include the development of handouts and fact sheets, table tents, bulletin boards, newsletters, infographics, digital screens, websites, blogs, and use of social media platforms such as Twitter, Instagram, Facebook, and Pinterest. Handouts and fact sheets are great tools for team nutrition seminars, training tables, fueling stations, weight rooms, training rooms, and athletic medicine waiting rooms. Some collegiate sports dietitians develop their own handouts based on the needs of their student-athlete population, whereas others purchase or download fact sheets from the Internet. It is crucial to review all purchased or downloaded materials for credibility and appropriateness of the message for the college student-athlete population. Fact sheets developed by RDNs through a collaboration between the NCAA, the Sports, Cardiovascular, and Wellness Nutrition (SCAN) dietetic practice group of the Academy of Nutrition and Dietetics, and the Collegiate and Professional Sports Dietitians Association (CPSDA) are available on the websites of the NCAA (www.ncaa.org), SCAN (http://scandpg.org), and CPSDA (http://sportsrd.org).

Table 13.2 Sports Nutrition Education Topics

Audience	Topic	Seminar Suggestions
Student athletes	Hydration	Weigh athletes privately before and after training. Inform athletes of their weight change, and discuss sweat rate and daily fluid requirements. Review ways to monitor hydration status, such as urine color and weight change before and after exercise.
	Dining out	Collect menus and nutrition information from the team's top restaurant choices at home and on the road when traveling for competitions. Discuss optimal meal choices and timing, along with specific menu options.

Continued on next page

Table 13.2: Sports Nutrition Education Topics (Continued)

Audience	Topic	Seminar Suggestions
Athletic trainers	Dietary supplements	Review the most recent NCAA[a] banned drugs list[16] and NCAA Bylaw 16.5.2[4] for lists of permissible supplement categories and impermissible ingredients. Discuss the NATA[b] position statements regarding evaluation of dietary supplements for performance nutrition and anabolic-androgenic steroids.[17,18] Bring samples of products to evaluate, including some that are banned, impermissible, and permissible.
	Athletes with type I diabetes	Review the American Diabetes Association Standards of Care[19] and the NATA position statement.[20] Apply to athlete case studies: the athlete's diabetes care plan; supplies for athletic training kits; preparticipation physical exams; recognition, treatment, and prevention of hypoglycemia and hyperglycemia; insulin administration; travel recommendations; athletic injury; and glycemic control.
Coaches	Recovery nutrition	Present evidence on nutrition for recovery. Show examples of foods, as well as permissible sports foods and supplements, that provide optimal carbohydrate, protein, and hydration for postexercise recovery.
	Weight management and body composition	Review departmental policies: how to refer athletes to the sports dietitian, what athletes can expect when working with the sports dietitian on weight loss or weight gain strategies, and how to identify athletes at risk for disordered eating and eating disorders.
Physicians	Iron screening protocol	Review which spots have athletes that are at highest risk of inadequate iron status and plan the best time to screen. Discuss iron cutoff levels and optimal nutrition plans with supplement dosage recommendations. Plan student-athlete education, follow-up, and reporting strategies.
Eating disorders team	Female athlete triad	Review current literature on the triad, including position statements from the Female Athlete Triad Coalition and the IOC.[c,8,9] Discuss ways to integrate education and prevention into nutrition, counseling, and medical services as a multidisciplinary team.

[a] NCAA, National Collegiate Athletic Association.
[b] NATA = National Athletic Trainers' Association
[c] IOC = International Olympic Committee

Collegiate sports RDNs can post high-visibility nutrition-themed articles or studies periodically on a bulletin board in a training room, weight room, fueling station, training table, or medical clinic waiting area as another way to highlight relevant sports nutrition information. Actions like posting recipes, resources, interactive quizzes, and contact information for the sports dietitian serves a dual purpose: These types of actions educate student-athletes and staff and function as as form of marketing services. Bulletin board topics that are timely and relevant to the student-athlete population are highlighted in Box 13.2. Placing table tents at the training table is a great way to capture the attention of student-athletes when they are most focused on food and nutrition. Box 13.3 lists suggested table-tent topics for training tables.

Many collegiate sports dietitians have turned low-tech handouts and bulletin boards into electronic newsletters or blog topics. Posting information about sports nutrition services, hours, contact information, and sports nutrition fact sheets on departmental websites is a great way to take advantage of the technology that student-athletes use today. Videos of supermarket tours and cooking demos can also be included. Some schools have password-protected Internet services available for their student-athletes; for other schools, this information will be available to student-athletes and the general population who may be browsing the school's website. Allowing public access to these materials can be a useful recruiting tool. The combination of print and digital sports nutrition education and information adds to the athletic department's culture of improving performance.

Box 13.2 Suggested Bulletin Board Topics for Each Academic Semester

Fall

- The Freshman 15: Is It Real?
- Meal Planning for Off-Campus Living
- Grocery Shopping 101
- Fueling for Preexercise
- Dining Out

Winter

- What's New for the New Year?
- Eating Disorders Awareness Week
- March Is National Nutrition Month
- Quick and Easy Snack Ideas
- Nutrition for Recovery

Spring/Summer

- Sports Foods and Supplements
- Breakfast Is for Champions
- Frequently Asked Questions
- Quick and Easy Meal Solutions
- Staying Hydrated in the Summer Heat

Box 13.3 Table-Tent Topics for Training Tables

Making the Best Choices at the Training Table

Are You Hydrated?

The Athlete's Plate

Hot Topics in Sports Nutrition

Snack Attack: How to Fill Nutrition Gaps

Get the Carbohydrate Edge

10 Tips for Fueling Like a Champion

Alcohol and Performance Do Not Mix

Fast-Food Facts

Reading Food Labels: What Athletes Need to Know

Dining Out—World Cuisine

Caffeine and Athletic Performance

Sports Nutrition Myths

Academic Responsibilities

In addition to being a clinician, educator, and administrator, the proficient and expert dietitian working on a college campus has a unique opportunity to serve as a teacher and academician. The collegiate sports dietitian is often invited to provide guest lectures or teach a class for credit. Establishing working relationships with academic departments on campus can yield opportunities for sports nutrition research and publication, as well as collaborative equipment purchases, such as a BOD POD system for air displacement plethysmography or a dual energy x-ray absorptiometry machine for body composition analysis. Additional academic opportunities include serving as a preceptor for students in dietetics or athletic training curricula, medical students in orthopedic rotations or sports medicine fellowships, and other sports medicine–related practicum experiences. As the demand for sports dietetics skills continues to increase, so does the need for additional training for this marketplace. Collegiate sports dietitians can establish and promote post graduate fellowships, internships, and immersion experiences as important training grounds for successful, industry-specific, skill development.

THE STUDENT-ATHLETE

Collegiate athletes are a diverse group of men and women ranging in age from 17 to 24 years. They are considered postadolescent young adults, or emerging adults.[21] Research suggests that this age group is still developing mentally and physically. They are known for taking more risks and being more self-centered and vulnerable to addiction and being less insightful or concerned about consequences than adults.[22] The student-athlete population at most NCAA institutions is typically diverse in terms of sex, race, culture, religion, nutrition knowledge, and socioeconomic status. Student-athletes are required to be full-time students during their years of athletic eligibility, but not all are awarded a full athletic scholarship that includes money for food, and many do not have access to a sports dietitian. Nutritional needs are constantly changing and evolve throughout the student-athlete's college career. Box 13.4 lists examples of typical nutritional concerns based on the athlete's year in school. In addition to learning about their sports nutritional requirements to augment training and improve athletic performance, many student-athletes learn valuable life skills regarding meal planning, grocery shopping, and proper food handling and storage, as well as nutrition guidelines for wellness and the prevention of chronic disease.

Box 13.4 Nutrition-Related Concerns of College Student-Athletes by Year of Eligibility

Freshman
- Transition to college life—dining-hall meal plan, alcohol, stress, time management
- Adapting to a new team and training program
- The "freshman 15"—weight management, body composition, body image
- Finding your social identity
- Increased competitiveness of collegiate sports
- Continued physical growth and development
- Emotional maturity and developing confidence

Sophomore
- Transition to off-campus living—menu planning, grocery shopping, and cooking skills
- Prevention of overtraining
- Training and nutritional periodization for year-round training and competition
- Balancing sports with academics and social life
- Perfecting the taper for endurance sports

Junior
- Moving out of dorms into house or apartment
- Easy meal-preparation ideas and recipes
- Preventing boredom or staleness with diet
- Nutritional variety and interest for the long haul
- Consistency with habits for continued success
- Growing demands of academic major

Senior or Fifth Year
- Leadership on and off the field of competition
- Life after college athletics
- Transition from collegiate athlete to professional athlete or recreational exerciser
- Increased focus on healthful eating for a lifetime

Nutrition Knowledge and Sources of Information

College athletes are often misinformed about their fueling requirements and arrive on campus with multiple sources of nutrition information, including parents, friends, teammates, coaches, magazines, and the internet. They are a captive audience, meaning that they typically use the sports medicine and nutrition services offered to them through the athletic department or campus health services. For many, these services are unlimited and available at no cost for the duration of their eligibility.

Not all college student-athletes have access to a collegiate sports dietitian to provide guidance on their performance training diet and a healthy lifestyle. Rosenbloom and colleagues assessed the nutrition knowledge of athletes at one NCAA Division I institution and found that many collegiate athletes have misconceptions about the roles of specific nutrients, such as carbohydrates, protein, vitamins, minerals, and supplements in sports performance. The students reported that their sources of sports nutrition information included coaches, athletic trainers, strength and conditioning staff, physicians, teammates, nutrition classes, sports dietitians, parents, and popular media. They concluded that athletes who make food choices based on inaccurate nutrition information could experience negative consequences in their performance.[23] Pawlak and colleagues found that athletes' daily schedules and their perception of a healthful diet's effects on their focus and concentration had the biggest impact on collegiate baseball players' intention to eat healthy food.[24] Another study reported the nutrition knowledge scores, nutrition choice scores, and nutrition practice scores for 185 players from 11 Mid-American Conference collegiate softball teams. Two-thirds had a failing knowledge score; their choice score suggested that they made poor nutrition choices—17% ate fast food every day or most days and over half said that they occasionally, rarely, or never have a set meal schedule. Respondents who said they ate using the USDA's Food Guide Pyramid graphic for guidance had healthier diets; only 10% indicated that they used the Food Guide Pyramid to make food choices every day or most days.[25] In 11 NCAA Division I volleyball players, nutrition knowledge scores ranged from 16 to 37 out of a possible 55 points before a nutrition intervention. At baseline, participants did not meet the sport-specific recommended requirements for energy (24.0 ± 8.6 kcal/kg/d vs the recommended 37 to 41 kcal/kg/d), carbohydrate (3.08 ± 1.1 kcal/kg/d vs the recommended 6 to 10 g/kg/d), protein (0.9 ± 0.3 kcal/kg/d vs the recommended 1.2 to 1.7 g/kg/d), or fat (77% of estimated needs). This was possibly due to meal skipping and the high number of subjects (50%) trying to lose weight. The athletes improved in all areas of knowledge and intake after the intervention.[26]

Personal Concerns

The student-athlete has a variety of personal, athletic, and health concerns that can affect his or her nutritional status and, in turn, success as a college student. Personal concerns include transitioning to college life; struggling with the increased time demands of collegiate academics and athletics; navigating new food resources; managing budgets (depending on scholarship status and family resources); managing multiple relationships with coaches, teammates, teachers, family, and friends; and experiencing lack of sleep. For many college athletes, this is the first time they have lived without parents or guardians and have been solely responsible for their own food choices. They bring with them 17 to 18 years of food and nutrition beliefs and behaviors, ranging from informed and sophisticated to misinformed and in line with the typical American diet. The *Dietary Guidelines for Americans 2015–2020* describes the average fruit, vegetable, dairy, and seafood intake as below recommended ranges for males and females age 14 to 30 years.[27] In 2013, the Centers for Disease Control and Prevention State Indicator Report on Fruits and Vegetables found that more than one-third of adolescents in the United States reported consuming fruits and vegetables less than once a day.[28] Once on campus, acclimating to dining hall food choices as a freshman and then possibly moving off-campus into a house or apartment in subsequent years and having to manage meal planning, grocery shopping, meal preparation, and food handling and storage for the first time may affect an athlete's nutritional status. Athletes who live off-campus but do not have transportation may have decreased access to food, which can make it challenging to follow a sound training diet. In addition, an athlete on a limited budget may opt to use food money for other purposes, leaving little money for meals.

Social pressures to use alcohol and drugs can jeopardize a student-athlete's athletic performance, health, and eligibility. Alcohol and drug use by college athletes is a major concern for athletic departments. Individuals involved in athletics are more likely to engage in a wide range of risky behaviors than are nonathletes.[29] Table 13.3 (page 277) reports NCAA findings regarding alcohol use by student athletes from 1993 to 2013, and Table 13.4 provides data on alcohol use by college students from the American College Health Association National College Health Assessment (ACHA-NCHA) II.[30-33] The NCAA National Study of Substance Use Habits of College Student-Athletes found that the overall use of alcohol by student-athletes increased between 2005 and 2009 but decreased in 2013 across all NCAA divisions.[31] Excessive drinking (five or more drinks for men; four or more drinks for women) is down since 2005 in male student-athletes from 63% to 44% and from 41% to 33% in female student-athletes. More than half of NCAA student-athletes reported that first-time use of alcohol occurred in high school or earlier.

Table 13.3 Alcohol Use by National Collegiate Athletic Association Student Athletes 1993–2013[30,31]

	Student Athletes Using Alcohol in Last 12 Months, %					
Division	1993	1997	2001	2005	2009	2013
Division I	86.3	79.2	80.5	74.3	81.7	78.4
Division II	89.1	79.7	78.8	74.9	81.5	79.3
Division III	93.2	82.6	83.3	81.6	85.3	83.3

The NCAA study reported that almost 60% of student-athletes continue to believe that their use of alcoholic beverages has no effect on athletic performance or on their general health, despite a push for educational programming provided to this population on the known risks of alcohol use in terms of athletic performance, academics, and health.[30] Box 13.5 describes the consequences of alcohol use on athletic performance.[34]

Box 13.5 Consequences of Alcohol Use on Athletic Performance[34]

Hydration: Alcohol is a powerful diuretic that leads to dehydration, which weakens the pumping force of the heart, impairs temperature regulation, and accelerates fatigue, all contributing to decreased aerobic and overall performance. Increased health risks during prolonged exercise in hot environments are also a concern.

Motor Skills: Alcohol slows reaction time and impairs precision, equilibrium, hand-eye coordination, accuracy, balance, judgment, information processing, focus, stamina, strength, power, and speed; impairments can last up to 72 hours after alcohol intake.

Strength, Power, and Sprint Performance: Alcohol leads to decreased strength, power, and sprint performance (eg, running and cycling times); decreased grip strength; decreased jump height; and faster time to fatigue during high-intensity exercise.

Recovery: Alcohol is a poor source of nutrients and may replace carbohydrates in the pre- and posttraining times, leading to poor training and recovery.

Risk of Illness and Injury: Athletes who drink alcohol have an elevated risk of injury. Regular alcohol consumption depresses immune function, increases swelling upon injury, and contributes to delayed healing.

Body Composition/Weight Management: Body-fat accumulation due to ethanol storage as fat and alcohol's appetite stimulation effect may lead to negative body composition changes and overall weight gain.

Effects of Heavy, Chronic Alcohol Consumption: Heavy alcohol consumption can cause nutritional deficiencies; altered digestion, absorption, and metabolism of nutrients; muscle damage, wasting, and weakness; and impaired ability to gain muscle mass and strength.

Long-Term Health: Long-term excessive alcohol consumption can cause pathological changes in liver, heart, brain, and muscle that can lead to disability; nutritional deficiencies; altered digestion, absorption, and metabolism of nutrients; muscle damage, wasting, and weakness; and impaired ability to gain muscle mass and strength.

While 19.3% of college student-athletes say they have never used alcohol, nearly half (49.3%) of college student-athletes report drinking alcohol during both the off-season and competitive season. Athletes attributed abstaining from alcohol mainly to concerns about health and athletic performance, to a desire to avoid alcohol's effects, or their beliefs and values. Excluding alcohol use, student-athletes are less likely to

Table 13.4 Reported Use of Alcohol, Tobacco, and Other Drugs Among College Students[32]

Frequency of use in past 30 days	Alcohol, %			Cigarettes, %		
	Males	Females	Total students	Males	Females	Total students
Never used	20.9	19.5	20.1	66.7	73.9	71.4
Used, but not in past 30 days	12.3	13.5	13.1	18.1	15.5	16.4
Used 1–9 days ago	47.5	52.9	50.8	8.6	6.0	6.9
Used 10–29 days ago	17.6	13.5	14.9	2.6	1.5	1.9
Used all 30 days ago	1.7	0.6	1.0	3.9	3.0	3.4
Any use within the past 30 days	66.8	67.0	66.8	15.2	10.5	12.2

Frequency of use in past 30 days	Marijuana, %			Other Drugs, %[a]		
	Males	Females	Total students	Males	Females	Total students
Never used	57.7	62.7	61.0	53.6	72.4	65.9
Used, but not in past 30 days	20.6	21.0	20.7	25.2	18.2	20.5
Used 1–9 days ago	12.2	11.4	11.7	14.4	7.3	9.7
Used 10–29 days ago	5.7	3.2	4.1	3.1	1.3	2.0
Used all 30 days ago	3.9	1.8	2.6	3.7	0.8	1.9
Any use within the past 30 days	21.7	16.3	18.3	21.2	9.4	13.6

[a] Includes cigars, smokeless tobacco, cocaine, methamphetamine, other amphetamines, sedatives, hallucinogens, anabolic steroids, opiates, inhalants, ecstasy, other club drugs, other illegal drugs. Excludes alcohol, cigarettes, tobacco from a water pipe, and marijuana.

engage in social drug use than other college students. Self-reported drug use is highest among student-athletes who are male, play men's lacrosse, or attend a Division III school.[30,31] Table 13.5 (page 278) shows how alcohol and other social drug use differs by team for both male and female collegiate student-athletes.[31]

The hazards of tobacco use are well known. The 2014 ACHA-NCHA Reference Group Executive Summary reported that 12.2% of college students had used cigarettes in the past 30 days.[32] Cigarette use among Division I student-athletes decreased from 16% to 10% between 2009 and 2013. Spit tobacco use is common among college athletes, despite the NCAA ban on the use of any tobacco product by all game personnel and all student-athletes during practice and competition. The NCAA study found that smokeless tobacco use over the past 12 months was greater in male than female athletes (24% and 2%, respectively) and highest in Division III athletes (18% in 2013), but it had decreased slightly from 17% to 16% among all Division I college athletes between the years 2009 and 2013.[31] About one-quarter of all men reported the use of spit tobacco in the past year, which is unchanged since 2005. The most frequent spit tobacco users are male athletes in ice hockey (49.4%), baseball (47.2%), lacrosse (40.0%), wrestling

Table 13.5 Division I College Athletes: Percentage of Social Drug Use Within the Previous 12 Months by Sport[30]

	Alcohol	Cigarettes	Cocaine	Spit Tobacco	Marijuana	Synthetic Marijuana
Male Athletes, %						
Baseball	85.8	13.6	1.7	49.6	19.0	2.5
Basketball	58.1	3.6	0.4	4.3	10.6	0.7
Football	70.9	7.0	1.2	19.2	17.4	1.9
Golf	90.0	17.4	0.5	30.3	15.0	0.0
Ice Hockey	98.0	16.2	4.2	39.5	19.9	0.5
Lacrosse	95.2	30.3	15.0	38.5	35.8	5.8
Soccer	82.3	11.0	3.1	10.4	16.4	1.0
Swimming	87.8	14.2	2.6	12.0	29.2	1.3
Tennis	82.1	12.8	2.8	13.6	21.0	1.4
Track	75.4	4.5	0.7	10.3	14.5	0.7
Wrestling	64.5	7.8	4.2	28.9	15.0	1.2
Female Athletes, %						
Basketball	65.8	2.1	0.0	1.2	10.1	0.6
Crew	84.4	3.7	0.0	0.0	19.3	0.9
Golf	77.5	5.8	0.0	1.9	7.2	0.5
Gymnastics	73.4	1.6	0.0	0.0	5.7	0.0
Lacrosse	98.5	16.9	0.8	2.3	23.1	0.0
Soccer	76.6	10.1	1.3	2.2	12.6	1.6
Softball	76.6	10.1	1.3	2.2	12.6	1.6
Swimming	88.7	3.0	1.0	0.0	21.1	0.3
Tennis	86.9	10.3	0.0	1.1	13.2	0.0
Track	73.0	2.1	0.8	2.4	11.5	0.5
Volleyball	86.0	2.7	0.0	0.8	13.6	0.8

(36.9%), golf (28.3%), and football (23.8%). In the same study, use of smokeless tobacco by Division I female student-athletes ranged from 0.0% (crew, gymnastics, swimming) to between 2.0% and 2.4% for soccer, softball, lacrosse, and track. Spit tobacco can lead to periodontal disease, loss of tooth structure, tooth staining, bad breath, and gum disease, as well an increased risk of oral cancer and leukoplakia.[35]

Tobacco education resources are available on the NCAA website (www.ncaa.org/health-and-safety/policy/drug-testing).

Performance Concerns

College athletes are concerned about nutrition as it relates to performance enhancement, prevention of fatigue, recovery from training and competition, use of dietary supplements, illness and injury, weight management, and altering or maintaining body composition.[36] Training and competing at the collegiate level may be vastly different for many athletes compared with high school, resulting in altered nutritional requirements. Wade and colleagues reported that when freshman student athletes arrive on campus, many have difficulty enduring collegiate sport training because they lack lower extremity and core strength, flexibility, proper training technique, and mental toughness, coupled with a lack of performance nutrition knowledge.[13] Educating student athletes about the nutritional demands of sport at the collegiate level is paramount.

FATIGUE PREVENTION

Nutritional causes of fatigue in athletes include inadequate energy intake, glycogen depletion, dehydration, and poor iron status. While iron deficiency can occur in both male and female athletes, approximately 60% of female college athletes are affected by iron deficiency.[37] Factors that contribute to iron loss in female athletes include menstruation, inadequate dietary iron intake, gastrointestinal bleeding, foot-strike hemolysis, sweat loss, and iron malabsorption. The consequences of iron deficiency are impaired athletic performance, immune function, and cognitive function. Cowell and colleagues reported that 24 of 55 NCAA Division I institutions (44%) screen their female athletes for iron deficiency. Twenty-two of those 24 institutions also provide nutrition advice to female student-athletes who are iron deficient, however. A great deal of variability existed among the institutions in terms of diagnostic criteria, treatment protocols, and follow-up procedures. The authors stated the need to develop standardized protocols for assessment and treatment of iron deficiency for female college athletes.[37] The following is a suggested protocol from Eichner[38]:
- Serum ferritin greater than 40 ng/mL: warrants no action
- Serum ferritin between 20 and 40 ng/mL: daily multivitamin with 27 mg elemental iron
- Serum ferritin less than 20 ng/mL: 325 mg ferrous sulfate once daily; follow-up after 100 tablets

RECOVERY

Emphasis on strategies for recovery from training and competition has increased. Strategies include stretching, nutrition, hydration, stress management, sleep, and the use of training-room modalities, including ice baths, contrast showers, massage, and foam roller exercises. Nutritional recovery is a term applied to the refueling and rehydration strategies in the immediate postexercise period to gain training adaptations and prevent fatigue in the next exercise sessions.[36]

It takes approximately 24 hours for the body to recover from a bout of training. For athletes training at low intensity once a day, no special recovery recommendations are required. However, for athletes who need speedy refueling (less than an 8-hour recovery between two fuel-demanding sessions), consuming carbohydrate (1.0–1.2 g/kg body weight) plus consuming protein (0.25 to 0.3 g/kg body weight) with adequate rehydration in the immediate postexercise period (within 60 minutes) improves glycogen resynthesis and muscle rebuilding and repair.[36] For more information on postworkout carbohydrate and protein recommendations see Chapters 2 and 3.

ERGOGENIC AIDS/DIETARY SUPPLEMENTS

Although many athletes understand the relationship between optimal nutrition and athletic performance, the pressure to use ergogenic aids and dietary supplements may be overwhelming and can lead to athletes choosing these products instead of food and fluid intake. Ergogenic aids are defined as external influences that enhance athletic performance and may include performance-enhancing drugs and dietary supplements. Athletes are a major target in the multibillion dollar supplement industry. The dietary supplement industry is underregulated by the US Food and Drug Administration, which has led to multiple reports of tainted supplements and athletes testing positive for banned substances. Many athletes use dietary supplements that claim to enhance athletic performance, gain muscle mass, lose body fat, or improve health and immune function.[31] The NCAA 2009 Survey of Member Institution's Drug-Education and Drug-Testing Programs reported that 22% of Division I, II, and III institutions provide nutritional supplements to their student-athletes, with 82% of Division I football schools providing nutritional supplements.[39] Froiland and colleagues reported on nu-

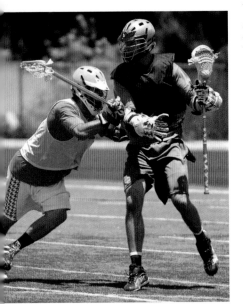

tritional supplement use among 203 college athletes (115 male and 88 female) and their sources of information. Eighty-nine percent of the student-athletes had used or were currently using nutritional supplements.[40]

Females were more likely to take calcium and multivitamins, and males had significant intake for ginseng, β-hydroxy β-methylbutyric acid, amino acids, glutamine, weight-gain products, and whey protein. The most frequently used supplements were energy drinks (73%), calorie-replacement products (61.4%), multivitamins (47.3%), creatine (37.2%), and vitamin C (32.4%). Females were more likely to obtain information from family members and males from nutrition store staff, fellow athletes, friends, or coaches. Female athletes were more likely to take supplements for their health or to make up for an inadequate diet; males took supplements to improve speed and agility or strength and power or to gain weight or muscle.[40] More recently, the 2013 NCAA Study of 21,000 student-athletes showed that 34.7% of NCAA student-athletes reported the use of nutritional supplements. The most commonly reported use overall was for multivitamins, creatine, and amino acid products. Products most commonly reported by men were testosterone boosters (ice hockey, football, baseball, and lacrosse athletes), creatine, and amino acids (ice hockey, football, baseball, lacrosse, and wrestling athletes).[31]

The US Anti-Doping Agency provides an online dietary supplement safety education and awareness resource called Supplement 411 (www.usada.org/substances/supplement-411), which can be adapted for use with NCAA student-athletes to help reduce their risk of taking a supplement contaminated with harmful or banned substances. More information on dietary supplements and ergogenic aids can be found in Chapter 7.

ILLNESS/INJURY PREVENTION/REHABILITATION

In 1982, the National Athletic Trainers' Association and the NCAA created an ongoing collegiate sports injury database called the NCAA Injury Surveillance Program.[41] Between 1988 and 2004, more than half of all athletic injuries to collegiate athletes were to the lower extremities. Preseason practice injury rates were two to three times higher than those recorded during the regular season; more injuries were reported during competition than practice during the regular season. Relatively few injuries occurred in weight rooms. Concussions and anterior cruciate ligaments injury rates increased significantly between 1988 and 2004, likely because of improved reporting and identification. Several sports showed decreased competition injury rates, including women's gymnastics, basketball, and field hockey. Spring football and women's basketball practice injury rates decreased. Sports involving collision and contact (eg, football and wrestling) had the highest injury rates in both games and practice, whereas men's baseball had the lowest rate of injuries in practice, and women's softball had the lowest rate in games. Sports considered noncontact, (eg, men's and women's soccer and basketball) still have a substantial number of injuries caused by player contact.

Special nutritional consideration must be paid to the injured athlete, including altered energy and protein needs, nutritional requirements pre- and postsurgery, and discontinuation of select dietary supplements before surgery. Additionally, the injured athlete may have increased concern about weight and body composition during periods of inactivity and rehabilitation. Wall and colleagues recommended dietary and rehabilitation goals that aim to limit the loss of muscle mass and strength following injury. Specific nutritional considerations include a daily dietary protein intake of 1.2 to 2.0 g/kg body weight with 0.3 g protein per kilogram body weight consumed every 3 to 5 hours spread across multiple meals to support muscle mass maintenance. Wall and colleagues suggested the use of quickly digested whey protein during the day and slowly digested casein protein before sleep.[42] Carbohydrate and fat requirements are determined on a case-by-case basis depending on each athlete's resting metabolic rate, daily activity level, and body composition goals.[42]

WEIGHT MANAGEMENT

Many student-athletes will consult with the sports dietitian about weight management—gain or loss. This is a great opportunity to evaluate the student-athlete's nutritional status and identify areas of need for sports nutrition education while counseling the athlete on appropriate weight management strategies. The position of the Academy of Nutrition and Dietetics, Dietitians of Canada, and the American College of Sports Medicine is stated as[36]:

> *Body weight and composition should not be the sole criterion for participation in sports; daily weigh-ins are discouraged. Optimal body fat levels depend on the sex, age, and heredity of the athlete and may be sport-specific. Body fat assessment techniques have inherent variability and limitations. Preferably weight loss (fat loss) should take place in the off-season or begin before the competitive season and involve a qualified sports dietitian.*

For weight loss, the sports dietitian must ensure adequate nutrient intake, provide a meal plan that minimizes loss of lean mass, and evaluate the student-athlete for risk of disordered eating. For weight gain, special care must be taken to help the athlete find ways to increase energy intake with calorically dense foods, ensure adequate nutrient intake, and avoid foods high in saturated fat and cholesterol that may increase risk of chronic disease. Athletes seeking to gain or lose weight are at risk of taking dietary supplements that may be tainted with harmful or banned substances. More information on weight management is found in Chapter 11.

BODY COMPOSITION

Body composition is a measure of the ratio of lean to fat mass. For a review of body composition techniques, see Chapter 9. Methods that have been used in the collegiate setting include hydrostatic weighing, skinfold measurements, air displacement plethysmography, bioelectrical impedance analysis, and dual-energy x-ray absorptiometry. All methods have a degree of error associated with them that must be considered when interpreting results. Although the assessment of body composition can be a useful tool in helping the student athlete track changes that may occur due to nutrition or training modifications, the *2014-15 NCAA Sports Medicine Handbook* points out the following factors to consider[43]:

- The weight on the scale does not tell an athlete what changes are occurring to his or her lean and fat mass.
- Comparing body composition with that of other athletes is not useful due to differences in age, weight, height, sex, and genetics and may lead to unhealthy nutrition and exercise practices.
- While achieving a body composition helps a student athlete achieve his or her best athletic performance, a very low body fat has serious consequences on health and performance. Minimum body composition standards exist for both male and female athletes.
- Changes in body composition occur slowly over time, and reassessment twice per year is sufficient except in rare circumstances.

There is no ideal body composition for any one athlete or sport. Providing athletes with goal ranges for body composition for their particular gender and sport, as well as tracking changes in lean and fat mass over time, can be useful. Many collegiate athletic departments have developed weight and body composition policies outlining who will do the measurements, how results will be presented to the athlete, who will have access to the data, how these data will be used, and how often measurements are repeated. These policies help to ensure that athletes are adequately educated about body composition assessment, that the data will not be abused or used punitively, and that the health and safety of the athlete are prioritized. For information on weight management for athletes refer to Chapter 11.

Table 13.6 Proportion of College Students Diagnosed or Treated by a Professional[a,32]

Health Problem	Diagnosed or Treated in Last 12 Months, %
Allergies	19.7
Sinus infection	16.9
Back pain	12.6
Strep throat	10.6
Urinary tract infection	10.0
Asthma	9.1
Migraine headache	7.8
Broken bone/fracture/sprain	7.7
Ear infection	7.0
Bronchitis	6.2
High blood pressure	3.1
Irritable bowel syndrome	2.9
High cholesterol	2.7
Repetitive stress injury	2.0
Mononucleosis	1.8
Diabetes	1.1
Chlamydia	1.1
Genital warts/human papillomavirus	1.0
Endometriosis	0.9
Genital herpes	0.7
Hepatitis B or C	0.3
Pelvic inflammatory disease	0.3
Gonorrhea	0.3
Tuberculosis	0.3
HIV infection	0.2

[a] n=79,266

Health Concerns

Health concerns for the student-athlete include gastrointestinal disorders, development of cardiovascular disease (CVD) risk factors, diabetes, disordered eating/eating disorders, and the female athlete triad. Although specific health assessment data on college athletes do not exist, health data reported in Table 13.6 (page 282) from the ACHA-NCHA II can help the collegiate sports RDN understand the variety of health problems experienced by college students, many of which are tied to nutritional status.[22]

GASTROINTESTINAL DISORDERS

Student-athletes may present with gastrointestinal issues, including gastroesophageal reflux, gastritis, nausea, constipation, diarrhea, irritable bowel syndrome, food sensitivities and intolerances, celiac disease, and inflammatory bowel diseases (eg, Crohn's disease, ulcerative colitis). The sports dietitian needs to be knowledgeable about MNT for these disorders and know how to balance an adequate training diet with the rigors of an academic and athletic training schedule.

CARDIOVASCULAR DISEASE RISK FACTORS

Although CVD risk factors, such as high cholesterol, high blood pressure, and diabetes, are not the first topic on the collegiate student-athlete's mind, it is well documented that heart disease is the number one cause of morbidity and mortality for all Americans.[44] Emerging science suggests that increased CVD risk is a reality for some collegiate student-athletes. The American Heart Association recommends screening college athletes for heart disease risk with the main goal of preventing sudden cardiac death and injury.[45] Muñoz and colleagues studied 135 NCAA Division II student athletes from 11 sports and found that a number of college athletes had one or more risk factors for CVD, including increased waist circumference, elevated blood pressure, high total cholesterol, and low high-density lipoprotein cholesterol, despite participation in sports. These factors may predispose college athletes to cardiac risk later in life when exercise regimens are reduced.[46] Borchers and colleagues reported that of 104 NCAA Division I football players, 21% were obese (body fat > 25%), 21% had insulin resistance, and 9% had metabolic syndrome. All of the study participants who were obese were offensive and defensive linemen, and they were at a significantly increased risk of insulin resistance and metabolic syndrome compared with other position players.[47] These data suggest that although Division I collegiate football players participate in high-intensity training, they are at risk of developing metabolic syndrome. Counseling and education on lifestyle modification, exercise, and diet for reduced CVD risk are needed for all athletes, especially as they transition from NCAA sports participation to life after college athletics.

DIABETES

Athletes with diabetes compete at the highest level in every sport. The sports dietitian should be part of the treatment team providing education and lifestyle strategies to optimize glycemic control.[20] The collegiate sports dietitian will more likely encounter type 1 diabetes because of the demographics of the college athlete and should be prepared to address those cases. Refer to Chapter 19 for detailed information on diabetes management in athletes.

DISORDERED EATING AND THE FEMALE ATHLETE TRIAD

College athletes, especially women, are at increased risk for disordered eating or pathogenic eating and weight-control behaviors. Disordered eating harms health and performance and may affect up to 25% of female collegiate athletes and 20% of male collegiate athletes competing in all sports. Reasons for this increased risk include the stress of transitioning to college; critical comments from coaches, parents, judges, peers, or teammates; increased academic demands; stress of losing scholarship or financial aid if they are injured or not able to participate in the sport; and pressures due to the technical, aesthetic, and other demands of sport. Eating disorders and disordered eating are associated with serious health problems, such as dehydration, electrolyte imbalance, depression, decreased bone density, and cardiac arrhythmia. The 2014 Female Athlete Triad Coalition Consensus Statement defines the female athlete triad as a medical

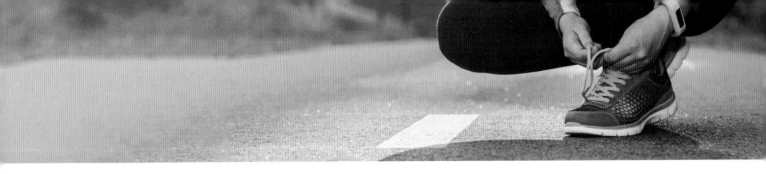

condition that involves three components: (1) low energy availability with or without disordered eating; (2) menstrual dysfunction; and (3) low bone mineral density.[8] Greenleaf and colleagues studied 204 female NCAA Division I college athletes from three universities across the United States and found that 25.5% were symptomatic (some symptoms reported but insufficient to warrant a clinical diagnosis) and 2% had eating disorders (anorexia nervosa, bulimia nervosa, subthreshold bulimia, menstruating anorexia, nonbingeing bulimia, and binge-eating disorder). These findings are consistent with other research on the prevalence of disordered eating and eating disorders in female college-athletes. There was no relationship between sport type and eating disorder classification, suggesting that eating disorders occur fairly consistently across sports.[48] The NCAA collected information on 1,445 male and female student-athletes from 11 NCAA Division I schools and reported that although rates of clinical eating disorders based on *Diagnostic and Statistical Manual-IV* criteria were low (0% for anorexia nervosa for both female and male athletes; 1.1% and 0% for bulimia for female and male athletes, respectively), the percentage of athletes at risk for disordered eating was significant (25% of female athletes and 9.5% of male athletes).[49] Eating disorders continue to be a problem that predominantly affects female athletes, but this study was unique in that it reported on the prevalence of eating disorders and risk of disordered eating in male college student-athletes as well.

Beals and Hill examined the prevalence of the female athlete triad as characterized by disordered eating, menstrual dysfunction, and low bone mineral density among 112 female college athletes in seven sports. They found that only one athlete met the criteria for all three disorders of the triad, but 28 athletes met the criteria for disordered eating, 29 athletes met the criteria for menstrual dysfunction, and 2 athletes had low bone mineral density.[50] Although the prevalence of clinical eating disorders is low in female college athletes, many are at risk for disordered eating, which places them at increased risk for menstrual irregularity and bone injuries. Collegiate athletic departments know that disordered eating and the triad may have begun during the high school years and gone undiagnosed and untreated until the athlete reaches college. Kroshus and colleagues found that only 19% of high school nurses in the United States were able to identify the three components of the female athlete triad, and only 25% said they work with coaches to help prevent health issues among female athletes.[51] When determining awareness and knowledge of the triad and its health implications among female high school athletes and their coaches, Brown and colleagues found that triad risk factors were prevalent among athletes, but coach knowledge of the triad was limited.[52] The 2014 IOC Consensus Statement: Beyond the Female Athlete Triad–RED-S discusses the impact of inadequate energy intake on health and performance for female athletes and potentially for male athletes, including metabolic rate, menstrual function, bone health, immunity, protein synthesis, cardiovascular health, and psychological health caused by relative energy deficiency. The consensus statement reviews screening, diagnosis, treatment, and return to play recommendations.[9] *The NCAA Coaches Handbook: Managing the Female Athlete Triad* is a useful tool for educating athletic department coaches and staff about prevention, detection, and treatment of the female athlete triad.[53] Refer to Chapter 18 for more information on eating disorders in athletes and the female athlete triad.

THE ATHLETIC DEPARTMENT

Stakeholders

Many services, operations, and personnel in and around the athletic department serve as strategic partners for the collegiate sports dietitian. Some key stakeholders are shown in Figure 13.1.

MEDICAL SERVICES

Medical services personnel, coaching staff, athletic administrators, support service staff, and academic faculty can all be important stakeholders in the success of sports nutrition services. Team physicians, orthopedic physicians, athletic trainers, and sport psychologists are important allies to the sports nutrition dietitian. The athletic trainers are an especially vital connection given their day-to-day involvement in student-athletes' medical care and overall team management. It is crucial to establish positive working relationships with these providers, who can subsequently support and facilitate the collegiate sports dietitian's work with the individual athletes and teams. Similarly, campus health services often have clinical laboratories and on-site pharmacies with staff members who can become valuable colleagues to collaborate with on nutrition-related biochemical screening protocols and over-the-counter dietary supplement or product purchasing. Some health centers may also have counseling and psychological services staff who can assist with initial assessments and diagnosis of athletes with disordered eating cases. These providers can help identify proper referral outlets and bridge short-term and long-term care as needed.

COACHES

Coaching staffs, consisting of head and assistant coaches, operations staff, and strength and conditioning coaches, are all obvious partners for the collegiate sports dietitian's work. Once these relationships have

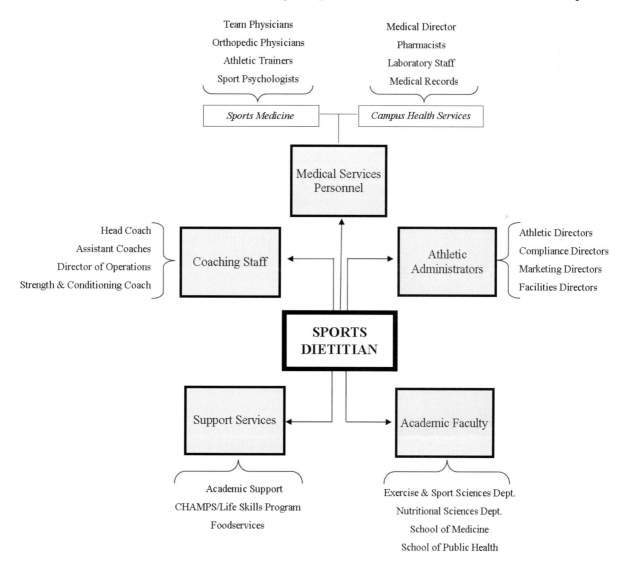

FIGURE 13.1 Stakeholders in College Athletes

been established, coaches will be more willing to allocate practice time to nutrition education, offer budgetary support toward nutrition priorities, and help facilitate a positive nutrition culture within the program. They can be vocal advocates of nutrition services and champion enhancement efforts to administration. In addition, coaches can promote sports nutrition in the recruiting process in an effort to set apart the comprehensive services offered by the college or university to their student-athletes. Parents are often impressed when a nutrition program is part of the athletic environment and is available to help support their children as they transition to campus life.

ADMINISTRATORS

Athletic administrators are key stakeholders in establishing and committing to nutrition services and including nutrition professionals in their department's philosophies. Athletic directors make the decision to invest in nutrition services and to offer them as part of the department's plan to carry out its mission. Compliance directors are important in interpreting and applying nutrition-related NCAA legislation at the campus level. They can also help identify available funding sources for special projects or needs (eg, student-athlete opportunity funds or NCAA grant monies). Marketing administrators can be especially valuable when considering contractual agreements with grocery, food retail, or supplement companies. Elements of these contracts can often be negotiated and structured to provide appropriate products or a level of support for nutrition services. These terms can potentially provide financial relief for team operating budgets, sports medicine supply lines, or nutrition department line items. Further, some administrators specifically oversee the construction or renovation of athletic facilities. The collegiate sports dietitian can suggest the inclusion of nutrition-related spaces, such as meal and training table spaces, easily accessible spaces for fueling stations, an area for cooking demonstrations, nutrition office and counseling space, or pre- and postworkout recovery spaces that include adequate food and product storage and food safety measures. Lastly, most athletic departments work with a fund-raising office and have a high-ranking administrator in the organizational structure that oversees the donor support relationships and funds. These administrators can identify potential program donors who may want to contribute to the development of nutrition-related projects or service growth.

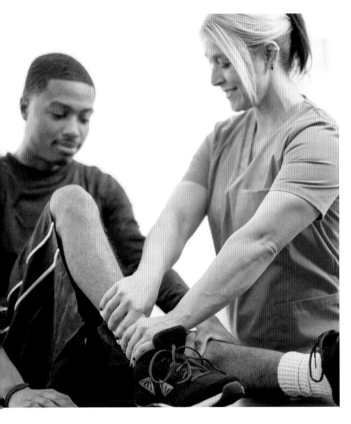

UNIVERSITY SUPPORT SERVICES

Connecting with support services, such as academic support, NCAA Life Skills, and campus foodservices, can enhance and assist the collegiate sports dietitian in his or her goal of educating and feeding the student-athlete. In 2014, the NCAA reached out to its membership to engage in collaborative efforts to renew the NCAA Life Skills program mission of student-athlete wellness. Nutrition knowledge, skill, and education are priorities in the personal enhancement component. Therefore, sports dietitians can support these institutional competencies by offering a variety of educational programming across classes and skill levels. Because planning and coordinating meals is a major function of a collegiate sports dietitian, the campus foodservice vendor is a clear collaborator for the sports RDN. The work of creating and implementing training tables and catered meals as well as purchasing and distributing other food provisions can be eased with strong relationships with foodservice personnel. The foodservice staff can also benefit from the RDN's involvement in providing expertise in recipe analysis and appropriate menu design.

ACADEMIC UNITS

Lastly, interfacing with academic units on campus can provide cooperative associations with many benefits. For example, the RDN may be interested in and able to teach a class, lecture, or serve as a preceptor for nutrition students in return for the opportunity to create internships, independent studies, or experiential learning experiences. The internships and other learning experiences can help the collegiate sports dietitian research special projects, create team education materials, manage fueling stations, and more. Further, the collegiate sports dietitian may be able to work collectively with the athletic and academic departments to create graduate assistant positions for students accepted in graduate degree programs and interested in gaining work experience as a sports dietitian. These positions help train aspiring sports dietitians and provide additional staff support for service delivery. All of these undergraduate and graduate experiences supplement dietetics curricula and improve industry-specific readiness.

National Collegiate Athletic Association Compliance

To work in the field of sports nutrition at the collegiate level, sports dietitians need an understanding of NCAA rules and regulations. The NCAA, through various committee structures, incorporates legislative actions into adopted operating and administrative bylaws. These rules and regulations govern the conduct of intercollegiate member institutions relating to athletic issues such as admissions, financial aid, eligibility, recruiting, and meals. Individual athletic departments are obligated to apply, adhere to, and enforce NCAA legislation. Each institution employs a compliance staff that oversees this function to ensure operational integrity. Most nutrition-related legislation falls within the financial aid, housing and meals, and banned drug list and nutritional supplement bylaws. Box 13.6 (page 288) outlines the major nutrition-related bylaws.

TRAINING TABLE AND MEALS

Significant changes in legislation surrounding athletes' meals took place in 2014. The NCAA lifted restrictions on meals and snacks, effectively deregulating many of the previous food limitations. Meals incidental to athletic participation for all student-athletes became allowable, as well as unlimited snacks. Regulations governing meals and snacks provided by the athletic department have been amended to offer more liberal use of whole foods to meet the unique nutritional needs of student-athletes. Meals used to be considered an extra benefit and limited to one meal per day, and snacks were limited to fruits, nuts, and bagels. Article 16 Awards, Benefits, and Expense for Enrolled Student-Athletes, Bylaw 16.5 Housing and Meals, includes and defines applications related to training table and meals.

Despite the additional meal classifications offered, the NCAA rule stating that institutions can provide one meal classified as a training table meal per day to student-athletes is still in effect.[4] The NCAA does not restrict the choice of meal, foods, or cost for the designated training table meal. This meal can be offered for breakfast, lunch, or dinner and can be specifically designed to meet the needs of the athletes. Each institution, team, or coach, in conjunction with the sports dietitian, should determine which meal provides the most nutritional benefit to the athletes while considering their academic, practice, and extracurricular schedules. The cost of the training table meal can exceed the regular on-campus dining hall rate; however, the difference between the rate and the actual cost of the training table meal must be paid by the athletic department or team budget. For example, if the actual cost of a training table dinner is $20 and the campus door rate for dinner is $14.50, then the athletic department or team is responsible for paying the $5.50 meal cost differential.

Scholarship, recruited nonscholarship, and walk-on athletes who are members of the team are all eligible to participate in the designated training table meal. However, any athlete without a room-and-board allowance must purchase their training table meals. They are eligible to purchase the meal at the board allowance rate vs the actual meal cost. For a scholarship athlete receiving board aid, the institution's determined meal cost is deducted from his or her room-and-board allowance.[4]

In addition to training table meals, institutions can now provide meals considered incidental to athletic participation. These meals do not need to be deducted from board allowances and can be received by any student-athlete not receiving scholarship aid. Collegiate sports dietitians should work with the local compliance staff to understand the application of this new provision. Additionally, if student-athletes miss a meal due to practice activities or an institutional committee meeting, they can still receive a training table meal from the institution provided that they previously paid for the same meal at the institution. Athletes can be provided with meals beginning the evening before a home competition through the time at which they are released at the close of competition. In conjunction with away competition, the NCAA also deregulated what institutions can offer as a snack, stating that institutions can provide snacks during vacation periods and that athletes are eligible to receive meals or the cash value of the meals. In 2014, the NCAA also regulated what institutions can offer as a snack, stating that institutions can provied snacks to student-athletes at any time. Fueling stations with whole foods, beverages, and grab-and-go type foods are now available in many locker rooms and central athletic facilities.

Subsidizing meal costs, training tables, meals incidental to participation, and unlimited snacks requires substantial investment from the athletic department, both financially and from a facility standpoint. Ideally, the training table meal would be served in an athletic facility convenient and accessible to athletes. However, if a specific athletic dining facility does not exist, training table or incidental meals can be catered and brought on-site or to any location. Often teams will have meals delivered to their locker room or team room. Meals can be provided by campus foodservice providers, outside caterers, or local restaurants or athletic departments can opt to support a self-operation foodservice. The landscape has certainly progressed since 1991, when the training table meal was limited to one per day, and from 2009, when the NCAA Housing and Meal Bylaw, Article 16.5, was amended to include provision of fruit, nuts, and bagels at any time. All of the legislative progress offers great flexibility and opportunity for appropriate, high-quality food choices. However, the legislative changes also bring potential operational and budgetary challenges to the athletic department and the collegiate sports dietitian. Armed with a sharp skill set and a full complement of knowledge, the collegiate sports dietitian is an excellent professional to assist in designing solutions to these food-related costs and challenges.

Box 13.6 Major Nutrition-Related Legislation by the National Collegiate Athletic Association[4]

Article 3.2.4 Active Membership. Conditions and Obligations of Membership

Bylaw 3.2.4.7 Drug-Testing Program and Consent Form. An active member shall administer annually, a drug testing consent form for each student-athlete (per Bylaw 12.02.13) pursuant to Bylaw 12.7.3 and shall ensure compliance with the following elements of the NCAA Drug-Testing Program:

(f) Designate an individual (or individuals) as the athletics department resource for questions related to NCAA banned drugs and the use of nutritional supplements; and

(g) Educate athletics department staff members who have regular interaction with student-athletes that:

(1) The NCAA maintains a list of banned drug classes and provides examples of banned substances in each drug class on the NCAA website;

(2) Any nutritional supplement use may present risks to a student-athlete's health and eligibility; and

(3) Questions regarding NCAA banned drugs and the use of nutritional supplements should be to the institution's designated athletics department resource individual (or individuals).

Article 5.3.2 Legislative Authority and Process. Amendment Process

Bylaw 5.3.2.1.2 Division I Legislative Process. Areas of Autonomy. The Atlantic Coast Conference, Big Ten Conference, Big 12 Conference, Pac-12 Conference and Southeastern Conference and their member institutions are granted autonomy in the following areas to permit the use of resources to advance the legitimate educational or athletics-related needs of student-athletes and for legislative changes that will otherwise enhance student-athlete well-being:

(j) Meals and Nutrition. Legislation related to meals and nutritional demands for student-athletes.

Article 15.2 Elements of Financial Aid

Bylaw 15.2.2 Room and Board. An institution may provide a student-athlete financial aid that includes the cost of room and board, based on the official allowance for a room as listed in the institution's official publication (eg, catalog) and a board allowance that consists of three meals per day or the institution's maximum meal plan that is available to all students, whichever is greater.

15.2.2.1 Room and Board Stipend. An institution may provide the student-athlete an amount equal to the institution's official on-campus room allowance as listed in its catalog, the average of the room costs of all of its students living on campus or the cost of room as calculated based on its policies and procedures for calculating the cost of attendance for all students. The institution also may provide the student-athlete an amount that is equivalent to the value of the maximum meal plan that is available to all students or the cost of meals as calculated based on its policies and procedures for calculating the cost of attendance for all students, excluding those meals provided as part of the training table. Meals provided on the training table shall be deducted at the regular cost figure from such a student-athlete's board allowance.

Continued on next page

15.2.2.1.5 Training Table Meals. The cost of meals provided on the institution's training table shall be deducted from a student-athlete's board allowance. In determining the cost figure to be deducted, the institution may use the actual meal costs listed in the institution's catalog or the average meal costs of its student-athletes living on campus.

15.2.2.1.6 Meals Incidental to Participation. The cost of meals and snacks provided as benefits incidental to participation in intercollegiate athletics need not be deducted from a student-athlete's board allowance. Such meals and snacks also may be received by a student-athlete who is not receiving athletically related financial aid inasmuch as they constitute a benefit incidental to athletics participation [see Bylaw 16.5.2-(d)].

Article 16.0 Awards, Benefits and Expenses for Enrolled Student-Athletes

Bylaw 16.5.2 Housing and Meals. Permissible. Identified housing and meal benefits incidental to a student's participation in intercollegiate athletics that may be financed by the institution are:

(c) Training Table Meals. An institution may provide only one training table meal per day to a student-athlete during the academic year on those days when regular institutional dining facilities are open (see Bylaw 15.2.2.1.5). A student-athlete who does not receive institutional athletically related financial aid covering the full cost of board, including a walk-on or partial scholarship recipient, may purchase one training table meal per day at the same rate that the institution deducts from the board allowance of student-athletes who receive athletically related financial aid covering board costs pursuant to Bylaw 15.2.2.1.5.

(d) Meals Incidental to Participation. An institution may provide meals to student-athletes as a benefit incidental to participation in intercollegiate athletics. An institution shall not provide student-athletes with a meal and cash for the same meal.

(1) Cash for Missed Meal Due to Practice Activities. An institution may provide to a student-athlete the cash equivalent of a meal missed due to practice activities only if he or she has previously paid for the meal (either individually or through the board element of a scholarship).

(2) Meals in Conjunction With Home Competition. All student-athletes are permitted to receive meals at the institution's discretion beginning with the evening before competition and continuing until they are released by institutional personnel. An institution shall not provide cash to student-athletes in lieu of meals during this time period. An institution, at its discretion, may provide a meal or cash (not to exceed $15), but not both, to student-athletes at the time of their release by institutional personnel.

(3) Meals in Conjunction With Away-from-Home Competition. An institution may provide meals to student-athletes in conjunction with away-from-home competition pursuant to one of the following options:

(i) All student-athletes are permitted to receive a pregame or postgame meal as a benefit incidental to participation in addition to regular meals (or meal allowances per institutional policy). An institution, at its discretion, may provide cash, not to exceed $15, in lieu of a postgame meal; or

(ii) All student-athletes are permitted to receive meals at the institution's discretion from the time the team is required to report on call for team travel until the team returns to campus. If a student-athlete does not use team travel to return to campus, he or she may receive meals at the institution's discretion up to the point he or she is released from team-related activities by the appropriate institutional authority. An institution shall not provide cash to student-athletes in lieu of meals under this option before their release. An institution may provide a meal or cash (not to exceed $15), but not both, to a student-athlete at the time of his or her release by the institutional authority, regardless of whether he or she uses team travel to return to campus.

(e) Snacks. An institution may provide snacks to a student-athlete at any time.

(g) Nutritional Supplements. An institution may provide permissible nutritional supplements to a student-athlete for the purpose of providing additional calories and electrolytes. Permissible nutritional supplements do not contain any NCAA banned substances and are identified according to the following classes: carbohydrate/electrolyte drinks, energy bars, carbohydrate boosters and vitamins and minerals.

Bylaw 16.8.2 Expenses Provided by the Institution for Practice and Competition. Nonpermissible

16.8.2.2 Conditioning Expenses Outside the Playing Season. An institution shall not provide expenses (eg, travel, lodging, meals) to student-athletes in conjunction with permissible conditioning activities that may occur outside the playing season during the academic year.

Bylaw 16.11 Benefits, Gifts and Services

16.11.1.5 Occasional Meals. A student-athlete or the entire team in a sport may receive an occasional meal in the locale of the institution on infrequent and special occasions from an institutional staff member. An institutional staff member may provide reasonable local transportation to student-athletes to attend such meals. A student-athlete or the entire team in a sport may receive an occasional meal from a representative of athletics interests on infrequent and special occasions under the following conditions:

(a) The meal may only be provided in an individual's home, on campus or at a facility that is regularly used for home competition and may be catered; and

(b) A representative of the institution's athletics interests may provide reasonable local transportation to student-athletes to attend the meal function only if the meal function is at the home of that representative.

DIETARY SUPPLEMENTS

Dietary supplement use, purchase, and provision are regulated by the NCAA. The bylaw states that only non–muscle-building supplements, without banned substances, can be provided for additional calories and electrolytes. When considering dietary supplements, products must be evaluated to ensure that they do not include banned substances. An updated banned substance list is released each year by the NCAA and can be accessed on the NCAA website in the drug testing information of the legislative and governance section. Stimulants, anabolic agents, and diuretics are examples of classes of banned substances.[16] The list also provides examples of banned substances in each class, but the list is not comprehensive. The NCAA maintains that student-athletes are responsible for anything they ingest. Therefore, in 2011, each institution was required to identify a resource person working on campus to answer dietary supplement (and banned drug) questions from student-athletes and staff and serve as the institutional designate. The NCAA provides access to the Resource Exchange Center for all member institutions. The collegiate sports dietitian can play a role in helping safeguard an individual's eligibility by establishing sound product evaluation and review processes and helping student-athletes assess their risk from the perspective of consuming a banned substance, as well as a health and safety perspective.

To purchase dietary supplements on behalf of the athletic department, collegiate sports dietitians must check whether supplements (or their ingredients) are permissible or impermissible to provide. The NCAA defines four classes of non–muscle-building permissible supplements that an institution can purchase to provide additional calories and electrolytes:

- Carbohydrate/electrolyte beverages
- Energy bars
- Carbohydrate boosters
- Vitamins and minerals

Impermissible supplements or ingredients are anything other than these four permissible classes. In 2000, the NCAA published a legislative assistance column and an official interpretation for member institutions, further explaining the intent and application of the supplement bylaw. In addition, a list of common impermissible ingredients identified by the NCAA Committee on Competitive Safeguards was published as examples but not to be used as an exhaustive list.[54] The following are examples of impermissible ingredients/supplements:

- Amino acids
- Conjugated linoleic acid
- Creatine
- Ginseng
- Green tea

The list is updated yearly by the NCAA (www.ncaa.org).

SUMMARY

The role of the sports dietitian at the collegiate level has evolved into a recognized, accepted, and desired component of enhancing performance, assisting in health care needs, and safeguarding the student-athlete's eligibility. The collegiate sports dietitian has a unique opportunity to become highly involved in the intercollegiate operation and the institution's academic environment. The skills and experience needed to carry out the responsibilities require an experienced RDN who is a proficient or expert practitioner. College sports dietitians often do more than provide nutrition services to student-athletes; they also assume administrative, foodservice, and academic duties. Student-athletes have personal and athletic concerns that are often at odds with optimal health. The collegiate sports dietitian can improve their nutrition knowledge and help them eliminate nutrition-related barriers to optimal training, performance, and health.

The athletic department houses many important stakeholders with whom collegiate sports dietitians need to collaborate to ensure success for nutrition services. The relationships established while working with these collegiate athletes are perhaps the most rewarding aspect of the job. The opportunity to contribute to their team and individual successes while becoming part of that team is personally and professionally rewarding.

FUTURE DIRECTIONS

Nearly 20 years ago, Clark wrote, "Opportunities for establishing strong sports nutrition positions at major universities are on the horizon."[2] Many of today's trends suggest that we may, in fact, be arriving at the horizon, and the time is right to move to establish a standard of excellence that will move sports nutrition services toward an unopposed position within colleges and universities. Many efforts have been successful in connecting with the NCAA and influencing legislative progress. The rise in participation and inclusion of additional sport programs likely means that increases in demands and scope of services will soon follow. Varying service models ranging from full-time positions to consulting sports dietitians are emerging; these are necessary to introduce athletic programs to the potential impact sports nutrition departments and individual dietitians can have. Further definition for these models could encourage member institutions across divisions to consider adding nutrition services. Postgraduate, expert-level training and experiences will be needed to keep pace with escalating opportunities and continue to strengthen the overall field. The administrative functions have seen recent rapid growth, and collegiate sports dietitians will want to seek out professional development in these areas.

As the market evolves and the field is able to produce a steady flow of effective, well-rounded practitioners ready to continue blazing these trails, industry standards need to be considered, along with additional advocacy efforts at broadening services, programs, and departments. As policies and procedures are put into place, sports dietitians can begin to assess and publish outcomes. Further research and validation in the areas of service impacts, delivery models, dietary patterns, and nutrition knowledge of today's collegiate athletes could all contribute to advancements. Interested dietitians should focus on becoming proficient experts to improve our abilities to implement evidence-based recommendations for the health and human performance of groups and individuals.

The demands of today's athletic environment have the potential to outpace our readiness and risk limiting our base of practice. Other areas fundamental to future developments are the need for nutrition operation coordinator positions, integration of culinary talent to assist with foodservices, an understanding of sport technology and wearable data interpretation, and examination of how sport science collaboratives can include the collegiate sports dietitian to further develop high-performing, elite athletes.

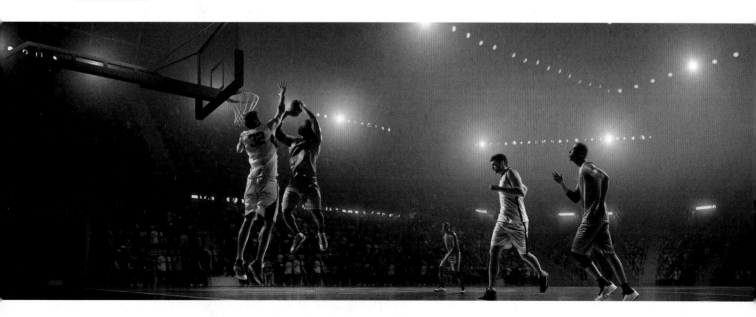

College sports nutrition opportunities are growing due in part to recognition of the discipline's impact on health, safety, and performance and the recent **NCAA** legislative changes that have brought about big foodservice opportunities and challenges, along with new options for athletic administrators. Effectively managing the full scope of need in this environment demands proficient and expert-level practitioners who can wear many hats.

Student-athletes tackle the typical academic, social, health, and personal life stage concerns just like other college students, in addition to managing their training and competition schedules. Either of these can independently or collectively create a continuum of nutritional risk. **RDNs** can be a resource while offering support and treatment for student-athletes.

Nutrition services can be more broadly implemented when the majority of athletic and campus stakeholder relationships are established and these individuals are engaged in the service's mission. Athletic trainers can be pivotal partners in the **RDN**'s work.

Many **NCAA** meal and nutritional supplement bylaws govern the boundaries of these provisions. Collegiate sports dietitians should familiarize themselves with these regulations so they can recommend and implement appropriate services.

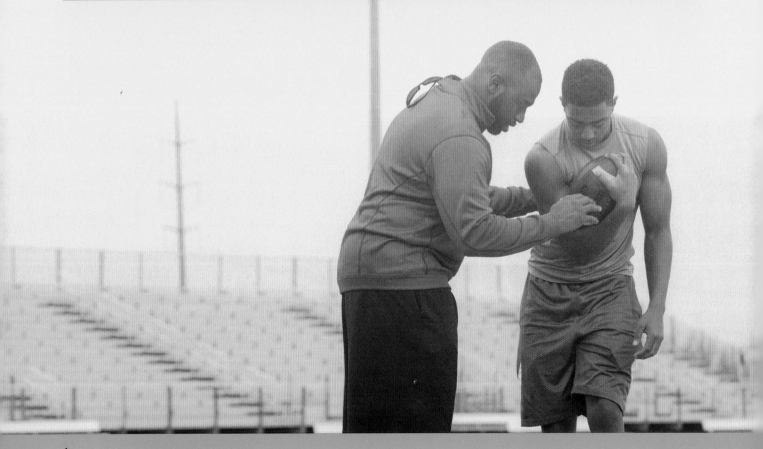

REFERENCES

1. Student-Athlete Participation: 1981-1982–2013-14 NCAA Sports Sponsorship and Participation Rates Report. www.ncaapublications.com/productdownloads/PR1314.pdf. Published October 2014. Accessed September 14, 2015.

2. Clark KL. Working with college athletes, coaches, and trainers at a major university. *Int J Sport Nutr.* 1994;4(2):135-141.

3. Steinmuller PL, Kruskall LJ, Karpinski CA, Manore MM, Macedonio MA, Meyer NL. Academy of Nutrition and Dietetics: revised 2014 standards of practice and standards of professional performance for registered dietitian nutritionists (competent, proficient, and expert) in sports nutrition and dietetics. *J Acad Nutr Diet.* 2014;114(4): 631-641.

4. National Collegiate Athletic Association. *2015-2016 NCAA Division 1 Manual.* Indianapolis, IN: NCAA; August 2015. www.ncaapublications.com/p-4388-2015-2016-ncaa-division-i-manual-august-version-available-august-2015.aspx. Accessed November 13, 2015.

5. The World Anti-Doping Code: The 2015 Prohibited List International Standard. World Anti-Doping Agency. https://wada-main-prod.s3.amazonaws.com/resources/files/wada-2015-prohibited-list-en.pdf. Published January 2016. Accessed March 1, 2016.

6. Quatramoni PA. Clinical observations from nutrition services in college athletics. *J Am Diet Assoc.* 2008;108(4):689-694.

7. McNulty KY, Adams CH, Anderson JM, Affenito SG. Development and validation of a screening tool to identify eating disorders in female athletes. *J Am Diet Assoc.* 2001;101(8):886-892.

8. DeSouza MJ, Nattiv A, Joy E, et al. 2014 Female Athlete Triad Coalition consensus statement on treatment and return to play of the female athlete triad: 1st international conference held in San Francisco, California, May 2012 and 2nd international conference held in Indianapolis, Indiana, May 2013. *Clin J Sports Med.* 2014;24(2):96-119.

9. Mountjoy M, Sundgot-Borgen J, Burke L, et al. The IOC consensus statement: beyond the female athlete triad–relative energy deficiency in sport (RED-S). *Br J Sports Med.* 2014;48(7):491-497.

10. Alaunyte I, Perry JL, Aubrey T. Nutritional knowledge and eating habits of professional rugby league players: does knowledge translate into practice? *J Int Soc Sports Nutr.* 2015;12:18.

11. Folasire OF, Akomolafe AA, Sanusi RA. Does nutrition knowledge and practice of athletes translate to enhanced athletic performance? Cross-sectional study amongst Nigerian undergraduate athletes. *Glob J Health Sci.* 2015;7(5):215-225.

12. Devlin BL, Belski R. Exploring general and sports nutrition and food knowledge in elite male Australian athletes. *Int J Sport Nutr Exerc Metab.* 2015;25(3):225-232.

13. Wade SM, Pope ZC, Simonson SR. How prepared are college freshman athletes for the rigors of college strength and conditioning? A survey of college strength and conditioning coaches. *J Strength Cond Res.* 2014;28(10):2746-2753.

14. Rockwell SM, Nickols-Richardson SM, Thye F. Nutrition knowledge, opinions, and practices of coaches and athletic trainers at a Division I university. *Int J Sports Nutr Exerc Metab.* 2001;11(2):174-185.

15. Torres-McGehee TM, Pritchett KL, Zippel D, Minton DM, Cellamare A, Sibilia M. Sports nutrition knowledge among collegiate athletes, coaches, athletic trainers, and strength and conditioning specialists. *J Athl Train.* 2012;47(2):205-211.

16. 2016-2017 NCAA Banned Drugs. NCAA website. www.ncaa.org/2016-17-ncaa-banned-drugs-list. Accessed October 13, 2016.

17. Buell JL, Franks R, Ransone J, Powers ME, Laquale KM, Carlson-Phillips A. National Athletic Trainers' Association position statement: evaluation of dietary supplements for performance nutrition. *J Athl Train.* 2013;48(1):124-136.

18. Kersey RD, Elliot DL, Goldberg L, et al. National Athletic Trainers' Association position statement: anabolic-androgenic steroids *J Athl Train.* 2012;47(5):567-588.

19. American Diabetes Association position statement: standards of medical care in diabetes—2015. *Diabetes Care.* 2015;38(suppl 1):24S-25S.

20. Jimenez CC, Corcoran MH, Crawley JT, et al. National Athletic Trainers' Association position statement: management of the athlete with type 1 diabetes mellitus. *J Athl Train.* 2007;42(4):536-545.

21. Arnett JJ. Emerging adulthood: a theory of development from the late teens to the twenties. *Am Psychol.* 2000;55(5):469-480.

22. Knox R. The teen brain: it's just not grown up yet. Broadcast on *Morning Edition*, National Public Radio. www.npr.org/templates/story/story.php?storyId=124119468. Broadcast March 1, 2010. Accessed August 3, 2016.

23. Rosenbloom CA, Jonnalagadda SS, Skinner, R. Nutrition knowledge of collegiate athletes in a Division I National Collegiate Athletic Association institution. *J Am Diet Assoc.* 2002;102(3):418-420.

24. Pawlak R, Malinauskas B, Rivera D. Predicting intentions to eat a healthful diet by college baseball players: applying the theory of planned behavior. *J Nutr Educ Behav.* 2009;41(5):334-349.

25. Hornstrom GR, Friesen CA, Ellery JE, Pike K. Nutrition knowledge, practices, attitudes and information sources of Mid-American Conference college softball players. *Food and Nutr Sci.* 2011;2:109-117.

26. Valliant MW, Emplaincourt HP, Wenzel RK, Garner BH. Nutrition education by a registered dietitian improves dietary intake and nutrition knowledge of a NCAA female volleyball team. *Nutrients*. 2012;4(6):505-516.

27. US Department of Agriculture, US Department of Health and Human Services. *Dietary Guidelines for Americans 2015-2020*. 8th ed. Washington, DC: US Government Printing Office; December 2015. www.cnpp.usda.gov/sites/default/files/dietary_guidelines_for_americans/PolicyDoc.pdf. Accessed September 23, 2015.

28. National Center for Chronic Disease Prevention and Health Promotion, Division of Nutrition, Physical Activity, and Obesity. *State Indicator Report on Fruits and Vegetables*. Atlanta, GA: Centers for Disease Control and Prevention; 2013. www.cdc.gov/nutrition/downloads/State-Indicator-Report-Fruits-Vegetables-2013.pdf. Accessed September 23, 2015.

29. Ford JA. Substance use among college athletes: a comparison based on sport/team affiliation. *J Am Coll Health*. 2007;55(6):367-373.

30. National Collegiate Athletic Association. NCAA study of substance use habits of college student-athletes 2005. Presented to: The National Collegiate Athletic Association Committee on Competitive Safeguards and Medical Aspects of Sports by the NCAA research staff, 2006. http://files.eric.ed.gov/fulltext/ED503214.pdf Accessed December 14, 2016.

31. National Collegiate Athletic Association. NCAA national study of substance use habits of college student-athletes final report 2014—NCAA research. www.ncaa.org/sites/default/files/Substance%20Use%20Final%20Report_FINAL.pdf. Revised August 2014. Accessed September 24, 2015.

32. American College Health Association. American College Health Association-National College Health Assessment II. Reference Group Executive Summary. Honover www.acha-ncha.org. Accessed September 25, 2015.

33. American College Health Association National College Health Assessment II: Spring 2014 Reference Group Executive Summary Spring 2014. Hanover, MD: American College Health Association; 2014. www.acha-ncha.org/docs/ACHA-NCHA-II_ReferenceGroup_ExecutiveSummary_Spring2014.pdf. Accessed September 25, 2015.

34. American College of Sports position statement on the use of alcohol in sports. *Med Sci Sports Exerc*. 1982;14:ix-xi.

35. Burak LJ. Smokeless tobacco education for college athletes. *J Phys Educ Recreat Dance*. 2001;72(1):37-45.

36. Thomas DT, Erdman KA, Burke LM. Position of the Academy of Nutrition and Dietetics, Dietitians of Canada, and the American College of Sports Medicine: nutrition and athletic performance. *J Acad Nutr Diet*. 2016;116(3):501-528.

37. Cowell BS, Rosenbloom CA, Skinner R, Summers SH. Policies on screening female athletes for iron deficiency in NCAA Division I-A institutions. *Int J Sports Nutr Exerc Metab*. 2003;13(3):277-285.

38. Eichner R. Anemia and female athletes. *Sports Med Dig*. 2000;22:57.

39. National Collegiate Athletic Association Committee on Competitive Safeguards and Medical Aspects of Sports. *NCAA 2009 Survey: Member Institution's Drug-Education And Drug-Testing Programs*. www.ncaa.org/sites/default/files/16.%20INstitutional%20DrugEducation%20and%20TestingSurvey2009.pdf. Accessed September 22, 2010.

40. Froiland K, Koszewski W, Hingst J, Kopecky L. Nutritional supplement use among college athletes and their sources of information. *Int J Sport Nutr Exerc Metab*. 2004;14(1):104-120.

41. Hootman JM, Dick, R Agel J. Epidemiology of collegiate injuries for 15 sports: summary and recommendations for injury prevention initiatives. *J Athl Train* 2007;42(2):311-319.

42. Wall BT, Morton JP, Van Loon LJC. Strategies to maintain skeletal muscle mass in the injured athlete: nutritional considerations and exercise mimetics. *Eur J Sport Sci*. 2015;15(1):53-62.

43. Assessment of body composition. In: *2014-15 NCAA Sports Medicine Handbook*. 25th ed. Indianapolis, IN: The National Collegiate Athletic Association; August 2014. www.ncaapublications.com/productdownloads/MD15.pdf. Accessed August 3, 2016.

44. Lloyd-Jones DM, Hong Y, Labarthe D, et al; American Heart Association Strategic Planning Task Force and Statistics Committee. AHA Special Report: Defining and setting national goals for cardiovascular health promotion and disease reduction; The American Heart Association's strategic impact goal through 2020 and beyond. *Circulation*. 2010;12(4)1:586-613.

45. Crawford M. Screening athletes for heart disease. *Heart*. 2007;93(7):875-879.

46. Muňoz L, Norgan G, Rauschhuber M, et al. An exploratory study of cardiac health in college athletes. *Appl Nurs Res*. 2009;22(4):228-235.

47. Borchers JR, Clem KL, Habash DL, Nagaraja HN, Stokley LM, Best TM. Metabolic syndrome and insulin resistance in Division I collegiate football players. *Med Sci Sports Exerc*. 2009;41(12):2105-2110.

48. Greenleaf C, Petrie TA, Carter J, Reel JJ. Female collegiate athletes: prevalence of eating disorders and disordered eating behaviors. *J Am Coll Health*. 2009;57(5):489-495.

49. Johnson C, Powers PS, Dick R. Athletes and eating disorders: the National Collegiate Athletic Association study. *Int J Eat Disord*. 1999;26(2):179-188.

50. Beals KA, Hill AK. The prevalence of disordered eating, menstrual dysfunction and low bone mineral density among US collegiate athletes. *Int J Sport Nutr Exerc Metab*. 2006;16(1):1-23.

51. Kroshus E, Fischer AN, Nichols JF. Assessing the awareness and behaviors of U.S. high school nurses with respect to the female athlete triad. *J Sch Nurs*. 2015;31(4):272-279.

52. Brown KN, Wengreen HJ, Beals KA. Knowledge of the female athlete triad and prevalence of triad risk factors among female high school athletes and their coaches. *J Pediatr Adolesc Gynecol*. 2014;27(5):278-282.

53. Sherman R, Thompson R; National Collegiate Athletic Association. *NCAA Coaches Handbook: Managing the Female Athlete Triad*. http://athletewellness.uncg.edu/wp-content/uploads/2014/05/Coaches-Handbook.pdf. Accessed August 3, 2016.

54. NCAA issues notice about nutritional-supplement provision. NCAA website. Published May 23, 2005. http://fs.ncaa.org/Docs/NCAANewsArchive/2005/Association-wide/index.html. Accessed August 3, 2016.

CHAPTER 14

MASTERS ATHLETES

Christine A. Rosenbloom, PhD, RDN, CSSD, FAND

INTRODUCTION

What do athletes do when they get older and are no longer competitive in the sport they love? Many of them are taking on a new title: masters athlete. Events for masters athletes can range from sanctioned events provided through formal governing bodies, such as USA Track & Field, to events such as the Huntsman World Senior Games held annually in Utah. In 2014, the World Senior Games hosted a record 10,856 athletes age 50 years and older competing in 27 sports representing 24 countries, a substantial increase from the 500 athletes who competed in the inaugural senior games were held in 1985. Almost every city and country in the world—from Auckland, New Zealand, to Vancouver, Canada—has an association devoted to masters athlete competitions. It is uncertain how many masters athletes there are worldwide, but almost every country has competitions designed for masters athletes. Box 14.1 provides an overview of some of the major organizations devoted to masters athletics.

Box 14.1 Examples of Masters Athlete Organizations

Organization	Description
National Senior Games: www.nsga.com	*History:* Originated as National Senior Olympics in 1985. Held first National Senior Olympics in 1987 with 2,500 competitors. Changed name to US National Senior Organization in 1990. Today known as National Senior Games. Athletes must be age 50 years or older and qualify through National Senior Games Association State Games.
	Sponsored activities: The Games is a 19-sport biennial competition for men and women and is the largest multisport event in the world for seniors.
International Masters Games Association (IMGA): www.imga.ch	*History:* First World Masters Games were held in 1985. Reorganized in 1995 as IMGA from member international federations to represent masters sports worldwide.
	Sponsored activities: World Masters Games, Winter World Masters Games, and European Masters Games are held every 4 years. The inaugural Americas Masters Games were held in 2016.
Huntsman World Senior Games: www.seniorgames.net	*History:* Began as World Senior Games in 1987. Today known as Huntsman World Senior Games. Open to any athletes age 50 years or older.
	Sponsored activities: Yearly competitions in St. George, Utah.
World Masters Athletics: www.world-masters-athletics.org	*History:* Begun by middle-aged road runners; first organized event was held in 1975. It has evolved into an international masters organization for track and field for those age 35 years or older.
	Sponsored activities: Sponsors area and world championships in both stadia (events held within a stadium, such as track-and-field and track running events) and nonstadia (events held on the road, such as cross-country and longer distance events).

WHO ARE MASTERS ATHLETES?

Many sports have masters divisions defined by the rules of the governing body (eg, USA Track & Field, World Masters Athletics, or National Senior Games Association) or a separate organization designed to meet the needs of retired professional athletes (eg, the Professional Golfers' Association Tour Champions and Association of Tennis Professionals Champions Tour). The age at which one becomes a "master" ranges from sport to sport and can be as young as 18 years (swimming) or as old as 50 years (golf). The World Masters Athletics organization defines the age for masters athletes as beginning at age 35 years for women and men. Competition is also age graded, usually in 5-year intervals. The website of the International Association of Athletics Federations displays records for masters events in age-graded categories up to the 95- to 99-year-old group. The focus of this chapter is on masters athletes who are age 50 years or older.

AGING IN THE UNITED STATES

The number of older people who will be competing at a masters level in athletics is unknown, but the population is aging, and it is a global phenomenon. In the United States, the number of people age 65 and older numbered 44.7 million in 2013, an increase of 8.8 million, or 24.7%, since 2003. In the US government-issued report *Profile of Older Americans: 2014* the following statistics are presented[1]:

- The number of Americans age 45 to 64 years who will reach 65 during the next 20 years had increased by 20.7% during the previous 10 years.
- More than one in seven, or 14.1%, of the population was older than 65 years.
- Individuals reaching age 65 had an average life expectancy of an additional 19.3 years (20.5 years for females and 17.9 years for males).
- There were more than 67,000 centenarians in 2013.

In 1900 there were 4.9 million persons age 60 years and older in the United States. That jumped to 45.8 million in 2000. It is projected that there will be 92.2 million older adults in 2030 and 112 million in 2050.[2]

The fitness industry is taking notice of the aging population. Gym and fitness memberships used to be concentrated in the 18- to 34-year-old range, but there is increased membership among those over age 50. Appealing to older adults has been called essential for gym franchises, and they have added such amenities as health maintenance services, including measuring and monitoring blood sugar, blood pressure, and bone density.[3]

Growth in masters competitions in recent years suggests increasing numbers in the future. In reviewing data for the New York City Marathon from 1983 through 1999, Joki and colleagues showed that older age groups had the largest relative increase in participation, and, as a group, masters athlete improved their performance times at a greater rate than younger athletes over the past 17 years.[4] Older women athletes outpaced older men in both participation and performance.

EXERCISE RECOMMENDATIONS AND BENEFITS OF EXERCISE IN ADULTS

In 1996, the US Surgeon General issued *Physical Activity and Health: A Report of the Surgeon General*, the first report of its kind. In the same year, the World Health Organization issued *The Heidelberg Guidelines for Promoting Physical Activity Among Older Persons*, stressing both the individual as well as the societal benefits of physical activity. The physical, mental, and societal benefits of a physically active lifestyle are summarized in Box 14.2 (page 298). These seminal reports concluded that regular physical activity induces higher cardiopulmonary fitness, which decreases overall mortality, reduces risk of coronary heart disease and high blood pressure, reduces the risk of colon cancer, protects against the development of type 2 diabetes mellitus, builds bone mass, increases muscle strength and balance, helps control body weight, relieves the symptoms of depression and anxiety, and improves mood.[5,6]

Box 14.2 Benefits of a Physically Active Lifestyle[5,6]

Physiological Responses

- Decreased resting blood pressure
- Increased cardiac output
- Increased blood flow to skeletal muscles and skin
- Increased maximal oxygen uptake (VO_2 max)
- Increased components of the immune system, such as natural killer cells and circulating T-lymphocytes and B-lymphocytes
- Increased bone mass
- Increased high-density lipoprotein cholesterol
- Increased strength and balance
- Normalized blood glucose levels

Health Benefits

- Decreased overall mortality
- Decreased risk of cardiovascular disease
- Decreased risk of hypertension
- Decreased risk of thrombosis
- Decreased risk of colon cancer
- Decreased risk of type 2 diabetes mellitus
- Decreased risk of obesity
- Decreased risk of falls and fractures in older adults
- Decreased symptoms of depression and anxiety
- Improved sleep
- Enhanced relaxation
- Enhanced mood state
- Increased psychological well-being
- Enhanced social and cultural integration

Societal Benefits

- Reduced health and social care costs
- Enhanced productivity of older adults
- A positive and active image of older adults

Since the initial government reports were released, the American College of Sports Medicine issued a position stand on exercise for older adults. The position stand concludes that older adults (most of the evidence was based on individuals over age 65, but younger adults were also included when relevant) benefit from four types of physical activity: aerobic exercise training, resistance exercise, flexibility exercise to extend range of motions in joints, and balance training to strengthen the lower body to reduce risk of falls.[7] The Centers for Disease Control and Prevention has expanded the recommendations to quantify that all adult Americans older than 65 years of age should get at least 150 minutes of moderate-intensity aerobic activity every week and perform muscle-strengthening activities that work the major muscles two or more times per week.[8] At every age, exercise induces beneficial physiological adaptations that improve functional abilities.

WHAT DO WE KNOW ABOUT AGING AND SPORT?

It is common to classify aging based on chronological age, but chronological age is a poor predictor of functional age. Someone may be 50 years old (chronological age) but, due to a sedentary lifestyle, may have difficulty performing activities of daily living (functional age). A 75-year-old who has been physically active throughout life may have better functional capacity than a much younger person who has not been active. For example, a 65-year-old masters athlete at may outperform a sedentary 25-year-old on measures of maximum oxygen consumption (VO_2 max), muscle strength, and flexibility.[9]

Peak performance in a sport depends on the key functional element required for success. For example, in sports such as gymnastics, for which flexibility is crucial, top athletes are usually in their teens. In aerobic sports, competitors usually peak in their mid-20s when training improvements and competition experience help athletes, but, in general, most champions are not older than mid to late 30s. In sports like golf, the best athletes are generally in their 30s or 40s.[9]

For some activities, aging may mean improved performance. For example, marathon times in older athletes have improved dramatically. In October 2011, an 80-year-old ran a 3:15:54 marathon—a remarkable feat when you consider that this 80-year-old averaged less than 7.5 minutes per mile for the 26.2 mile course. Lepers and Cattagni analyzed running times in the New York City Marathon from 1980 through 2009 and found that during that period not only did the participation of masters runners increase but the times of older runners also significantly improved (for men older than 64 years and women older than 44 years).[10] The authors concluded that master runners have "probably not yet reached their limits in marathon performance." As another example, Akkari and colleagues studied running and swimming times of masters athletes, using data from masters organizations databases from 1975 through 2013. Age groups were separated into eight 5-year segments, spanning ages 40 to 79. A progressive improvement in athletic event time was significantly greater as age increased, leading to the conclusion that not only is participation in masters competition increasing but the performance also continues to improve.[11]

AGE-RELATED PHYSIOLOGICAL CHANGES

This section will review some age-related physiological changes and how the changes are attenuated in masters athletes. Research on masters athletes is frequently conducted on endurance athletes, and the physiological benefits of aerobic exercise are found in almost every body system. In general, the research on masters athletes shows that participation in competition at the masters level confers physical and psychological benefits.[12-16] Data are limited on many aspects of age changes in older athletes, but examples from the literature are cited when available.

Oxygen Uptake and Aerobic Capacity

Maximum oxygen consumption decreases by about 10% per decade in healthy adults beginning at about age 30 years. In older endurance athletes, the decline is still evident, but it occurs at a slower rate of about 5% per decade.[17] Researchers note that it is hard to determine how much of this loss is due to the normal aging process or to the adoption of a more sedentary lifestyle. In a longitudinal study of 42 athletes, Katzel and colleagues found a 22% decrease in VO_2 max in older endurance athletes during an 8-year follow-up period. The greatest decrease in VO_2 max occurred in athletes who could not maintain a high volume of training, suggesting that the decrease in VO_2 max is related less to aging and more to an inactive lifestyle. In this study, only 7 athletes (17% of study participants) were still training at high volume at the end of the study. The authors concluded that maintaining a high level of aerobic fitness, even for a highly motivated athlete, becomes more difficult with advancing age.[18] Exercise can improve oxygen uptake, but even the most fit masters athlete will see some decline in oxygen uptake as he or she ages.

Muscle Quantity and Quality

Muscle strength declines with age. The average strength of individuals in their 80th decade is about 40% less than those in their 20s.[19] This is important because muscle strength is a strong predictor of several detrimental outcomes: slower gait speed, increased risk of falls, and increased risk of hospitalization and mortality. Compared with older adults with high muscle strength, older adults with low muscle strength have a 4.3-fold greater risk for slow gait speed and a 2.6-fold greater risk for severe mobility problems. Many changes at both the cellular and molecular level appear to contribute to changes in aging muscle. These include a decrease in size and number of type II muscle fibers, a shift from fast to slow fiber type, reduced number of mitochondria, reduced number of satellite cells, infiltration of fat into muscle, reduction in myosin and protein content and function, and reduced elasticity of muscle.[20] Melov and colleagues reported that a 6-month resistance training program can reverse muscle weakness and improve muscle strength in healthy older adults.[21] The Cochrane Review of 121 randomized control trials including 6,700 participants shows that progressive resistance strength training is an effective intervention for improving physical functioning of older adults.[19] How these data relate to nutritional interventions will be covered later in this chapter.

Body Composition

"Aging is a process that has deleterious effects in nearly every facet of human body composition."[22] In general, aging results in:

- increases in belly (abdominal) fat;
- increases in fat deposits in skeletal and heart muscle, liver, and bone marrow;
- increases in body weight up until about the age of 70 in both women and men; and
- redistribution of body fat with increase in visceral fat and decreases in peripheral fat stores.

Many of these changes cannot be assessed with the typical anthropometric measures commonly available in outpatient settings (ie, body weight, waist circumference, skinfold measurements). What is unclear is if these changes are due to lifestyle or a combination of age-related physiological metabolic processes. It is beyond the scope of this chapter to discuss sex, racial, or ethnic differences in body composition. See Kuk and colleagues for a thorough review of the literature.[22]

Researchers have not yet clearly demonstrated if exercise erases all of these body composition changes, because that is not directly reported in the masters athlete literature. However, many studies on masters athletes designed to assess other physiological changes frequently report weight, percent body fat, and percent lean mass as demographic information. From these studies, it is clear that body weight of masters athletes is more likely than that of nonathletes to remain in the healthy range of body mass index (BMI) of 18.5 to 24.9 kg/m².[12,14,15,18]

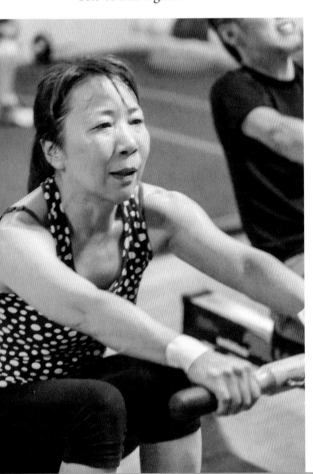

In addition to increases in adiposity with aging, a decrease in muscle mass is also observed. Wroblewski and colleagues wanted to know if chronic exercise, such as practiced by masters athletes, could attenuate changes in body composition. The researchers recruited 20 men and 20 women who trained for masters competitions four or five times or more per week. The athletes ranging in age from 40 to over 70 years (five men and five women in each 10-year age group of 40 through 49, 50 through 59, 60 through 69, and 70 and older). In this population, chronic exercise training preserved lean muscle mass while preventing fat infiltration into other tissues. Not all body composition changes were attenuated; there was a slight increase in total body fat, but it appears that exercise training can help prevent some of the deleterious changes in body composition with aging.[23]

Cardiovascular Health and Disease Risk

For years, aerobic exercise has been recommended to lower risk of cardiovascular disease. Seals and colleagues found that endurance-trained masters athletes have more favorable lipid profiles compared with both younger men and older sedentary men.[13] Specifically, high-density lipoprotein cholesterol was significantly higher in the masters athletes, which may confer a reduced risk for coronary artery disease.[17]

A longitudinal study on coronary heart disease (CHD) risk factors in older track athletes was reported by Mengelkoch and colleagues. Twenty-one participants, age 60 to 92 years, were assessed at three evaluation points (initial, 10 year, and 20 year). Measurements included smoking history, blood pressure, resting electrocardiogram, total cholesterol, plasma glucose, body weight, percentage body fat, BMI, waist-to-hip ratio, and VO$_2$ max. All CHD risk factors remained low, and even after 20 years, all values for variables measured were within normal limits. In this study, the prevalence of CHD risk factors remained low into old age in masters athletes, indicating that regular activity has a favorable effect on physical measurements that impact chronic disease risk.[14]

However, while exercise appears to offer benefits on lipid levels into old age in masters athletes, a hiatus from training of just 2 months resulted in a reversal of the favorable lipid profile found in trained cyclists. Like the decreases in VO$_2$ max found with decreased training volume, it seems that continued exercise is necessary to maintain a favorable lipid profile in older athletes.[15]

Impaired glucose tolerance is also associated with metabolic syndrome, a set of risk factors tied to increased risk of heart disease. Seals and colleagues compared endurance-trained masters athletes (mean age = 60 years) with young endurance-trained men (mean age = 26 years) and found that the masters athletes had a significantly blunted insulin response after the glucose challenge similar to that of the young athletes when given an oral glucose tolerance test.[16] These data suggest that deterioration of glucose tolerance is not a consequence of the normal aging process and that regular, vigorous physical activity can prevent the deterioration of glucose tolerance and insulin sensitivity.[17] Exercise is a top-line recommendation to improve glucose disposal, moderate blood sugar levels, and blunt insulin levels.[24] Higher levels of physical activity are also related to lowering hemoglobin A1C (HbA1c) in both younger and older adults.[25]

Bone Health

There is increasing interest in bone health in the older population, and osteoporosis is considered a major public health concern. According to the National Osteoporosis Foundation, approximately 54 million Americans over 50 years of age are affected by low bone mass or osteoporosis. Currently, 10.2 million individuals have osteoporosis, and an estimated 43.4 million individuals have been diagnosed with osteopenia (low bone mass). Eighty percent of those affected by osteoporosis are women.[26]

Exercise, especially weight-bearing exercise, confers benefits to bone mineral density (BMD). Loading the skeleton with weight improves the strength and density of bones.[2] Research with masters athletes has found that habitual physical exercise throughout life can help preserve bone health. Florindo measured BMD in more than 300 Brazilian athletes over the age of 50 and found significant positive associations between physical activity and bone mass density in older men.[27]

Non–weight-bearing exercise, like swimming, is thought to be less effective in protecting bone, but female runners and swimmers recruited from the 2005 National Senior Olympics were found to have *z* scores well above the national average for their age and sex, suggesting that exercise has a positive effect on mediating bone loss in older women.[28]

Summary of Physiological Changes with Aging Overview

Currently, there is not abundant research on all body systems and the benefits of physical activity in masters athletes. Most of the studies involve athletes competing in endurance events (predominantly running and cycling), but research shows clearly that people who maintain an active lifestyle reap many physical health benefits. Chronic diseases such as cardiovascular disease, hypertension, and diabetes are less prevalent in masters athletes compared with age-matched sedentary persons. Changes considered a typical consequence of aging, such as reduced muscle mass and strength, reduced aerobic capacity, bone loss, and deterioration of the insulin response to a glucose challenge, seem to be minimized in masters athletes because of their lifelong habit of physical activity. These athletes might very well use it and not lose it.

It is unfortunate that practitioners and specialists have so few studies on energy and macronutrient and micronutrient intakes of masters athletes. Sports dietitians and researchers in the field of sports medicine will find this area ripe for study to add to the scant body of literature. This section gives an overview of what we know.

Energy Intake and Expenditure and Exercise

There is evidence to suggest that energy needs decrease with age. Approximately one-third of the decrease in energy needs is related to a decrease in basal metabolic rate (BMR) and the remainder to decreases in physical activity. However, most research on BMR in older adults does not include individuals who vigorously exercise. Even so, Van Pelt and colleagues concluded that resting metabolic rate (RMR) decreases with age, even in highly active older men, but the decrease is related to age-associated decreases in exercise training volume and intensity.[29]

The Dietary Reference Intakes (DRIs) for energy and macronutrient intakes established estimated energy requirements (EERs) at four levels of energy expenditure. But, even the category of active physical activity level, as described by the DRI report, may be too low for a masters athlete. Table 14.1 shows EERs for active older adults, which may be used to determine individualized energy needs.[30]

Table 14.1 Estimated Energy Requirements for Active Older Adults[26]

Age Group, y	Men, kcal/d	Women, kcal/d
50–59	2,757	2,186
60–69	2,657	2,116
70–79	2,557	2,046
80–89	2,457	1,976

Few studies have assessed energy needs of older exercisers. In the studies that have tried to quantify energy needs, results have shown that energy needs do not differ for masters athletes compared with younger athletes.[31,32] The main factor predicting energy needs is the volume of exercise, not aging, per se. One review of energy expenditure and aging concluded that regular participation in physical activity (aerobic activities, primarily running) may attenuate the age-related decrease in RMR.[33]

Even fewer studies have assessed energy needs of masters athletes engaged in strength-training. Campbell and colleagues studied the effects of 12 weeks of progressive resistance training on energy balance in sedentary, healthy older adults (eight men and four women, ages 56 to 80 years). At the end of 12 weeks of strength-training, muscular strength increased, fat-free mass increased, fat mass decreased, and mean energy intake needed to maintain body weight increased by approximately 15% during the resistance-training program.[34]

Studies have reported that exercise training increases the thermic effect of food (TEF) in older people. Lundholm and colleagues studied active, well-conditioned men (mean age = 70 years) participating in aerobic exercise three to five times per week for at least 1 hour. Case controls were used for comparison. Participants were fed a liquid formula containing 500 kcal (56% carbohydrate, 24% protein, 20% fat), and BMR was measured. Higher oxygen uptake was found in the well-trained men compared with the sedentary control group, and the TEF was significantly increased (approximately 56%). The authors concluded that, in this study, physical activity seemed to have a potentiating effect on TEF in older people.[35]

Although scant research exists on energy needs of masters athletes, practitioners can use the same energy equations they use for younger athletes in assessing energy needs. It is important to accurately quantify activity because training tends to decrease in older athletes, and, therefore, based on training volume, energy expenditure might not be as high. For more detail on energy balance, see Chapter 10.

Carbohydrate

Carbohydrate should provide the major source of energy in any athlete's diet (see Chapter 2). DRIs suggest a carbohydrate range of 45% to 65% of total energy.[30] Although no ideal level of carbohydrate consumption has been defined for masters athletes, the guidelines used for younger athletes should be recommended: 3 to 5 g/kg/d for very light, low-intensity skill exercise, 5 to 7 g/kg/d for moderate-intensity exercise or those training for about an hour a day, and 6 to 10 g/kg/d for endurance athletes who train at moderate intensity for 1 to 3 h/d. Flexibility is important in establishing carbohydrate goals, recognizing that individual preferences, as well as training and competition schedules, may necessitate adjustment of carbohydrate intake. To meet fuel needs and general nutrition goals, athletes who exercise less than 1 h/d with moderate-intensity activity or several hours with low-intensity exercise should aim for 3 to 5 g/kg/d.[36] Currently, there is no reason to believe that masters athletes would not benefit from the same carbohydrate recommendations, based on studies of younger adult athletes.[37]

Many masters athletes may be confused about the role of carbohydrate in sport because they are exposed to media messages that promote protein as good and carbohydrate as bad. Drastically cutting carbohydrate intake while increasing protein foods may diminish the athlete's performance. Aiming for quality carbohydrates (whole grains, fruits, vegetables, and reduced-fat dairy), while decreasing refined carbohydrates and sugar-rich foods, is one strategy to help athletes consume adequate carbohydrate to meet the demands of training and competition, maintain energy balance, and reduce risk for some chronic diseases.

Protein

The debate about protein needs of exercising individuals is not new, but the context of aging poses the question: What are the dietary protein requirements of masters athletes? Due to insufficient research and individual variation, it is impossible to answer this question, and there may never be an answer. When conducting research on protein requirements for older adults, the definition of older adult often used is someone aged 65 year or older. Nutrition and resistance exercise are both needed to stimulate muscle protein synthesis (MPS); however, older adults may need higher intakes of protein than younger adults to stimulate MPS.[38-40] The term *anabolic resistance* is used to describe the decreased sensitivity of muscle to small amounts of dietary protein in aging individuals.[38]

There is mounting evidence, supported by several consensus statements, that the Recommended Dietary Allowance for protein (0.8 g/kg body weight) is inadequate to promote optimal health in older adults. Recent research indicates that the timing and distribution of protein throughout the day is important for stimulating MPS and maintaining muscle mass and function in older adults.[38,41,42]

In young men, 20 g protein is the suggested amount per meal to stimulate MPS, but in older adults, it appears to be greater, at about 35 to 40 g protein per meal.[40] Moore and colleagues suggest 0.4 g protein per kilogram per meal or 1.2 g protein per kilogram per day, along with resistance exercise to overcome anabolic resistance.[38] Ingesting specific quantities of protein at each meal, equally spaced throughout the day, appears to confer the greatest advantage for older adults. Most adults consume less than 15 g protein at breakfast, while the evening meal typically contains more than 60% of daily protein.[39]

The European Union Geriatric Medicine Society appointed an international study group to review dietary protein needs with aging. The PROT-AGE Study Group made the following recommendations:

- To maintain and regain muscle, older adults (>65 years) should consume 1.0 to 1.2 g protein per kilogram body weight per day.

- Premeal anabolic threshold of dietary protein and amino acids intake is higher in older adults compared with younger adults, and recommended intake is 25 to 30 g protein per meal with 2.5 to 2.6 g leucine.[43]

For more information on protein and the amino acid leucine as they relate to athletes, see Chapter 3.

Fat

The recommended daily intake of fat for athletes is approximately 1 g/kg. Recommended fat intake for older active people does not differ from that for younger people. An intake of 20% of energy from fat ensures adequate intake of essential fatty acids, with 30% to 35% of energy from fat as the upper limit recommended by most professional health organizations.[44] DRIs suggest fat ranges of 20% to 35% of total energy.[30] The *Dietary Guidelines for Americans 2015–2020* recommends limiting saturated fats to 10% of calories and replacing saturated fats with unsaturated fats. The limits on dietary cholesterol are not emphasized; however, dietary cholesterol should be considered within the context of a healthy eating plan. Many foods high in cholesterol are also high in saturated fats; two exceptions are eggs and shellfish. While high in cholesterol, they are low in saturated fats and provide good sources of high-quality protein for aging athletes.[45]

Micronutrients Overview

Ideal vitamin and mineral requirements for older individuals have yet to be established. DRIs recognize the increased need for some micronutrients in people older than age 50 years.[44] DRIs for vitamins D, B-6, and B-12 and the mineral calcium are higher for older adults, and DRI for iron is decreased for older women. Deficiencies in micronutrients can impair exercise tolerance, but little is known about the dietary intakes or requirements of masters athletes.

Only a few studies have assessed nutrient intakes in masters athletes, and nothing current is found in the literature. Nieman and colleagues studied completed 3-day food records from 291 masters men and 56 masters women who participated in the 1987 Los Angeles Marathon. The masters men marathoners averaged 2,526 kcal/d, and the masters women marathoners averaged 1,868 kcal/d. In this study, the marathoners consumed a greater percentage of their energy from carbohydrate and a smaller percentage of energy from fat compared with data for the general population. Nieman and colleagues found that the women runners had low intakes of vitamin D and zinc compared with the recommended daily allowance.[46]

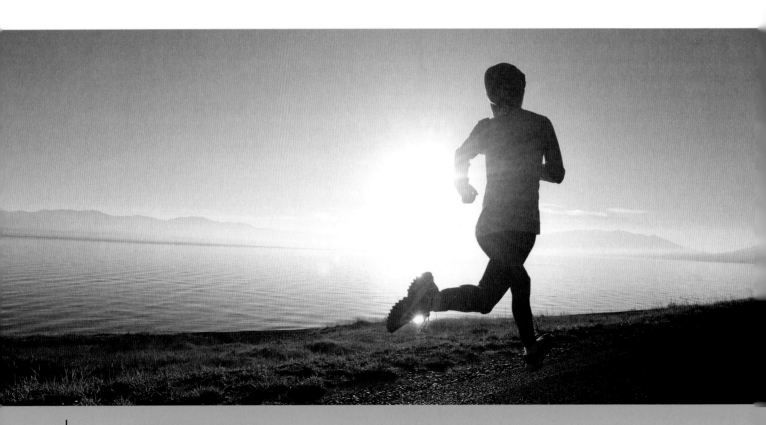

A handful of other studies have found that while masters athletes consume more calories than sedentary age-matched individuals and more than predicted energy intakes based on the national dietary guidelines, masters athletes are not meeting all of the nutrient intake targets. Specifically, they have low intakes of vitamins D and E, folic acid, calcium, zinc, and magnesium.[47,48]

We could benefit from additional studies to assess micronutrient intakes in masters athletes, but at this time there is paucity of research.

CLOSER LOOK AT CALCIUM AND VITAMIN D

Two micronutrients warrant special mention for older adults: vitamin D and calcium. Vitamin D is important for many biological functions, but its role in maximizing bone health and muscle function are of critical importance for older adults. Without vitamin D, only 10% to 15% of calcium is absorbed.[49] Aging decreases the ability of the skin to produce vitamin D-3. The Endocrine Society Clinical Guidelines suggest the following:

- Measure serum circulating a 25(OH)D to evaluate vitamin D status. (This is the major circulating form of vitamin D.)
- Vitamin D deficiency is defined as a 25(OH)D level of less than 20 ng/mL.
- Vitamin D insufficiency is defined as a 25(OH)D level of 21 to 29 ng/mL.
- Adults aged 50 to 70 years require at least 600 IU vitamin D per day; adults over age 70 need 800 IU per day.
- To raise levels consistently above 30 ng/mL, adults may need 1,500 to 2,000 IU vitamin D per day.[49]

In addition to vitamin D, calcium is critical to maintaining bone mass in older adults. Calcium requirements increase with age to 1,200 mg/day for women over 51 years of age and for men over 71 years of age.[44] While most of the research on calcium intake and BMD is focused on older women, Reid and colleagues wanted to know if calcium supplementation could improve BMD in older men. In a randomized, double-blind controlled trial, 323 men (average age = 57 years) were randomized to placebo, 600 mg, or 1,200 mg of calcium for 2 years. At the end of the study, BMD increased in hip and total body (stated endpoints) by 1% to 1.5% for the 1,200 mg group compared with placebo and 600 mg calcium supplementation. The authors concluded that 1,200 mg of supplemental calcium has effects on BMD in men comparable to results found in postmenopausal women.[50]

Reports that calcium supplementation caused calcium deposition in coronary arteries frightened many older adults and kept them from taking calcium supplements to ensure achieving the levels recommended by the Institute of Medicine. However, data from the Framingham Offspring Study does not support the finding that dietary calcium contributes to calcium deposition in arteries. In an observational prospective study of 669 women and 532 men (average age = 60 years), calcium intake was not associated with increased coronary artery calcification.

Participants completed food frequency questionnaires at clinic visits between the years 1998 and 2001 and then underwent computed tomography scans to determine calcification of coronary arteries. The researchers concluded that dietary or supplemental calcium neither decreased nor increased coronary artery calcification.[51] The take-home message is that men and women should get adequate calcium in their diets to protect bone health, but more is not better. A food-first approach is always best, but when dietary intake cannot achieve the recommended calcium intake, small amounts of supplemental calcium can be used to fill the gap between dietary intake and recommended intakes. The International Osteoporosis Foundation has developed an online calculator that can be used to determine usual calcium intake (www.iofbonehealth.org/calcium-calculator).

Although limited studies have shown that masters athletes have increased energy intake, masters athletes assume that higher energy intakes will result in improved nutrient intakes. However, that is not always true. Professionals working with masters athletes should pay close attention to vitamins D, E, B-12, folate, riboflavin, pyridoxine and the minerals calcium, magnesium, and zinc when assessing diet and performance. Masters athletes older than 60 years may benefit from synthetic forms of vitamins D and B-12 because absorption and utilization of natural forms may be impaired in aging.

Much remains to be learned about the effects of aging and activity on micronutrient intakes. Blumberg and Meydani point out that there is little evidence to support an ergogenic effect of increased intakes of vitamins or minerals; however, optimal intakes of nutrients show promise to reduce tissue injury resulting from exercise.[52]

DIETARY SUPPLEMENTS

Dietary supplements are often marketed to older adults for a variety of reasons, mainly to fight aging. No dietary supplement is antiaging, but a few supplements may be helpful to some masters athletes.

Antioxidant supplements are frequently touted to improve performance and help reduce oxidative damage resulting from exercise. If there is a downside to exercise, it is the production of free radicals during strenuous activity. Although the body increases its natural antioxidant defense systems in the face of activity, it is not clear if it is sufficient to fight free-radical production without additional antioxidants obtained from supplements.[53,54] Increasing antioxidant-rich foods in the diet is one way to increase these nutrients, but for vitamin E, a fat-soluble vitamin, it is often difficult to get the DRI of 15 mg without including plant oils, seeds, and nuts. Although the evidence for using antioxidant supplements to combat free-radical production is equivocal, using the Tolerable Upper Intake Level established in the DRIs (2,000 mg of vitamin C and 1,000 mg of vitamin E), can provide guidance for a sports dietitian working with masters athletes.[44-55]

Creatine is a popular dietary supplement with athletes (see Chapter 7). Some evidence supports adding creatine to strength training to augment physiological adaptations to exercise in older adults.[56] Lower levels of creatine and phosphocreatine in skeletal muscle occur with aging, and phosphocreatine regeneration following exercise falls about 8% per decade after the age of 30.[57] Candow and colleagues conducted a meta-analysis on creatine supplementation during resistance training in people over the age of 50. They concluded that creatine supplementation resulted in greater training capacity leading to muscle accretion and strength gains in older adults who strength train. Combining creatine with resistance training could be an effective lifestyle intervention to combat sarcopenia of aging.[56] While not all studies show a benefit and not all athletes respond to creatine supplementation by increasing training capacity or muscle accretion, Phillips suggests that 5 g creatineper day ingested with some carbohydrate plus a progressive resistance exercise training program could have beneficial results for some older athletes.[40]

An area of emerging research is supplementation with n-3 fatty acids. Sarcopenia is thought to be associated with chronic low-level inflammation, and n-3 fatty acid supplementation can reduce inflammation.[40] Whether supplementation will help older athletes maintain or build muscle has yet to be established, and supplementation with n-3 fats in prevention of inflammatory disorders has shown disappointing results, but there is a theoretical basis for supplementation.

In a 2011 study with a small sample size (n = 16), healthy older adults (> 65 years) were randomized to receive 4 g of Lovaza (1.86 g eicosapentaenoic acid and 1.5 g docosahexaenoic acid) or corn oil. The rate of muscle protein synthesis and anabolic signaling pathways were evaluated before and after the 8-week study. The group receiving the n-3 fatty acids had hyperaminoacidemia and an increase in the activation of muscle signaling pathways.[58] More research needs to be conducted before supplementation is recommended, but this could be a relatively inexpensive way to help maintain muscle mass with aging.

Banned Substances

It is important to know that some governing bodies have begun testing masters athletes for banned substances. This is not without controversy because many of the drugs on the banned substances lists are medications commonly used by older adults to treat disease. Aromatase inhibitors, including letrozole (Femara) and anastrozole (Arimidex), and selective estrogen receptor modulators, including tamoxifen, are on the banned substances list. These drugs are used by breast cancer survivors, and although athletes can apply for a therapeutic use exemption, many may not realize that a drug prescribed by a physician could be considered doping to gain an advantage in sport. For a complete list of banned substances, see the World Anti-Doping Agency website (www.wada-ama.org).

FLUIDS

There are several reasons to be concerned about hydration status in masters athletes. First, older adults have less body water. Body water decreases to about 60% to 70% in older adults, from a high of 80% in infancy.[59] Second, thirst sensation decreases with age with a blunting of thirst in response to dehydration. Body water regulation relies on thirst to control water intake. Third, after the age of 40, renal mass declines with a subsequent decrease in renal blood flow. The ability an older person's kidneys to concentrate urine decreases, meaning more water is needed to remove waste products.[60] In addition, sweat glands change as the skin ages, with less sweat produced per gland with aging.[61] Lastly, there is an increase in plasma osmolality at rest, and it takes more time to restore body fluids in the face of dehydration.[60] Normal age-related changes in thirst and fluid regulation, coupled with the increased need for fluids in the exercising individual, make this a topic of paramount concern to masters athletes.

In addition to normal age changes in hydration status, common medications used by older adults may affect total body water. Nonsteroidal anti-inflammatory drugs, commonly used for mild to moderate pain, not only inhibit prostaglandins involved in pain and inflammation but also those involved in normal renal function. Some medications may blunt the thirst effect (such as selective serotonin reuptake inhibitors), and some drugs and herbal supplements increase urinary output (eg, thiazide diuretics, ginseng, saw palmetto, St John's wort, and wheatgrass).[62] Masters athletes should be aware of the effects of medications on hydration.

Kenney and Anderson conducted several studies on the effect of exercise and fluid needs in older individuals. They studied 16 women (8 older women and 8 younger women) exercising in hot, dry environments and warm, humid environments. Participants exercised on a treadmill for 2 hours at relatively low intensity

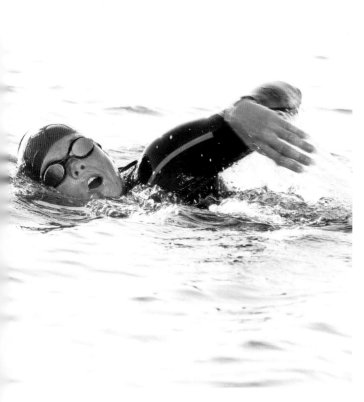

and were not allowed to consume fluids during the trials. Four of the older women were unable to complete either the hot-dry or warm-humid exercise trials. In the warm-humid environment, older women sweat at a rate equal to that of young women, but in the hot-dry environment the older women sweat less. The authors suggest that older women retain the ability to produce high sweat rates, but the sweat rate may be altered if adequate hydration is not available.[63]

Zappe and colleagues studied active older men and younger men to assess whether older active men showed an expansion of fluid volume after repeated exercise, as has been found in younger men. During 4 days of exercise, older men were able to maintain body fluid and electrolyte balance in a manner similar to that of the younger men. However, unlike younger men, older men did not have increased plasma volume. Older men had a blunted thirst effect in the face of loss of body water.[64]

Kenney noted that older athletes can exercise in hot environments and can tolerate heat stress as well as younger athletes of similar VO$_2$ max, acclimatization state, body size, and composition. However, there are subtle age-related differences in the blood flow to the skin and body fluid balance. Masters athletes who are well-conditioned and acclimatized to the heat should not suffer adverse effects associated with normal aging.[65] In a later study, Kenney suggested that the ability to exercise in warm environments is less a function of aging than of physiological health and functional capacity.[66] Box 14.3 gives tips for older athletes exercising in hot or humid conditions.

Box 14.3 Fluid Tips for Older Athletes in Hot or Humid Conditions[55]

Acclimate. Perform about half of your usual exercise on the first few days of hot weather. Decrease the duration or slow the pace, then gradually build it back up.

Hydrate. Drink approximately 16 ounces of fluid 30 to 40 minutes before exercise and at least 8 ounces every 15 minutes during exercise. Weigh yourself before and after exercise. After exercise, drink enough fluid to get back to, or near, the preexercise weight over a 2-hour period. Eat foods with high water content. Use a sports drink to restore lost electrolytes and keep the "drive to drink" alive.

Use common sense. If you are concerned that it is too hot to exercise, it probably is.

Learn about exercise in the heat. Pay attention to warning signs and symptoms of dehydration, heat exhaustion, and heat stroke.

FEATS OF AGING ATHLETES

The aging of the population brings challenges and opportunities to athletes. Today, older people run marathons, climb mountains, skydive, swim competitively, and hike the 2,160-mile Appalachian Trail. Consider these feats by masters athletes:

- Diana Nyad, at the age of 64, swam 110 miles from Cuba to Florida; 53 hours of nonstop swimming after four previous failed attempts.
- Tom Watson finished second at the 2009 British Open, at the age of 59, losing by one stroke in a playoff.
- Dara Torres is the first ever US swimmer to compete in five Olympic Games, and she medaled three times in the 2008 Beijing Olympics at the age of 41.
- Eamonn Coghlan, a dominating indoor runner in the mid-1970s and 1980s, was the first man older than 40 to break the 4-minute mile.
- Randy Johnson, a pitcher for the Arizona Diamondbacks, threw a perfect game at the age of 40—the oldest player to do so. His last pitch was clocked at 98 miles per hour.
- Priscilla Welch, a 58-year-old lifelong marathoner, was named the best female masters marathoner in history by *Runner's World*. At age 42 she won the overall women's title at the New York City Marathon, the oldest woman to claim that honor.
- Nolan Ryan played major league baseball for 27 seasons and was still hurling his fastball at more than 95 miles per hour at the age of 45.
- Boxer George Foreman won the world heavyweight championship 2 months shy of his 46th birthday.
- Haile Sataylin of Israel made history when he competed in the 2008 Olympic Games in the men's marathon at the age of 53.
- Sister Madonna Buder, known as the "Iron Nun," is the oldest person to finish an Ironman Triathlon in under the 17-hour time limit in 2008, at the age of 77.
- Yuichiro Miura of Japan became the oldest person to summit Mount Everest at the age of 80 in 2013.

KEY TAKEAWAYS

The evidence is clear that many older people can maintain a vigorous lifestyle. Although there is minimal research on the nutritional needs of masters athletes, several conclusions can be drawn. Health professionals working with masters athletes should consider these key points:

Aging has deleterious effects on almost all body systems, but regular physical activity appears to lessen most of these age-related changes.

Metabolic rate is driven by lean tissue and physical activity.

Older adults who remain physically active have the same needs for energy as active younger athletes. Energy intake should be adjusted when training volume decreases.

Fluid may be the most important nutrient for masters athletes—a programmed schedule of drinking can reduce the risk for dehydration without overconsumption of fluids.

Carbohydrate and fat recommendations are the same for older athletes as for younger athletes, and adjustment should be made based on duration and intensity of exercise.

Protein needs appear to be higher in older adults, and distributing protein intake throughout the day with approximately equal intakes at each meal may provide an anabolic environment of muscle and help to overcome the anabolic resistance of aging muscle.

Older adults should pay special attention to vitamin and mineral intakes. A multivitamin and mineral supplement formulated for seniors may be a good addition to supplement dietary intake. Senior-formulated vitamin and mineral supplements contain less iron and more vitamins B-12, B-6, and D compared with a supplement targeted for younger adults.

Masters athletes in competition may be drug tested for banned substances. Several drugs commonly used to treat chronic diseases are on the banned substance list, so masters athletes may need a therapeutic use exemption if they take certain prescription medications.

REFERENCES

1. Administration on Aging. *Profile of Older Americans: 2014.* www.aoa.acl.gov/Aging_Statistics/Profile/2014/2.aspx. Updated October 7, 2014. Accessed July 21, 2015.

2. Administration on Aging. Projected future growth of the older population. www.aoa.acl.gov/Aging_Statistics/future_growth/future_growth.aspx. Updated October 7, 2014. Accessed September 8, 2015.

3. FranchiseHelp. Fitness industry analysis—cost & trends. www.franchisehelp.com/industry-reports/fitness-industry-report/. Accessed September 8, 2015.

4. Joki P, Sethi PM, Cooper AJ. Master's performance in the New York City Marathon 1983-1999. *Br J Sports Med.* 2004;38(4):408-412.

5. US Department of Health and Human Services. *Physical Activity and Health: A Report of the Surgeon General.* Atlanta, GA: US Department of Health and Human Services, Centers for Disease Control and Prevention, National Center for Chronic Disease Prevention and Health Promotion; 1996.

6. World Health Organization. *The Heidelberg Guidelines for Promoting Physical Activity Among Older Persons.* Geneva, Switzerland: World Health Organization; 1996.

7. American College of Sports Medicine, Chodzko-Zajko WJ, Proctor DN, et al. American College of Sports Medicine position stand. Exercise and physical activity for older adults. *Med Sci Sport Exerc.* 2009;41(7):1510-1530.

8. Centers for Disease Control and Prevention. How much physical activity do older adults need? www.cdc.gov/physicalactivity/basics/older_adults/index.htm. Updated June 4, 2015. Accessed July 21, 2015.

9. Shephard RJ. Aging and exercise. In: Fahey TD, ed. *Encyclopedia of Sports Medicine and Science.* 1998. Internet Society for Sport Science. www.sportsci.org/encyc/agingex/agingex.html. Accessed July 27, 2015.

10. Lepers R, Cattagni T. Do older athletes reach limits in their performance during marathon running? *Age (Dordr).* 2012;34(3):773-781. www.ncbi.nlm.nih.gov/pmc/articles/PMC3337940/. Accessed July 21, 2015.

11. Akkari A, Machin D, Tanaka H. Greater progression of athletic performance in older masters athletes. *Age Ageing.* 2015;44(4):683-686.

12. Shephard RJ, Kavanagh T, Mertens DJ, Qureshi S, Clark M. Personal health benefits of masters athletic competition. *Br J Sports Med.* 1995;29(1):35-40.

13. Seals DR, Allen WK, Hurley BF, Dalsky GP, Ehsani AA, Hagberg JM. Elevated high-density lipoprotein cholesterol levels in older endurance athletes. *Am J Cardiol.* 1984;54(3):390-393.

14. Mengelkoch LJ, Pollock ML, Limacher MC, et al. Effects of age, physical training, and physical fitness on coronary heart disease risk factors in older track athletes at twenty-year follow-up. *J Am Geriatr Soc.* 1997;45(12):1446-1453.

15. Giada F, Vigna GB, Vitale E, et al. Effect of age on the response of blood lipids, body composition, and aerobic power to physical conditioning and deconditioning. *Metabolism.* 1995;44(2):161-165.

16. Seals DR, Hagberg JM, Allen WK, Dalsky GP, Ehsani AA, Holloszy JO. Glucose tolerance in young and older athletes and sedentary men. *J Appl Physiol.* 1984;56(6):1521-1525.

17. Maron BJ, Araújo CGS, Thompson PD, et al. Recommendations for preparticipation screening and the assessment of cardiovascular disease in masters athletes. *Circulation.* 2001;103(2):327-334.

18. Katzel LI, Sorkin JD, Fleg JL. A comparison of longitudinal changes in aerobic fitness in older endurance athletes and sedentary men. *J Am Geriatr Soc.* 2001;49(12):1657-1664.

19. Liu CJ, Latham NK. Progressive resistance strength training for improving physical function in older adults (review). *Cochrane Database Syst Rev.* 2009;8(3):CD002759.

20. Miljkovic N, Lim JY, Miljkovic I, Frontera WR. Aging of skeletal muscle fibers. *Ann Rehabil Med.* 2015;39(2):155-162.

21. Melov S, Tarnopolsky MA, Beckman K, Felkey K, Hubbard A. Resistance exercise reverses aging in human skeletal muscle. *PLoS ONE.* 2007;2(5):e465. doi:10.1371/journal.pone.0000465.

22. Kuk JL, Saunders TJ, Davidson LE, Ross R. Age-related changes in total and regional fat distribution. *Ageing Res Rev.* 2009;8(4):339-348.

23. Wroblewski AP, Amati F, Smiley MA, Goodpaster B, Wright V. Chronic exercise preserves lean muscle mass. *Phys Sportsmed.* 2011;39(3):172-178.

24. American Diabetes Association. Diabetes mellitus and exercise. *Diabetes Care.* 2002;25(suppl 1):64S-68S.

25. Gay JL, Buchner DM, Schmidt MD. Dose-response association of physical activity with HBA1c: intensity and bout length. *Prev Med.* 2016;86:58-63.

26. General facts . National Osteoporosis Foundation website. www.nof.org/prevention/general-facts/. Accessed August 26, 2016

27. Florindo AA, Latorre Mdo R, Jaime PC, Tanaka T, Pippa MG, Zerbini CA. Past and present habitual physical activity and its relationship with bone mineral density in men aged 50 years and older in Brazil. *J Gerontol Med Sci.* 2002;57(10):M654-M657.

28. Velez NF, Zhang A, Stone B, Perera S, Miller M, Greenspan SL. The effect of moderate impact exercise on skeletal integrity in master athletes. *Osteoporosis Int.* 2008;19(10):1457-1464.

29. Van Pelt RE, Dinneno FA, Seals DR, Jones PP. Age-related decline in RMR in physically active men: relation to exercise volume and energy intake. *Am J Physiol Endocrinol Metab.* 2001;281(3):E633-E639.

30. Institute of Medicine. *Dietary Reference Intakes for Energy, Carbohydrates, Fiber, Fat, Protein, and Amino Acids (Macronutrients)*. Washington, DC: National Academy of Sciences Press; 2002. www.nap.edu/books. Accessed September 8, 2015.

31. Bunyard LB, Katzel LI, Busby-Whitehead MJ, Wu Z, Goldberg AP. Energy requirements of middle-aged men are modifiable by physical activity. *Am J Clin Nutr*. 1998;68(5):1136-1142.

32. Wilmore JH. Stanforth PR, Hudspeth LA, et al. Alterations in resting metabolic rate as a consequence of 20 wk of endurance training: the HERITAGE Family Study. *Am J Clin Nutr*. 1998;68(1):66-71.

33. Starling RD. Energy expenditure and aging: effects of physical activity. *Int J Sport Nutr Exerc Metab*. 2001;11(suppl):208S-217S.

34. Campbell WW, Crim MC, Young VR, Evan WJ. Increased energy requirements and changes in body composition with resistance training in older adults. *Am J Clin Nutr*. 1994;60(2):167-175.

35. Lundholm K, Holm G, Lindmark L, Larrson B, Sjostrom L, Bjorntop P. Thermogenic effect of food in physically well-trained elderly men. *Eur J Appl Physiol*. 1986;55(5):486-492.

36. Burke LM, Hawley JA, Wong J, Jeukendrup AE. Carbohydrate for training and competition. *J Sports Sci*. 2011;29(suppl 1):17S-27S.

37. Tarnopolsky MA. Nutritional consideration in the aging athlete. *Clin J Sport Med*. 2008;18(6):531-538.

38. Moore DR, Churchward-Veane TA, Witard O, et al. Protein ingestion to stimulate myofibrillar protein synthesis requires greater relative protein intake in healthy older versus younger men. *J Gerontol A Biol Sci Med Sci*. 2015;70(1):57-62.

39. Layman DK, Anthony TG, Rasmussen BB, et al. Defining meal requirements for protein to optimize metabolic roles of amino acids. *Am J Clin Nutr*. 2015;101(suppl):1330S-1338S.

40. Phillips SM. Nutritional supplements in support of resistance exercise to counter age-related sarcopenia. *Adv Nutr*. 2015;6(4):452-460.

41. Deer RR, Volpi E. Protein intake and muscle function in older adults. *Curr Opin Clin Nutr Metab Care*. 2015;18(3):248-253.

42. Padden-Jones D, Campbell WW, Jacques PF, et al. Protein and healthy aging. *Am J Clin Nutr*. 2015;101(suppl):1339S-1345S.

43. Bauer J, Biolo G, Cederholm T, et al. Evidence-based recommendations for optimal dietary protein intake in older people: a position paper from the PROT-AGE Study Group. *J Am Med Dir Assoc*. 2013;14(8):542-559.

44. Institute of Medicine. *Dietary Reference Intakes: Recommended Intakes for Individuals*. Washington, DC: National Academy Press; 1998.

45. US Department of Health and Human Services and US Department of Agriculture. *2015–2020 Dietary Guidelines for Americans*. 8th ed. December 2015. http://health.gov/dietaryguidelines/2015/guidelines/. Accessed February 3, 2016.

46. Nieman DC, Butler JV, Pollett LM, Dietrich SJ, Lutz RD. Nutrient intake of marathon runners. *J Am Diet Assoc*. 1989;89(9):1273-1278.

47. Chatard JC, Boutet C, Tourny C, Garcia S, Berthouze S, Guezenee CY. Nutritional status and physical fitness in elderly sportsmen. *Eur J Appl Physiol*. 1998;77(1-2):157-163.

48. Beshgetoor D, Nichols JF. Dietary intake and supplement use in female master cyclists and runners. *Int J Sport Nutr Exerc Metab*. 2003;13(2):166-172.

49. Holick MF, Binkly NC, Bischoff-Ferrari HA, et al. Evaluation, treatment, and prevention of vitamin D deficiency: an Endocrine Society clinical practice guideline. *J Clin Endocrinol Metab*. 2011;96(7):1911-1930.

50. Reid IR, Ames R, Mason B, et al. Randomized controlled trial of calcium supplementation in healthy, nonosteoporotic older men. *Arch Intern Med*. 2008;168(20):2276-2282.

51. Samelson EJ, Booth SL, Fox CS, et al. Calcium intake is not associated with increased coronary artery calcification: the Framingham Study. *Am J Clin Nutr*. 2012;96(6):1274-1280.

52. Blumberg JB, Meydani M. The relationship between nutrition and exercise in older adults. In: Lamb DR, Gisolfi CV, Nadal E, eds. *Exercise in Older Adults: Perspectives in Exercise Science and Sports Medicine*, vol 8. Carmel, IN: Cooper Publishing Group; 1995:353-394.

53. Powers SK, Criswell D, Lawler J, et al. Rigorous exercise training increases superoxide dismutase activity in ventricular myocardium. *Am J Physiol*. 1998;265(6 pt 2):H2094-H2098.

54. Clarkson PM, Thompson HS. Antioxidants: what role do they play in physical activity and health? *Am J Clin Nutr*. 2000;72(suppl 2):637S-646S.

55. Brisswalter J, Louis J. Vitamin supplementation benefits in master athletes. *Sports Med*. 2014;44(3):311-318.

56. Candow DG, Chilibeck PD, Forbes SC. Creatine supplementation and aging musculoskeletal health. *Endocrine*. 2014;45(3):354-361.

57. Fleischman A, Makimura H, Stanley TL, et al. Skeletal muscle phosphocreatine recovery after submaximal exercise in children, young and middle-aged adults. *J Clin Endocrinol Metab*. 2010;95 (9):E69-E74.

58. Smith GI, Atherton P, Reeds DN, et al. Dietary omega-3 fatty acid supplementation increases the rate of muscle protein synthesis in older adults: a randomized controlled trial. *Am J Clin Nutr*. 2011;92(2):402-412.

59. Institute of Medicine. *Dietary Reference Intakes for Water, Potassium, Sodium, Chloride, and Sulfate.* Washington, DC: National Academies Press; 2004. www.nap.edu. Accessed February 2, 2016.

60. Sawka MN, Burke LM, Eichner ER, Maughan RL, Montain SJ, Stachenfled NS. Exercise and fluid replacement. *Med Sci Sport Exerc.* 2007;39(2):377-390.

61. Kenney WL, Fowler SR, Methylcholine-activated eccrine sweat gland density and output as a function of age. *J Appl Physiol.* 1988;65(3):1082-1086.

62. Walter AN, Lenz TL. Hydration and medication use. *Am J Lifestyle Med.* 2011;5(4):332-335.

63. Kenney WL, Anderson RK. Responses of older and younger women to exercise in dry and humid heat without fluid replacement. *Med Sci Sports Exerc.* 1988;20(2):155-160.

64. Zappe DH, Bell GW, Swartzentruber H, Wideman RF, Kenney WL. Age and regulation of fluid and electrolyte balance during repeated exercise sessions. *Am J Physiol.* 1996;270(1 pt 2):R71-R79.

65. Kenney WL. Are there special hydration requirements for older individuals engaged in exercise? *Austral J Nutr Diet.* 1996;53(suppl):43S-44S.

66. Kenney WL. Dietary water and sodium requirements for active adults. *Sports Sci Exch 92.* 2004;17(1). www.gssiweb.org/en/Article/sse-92-dietary-water-and-sodium-requirements-for-active-adults. Accessed November 6, 2015.

INTRODUCTION

The usual working definition of *elite* is "the best" or "the chosen few." This chapter addresses the nutritional needs of athletes who have reached the professional, world-class, or Olympic rank in their respective sports. These athletes have special nutritional requirements or challenges as a result of their extreme levels of training and competition, as well as the lifestyle that underpins their sporting involvement.

Sports dietitians are drawn to work with top athletes for many reasons, including the following:

- These athletes are often operating at the extremes of human nutrition and physiological capacity. It is fascinating to see what the human body can achieve and how it must be fueled to reach this level of operation.
- Elite athletes represent a motivated group of clients who seek and appreciate the nutrition advice that they are offered and usually adhere to recommendations.
- Sports dietitians have the opportunity to work with famous people and in high-profile situations, which can seem glamorous and can publicize a private practice.
- Sports dietitians are surrounded by inspired and inspiring people. They become participants in the excitement and emotion of high-level sports competitions.
- The work can provide opportunities to travel.
- Sports nutrition is a precise discipline with tangible benefits. The athlete and the sports dietitian receive short-term rewards and rapid feedback about the success of their nutrition strategies.
- The work draws on the sports dietitian's creativity and ingenuity to find practical strategies to address the athlete's unique nutritional challenges. Finding individualized solutions to these problems is interesting and demanding.

Of course, these and other ideas about working with elite athletes are usually just perceptions, and some ideas are ill founded. For example, many dietetics students are interested in sports nutrition as an alternative to a career in weight-loss counseling. Yet, the most common reason for athletes to seek the help of a sports dietitian is to reduce weight or body fat. This chapter will provide an overview of some of the nutritional issues that are important to top-level athletes, as well as strategies for the sports dietitian to work successfully with such clients.

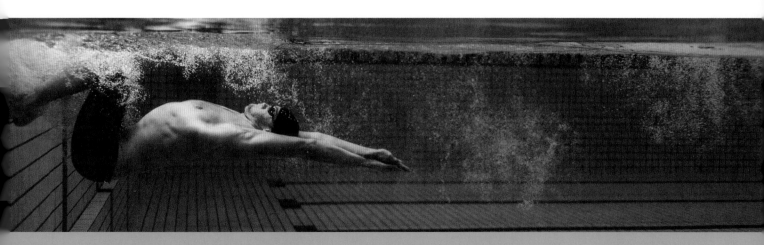

THE STRUCTURE OF HIGH-LEVEL SPORT—IMPLICATIONS FOR NUTRITIONAL NEEDS AND PRACTICE

There are several characteristics of high-level sports that create special nutritional needs or challenges for the athletes involved. These include:

- heavy training load,
- demanding competition schedule,
- frequent travel,
- unusual environments for training adaptations or competition preparation (heat, altitude),
- the culture of sport (the price and rewards of fame and publicity), and
- the influence and power of coaches and other personnel involved with the athlete.

Although there are clear differences among sports, the training program of an elite or professional athlete typically involves 15 to 30 hours of highly periodized and specialized exercise sessions each week. Other activities related to recovery, injury treatment and prevention, or team play and preparation may also be in the weekly schedule. The training program is likely to change but often calls for high energy requirements and targeted needs for carbohydrate and protein around key sessions to support high-quality training and recovery and adaptation, respectively. There may be increased requirements for some nutrients and the need to address substantial losses of fluids and electrolytes through sweating. At this level of sport, athletes would be expected to have the support and incentive to implement cutting-edge sports nutrition practices, including many of the evolving themes in sports nutrition,[1] such as awareness of the benefits of periodizing nutrition strategies and nutrient intake,[2,3] as well as the strategic timing of nutrient intake in relation to exercise or postexercise recovery and adaptation.[4] To meet such goals, an athlete will need access to a supply of suitable foods or tailor-made sports products providing these nutrients and will also need an opportunity and appetite to consume them in sufficient amounts. Several factors can challenge these goals, particularly during travel; this will be discussed separately in this chapter.

Elite Athlete Competition Schedules

The competition schedule of the elite athlete usually presents a set of nutritional and lifestyle challenges that differ from the training situation. In general, athletes organize their training to peak at one to three major competitions each year; however, most will compete in many other events each year. Athletes use these lesser competitions to practice and fine-tune their strategies for key events or to provide high-quality

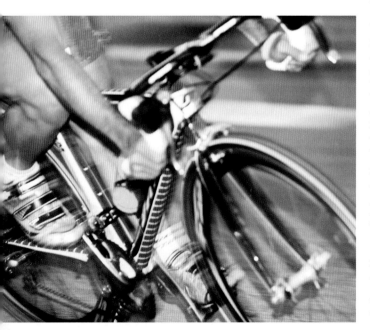

training sessions for more important competitions. In addition, each competition may involve more than one round of events (ie, heats, semifinals, and finals) that ultimately decide the outcome. Some sports, particularly team sports, can be played in a tournament format with a series of games every 24 to 72 hours. Team sports played seasonally, traditionally with a weekly game, have evolved to have even more demanding competitive schedules at the elite level. In fact, it is not unusual for professional soccer, baseball, and basketball players to play a match every 2 or 3 days, especially when the player or the team is entered into more than one association or league.[5]

During each competition phase, athletes are usually focused on acute issues of refueling and rehydration—undertaking special eating strategies before, during, and after an event to meet the needs of their event.[6,7] Travel and other factors that limit food availability can often challenge the athlete to meet immediate nutritional goals, not to mention big picture issues of energy balance and overall macronutrient and micronutrient needs. The sports dietitian needs to be creative in helping the athlete achieve such strategies as carbohydrate loading, an optimal pre-event meal, food and fluid intake during an event, and proactive recovery eating. However, when competition makes up a substantial proportion of the elite athlete's life and total eating patterns—for example, professional cyclists who compete approximately 100 days each year and ride in stage races lasting up to 3 weeks[8]—there is a need for competition nutrition strategies that also include all dietary goals.

Elite Athlete Lifestyles

The lifestyle of most top-level athletes is busy and irregular. At the entry point into an elite sport, many younger athletes juggle training and events around the commitments of high school and college. Because many sports are not wholly professional or financially rewarding, some top-class athletes must continue to work part-time or full-time in addition to keeping their sporting commitments. Meals and snacks eaten during the day must fit into their lifestyles (eg, work, school, and family commitments). A chaotic or displaced eating pattern may challenge some athletes to meet the high energy and nutrient requirements associated with maturational and muscular growth, training, and recovery—in particular, prolonged sessions of high-intensity work or resistance-training programs designed to increase muscle size and strength.

Professional (or otherwise full-time) athletes generally have the luxury of spreading their training schedule and other commitments, such as medical and testing appointments or team activities, over the day. However, sometimes during periods of multiple daily practices, training camps, or competition travel, the athlete is faced with a busy timetable that interferes with a normal eating schedule. At other times, they are left with a considerable amount of free time during the day. In some situations, eating becomes a form of entertainment, which can lead to nutritional problems such as eating unnecessary amounts of food or making inappropriate food choices. In both situations, it is important for athletes to have a clear understanding of their nutritional goals and to formulate an eating program that can achieve such goals.

The elite level of sport is a specialized environment, which includes not only the physical aspects of club rooms and training or competition venues but also the culture of each sport. The pressure to win often means that the athlete is desperate to find dietary shortcuts or magic bullets, becoming an easy target for the unsupported claims made about fad diets, dietary supplements, and other unusual eating strategies. The athlete is often susceptible to and specifically targeted by companies and individuals who recognize the benefits of being associated with a high-profile individual or team. Many sports provide an insular world where high-level athletes swap ideas and theories with their peers, trainers, and coaches or are influenced by material on the internet and in sports magazines, without necessarily checking the credibility of their information sources. Sports dietitians need to break into these circles to be aware of the latest trends and ideas. They must also contend with a wide array of other, often influential sources of nutrition advice directed at the athlete. They may have to fight for the athlete's time, concentration, or resources, which are often limited and must be shared with other sports science and medical professionals, managers, coaching and training staff, and the media. On the positive side, most top-level athletes take a professional approach to preparing for their sport and will make effective use of information and practical advice. The structure of many high-level teams and sporting organizations is to surround their athletes with a group of professionals specializing in sports science and medicine and as well as training and conditioning. It is both efficient and rewarding to be part of such a support network, and the sports dietitian should find ways to optimize his or her interaction in the multidisciplinary team.[9]

NUTRITIONAL ISSUES

In an ideal world, elite athletes would meet their increased energy needs and nutrient requirements with well-chosen and varied diets. However, this may not always to be the case. Very few studies have been conducted on the dietary practices of the world's top athletes, and much of the available literature fails to address the potential for biased data due to the limitations of dietary survey methodology. Even fewer studies have measured indexes of nutritional status among top athletes. Nevertheless, it seems most elite male athletes have the potential to consume diets that meet the guidelines for sports nutrition. Elite female athletes are at greater general risk of suboptimal intakes of a range of nutrients due to their apparent restriction of energy intakes and pursuit of fad diets because of concerns about body mass and body fat.[10] Other athletes at risk are those involved in weight-controlled or weight-division sports, such as boxing, wrestling, weight lifting, and lightweight rowing, for which preparation for competition often involves severe energy restriction.[11]

Meeting Energy and Fuel Needs Across a Range of Extremes

An athlete's energy intake is of interest for several reasons[12]:

- It sets the potential for achieving the athlete's requirements for energy-containing macronutrients (especially protein and carbohydrate) and the food needed to provide vitamins, minerals, and other non–energy-containing dietary compounds required for optimal function and health.
- It helps the athlete manipulate muscle mass and body-fat levels to achieve the specific body composition ideal for athletic performance.
- It affects the function of many body systems related to health and performance.
- It challenges the practical limits to food intake set by such issues as food availability and gastrointestinal comfort.

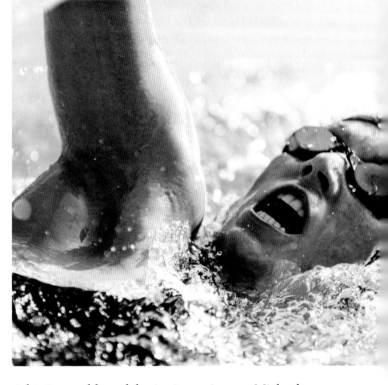

The total energy expenditure of each athlete is unique, arising from the contribution of basal metabolic rate, the thermic effects of food and exercise, and, in some cases, growth. Energy expenditure is increased by high levels of lean body mass, growth (including the desired adaptations to a resistance-training program), and a high-volume training program. (For more information on energy balance, see Chapter 10.) For some elite athletes, these three factors coexist to create very large energy demands—for example, the male swimmer or rower who faces an increase in training commitment during periods of adolescent growth spurts. Other elite athletes have very large energy requirements due to the extraordinary fuel demands of their competition programs. The energy and fuel costs of very strenuous exercise programs are impressively high. For example, professional cyclists in the Grand Tours have been reported to consume mean daily intakes exceeding 5,500 kcal and 12 g carbohydrate/kg body weight for periods of 3 weeks during competition.[13,14] During the 2008 Beijing Olympic Games, media sources reported that eight-time gold-medal-winning swimmer Michael Phelps consumed approximately 12,000 kcal/d. This news created considerable awe among the public but caused skepticism among sports nutrition experts. Phelps denied this information in his subsequent autobiography, claiming his true intake may be up to 8,000 to 10,000 kcal/d.[15] These figures may be estimates of his heaviest days of intake rather than a true average but nevertheless illustrate the potential for high energy needs among athletes with heavy training loads.

At such extreme levels of energy demand, lack of nutrition knowledge, limited access to suitable foods, gastrointestinal discomfort, or inadequate time for preparing or eating food can prevent the athlete from consuming sufficient food or fluid over the day to meet his or her energy needs. Indeed, this scenario is now recognized as a cause of low energy availability, which can lead to the range of health and performance concerns generally noted to occur in relation to deliberate food restriction or disordered eating.[16] Even when overall energy needs can be met, the athlete may experience difficulty in achieving intake goals of specific nutrients (eg, carbohydrate and protein) around exercise sessions. Here, there may be a need to consume foods and drinks in greater quantities than would be provided in an everyday diet or dictated by appetite and thirst. Again, the availability of foods and fluids, or opportunities to consume them, may be limited, and the athlete may be distracted by other activities (eg, media commitments, drug testing, performance debriefs). To meet these challenges, the athlete will need to plan ahead to meet nutrient goals from foods convenient to store, prepare, and eat. Specialized advice from a sports dietitian is therefore useful to help address energy intake challenges athletes face. See Box 15.1 for suggestions for increasing energy intake, and refer to Chapter 11 for additional information relevant to this topic.

Box 15.1 Guidelines to Help Elite Athletes Achieve High Energy Intakes[8]

Meal Spacing
- Use a food diary to identify *actual* intake rather than perceived intake.
- Consume carbohydrate during prolonged exercises to provide fuel and additional energy.
- Eat a carbohydrate and protein snack after exercise to enhance recovery and increase total daily energy intake.

Food Availability
- Shop for food and prepare meals in advance of hectic periods.
- Overcome postexercise fatigue by preparing meals and snacks in advance.
- When traveling, take snacks that can be easily prepared and eaten (eg, cereal and powdered milk, granola and sports nutrition bars, liquid meal supplements, and dried fruit and nuts).
- Have snacks and light meals available at home (eg, fruit, fruit smoothies, yogurt, and sandwiches).
- Consider specialized products such as sports drinks, gels, and bars during exercise and sports nutrition bars and liquid meal supplements after exercise. (In most training situations, athletes will need to provide their own products.)

Appetite Management and Gastric Comfort
- Reduce gastric discomfort with small, frequent meals.
- Drink liquid meal supplements, flavored milk, fruit smoothies, sports drinks, soft drinks, and juices to provide energy, nutrients, and fluids.
- Choose energy-dense meals and snacks, including sugar-rich foods.
- Avoid excessive intake of high-fiber foods, which may limit total energy intake or lead to gastrointestinal discomfort.
- Overcome appetite suppression with small pieces of food or easy-to-eat foods that do not require considerable cutting and chewing (eg, fruit, sandwiches served as finger foods, or a stir-fry).
- Consider postexercise environmental conditions. Heat and dehydration may be matched by cool and liquid-based choices such as fruit smoothies, yogurt, or ice cream. In cold conditions, warm soup, toasted sandwiches, or pizza may be more appetizing.

The Ideal Body Composition for Optimal Performance

Physical characteristics, including height, limb lengths, total body mass (weight), muscle mass, and body fat, can all play roles in sports performance. Many elite athletes are subjected to rigid criteria for an ideal physique based on the characteristics of other successful competitors. The pressure to conform to such an ideal comes from the athlete's own perfectionism and drive to succeed, as well as the influence of coaches, trainers, other athletes, and the media. Although athletes at all levels may battle to achieve their desired weight and body-fat level, a disadvantage of being an elite athlete is that this battle may be played out in the public arena; via commentary on websites, newspapers, and magazines; and in the discussion of sports reporters. Wearing tight-fitting clothing (such as you might find in a team uniform) in public has been identified as a risk factor for the development of disordered eating among athletes.[17] Imagine how this stress is amplified when the (largely sedentary) audience (measured in the millions) feels justified in criticizing an athlete for perceived pockets of fat made apparent by tight-fitting spandex. Many well-known female swimmers, tennis players, and gymnasts have suffered such humiliation.[18]

Although information about the physique of elite athletes is a source of fascination for the community, as well as other athletes, we should be cautious about making rigid prescriptions about the ideal physique based on the anthropometrics of successful competitors. The concept of a single ideal fails to take into account the considerable variability in the physical characteristics of people, even among individuals in the same sport. Furthermore, athletes sometimes need many years of training and maturation to finally achieve their optimal shape and body composition. In addition, these features are not static but change over the course of the periodized year. Finally, because a wide variety of techniques are used to assess characteristics such as body fat or lean mass, it is impractical to generalize an ideal body type from available data about specific athletes. Clinical experience shows a range of values for body fat and body weight consistent with long-term good performance and health within each sport. Sequential profiling of an athlete can monitor the development of physical characteristics associated with good performance for that individual, as well as identify the changes in physique expected over a season or period of specialized training. For additional information on nutrition assessment and body composition, see Chapters 8 and 9.

However, in many sports in which a low body-mass or body-fat level offers distinct advantages to performance, fat loss has become a focus or even an obsession. The benefits of leanness can be seen in terms of the energy cost of movement (eg, distance running, cycling), the physics of movement in a tight space or against gravity (eg, gymnastics, diving, cycling uphill), or aesthetics (eg, gymnastics, bodybuilding). In many such weight-conscious (or body-fat-conscious) sports, elite athletes strive to achieve minimum body-fat levels; some athletes try to reduce their body fat to levels less than what is considered natural or healthy. In the short term, this may improve performance. However, the long-term disadvantages include outcomes related to having very low body-fat stores, as well as the problems associated with unsound weight-loss methods. Excessive training, chronically low intakes of energy and nutrients, and psychological distress are often involved in fat-loss strategies and may cause long-term damage to health, well-being, or performance.[19] There is now clear recognition of the problems of low energy availability, characterized by the syndrome known as relative energy deficiency in sport (RED-S), whereby energy intake fails to meet the requirements for basal activities related to health and function once the energy cost of exercise is taken into account.[16]

Techniques for early recognition and treatment of RED-S should be put into place in the elite athlete environment. Ironically, this may sometimes be challenging to implement in high-performance sports, despite the growing evidence that low energy availability impairs performance as well as health.[20] The perceived or real benefits of achieving very low levels of body fat and body mass have become so engrained in some elite sports that unhealthy patterns of restrained eating are normalized or even regarded as heroic. Many biographies of the careers of elite athletes reveal stories of extreme eating behaviors that were considered simply part of their sport. For example, road cyclist Tyler Hamilton noted a range of weight-loss techniques he used in his constant battle to be as lean as possible, including a strategy shared by other riders: "come home from a training ride, chug a big bottle of fizzy water and take two or three sleeping pills. By the time you woke up, it would be dinner, or if you were lucky, breakfast."[21] Road cyclist Michael Rasmussen became obsessed with removing any excess weight (down to the milligram), such as peeling off unnecessary stickers from his bike; this carried over to his training diet. He was "famous for counting each grain of rice before eating and taking water—not milk—with his breakfast cereal."[22] There is a clear need for a change in the culture around weight and body fat within many elite sports. A more sensible approach to weight management is covered in greater detail in Chapter 11.

The Special Challenges of Travel

Travel plays a major role in the lifestyle of the elite athlete, and most world-class athletes often travel within their own state or country as well as internationally for competition or specialized training opportunities. The various challenges imposed by travel, intenational or domestic, are summarized in Box 15.2.[23] They include disruption to the athlete's normal eating routine and access to their preferred foods, as well as exposure to a different standard of food and water hygiene. The process of travel itself is also problematic, exposing the athlete to jet lag, interruption of the normal training program, and boredom eating when confined during travel.

Box 15.2 Challenges and Solutions for the Traveling Athlete[23]

Challenges of Traveling

- Disruptions to the normal training routine and lifestyle while the athlete is en route
- Changes in climate and environment that create different nutritional needs (this is especially the case during training camps at altitude or where heat acclimatization is necessary)
- Jet lag
- Changes to food availability, including absence of important and familiar foods
- Reliance on hotels, restaurants, and takeout food instead of home cooking
- Exposure to new foods and eating cultures
- Temptations of all-you-can-eat meal options in some athletic settings
- Risk of gastrointestinal illnesses due to exposure to food and water with poor hygiene standards
- Excitement and distraction of a new environment

Strategies to Cope with the Challenges of Traveling

1. Planning ahead
- Before leaving home, the athlete should investigate food issues on travel routes (eg, airlines) and at the destination. Caterers and food organizers should be contacted well ahead of the trip to let them know meal timing and menu needs.

2. Supplies to supplement the local fare
- A supply of portable, nonperishable foods should be taken or sent to the destination to replace important items that missing. Useful items include breakfast cereal, cereal bars and crackers, dried fruit, and specialized sports products, such as powdered liquid meals and sports drinks.
- The athlete should be aware that many catering plans only cover meals. Since the athlete's nutritional goals are likely to include well-timed and well-chosen snacks, supplies should be taken to supplement meals en route and at the destination.

3. Eating and drinking well en route
- Many athletes will turn to boredom eating when confined. Instead, they should eat according to their real needs, taking into account the forced rest while traveling.
- When moving to a new time zone, the athlete should adopt eating patterns that will suit the destination as soon as the trip starts. This will help the body clock to adapt.
- Unseen fluid losses in air-conditioned vehicles and pressurized plane cabins should be recognized, and a drinking plan should be organized to keep the athlete well hydrated.

4. Taking care with food and water hygiene
- It is important to find out whether the local water supply is safe to drink. Otherwise, the athlete should stick to drinks from sealed bottles or hot drinks made from well-boiled water. Ice added to drinks is often made from tap water and may be a problem.
- In high-risk environments, the athlete should eat only at good hotels or well-known restaurants. Food from local stalls and markets should be avoided, however tempting it is to have an authentic cultural experience.
- Food that has been well cooked is the safest; it is best to avoid salads or unpeeled fruits that have been in contact with local water or soil.

5. Adhering to the food plan
- The athlete should choose the best of the local cuisine to meet nutritional needs, supplementing his or her own supplies where needed.
- The athlete should be assertive in asking for what he or she needs at catering outlets, for example, low-fat cooking styles or an extra carbohydrate choice.
- The challenges of all-you-can-eat dining should be recognized. The athlete should stick to his or her own meal plan and resist the temptation to eat what is there or what everyone else is eating.

Elite athletes need to become organized travelers, identifying the challenges of their intended locations before the trip and planning to circumvent potential problems (see Box 15.2).[23] During travel, athletes should adjust their eating to suit a period of inactivity, as well as any increases in fluid losses due to a dry atmosphere. They should also switch to a meal routine based on the time zone of their country of destination to assist with the change in body clock. The travel plan may include organizing catering needs and menus before the trip. In addition, supplies of special foods and drinks may be taken on the trip to complement these catering plans or to make up for the absence of key nutrients or favorite foods.

Of course, these plans must be implemented with an understanding of some of the practical constraints involved. For example, quarantine laws in some countries or states may prevent the importation of some food products. In addition, the athlete should be aware that heightened security regulations and the increase in ticket prices have made travel more challenging. Tighter weight restrictions on checked luggage make it difficult for the athlete to include his or her own specialized sporting equipment, let alone food supplies, and large containers of liquids may not be carried onto a flight. Strategies to address these challenges include removing packaging from foodstuffs, taking powdered versions of sports foods to lighten luggage, and organizing supplies to be freighted over or delivered directly to travel destinations rather than transported with the athlete. Elite athletes can sometimes be fortunate to have personal or team-based sponsorships with airlines or other travel agencies that can facilitate the transport of their luggage. Being famous can be beneficial when presenting at check-in with special needs, but a good travel plan should not rely on special last-minute help. If sports foods or supplements are sourced from a local supplier, the athlete should take special caution regarding the potential for contamination with banned substances (see the supplements section later in this chapter).

Often, competitions or specialized training protocols occur in physiologically challenging environments, such as a hot climate or moderate altitude. For example, the summer Olympic Games were held in very hot weather in Atlanta (1996), Athens (2004), and Beijing (2008), and soccer matches during the 2010 World Cup in Johannesburg were played at an altitude of approximately 1,700 m. In such cases, the athlete usually undertakes acclimatization in a similar environment or in a chamber that can simulate the characteristics of the competition site. This is done as final preparation for the competition. However, on other occasions the athlete may choose to train in hot conditions or at a high altitude (or simulated altitude) to gain physiological adaptations that can be applied to moderate weather or a sea-level environment. Nutritional requirements during these specialized periods will reflect both the type of training, ranging from a precompetition taper to a period of intensified training, as well as the additional needs posed by heat or altitude. In both hot and moderate- to high-altitude environments, the athlete can expect to incur an increase in needs for nutrients, including energy, fluid, carbohydrate, and protein.[24]

Finally, some sporting competitions or environments involve cultural, religious, or practical limitations on the food supply that athletes must plan for. Athletes traveling to Muslim-based countries may find that they are unable to access pork products on menus; in deference to Hindu populations, beef may not be served, as was the case in the athletes' dining hall at the 2010 Commonwealth Games in New Delhi, India. Around the world, many institutions enact a ban on nuts or other high-risk food allergens. When these foods play a large role in the athlete's diet, it can be difficult to find a sufficient range of alternative choices. The 2012 London Olympic Games overlapped with the month of Ramadan. Fasting during Ramadan, the ninth month of the lunar calendar, is one of the five pillars of the Islamic faith and involves abstention from all fluid and food intake from first light to sunset, as well as prayer and food rituals involved with the breaking of the fast at sunset and throughout the night. Although Ramadan is an annual event that coincides with various sporting competitions each year, the London Olympics brought this to the attention of many athletic and spectating communities for the first time and required a range of special catering activities and education strategies.[25]

Do the Results of Studies on Recreational Athletes Apply to Elite Athletes?

Some think that sports foods and supplements or sports nutrition strategies such as carbohydrate-loading are targeted at the elite athlete. It is true that the pressures and rewards for optimal performance are greater at this level and may justify the expense or effort involved in addressing special nutritional needs. However, the majority of studies on sports nutrition strategies involve subjects throughout the spectrum, from recreationally active to well-trained. In fact, few intervention studies have involved world-class or elite athletes. This is understandable, of course, because by definition elite athletes are a scarce resource, and it is difficult to arrange a study that does not conflict with their commitments to training and competition.[26] However, elite athletes almost certainly have genetic endowment, as well as acquired traits gained from their training history and training programs, that differ from those of nonelite athletes. Because the results of a research study apply with reasonable certainty only to populations that have similar characteristics to the sample involved in the investigation, it is not clear whether elite athletes will respond to strategies that have been tested on nonelite or recreational competitors in the same way. An elite athlete may benefit from something that has no detectable effect on recreational athletes. Conversely, strategies that enhance the performance of a recreational performer may not benefit the elite athlete.

This issue has been recently examined in relation to the hypothesis that beetroot juice/nitrate supplementation is less effective in enhancing the performance of elite competitors than lower-level athletes. The commentaries on this topic are interesting in their specific application to this reasonably new supplement as well as their potential extension to other nutrition strategies.[27,28] Some evidence for the hypothesis that nitrate supplementation provides a smaller benefit to high-caliber athletes has been provided by cross-sectional studies,[29] as well as a meta-analysis of the available literature.[30] As usual, issues with the robustness of this literature makes it dangerous to make firm conclusions. However, some theories explain why differ-

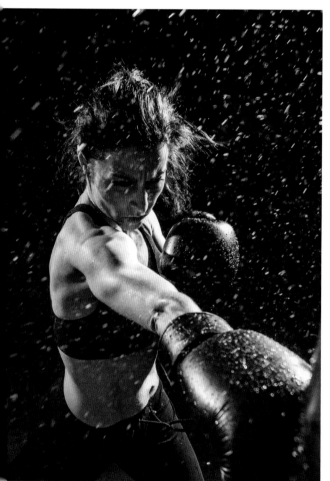

ences in responsiveness might occur according to the training status of the athlete. For example, compared with moderately trained individuals, experts speculate that elite athletes have different composition of muscle fiber type, greater muscle capillarization and adaptation (which reduces the development of hypoxia and metabolic acidosis), and a more developed pathway to produce nitric oxide (NO) from arginine; these conditions may reduce the benefit of an enhanced activity of the nitrate-nitrite-NO pathway.[31]

Does this mean that elite athletes should not bother to experiment with beetroot juice supplements? A cost-benefit analysis would err on the side of the potential benefits. Given that responders are still apparent in studies involving elite cohorts and that few side effects other than pink urine or stools following beetroot juice ingestion have been reported, nitrate consumption may be a useful nutrition strategy for high-caliber athletes.[27] The efficacy of this strategy is likely to be associated with the specific conditions of the sporting event. Athletes may benefit more in shorter, high-intensity sports due to the greater hypoxic and acidic stress favoring the nitrate-nitrite-NO pathway and the relatively greater involvement of type II fibers. In particular, the localization of these conditions in smaller muscle groups may favor effects during upper-body dominant exercise,[28] which explains observations of benefits to competitive athletes in kayaking and rowing.[32,33] Applying this strategy to situations of hypoxia, such as altitude training or competition in high-altitude environments

(eg, cross-country skiing, mountainous cycling stages) where O_2 availability is challenged, also bears consideration and further study.[28] Therefore, even if there is general evidence that nitrate supplementation is valuable to lesser-trained or lower-caliber athletes, there are perhaps certain sports, events, and conditions where it may assist elite competitors.

With some strategies, variations should be expected in outcomes in the field: Real-life practices of elite athletes do not conform to the conditions used when the nutrition practice was tested in the laboratory. For example, many studies are done with subjects in a fasted state, with the athlete drinking only water during an exercise session. The results may be different when the same nutrition practice is conducted in real life after a carbohydrate-rich meal.[34] At other times, elite athletes may choose or be forced by the circumstances of their event to follow the existing sports nutrition guidelines in a different way. For example, world-class marathon runners typically drink at rates of approximately 200 to 600 mL/h during races and can become significantly dehydrated,[35] despite guidelines that promote higher rates of intake to better match sweat losses.[36] These runners often take a calculated risk in balancing the benefits of fluid intake against the potential for gut discomfort or the time taken to grab and consume drinks while running at approximately 20 km/h. Their cost-benefit analysis of this nutrition strategy would differ from that of a recreational athlete who is moving slower and has less need to count every second during a run.

In summary, there is currently insufficient information to make different recommendations for elite athletes regarding sports nutrition practice other than to recognize that the rules and conditions of their events may provide logistical challenges to fulfilling the existing guidelines. However, sports scientists are encouraged to conduct research with elite athletes and the real-life conditions under which their sports are played so that recommendations can be fine-tuned.

What Magnitude of Performance Change Is Important to an Elite Athlete?

In many sports, the outcomes are decided by milliseconds, millimeters, a single fumble, or an expert action; the difference between winning and losing is measured in millions of dollars and everlasting fame. Hallmarks of traditional intervention studies in sports nutrition—small sample sizes, performance protocols of modest reliability, and traditional probability statistics—make it unlikely to detect differences or changes in performance that could be worthwhile to the athlete.[25] Indeed, most scientific investigations of nutrition strategies, particularly supplement use, are biased toward rejecting the hypothesis that the product or tactic enhances performance.

Many elite athletes take a favorable attitude to unproven supplements on the basis that even a miniscule effect is worth the investment. This concept is often confirmed by the discussion in newer research papers in which the performance difference due to an intervention is directly compared with the outcome of a sporting event. For example, the researchers may note that the mean improvement in performance with Supplement X was 2.3%, which would span the difference between the first-place winner and the eighth finisher in a particular race. There is often an inference or misunderstanding that if the eighth athlete in this race used Supplement X, his or her performance would be elevated to winning status. However, this simplistic approach misrepresents the real nature of sports performance because it focuses only on interindividual differences rather than the equally important issue of intraathlete variability or reliability. More specifically, it neglects the reality that the day-to-day performance of athletes varies across a range that overlaps with that of their fellow competitors, such that the rerunning of an event would likely lead to a different outcome without any intervention being applied.

Hopkins and colleagues have discussed alternative ways to detect worthwhile performance enhancements in elite sports, taking into account the margins in performance between and within highly competitive athletes. After modeling the results of various sporting events, they suggest that worthwhile changes to the outcome of most events require a performance difference equal to approximately 0.3 to 0.5 times the variability (coefficient of variation [CV]) of performance for that event.[26] Furthermore, across a range of events, the CV of performance of top athletes is usually within the range of 0.5% to 3%, with differences according to the type of effect and the caliber of the performer.[37] However, an improvement of approximately 0.5% of the event CV does not guarantee clear movement of the athlete from finalist to winner but may increase their likelihood of winning by about 10%. Such a difference is still outside the realm of detection for many of the studies commonly published in scientific journals. Nevertheless, scientists can interpret their results meaningfully by reporting the outcome as a percentage change in a measure of athletic performance

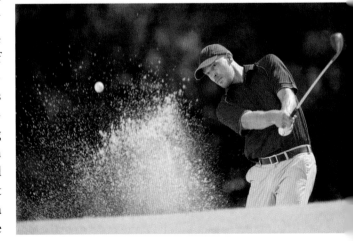

and using 90% to 95% confidence limits to describe the likely range of the true effect of the treatment on the average athlete represented in the study.[26]

Many investigations of sports nutrition interventions now also report the results of individual subjects as well as the mean group outcome and show that even when the mean response suggests a worthwhile improvement in performance, the experiences of individual subjects can range from a negative effect to a very large performance gain. The occurrence of side effects can also be an individual experience. Such differences in response to the same intervention are often interpreted as evidence of a responder vs nonresponder phenomenon. While this outcome undoubtedly occurs in the case of some products and individuals, some care should be taken in distinguishing it from the previously discussed day-to-day variability in performance.

Part of the modern landscape of health and medicine includes the gathering appreciation that genetic differences may also account for a large fraction of the variability in health responsiveness. For example, some studies have shown that genetic differences affect caffeine's ability to enhance sports performance. For example, a study of cyclists subdivided the group according their expression of a single nucleotide polymorphism of a gene associated with cytochrome P450 (CYP1A2), a family of proteins that metabolize drugs in the liver. Overall, athletes who carried the AA version of the gene achieved a 5.9% improvement in 40-km time ($P < 0.001$) while athletes who carried the C allele achieved only a 1.8% improvement ($P = 0.04$).[38]

Various sources of information should be used to explore or confirm the concept of individual responsiveness to a sports nutrition intervention. Within research scenarios, the starting point is to control the situation so that the intervention is the only variable changing. Additional techniques include looking for a correlation between markers of altered biochemistry or physiology associated with an intervention and change in performance. Including large numbers of subjects and undertaking covariate analysis of various characteristics—including genetic profiling—provide a sophisticated, albeit resource intensive, tactic. A simpler strategy is to undertake repeated interventions of the strategy within the trial to look for a consistent response.

Within real-life practice, elite athletes who receive sports science support may have access to information about their specific physiological or biochemical responses to certain nutrition interventions to enable them to identify successful strategies or tweak characteristics. In the future, it may become possible to receive a genetic profiling report that could identify potential responsiveness to different kinds of strategies. For the moment, the most pragmatic way for an athlete to investigate a sports nutrition intervention is to consider best-practice guidelines as a starting point that will cover most individuals. Further, they may identify if they are a nonresponder or responder to the intervention via trial and error, aided by standardized application and systematic reporting of the outcomes of their activities.

STRATEGIES FOR WORKING WITH ELITE ATHLETES

A successful practice with elite athletes requires the sports dietitian certain strategies and personal characteristics. The following ideas can help the sports dietitian develop a rewarding career.

Getting Started

Be prepared to start at the bottom to gain experience. Look for opportunities to start with local teams and athletes rather than expecting to start with a job with a national sporting organization or major professional team.

Use your contacts and involvement in sports to develop a knowledge base and experience. Your own sporting experiences can earn credibility with athletes and coaches and provide an intimate understanding of what it is like to be an athlete.

Find a mentor. Set a professional development program for yourself that includes regular journal reading and conference attendance. Stay up to date with both the science and practice of sports nutrition.

Learn About a Sport and Its Special Features

Learn all you can about how a sport influences nutritional needs of competitors, as well as current nutrition practices and beliefs. Get specific information about training practices, competition programs, and lifestyle patterns, including individual differences among players on a team and among different sports.

Attend training sessions and events to better understand the culture and experiences of athletes, coaches, and other team members. Let the athletes know that you are interested in their activities.

Stay informed about supplements used or promoted within a sport. To stay abreast of current ideas and practices, monitor information from the internet, sports magazines, health-food shops, and supplement stores, as well as the general talk among players.

Be a Team Player

Identify all the people who work with an individual athlete or team to provide their nutrition ideas or achieve their nutrition practice. This will include people in the organized support structure and in the personal network that each athlete may develop. Be prepared to listen to the approaches and input of these people, and find a niche in which your services and ideas will be appreciated.

Know when to stand your ground (you are the nutrition expert) and when to be flexible (a compromise of your ideas may be necessary for athletes to accept). Look for middle ground. For example, a coach or trainer may insist that the athlete consume branched-chain amino acids after a training session to promote recovery. Rather than debating whether the present literature provides support for benefits of postexercise supplementation with amino acid supplements, consider setting up recovery snacks for the team, including fruit smoothies, flavored yogurt, and cereal with milk. Provide educational material showing the coach and athletes that these snacks provide a good source of branched-chain amino acids (similar to amounts found in supplements), as well as carbohydrate and fluid for refueling and rehydration.

Participate (when invited) in all activities of the athlete or team support network, even if these do not seem to directly involve nutrition. Cultivate relationships among other professionals or team support personnel so they are aware of what you can do and will provide early referrals of athletes for your specialty services and support your nutrition plan when you are not present (eg, during team travel).

Be Creative with Nutrition Activities

Create educational resources that target the needs and interests of your individual athletes and teams. Use innovative ways to provide information rather than relying on standard lectures or interview and consultation formats. Be prepared to put information or activities into bite-size chunks or address the issues that are of immediate interest to your athletes rather than following a standard script.

Plan interactive activities, such as cooking classes, supermarket tours, or installation of recovery snacks at training or competition venues. These activities provide tangible outcomes. Many people learn better through practical activities.

Remember, It Is Not All About You

Many people who become involved in the preparation of elite athletes start to identify closely with the success of these athletes. Although it is rewarding to feel that you contributed to a successful outcome or were part of a valued support team, it is important to maintain perspective about your role. High-level sports and high-profile athletes attract an entourage of people, many of whom use a cult of personality to make themselves seem indispensable. In some cases, members of this entourage can become as famous (or infamous) as the athlete. Although it is often important to be able to sell your message in a memorable way, it is more important to maintain an appropriate and ethical profile.

Stay Ethical

Sport is all about rules and regulations. There is a professional code of conduct that covers your role as nutrition adviser or therapist. Sometimes you may feel pressured to assist an athlete in a dangerous or unethical practice, such as excessive loss of body fat or weight or use of a supplement containing prohibited substances (see Chapter 7). Stay true to professional standards, even when the athlete threatens to undertake the practice without your assistance.

In addition, maintain confidentiality in your work with high-profile athletes. Even when opinions or information seem to be discussed as public conversation, guard your knowledge about the athletes with whom you work. This includes the nature of your nutrition work as well as other information, such inside knowledge of injuries or other problems. At best, breaches of this information are an invasion of the athlete's privacy. At worst, they may be considered insider trading in a world where betting on sports is a highly lucrative industry.

Tips for Survival in a High-Pressure Environment

Be organized and have definite goals for your activities. Set up a contract with the appropriate person (medical director, head coach, athlete) in which the range of services you can provide is discussed and agreed upon. Provide feedback or summary information on completed services so that your input is documented and appreciated.

Do not forget to build in ways of assessing and rewarding your own progress and achievement of goals. It is easy to overlook your own performance when the focus is on the athlete's.

Finally, make sure you look after your own health and well-being. Sometimes, the service of athletes requires long hours and the elevation of their needs above your own. Be prepared for the politics of high-level sport. Coaches and medical staff are frequently abandoned by their athletes, often for no fault of their own. Expect that this will happen to you. Be prepared to pick yourself up and develop a new plan.

SUMMARY

Working with elite athletes provides an opportunity for the sports dietitian to test his or her sports science knowledge and creativity in solving practical challenges faced by athletes pushing to their extreme limits. The elite environment can be both high pressure and high return. The sports dietitian will need to remain up to date with the latest scientific information and adhere to a code of conduct that includes understanding of the ethics of sport, respect for confidentiality, and care for his or her own well-being. It can be rewarding to see that nutrition plays a role in the achievement of the highest levels of success in sport. However, the role is often specific to the needs of a gifted individual and a unique situation.

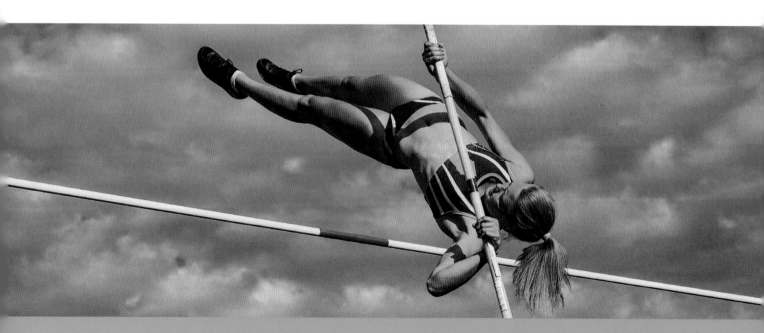

Elite athletes train and compete at high intensity and undertake multiple training sessions; for most elite athletes this is their job.

Elite athletes are highly motivated; they seek and appreciate the nutrition advice that they are offered and usually adhere to recommendations.

Fueling strategies should focus on energy and carbohydrate availability.

During competition, the athlete is most focused on acute issues of fueling and hydration before, during, and after an event.

Travel plays a major role for the elite athlete; domestic and international competitions disrupt the athlete's usual eating routine and access to their preferred foods and expose them to a different standard of food and water hygiene.

Sports dietitians who work with elite athletes should practice ethical behaviors in all dealings with the athletes.

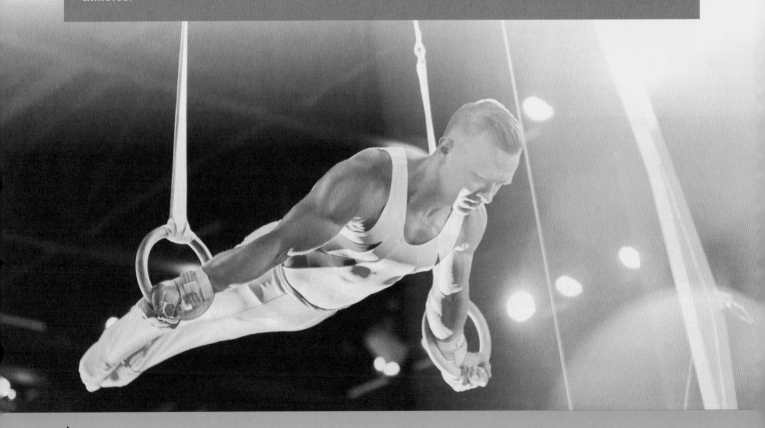

REFERENCES

1. Thomas DT, Erdman KA, Burke LM. Position of the Academy of Nutrition and Dietetics, Dietitians of Canada, and the American College of Sports Medicine: nutrition and athletic performance. *J Acad Nutr Diet.* 2016;116(3):501-528.

2. Stellingwerff T. Contemporary nutrition approaches to optimize elite marathon performance. *Int J Sports Physiol Perform.* 2013;8(5):573-578.

3. Mujika I, Stellingwerff T, Tipton K. Nutrition and training adaptations in aquatic sports. *Int J Sport Nutr Exerc Metab.* 2014;24(4):414-424.

4. Burke L. Nutrition for recovery after training and competition. In: Burke L, Deakin V, eds. *Clinical Sports Nutrition.* 5th ed. Sydney, Australia: McGraw-Hill; 2015:420-562.

5. Reilly T. Football. In: Reilly T, Secher N, Snell P, Williams C, eds. *Physiology of Sports.* London, United Kingdom: E & FN Spon; 1990:371-426.

6. Burke L. Preparation for competition. In: Burke L, Deakin V, eds. *Clinical Sports Nutrition.* 5th ed. Sydney, Australia: McGraw-Hill; 2015:346-376.

7. Jeukendrup A. Carter J, Maughan R. Competition fluid and fuel. In: Burke L, Deakin V, eds. *Clinical Sports Nutrition.* 5th ed. Sydney, Australia: McGraw-Hill; 2015:377-419.

8. Mujika I, Padilla S. Physiological and performance characteristics of male professional road cyclists. *Sports Med.* 2001;31(7):479-487.

9. Burke LM. Practical and cultural factors. In: *Practical Sports Nutrition.* Champaign, IL: Human Kinetics; 2007:27-39.

10. Burke LM, Cox GR, Cummings NK, Desbrow B. Guidelines for daily carbohydrate intake: do athletes achieve them? *Sports Med.* 2001;31(4):267-299.

11. Walberg-Rankin J, Gibson J. Making weight. In: Burke L, Deakin V, eds. *Clinical Sports Nutrition.* 5th ed. Sydney, Australia: McGraw-Hill; 2015:191-212.

12. Burke LM. Energy needs of athletes. *Can J Appl Physiol.* 2001;26(suppl):202S-219S.

13. Garcia-Roves PM, Terrados N, Fernandez SF, Patterson AM. Macronutrients intake of top level cyclists during continuous competition—change in feeding pattern. *Int J Sports Med.* 1998;19(1):61-67.

14. Saris WHM, van Erpt-Baart,MA, Brouns F, Westerterp KR, ten Hoor F. Studies on food intake and energy expenditure during extreme sustained exercise: the Tour de France. *Int J Sports Med.* 1989;10(suppl):26S-31S.

15. Phelps M, Abrahamson A. *No Limits: The Will to Succeed.* Sydney, Australia: Simon and Schuster; 2008.

16. Mountjoy M, Sundgot-Borgen J, Burke L, et al. The IOC consensus statement: beyond the Female Athlete Triad—Relative Energy Deficiency in Sport (RED-S). *Br J Sports Med.* 2014;48(7):491-497.

17. Nattiv A, Loucks AB, Manore MM, Sanborn CF, Sundgot-Borgen J, Warren MP. American College of Sports Medicine position stand. The female athlete triad. *Med Sci Sports Exerc.* 2007;39(10):1867-1882.

18. Burke LM. Swimming and rowing. In: *Practical Sports Nutrition.* Champaign, IL: Human Kinetics; 2007:141-167.

19. Sundgot-Borgen J, Meyer NL, Lohman TG, et al. How to minimise the health risks to athletes who compete in weight-sensitive sports review and position statement on behalf of the Ad Hoc Research Working Group on Body Composition, Health and Performance, under the auspices of the IOC Medical Commission. *Br J Sports Med.* 2013;47(16):1012-1022.

20. Vanheest JL, Rodgers CD, Mahoney CE, De Souza MJ. Ovarian suppression impairs sport performance in junior elite female swimmers. *Med Sci Sports Exerc.* 2014;46(1):156-66.

21. Hamilton T, Coyle D. *The Secret Race: Inside the Hidden World of the Tour de France: Doping, Cover-ups, and Winning at All Costs.* London, United Kingdom: Bantam Press, 2012.

22. Saddles B. Rasmussen blows whistle on a decade of dope. Eurosport website. www.eurosport.com/cycling/rasmussen-blows-whistle-on-a-decade-of-dope_sto4706268/story.shtml. Published January 2, 2013. Accessed December 16, 2016.

23. Burke LM. Sports nutrition: practical guidelines for the sports physicians. In: Schwellnus MP, ed. *Olympic Textbook of Medicine in Sport.* Oxford, United Kingdom: Blackwell Publishing Ltd; 2008:508-600.

24. Ross M, Martin D. Nutritional issues for special environments: training and competing at altitude and in hot climates. In: Burke I., Deakin V, eds. *Clinical Sports Nutrition.* 5th ed. Sydney, Australia: McGraw-Hill; 2015:767-791.

25. Burke L. Fasting and recovery from exercise. *Br J Sports Med.* 2010;44(7):502-508.

26. Hopkins WG, Hawley JA, Burke LM. Design and analysis of research on sport performance enhancement. *Med Sci Sports Exerc.* 1999;31(3):472-485.

27. Jonvik KL, Nyakayiru J, van Loon LJ, Verdijk LB. Viewpoint: can elite athletes benefit from dietary nitrate supplementation? *J Appl Physiol (1985).* 2015;119(6):759-761.

28. Hultström M, Amorim de Paula C, Antônio Peliky Fontes M, et al. Commentaries on Viewpoint: can elite athletes benefit from dietary nitrate supplementation? *J Appl Physiol (1985).* 2015;119(6):762-769.

29. Porcelli S, Ramaglia M, Bellistri G, et al. Aerobic fitness effects the exercise performance responses to nitrate supplementation. *Med Sci Sports Exerc*. 2015;47(8):1643-1651.

30. Hoon MW, Johnson NA, Chapman PG, Burke LM. The effect of nitrate supplementation on exercise performance in healthy individuals: a systematic review and meta-analysis. *Int J Sport Nutr Exerc Metab*. 2013;23(5):522-32

31. Jones AM. Dietary nitrate supplementation and exercise performance. *Sports Med*. 2014;44(suppl 1):35-45.

32. Hoon MW, Jones AM, Johnson NA, et al. The effect of variable doses of inorganic nitrate-rich beetroot juice on simulated 2,000-m rowing performance in trained athletes. *Int J Sports Physiol Perform*. 2014;9(4):615-620.

33. Peeling P, Cox GR, Bullock N, Burke LM. Beetroot juice improves on-water 500 m time-trial performance, and laboratory-based paddling economy in national and international-level kayak athletes. *Int J Sport Nutr Exerc Metab*. 2015;25(3):278-284.

34. Burke LM, Claassen A, Hawley JA, Noakes TD. Carbohydrate intake during prolonged cycling minimizes effect of glycemic index of preexercise meal. *J Appl Physiol (1995)*. 1998;85(6):2220-2226.

35. Beis LY, Wright-Whyte M, Fudge B, Noakes T, Pitsiladis YP. Drinking behaviors of elite male runners during marathon competition. *Clin J Sport Med*. 2012; 22(3):254-261.

36. American College of Sports Medicine, Sawka MN, Burke LM, Eichner ER, Maughan RJ, Montain SJ, Stachenfeld NS. American College of Sports Medicine position stand. Exercise and fluid replacement. *Med Sci Sports Exerc*. 2007;39(2):377-390.

37. Malcata RM, Hopkins WG. Variability of competitive performance of elite athletes: a systematic review. *Sports Med*. 2014;44(12):1763-1774.

38. Womack CJ, Saunders MJ, Bechtel MK, et al. The influence of a CYP1A2 polymorphism on the ergogenic effects of caffeine. *J Int Soc Sports Nutr*. 2012;9(1):7.

CHAPTER 16

VEGETARIAN ATHLETES

D. Enette Larson-Meyer, PhD, RDN, CSSD, FACSM

INTRODUCTION

Athletes may elect to follow vegetarian diets for health, ethical (animal rights), ecological, environmental, religious, or spiritual reasons. Although the exact number of athletes who follow strict vegetarian eating patterns is unknown, recent evidence suggests that as many as 8% of athletes surveyed at the 2010 Commonwealth Games followed vegetarian diets, and 1% of those were vegan.[1] Well-planned vegetarian diets are nutritionally adequate, appropriate for athletes at all levels—from recreational to elite—and provide health benefits in the prevention and treatment of chronic diseases.[2-5] Like most athletes, vegetarian athletes may benefit from education about food choices to optimize their health and peak performance.

This chapter reviews the energy, macronutrient, vitamin, and mineral requirements of the vegetarian athlete and provides tips for meeting nutritional needs with a vegetarian diet. The chapter also discusses nutrition recommendations before, during, and after exercise and tips for the sports dietitian working with vegetarian athletes.

SPORTS NUTRITION CONSIDERATIONS: ENERGY AND MACRONUTRIENTS

Energy

The energy needs of athletes and active individuals vary considerably and are dependent on body size, body composition, sex, training regimen, and nontraining physical activity patterns; vegetarian athletes have the same energy needs. Energy expenditure is estimated to range from 2,600 kcal/d in female swimmers to 8,500 kcal/d in male cyclists participating in the Tour de France bicycle race.[6]

In practice, total daily energy expenditure (TDEE) of individual athletes can be estimated using a variety of methods (see Chapter 10). The most straightforward method is to use the predictive equations from the Dietary Reference Intakes (DRIs) to estimate resting energy expenditure (REE) and multiply estimated REE by an activity factor between 1.4 and 2.5 depending on the physical activity level of the athlete (Box 16.1 on page 330).[7-9] Another method is to sum the estimates of the components of TDEE, which include REE, the energy cost of training or organized physical exercise, and the energy cost of occupational and spontaneous physical activity (nontraining energy expenditure), as outlined in Box 16.1.[10] Although estimating TDEE from its components may be more cumbersome, it accounts for more variation in training and daily activity patterns and can serve as an educational tool when calculated in the athlete's presence. Estimates of TDEE may be useful when developing meal plans and when evaluating adequacy of energy intake (along with body weight changes and dietary intake assessments).

Meeting energy needs is a nutrition priority for all athletes. Inadequate energy intake relative to energy expenditure negates the benefits of training and compromises performance. While some athletes who follow vegetarian and vegan diets may have difficulty meeting energy requirements due to the high fiber or low energy density of plant-based diets, sports dietitians are likely to encounter vegetarian athletes with a variety of energy needs.[7] Some will need to consume six to eight meals and snacks per day and avoid excess dietary fiber to meet energy needs and maintain body weight. Others may require lower energy intakes

Box 16.1 Calculating Range of Total Daily Energy Needs[7-10]

Total daily energy needs = TDEE[a] + TEF[b]

TDEE = REE[c,d] + NEAT[e] + ExEE[f]

- REE = 22 × fat-free mass (kg)
- NEAT = Physical activity level × REE
  - Light activity = 0.3 × REE
  - Moderate activity = 0.5 × REE
  - Heavy activity = 0.7 × REE
- To determine ExEE, refer to physical activities charts (found in many nutrition or exercise physiology texts)
- TEF = 6% to 10% of TDEE
  - TEF = 0.06 × TDEE
  - TEF = 0.10 × TDEE

Example 1

Female college soccer player who practices for 90 minutes and weight-trains for 30 minutes

- Weight = 60 kg with 20% body fat (lean body weight = 48 kg)
- Assume light occupational activity (student)
- A 60-kg female athlete uses ~8.0 kcal/min for soccer practice and 6.8 kcal/min for weight-training

REE = 22 × 48 = 1,056 kcal

NEAT = 0.3 × 1,056 kcal = 317 kcal

ExEE = (8.0 kcal/min × 90 min) + (6.8 kcal/min × 30 min) = 720 kcal + 204 kcal = 924 kcal

TDEE = 1,056 + 317 + 924 = ~2,297 kcal

TEF = 0.06 × 2,297 = ~138 kcal

TEF = 0.10 × 2,297 = ~230 kcal

Total daily energy needs (lower) = 2,297 + 138 = 2,435 kcal

Total daily energy needs (upper) = 2,297 + 184 = 2,527 kcal

Example 2

Male recreational runner who works as a musician and runs 35 miles/wk (average of 43 min/d at a 7 mph pace).

- Weight = 75 kg
- Body fat = 16% (lean body weight = 63 kg)
- Assume moderate occupational activity (stands, moves, loads/unloads equipment regularly, some sitting)
- A 75-kg male athlete uses ~14.1 kcal/min when running at a steady 7-mph pace

REE = 22 × 63 = 1,386 kcal

NEAT = 0.5 × 1,386 kcal = 693 kcal

ExEE = 14.1 × 43 min = 606 kcal

TDEE = 1,386 + 693 + 606 = ~2,685 kcal

TEF = 0.06 × 2,685 = ~161 kcal

TEF = 0.10 × 2,685 = ~268 kcal

Total daily energy needs (lower) = 2,685 + 161 = 2,846 kcal

Total daily energy needs (upper) = 2,685 + 268 = 2,953 kcal

---

[a] TDEE = total daily energy expenditure

[b] TEF = thermic effect of food

[c] REE = resting energy expenditure

[d] The Cunningham equation for estimating REE has been shown to more closely estimate the actual REE of endurance-trained men and women than other available equations.[10]

[e] NEAT = nonenergy activity thermogenesis (energy expenditure during nontraining activities)

[f] ExEE = energy expenditure during training

to promote weight reduction for health or performance. Sports dietitians should work with each athlete to help meet his or her individual energy needs by consuming a variety of foods, including whole grains, fruits, vegetables, legumes, nuts, seeds, and (if desired) dairy products and eggs.[2] Both MyPlate, which has adjustments of energy requirements and tips for vegetarians, and the guidelines developed by Larson-Meyer specifically for vegetarian athletes may be useful in educating athletes about healthy eating patterns.[3,11] Eating plans developed for individuals who consume vegetarian or vegan diets may also provide a useful framework if the number of servings is increased appropriately.[12,13]

Box 16.2 (page 332) contains sample menus for a 3,000-kcal vegetarian diet and a 4,600-kcal vegan diet. These energy levels may be required to meet the needs of individuals who train or exercise regularly. Vegetarian athletes who struggle to consume adequate energy may benefit from consuming only one-third to one-half of their grains and fruit in the whole, unprocessed form.[3] This will reduce excessive fiber intake and reduce early onset of satiety. Additionally, vegetarian athletes struggling to meet energy demands may benefit from selecting more energy dense foods, such as nuts, seeds, and avocados, and decreasing the amount of fiber in the diet.

Carbohydrate

Carbohydrates should make up the bulk of the athlete's diet. Adequate carbohydrate intake maintains muscle and liver glycogen stores from day to day.[7,14-17] Further, it optimizes mood and performance during prolonged, moderate-intensity exercise and intermittent, short-duration, high-intensity exercise.[18-26] Thus for many athletes, maintaining sufficient carbohydrate intake during training will result in a delayed time to fatigue during training or competition or better sprinting potential at the end of a race or sporting event. The benefit of carbohydrate consumption, however, is not limited to the maintenance of muscle and liver glycogen stores. Dietary carbohydrate may also be important for maintenance of the tricarboxylic acid cycle (also known as Krebs cycle) intermediates and preservation of the bioenergetic state of muscle during intense exercise, factors also important for optimal muscle function and performance.[20,24] (For more information on carbohydrate, refer to Chapter 2.)

The carbohydrate needs of active individuals are easily met on a vegetarian diet by consuming a variety of sources such as cereals, grains, legumes, starchy vegetables, fruits, and some meat analogues such as tempeh. The carbohydrate recommendations for athletes range from as low as 3 to 5 g/kg body weight per day to as high as 12 g/kg body weight per day.[7,27] The amount recommended within this range depends on the athlete's TDEE, training intensity and training periodization, and training goals. For example, college, elite, or other competitive athletes undergoing extreme training (> 4 h/d) may benefit from a higher carbohydrate intake and should strive for the higher recommended range of 8 to 12 g/kg body weight per day. Conversely, athletes participating at a level that demands less training (eg, skill-based activity or recreational exercisers) or those attempting to reduce body weight or fat stores may require only 3 to 5 g/kg body weight per day.[27,28] Sports dietitians may find that the concept of carbohydrate exchanges and label-reading exercises are useful for educating athletes about meeting their carbohydrate needs.[3] Knowledge of carbohydrate sources is also useful in planning carbohydrate intake before, during, and after exercise.

Protein

The protein needs of athletes vary according to the sport or activity, intensity of training, and level of experience.[28] Protein needs of active vegetarians who engage in light to moderate activity several times per week are likely met by the Recommended Dietary Allowance (RDA) of 0.8 g/kg body weight per day. The protein requirements of those who train more intensely may be higher than the RDA to support positive nitrogen balance and promote muscle protein synthesis postexercise. The protein recommendation for athletes ranges from 1.2 to 20 g/kg body weight per day.[7] Additional protein and essential amino acids are needed during routine endurance and strength training to cover increased protein utilization as an auxiliary fuel during exercise and enhanced protein deposition during muscle development.[29] Furthermore, inadequate intake of total energy or carbohydrate increases protein needs. During prolonged endurance activity, for

Box 16.2 Sample 3,000-kcal Vegetarian Menu and 4,600-kcal Vegan Menu[a]

3,000 kcal[b] Vegetarian Menu

Breakfast

1 cup raisin bran

1 cup fat-free milk

2 slices mixed-grain toast

2 tsp margarine

1 medium banana

8 oz fruit juice

Lunch

Whole-wheat pita stuffed with shredded spinach, sliced tomato, 2 oz feta cheese, 2 Tbsp olive oil

1 large apple

2 small oatmeal cookies

Snack

Sesame seed bagel

1 Tbsp peanut butter

1 Tbsp jam

Dinner

Lentil spaghetti sauce (1 cup cooked lentils, ½ onion, 1½ cups canned tomatoes, 1 Tbsp olive oil)

3 oz dry pasta, cooked

1 Tbsp parmesan cheese

2 (1-oz) slices french bread dipped in 1 Tbsp olive oil

1 cup steamed broccoli

Snack

1 cup fruit yogurt

4,600 kcal[c] Vegan Menu

Breakfast

1½ cups raisin bran

1 cup fortified soy milk

3 slices mixed-grain toast

3 tsp margarine

1 medium banana

8 oz fruit juice

Lunch

Tofu salad on a 4-oz hoagie roll (1 cup firm tofu, 2 tsp mustard, 2 tsp soy mayonnaise, lettuce, tomato)

1 large apple

3 small oatmeal cookies

8 oz carrot juice

Snack

Sesame seed bagel

1 Tbsp peanut butter

1 Tbsp jam

1 cup fortified soy milk

Dinner

Lentil spaghetti sauce (1½ cup cooked lentils, ½ onion, 1½ cups canned tomatoes, 1 Tbsp olive oil)

4 oz dry pasta, cooked

3 (1-oz) slices french bread dipped in 2 Tbsp olive oil

1½ cups steamed collards

Snack

1 cup fruit sorbet

1 oz toasted almonds

[a] Both menus assume that grain products are made from enriched flour.

[b] Vegetarian menu: 3,066 kcal, 106 g protein, 469 g carbohydrate, 85 g fat (14% protein, 25% fat, 61% carbohydrate), 1,600 mg calcium, 29 mg iron, 14 mg zinc.

[c] Vegan menu: 4,626 kcal, 146 g protein, 704 g carbohydrate, 136 g fat (13% protein, 26% fat, 61% carbohydrate), 1,133 mg calcium, 60 mg iron, 15 mg zinc.

example, athletes with low glycogen stores metabolize twice as much protein as those with adequate stores, primarily due to increased gluconeogenesis.[30] Recent research also suggests that dietary protein—particularly the amino acid leucine—may play a role beyond the supply of building blocks and energy and serve as an important trigger for muscle protein synthesis induced by training.[28] More specifically, increases in leucine concentration to a critical threshold after a meal are thought to turn on muscle protein synthesis (see Chapter 3 for additional details). Research further shows that the peak in leucine concentration varies by content and absorbability of leucine in individual proteins (see Table 16.1). Whey, for example, induces

Table 16.1 Approximate Leucine, Valine, and Isoleucine Content of Selected Vegetarian Protein Sources

Food	Portion	Protein, g	Leucine, g	Valine, g	Isoleucine, g
Cheese, Brie	1 oz	5.9	0.55	0.38	0.29
Cheese, cheddar	1 oz	7.1	0.68	0.47	0.44
Cheese, Swiss	1 oz	7.6	0.84	0.67	0.44
Cottage cheese, 2%	½ cup	13.4	1.34	0.90	0.71
Egg, whole	1 large	6.3	0.54	0.43	0.34
Black beans	½ cup	7.6	0.61	0.40	0.34
Garbanzo beans	½ cup	7.3	0.52	0.31	0.31
Lentils	½ cup	8.9	0.65	0.44	0.39
Pinto beans	½ cup	7.7	0.65	0.45	0.36
Soy beans, mature	½ cup	14.3	1.17	0.72	0.69
Soy beans, green	½ cup	12.4	0.80	0.49	0.49
Tofu, firm	½ cup	19.9	1.51	1.00	0.99
Tofu, soft	½ cup	8.1	0.62	0.40	0.41
Soy protein isolate	1 oz	22.9	1.9	1.2	1.2
Peanut butter	2 Tbsp	8.0	0.49	2.46	0.19
Milk, nonfat (skim)	1 cup	8.3	0.80	0.44	0.37
Milk, reduced-fat (2%)	1 cup	8.1	0.81	0.53	0.45
Yogurt, low-fat vanilla	1 cup	12.1	1.2	1.0	0.66
Whey, sweet fluid	1 cup	2.1	0.19	0.11	0.12
Whey, sweet dry	4 Tbsp	3.9	0.36	0.21	0.22

Adapted from the US Department of Agriculture National Nutrient Database for Standard Reference (Release 28, revised May 2016).

a much greater spike in plasma leucine than do soy or casein proteins. Soy, particularly fiber-free isolated protein, is a rich source of leucine, as are most legumes. The leucine in these products is not as absorbable as the leucine in whey and is therefore not thought to trigger muscle protein synthesis as rapidly as whey. A recent study, however, found that consumption of pea protein was just as effective as consumption of whey in promoting gains in muscle mass and strength during 12 weeks of resistant training.[31]

There is no research to suggest that protein recommendations are different for athletes following a vegetarian diet than for those on an omnivorous diet. While it has been suggested that vegetarians may need approximately 10% more protein than omnivores to account for the lower digestibility of plant proteins compared with animal proteins, the Institute of Medicine does not think there is sufficient evidence to support an additional protein requirement for vegetarians consuming complementary plant proteins.[7,32,33] In support, a meta-analysis of nitrogen-balance studies found that the source of dietary protein did not significantly affect the protein needs of healthy individuals.[34] However, sports dietitians should be aware that protein needs might be slightly higher in athletes whose dietary protein sources are mainly from plant sources that are more difficult to digest, such as legumes and some cereal grains, rather than plant sources that are easier to digest, including soy protein.[35]

Vegetarian athletes can easily meet their elevated protein needs if their diets are adequate in energy and contain a variety of plant-based protein foods, such as legumes (including soy foods), nuts, seeds, and grains (see Table 16.2). Based on extensive research, Young and Pellett have emphasized that vegetarians do not need to be overly concerned with protein complementing—or eating specific combinations of plant-based proteins in the same meal—as was once believed, but they should strive to consume a variety of plant foods during the course of a day.[36] This pattern should provide all essential amino acids and ensure adequate nitrogen retention and utilization in healthy adults.[2,36] Emphasizing amino acid balance at individual meals is not necessary because limiting amino acids in one meal is buffered by amino acid pools found primarily in skeletal muscle and supported by turnover of endogenous gut proteins.[36,37] Furthermore, although some plant foods tend to be low in certain amino acids—including methionine and lysine—usual combinations of protein, such as beans and rice, tend to be complete.[36] It is important to note, however, that because cereals tend to be low in lysine, athletes who do not consume dairy or eggs should incorporate beans and soy products into their diets to ensure adequate lysine intake.[36]

Vegetarian diets contain an average of 12.5% of energy from protein, whereas vegan diets contain 11%.[12] Thus, an 80-kg male athlete consuming 3,600 kcal, for example, would receive 1.41 and 1.2 g protein/kg body weight from the average vegetarian and vegan diets, respectively. Similarly, a 50-kg female gymnast consuming 2,200 kcal would receive 1.38 g/kg body weight from a vegetarian diet and 1.21 g/kg from a vegan diet. Most vegetarian athletes, therefore, meet the lower range of the recommendation without special meal planning. Strength-training athletes (weight lifters, football players, wrestlers), athletes in high-frequency or interval training, or athletes actively restricting energy intake may need to focus on the including more protein-rich foods if protein intakes in the upper range of the recommendation (ie, 1.7–2.0 g/kg) are desired.[28] This is easily accomplished by encouraging athletes to incorporate protein-rich vegetarian foods in their regular meals or snacks. Specific examples include adding soy milk to a fruit snack, lentils to spaghetti sauce, tofu to stir-fry, garbanzo beans to salad, or cottage cheese or Greek yogurt to a fruit snack. Athletes should also be educated that not all milk alternatives (ie, almond and rice milks) are rich sources of proteins. Furthermore, there may be additional benefit to protein consumption in proximity to strength or endurance exercise and to spreading protein throughout the course of the day (ie, consuming 20 to 25 g at regular meals and snacks vs all in an evening meal).[38,39] Both may enhance maintenance of and net gains in skeletal muscle.[38,40]

Fat

Dietary fat should make up the remainder of energy needs after carbohydrate and protein requirements are met. The Academy of Nutrition and Dietetics, the American College of Sports Medicine, and Dietitians of Canada recommend that fat intake guidelines align with the Dietary Guidelines for Americans.[7] Consumption of less than 20% of energy from fat, however, is not recommended and has the potential to impair endurance performance, unfavorably alter lipid profile, and interfere with normal menstrual function in female athletes.[7,41-48] Fat is particularly important in an athlete's diet because it provides energy, essential fatty acids, and other essential elements of cell membranes and is needed for absorption of fat-soluble vitamins. Research also suggests that dietary fat may be necessary for maintaining intramyocellular triglyceride stores, which serve as an important fuel source during prolonged, moderate-intensity exercise.[45,49-51] Studies to date, however, have not demonstrated that low intramyocellular triglyceride stores are responsible for the reduced performance associated with very-low-fat diets.[46]

Careful assessment of the amount and type of fat consumed may be useful. Some vegetarian athletes, particularly endurance-trained athletes (runners and triathletes), may consume excessive carbohydrate and

Table 16.2 Approximate Protein Content of Selected Vegetarian Food Sources

Food	Portion	Protein, g/portion
Bread, most types	1 oz (1 slice)	2–3
Rice, pasta, other grains, cooked	⅓–½ cup	2–3
Cheese, medium to hard	1 oz	7
Cheese, cottage	½ cup	16
Egg, whole	1 large	7
Legumes (most beans, peas, and lentils)	½ cup	7
Milk, all types	1 cup	8
Nuts, most types	2 Tbsp	7
Peanut butter	2 Tbsp	7
Tempeh	½ cup	15
Tofu, firm	1 cup	20
Tofu, soft	1 cup	10
Vegetables, most	½ cup	2–3
Vegetarian "burgers"	1 patty (71 g)	6–16
Vegetarian "chicken"	1 patty (71 g)	9–12
Vegetarian "dogs"	1 dog	9–12
Yogurt, most types	1 cup	8–10

Adapted from the US Department of Agriculture National Nutrient Database for Standard Reference (Release 28, revised May 2016) and selected food labels.

inadequate fat, often with the misconception that dietary fat increases body fat and impairs performance. Similarly, recreational athletes with cardiovascular disease or type 2 diabetes (eg, an active vegetarian following a heart attack) may be following extremely low-fat vegetarian diet plans (<10% energy from fat) recommended by Ornish and Barnard, which are shown to promote regression of coronary atherosclerosis and improve glycemic control.[52-56] Such low-fat diets, however, may be too restrictive for athletes during heavy training. On the other hand, other vegetarian athletes may have jumped on the low-carbohydrate bandwagon and started consuming diets that lack carbohydrates or are too rich in saturated fat, possibly from bakery products or processed foods.

The type of fat included in the diet of vegetarian athletes is also important. The proportion of energy from the various fatty acids should be in accord with national guidelines and contain approximately 10% of energy from polyunsaturated fat, at least 10% as monounsaturated fat, less than 10% from saturated fat, and little to no *trans* fats and should meet the DRI of 1.6 and 1.1 g/d of α-linolenic acid (ALA) for men and women, respectively.[8,57-60] Vegetarian diets are generally rich in sources of n-6 polyunsaturated fatty acids but may be low in n-3 fatty acids.[5] Because n-3 fatty acids may be important for controlling inflammation, vegetarian athletes may benefit from incorporating more foods rich in n-3 fatty acids (walnuts; flaxseed;

and ancanola, flax, hemp, and walnut oils) into the diet in place of some oils rich in n-6 fatty acids (corn, cotton seed, sunflower, and safflower).[61] Although less than 10% of ALA is elongated to eicosapentaenoic acid (EPA) in humans, its conversion may be improved when n-6 concentrations in diet or blood are not high or excessive.[62] Athletes who may benefit from increased n-3 consumption, including pregnant athletes and those with chronic inflammatory injuries or cardiovascular disease, may want to consider microalgae supplements rich in docosahexaenoic acid (DHA).[63] These supplements are well absorbed and positively influence blood concentrations of both DHA and EPA.[64]

SPORTS NUTRITION CONSIDERATIONS: MINERALS AND VITAMINS

Calcium and Vitamin D

CALCIUM

Regular exercise has not been shown to increase calcium requirements.[8] Thus, athletes and active individuals should strive to meet the DRI of 1,000 mg for those between ages 19 and 50 years, 1,200 mg for those older than 50, and 1,300 mg for those younger than 18.[8] Limited evidence also suggests that athletes with amenorrhea may benefit from an additional 500 mg of calcium per day to retain calcium balance.[65] Low dietary calcium levels, along with reduced vitamin D status, are associated with decreased bone density and increased risk for stress fractures, particularly in amenorrheic athletes.[66-68] One recent study found that 8 weeks of supplementation with 800 IU of vitamin D plus 2,000 mg calcium reduced incidence of stress fracture in female naval recruits by 20%.[69]

In general, vegetarian athletes who are eumenorrheic can meet calcium requirements by including eight servings of calcium-containing plant foods or several servings of dairy daily (see Box 16.3). Nondairy foods rich in well-absorbed calcium include low-oxalate green leafy vegetables (kale; broccoli; Chinese cabbage; and collard, mustard, and turnip greens), calcium-set tofu, textured vegetable protein, fortified rice and soy milks, tahini, certain legumes, fortified orange juice, blackstrap molasses, and, possibly, calcium-fortified cereals.[2,13] Laboratory studies determined that calcium bioavailability of most of these plant foods is as good as or better than cow's milk, which has a fractional absorption of 32%.[70-73] The exceptions include soy milk fortified with tricalcium phosphate, most legumes, nuts, and seeds, which have a fractional absorption of 17% to 24%.[73] Other plant foods, including beet greens, rhubarb, spinach, and swiss chard, are not well-absorbed sources of calcium due to their high oxalate or phytate content. A clinical study also found that young vegetarians maintained positive calcium balance and appropriate bone resorption (measured by urinary deoxypyridinoline) when calcium was provided from dairy products or plant foods, despite a lower calcium intake on the plant-based diet (843 ± 140 mg) compared with the dairy-containing diet (1,322 ± 03 mg).[74]

Although it is possible to maintain calcium balance on a plant-based diet in a Western lifestyle, some athletes may find it convenient to use fortified foods or calcium supplements to achieve calcium balance, particularly when requirements are elevated due to amenorrhea or menopause.[2,13,71]

Because vitamin D is also required for adequate calcium absorption and promotion of bone health, a calcium supplement containing vitamin D is advised. Research has shown that only 10% to 15% of dietary calcium is absorbed in the vitamin D–deficient state, whereas 30% to 35% is absorbed when vitamin D status is sufficient.[75,76] Higher bioavailability with higher vitamin D status is promoted by vitamin D–induced expression of calbindin (an intestinal calcium-binding protein) and an epithelial calcium channel protein that increases the efficiency of calcium and phosphorus absorption by active transport across the intestinal mucosa.[77]

VITAMIN D

Recent research has revealed that, beyond bone health, vitamin D is involved in many physiological functions important to an athlete's health and performance, including immune function, inflammatory modulation, and skeletal muscle function.[78-84] Athletes living at northern or southern latitudes (> 32°) with dark pigmented skin or excess body fat or who train primarily indoors or in the early morning or late afternoon throughout the year are at risk for poor vitamin D status.[78,79,85-87] These athletes would benefit from supplementation with enough vitamin D to maintain serum calcium concentrations within the optimal range of 40 to 70 ng/mL.[81] Both vitamin D-3 (cholecalciferol) and D2 (ergocalciferol) are used in supplements and to fortify foods, including cow's milk and some brands/types of soy and rice milks, orange juice, breakfast cereals, margarines, and yogurt. Vitamin D-3, obtained through ultraviolet radiation of 7-dehydrocholesterol from lanolin, is not vegan. Vitamin D-3 derived from lichen and vitamin D-2 produced from irradiation of ergosterol from yeast are acceptable to vegans.[76,88] Research has suggested that vitamin D-2 is as effective as vitamin D-3 at lower doses (ie, 1,000 IU) but less effective at increasing and maintaining endogenous 25(OH)D concentrations when taken in higher doses (> 4,000 IU).[89-91] Natural and fortified sources of vitamin D are listed in Box 16.3. (See Chapter 5 and reference 78 for additional information on vitamin D assessment and needs of athletes.)

Box 16.3 Vegetarian Sources of Selected Vitamins and Minerals

Nutrient	Good Food Choices
Calcium	Calcium-set tofu, calcium-fortified beverages (orange juice and other fruit juices, soy and rice milks), broccoli, Chinese cabbage, kale, collard greens, mustard greens, turnip greens, almonds, tahini, texturized vegetable protein, blackstrap molasses, cow's milk, certain cheeses, and legumes
Iron	Legumes, nuts and seeds, whole/enriched grains, enriched/fortified cereals and pasta, leafy green and root vegetables, and dried fruits
Iodine	Iodized salt and sea vegetables (kombu, arame, dulse, and other types of seaweed)
Magnesium	Legumes, nuts and seeds, whole grains, green leafy vegetables, blackstrap molasses
Riboflavin	Whole-grain and fortified breads and cereals, legumes, tofu, nuts and seeds, tahini, bananas, asparagus, figs, dark-green leafy vegetables, avocado, most sea vegetables (kombu, arame, dulse and other types of seaweed), and dairy products
Vitamin B-12	Yeast flakes, fortified foods such as ready-to-eat cereal, meat analogues, some types/brands of soy and rice milks, dairy products, and eggs
Vitamin D[a]	Fatty fish (salmon, sardines, mackerel), fortified foods (cow's milk, some types/brands of soy and rice milks), orange juice, ready-to-eat breakfast cereals, margarines, yogurt, egg yolks, and sun-dried mushrooms
Zinc	Legumes, nuts and seeds, whole-grain products, fortified ready-to-eat cereal, soy products, commercial meat analogues, and hard cheeses

[a] Sun exposure (~5–30 min on the arms and legs between 10 AM and 2 PM non–daylight savings time, several times a week) is another source of vitamin D.

Adapted from the US Department of Agriculture National Nutrient Database for Standard (Release 28, revised May 2016) and reference 6.

Iron

Iron depletion is one of the most prevalent nutrient deficiencies in athletes—especially female athletes.[92-94] Iron depletion with anemia (stage III) and without anemia (stage II) can impair muscle function and maximal oxygen uptake and can decrease endurance.[95-97] Whereas iron depletion among athletes is most commonly attributed to insufficient energy or low iron intakes, other factors can affect iron status, including vegetarian diets, periods of rapid growth, training at altitude, acute inflammation, and increased iron losses through gastrointestinal bleeding, heavy sweating, foot strike, intravascular hemolysis, chronic disease, hematuria, or heavy menstrual blood losses.[7,92,98-102]

Most of the iron in a vegetarian diet is nonheme iron, which has a lower absorption rate (2% to 20%) than heme iron (15% to 35%) and is sensitive to inhibitors and enhancers of iron absorption.[103] Inhibitors

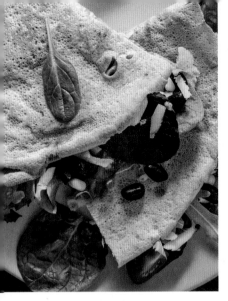

of iron absorption include phytates, calcium, and the polyphenolics (including tannins) in tea, coffee, herb teas, and cocoa.[2] Fiber has only a slight impact on impairing iron absorption.[104]

Oxidating Fe^{3+} (reducing it to Fe^{2+}) means that vitamin C, and other organic acids (citric, malic, lactic, and tartaric acids) can significantly enhance iron absorption and reduce the inhibitory effects of tannins and phytates, as can allium spices, including onions and garlic.[8,105-107] Furthermore, individuals with low iron stores or a higher physiological need for iron will tend to absorb more iron and excrete less. Iron absorption may also be impacted by conditions affecting the absorptive capacity of enterocytes (eg, celiac disease and gastric bypass surgery). Due to increased iron losses and the lower bioavailability of iron from a vegetarian diet, there is some indication that vegetarian athletes have higher iron needs. The recommended intake may be 1.3 to 1.8 times higher than the RDA, respectively.[8] Therefore, it may be prudent for vegetarian athletes to aim for iron intakes that are slightly higher than the RDA.

In most cases, vegetarians who eat a varied and well-balanced diet rich in whole grains, legumes, nuts, seeds, dried fruits, iron-fortified cereals, and green leafy vegetables can achieve adequate iron status without iron supplementation. Studies of vegetarian athletes and nonathletes have found that vegetarians have average iron intakes, similar to or higher than that of nonvegetarians, yet they often have lower iron status.[12,106,108,109] Vegetarian athletes should, therefore, be educated about plant sources of iron (see Box 16.3), along with factors that enhance and interfere with its absorption. For example, an athlete who drinks coffee, tea, or milk with legume-containing meals should be advised to drink citrus fruit juice instead to enhance the iron absorbed from that meal. While supplementation has been shown to improve energy efficiency and endurance performance in iron-depleted athletes who are not anemic, supplements should be recommended only for those with compromised stores, as indicated by a low serum ferritin level, elevated total iron binding capacity, or elevated serum transferrin receptor (see Chapter 5 for further information).[94,110,111] Reduced hemoglobin, hematocrit, or red blood cell concentrations in athletes are not good indicators of iron status in endurance athletes due to exercise-induced plasma volume expansion.[7,112] Athletes taking iron supplements should have iron status monitored because of the prevalence of hereditary hemochromatosis and other iron overload abnormalities in the United States and the potential association between iron status and chronic disease.[8,113]

Zinc

Vegetarian athletes, female athletes, and athletes in heavy training commonly have serum zinc concentrations on the lower end of the normal range or below the recommended level.[114,115] In vegetarians, lower zinc status is most likely due to the reduced bioavailability of zinc from plant foods compared with animal foods but may also be related to the selection of zinc-poor foods.[2,8,107] Lower bioavailability in vegetarian diets is due mainly to the higher phytic acid content of many plant foods, including phytate-rich unrefined grains and legumes.[116] Lower bioavailability may increase the dietary zinc requirement by 50%.[8] While overt zinc deficiency is typically not present in Western vegetarians, the significance of marginal deficiency is unknown due to the difficulty of evaluating zinc status.[2] Serum zinc concentrations, for example, are often altered by increases in training intensity and may not reflect tissue zinc stores or zinc status.[114,117,118] Although more research is needed, zinc supplementation has not been shown to influence serum zinc concentrations during training or offer performance benefits.[117-119]

Due to potential negative effects of zinc status on health and performance, sports dietitians should work with vegetarian athletes to ensure that the RDA for zinc is met or exceeded through consumption of zinc-containing plant foods. Consumption of zinc-containing foods with organic acids, including citric acid (found in many fruits and vegetables), may enhance zinc absorption.[120] In support of this recommendation, a study from the US Department of Agriculture found that nonathletic women consuming a diet containing legumes and whole grains for 8 weeks maintained zinc status within normal limits, even though the diet was lower in total zinc and higher in phytate and fiber than a control omnivorous diet.[121] To maintain adequate zinc status, the authors advised that legumes and whole grains be consumed regularly. Another study of women who habitually followed a plant-based diet found that adding milk and yogurt to a plant-based diet high in phytate increased zinc bioavailability by more than 70% without altering iron bioavailability.[122] Soaking and sprouting beans, grains, nuts, and seeds are other methods that can improve zinc bioavailability by reducing binding to phytic acid.[2] The zinc content of selected protein-containing plant foods is shown in Box 16.3.

Iodine

Iodine status has not generally been a concern for athletes living in industrial countries. Evidence is mounting, however, that some vegetarians and vegans may be at increased risk for iodine deficiency.[4,123-126] One study that assessed the iodine status of 81 nonathletic adults found that 25% of the vegetarians and 80% of the vegans had iodine deficiency (urinary iodine excretion value below 100 µg/L) compared with 9% in nonvegetarians.[123] The higher prevalence of iodine deficiency among vegetarians is thought to be a consequence of prevailing (or exclusive) consumption of plant foods grown in soil with low iodine content, limited consumption of cow's milk, little or no intake of fish or sea products, and reduced use of iodized salt.[123-125] These studies have exposed a need for more research, looking especially at the possible effects of iodine deficiency on the health and performance of athletes. Vegetarian athletes can ensure adequate iodine status by consuming one-half teaspoon of iodized salt in the diet daily.[127] Sea salt, kosher salt, and salty seasonings such as tamari are generally not iodized. Neither are most high-sodium processed foods. Finally, while plant foods such as cruciferous vegetables, sweet potatoes, and soybeans naturally contain goitrogens, these foods have not been associated with hypothyroid or thyroid insufficiency if iodine status is adequate.[128]

Magnesium

Suboptimal magnesium status is thought to be widespread in the United States.[129] Athletes participating in sports requiring weight control (eg, wrestling, ballet, and gymnastics) are especially vulnerable to an inadequate magnesium status.[7,130] Athletes participating in strenuous exercise may also be at risk due to increased magnesium losses in urine and sweat that may increase magnesium requirements by 10% to 20%. Marginal magnesium deficiency impairs exercise performance and amplifies the negative consequences of strenuous exercise including oxidative stress. In athletes with suboptimal status, increased dietary intake of magnesium or magnesium supplementation will have beneficial effects on exercise performance.[130] Foods rich in magnesium, which come mostly from unprocessed plant-based sources, are listed in Box 16.3.

B Vitamins

Vegetarian diets can easily provide the requirements for most B vitamins.[2,131] Diets containing little to no eggs or dairy and those low in energy, however, may not supply adequate vitamin B-12 and riboflavin.[132]

VITAMIN B-12

Cobalamin, the active form of vitamin B-12, is found almost exclusively in animal products.[133] Vegan athletes should, therefore, make the effort to consume vitamin B-12–fortified foods daily or take a multivitamin containing vitamin B-12. Food sources of vitamin B-12 include yeast flakes, soy milk and other fortified plant-based milks, breakfast cereals, and meat analogues that are vitamin B12–fortified.[2] Although some discussion in the lay literature suggests that fermented soy products and nori and chorella seaweeds can supply bioavailable vitamin B-12, research does not consistently support this concept, which arose because the standard assay for determining vitamin B-12 content does not distinguish between biologically active forms and analogues.[134-136]

Vegetarians who consume dairy products or eggs are likely to have adequate intakes of vitamin B-12; however, both vegans and vegetarians may be at risk for low B-12 status.[2,133,137] Because of the irreversible neurologic damage that can occur with vitamin B-12 deficiency, markers of vitamin B-12 status (homocysteine, methylmalonic acid, and holotranscobalamin II) should be measured if there is concern that the athlete's diet may be lacking in reliable sources of vitamin B-12.[133] The typical manifestation of vitamin B-12 deficiency as macrocytic anemia can be masked by high folate intake, a probable finding in vegan or vegetarian athletes who consume ample legumes and dark green leafy and other vegetables.

RIBOFLAVIN

Riboflavin intake may be low in athletes who avoid dairy products, particularly when energy intake is restricted to promote weight loss.[7,131] There is some evidence that riboflavin needs may be increased in individuals who are habitually physically active and in those who begin an exercise program, particularly if riboflavin status was marginal prior to exercise initiation.[8,138,139] Because dairy products are rich sources of riboflavin, education on the plant sources of riboflavin may help ensure adequate intake. Good plant sources of riboflavin are shown in Box 16.3(page 337).

SPORTS NUTRITION CONSIDERATIONS: SUPPLEMENTS

Vegetarian athletes, like other athletes, may inquire about nutritional supplements or ergogenic aids to assist their athletic training and performance. Like all athletes, vegetarian athletes should first be encouraged to follow a balanced diet before considering supplements. Vegetarian and vegan athletes might be concerned about whether the ingredients are animal or plant derived, which may vary by manufacturer (see *Vegetarian Journal's Guide to Vegetarian and Vegan Restaurants in the US and Canada* in the Vegetarian Resources section at the end of this chapter). An extensive discussion of supplements can be found in Chapter 7, but supplements of particular interest to vegetarian athletes—protein, creatine, and carnitine—are briefly discussed here.

Protein Supplements

Protein from supplements is not needed if the athlete is consuming adequate energy and making proper food choices.[28] For convenience, protein-containing sports beverages and bars can be used occasionally to supplement the diet. Recent research has suggested that supplemental beverages that contain only soy protein are not as effective as milk at promoting postexercise muscle protein synthesis over the short term, but long-term studies are not available.[140-143]

Creatine and Carnitine

Creatine and carnitine are supplied by meat and other animal products in the diet. Even though these molecules can be endogenously synthesized from amino acid precursors, serum concentrations of creatine and carnitine and skeletal muscle concentrations of creatine are lower in those following vegetarian diets.[144-149] Substantial evidence suggests that supplementation with creatine monohydrate can increase skeletal muscle creatine content and improve performance in repeated bouts of maximal and endurance sprinting and can provide potential gains in fat-free mass, muscle force, and power output with resistance training. Several, but not all, studies have noted that vegetarians who take creatine supplements experience greater increases in skeletal muscle total creatine, phosphocreatine, lean tissue mass, and work performance during weight-training and anaerobic bicycle performance than their nonvegetarian teammates.[146,149-151] There is no evidence, however, that vegetarians benefit from carnitine supplementation. Furthermore, although a plant-based diet does not seem to negatively affect muscle buffering capacity due to the lower carnosine content.[152] However, supplementing with β-alanine has been shown to effectively buffer muscle pH in athletes.[153] This is not expected to differ in athletes following a plant-based diet, although research is needed.

Preexercise Nutrition

Eating before exercise has been shown to improve performance.[7] The meal or snack eaten before a competition or exercise session should be high in carbohydrate (to maintain blood glucose and top off glycogen stores), provide fluids, and prevent hunger and gastrointestinal distress. Studies show that intake of 1 to 4 g carbohydrate per kilogram body weight approximately 1 to 4 hours before endurance exercise has the potential to improve endurance performance by as much as 14% and is also thought to benefit high-intensity activity lasting several hours.[154-156] Athletes should be encouraged to consume familiar, well-tolerated, high-carbohydrate meals low in fiber, simple sugars, and sodium.[7] Smaller meals should be consumed in proximity to exercise or a sport event to allow for gastric emptying, whereas larger meals maybe consumed when more time is available.[7] As a guideline, aim for 1 to 4 g of carbohydrate per kilogram body weight in the pre-event meal 1 to 4 hours before exercise.[27] In general, smaller amounts, such as 1 to 2 g carbohydrate per kilogram body weight, are suggested closer to exercise.[19] Vegetarian athletes accustomed to eating gas-producing foods such as legumes, not typically recommended in the pre-event meal, may tolerate these foods without complications. Athletes who experience gastrointestinal distress may find liquid meals, such as fruit smoothies, more tolerable before exercise. While some studies suggest that emphasizing low glycemic index foods compared with high glycemic index foods (eg, lentils vs mashed potatoes) may offer a performance advantage, particularly during prolonged submaximal exercise; however, other studies have found no performance advantages.[157,158] Athletes interested in trying new pre-event regimens should experiment with new foods and beverages during practice sessions.

In addition, vegetarian athletes should follow the recommended guidelines for fluid consumption to avoid beginning exercise in a dehydrated state. These include maintaining adequate hydration in the 12- to 24-hour period before exercise and consuming 5 to 7 mL of water or other fluidsper kilogram body weight at least 4 hours before exercise.[158] Fluid ingestion too close to exercise increases the likelihood that the athlete may need to urinate before or during training or competition. Chapter 6 provides more information on hydration for athletes.

Nutrition During Exercise

Ingesting between 40 to 75 g carbohydate per hour has been shown to benefit performance during both prolonged, moderate-intensity exercise lasting 2 hours or more and variable-intensity exercise of shorter duration, such as soccer and other team sports.[19,159-162] This performance benefit presumably results from maintenance of blood glucose concentrations and preservation of carbohydrate oxidation, which decreases as glycogen stores become depleted.[163] Ingesting fluid-replacement beverages at the recommended carbohydrate concentration of 6% to 8% provides carbohydrate while simultaneously meeting fluid needs; this approach may be beneficial to performance in events lasting 1 hour or less, particularly when exercise is initiated in the fasting or near-fasting state.[7,164] For longer events, consuming between 30 to 60 g carbohydrate per hour has unequivocally been shown to improve performance.[7]

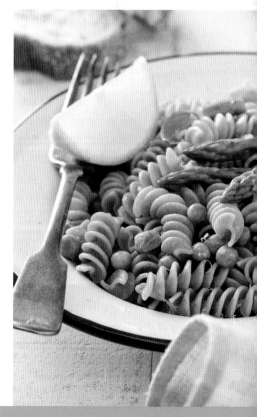

Based on recent research gindings, ingesting up to 136 g carbohydrate per hour in the form of mixed sugars (ie, glucose plus fructose) provides benefits for events lasting longer than 2 to 3 hours, ingesting up to 90 g of carbohydrate is now the suggested fueling strategy for ultraendurance events lasting longer than 2.5 to 3 hours.[27,165,166] Mixed sugars use different intestinal transporters and allow for increased absorption and oxidation of exogenous sugars. Additionally, current research indicates that mouth rinsing with a carbohydrate-containing solution may enhance performance in some events via central nervous system effects.[27,167]

Adequate fluid intake is also essential for maintaining endurance performance and, along with carbohydrates, has a cumulative effect on enhancing performance.[161] Intake of carbohydrate and fluid should be initiated shortly after the start of exercise to maximize time for sugar and nutrients to reach the bloodstream. Fluid replacement goals depend on the athlete's sweat rate, exercise intensity, exercise duration, and environmental temperatures.[168] In general, however, enough fluid should be consumed during exercise to avert a fluid deficit in excess of 2% of body weight.[7,164,168] (See Chapter 6 for additional information on hydration.)

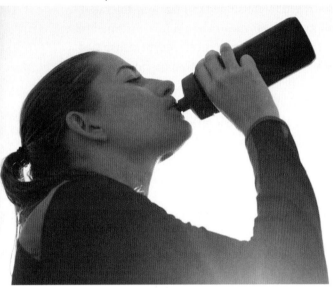

Although commercial sports drinks and gels consumed with water work well for delivering easily absorbed carbohydrate, some vegetarian athletes may prefer natural or noncommercial sources of carbohydrate.[169] In this case, fruit juices diluted with water (4 ounces juice in 4 ounces water = 6% solution); low-sodium vegetable juices, such as carrot juice (7% solution); and honey or solid foods ingested with water (8 ounces for every 15 g carbohydrate = 6.3%) may be appropriate. Research has shown that solid food and honey are as effective as liquids for increasing blood glucose and enhancing performance and are easily digested.[170-173] Thus, providing a range of drinks and sports products can help athletes meet the recommended carbohydrate intake during exercise and gives athletes many options to choose from.[27] A pinch of table salt can also be added to juices or low-sodium solids as necessary for events lasting longer than 3 to 4 hours.[174] Although there is some evidence that adding protein to fluid replacement beverages may benefit performance or postexercise recovery, more research is needed.[175-179] As a final point, note that although many vegetarians may be interested in honey because it is perceived as natural sugar, vegans may be opposed to it because it is an animal product.[180]

Postexercise Nutrition

All athletes—including vegetarian athletes—should consume a mixed meal or snack providing carbohydrates, protein, and fat soon after a strenuous competition or training session. This may be particularly beneficial following prolonged or strenuous exercise when athletes should make an effort to consume carbohydrate and possibly protein immediately after exercise to promote recovery, particularly if exercise training is to be resumed the following day.[27,28]

Carbohydrate intake between 1 and 1.2 g per kilogram body weight per hour for the first 4 hours after exercise is recommended to replace muscle glycogen and ensure rapid recovery.[7,27] Foods with a high glycemic index or those containing both carbohydrate and protein (approximately 1 g protein to 3 g carbohydrate) may promote a more rapid rate of muscle glycogen storage after exercise by stimulating greater insulin secretion.[158,181-183] Evidence suggests that consuming protein along with carbohydrate after endurance or resistance training may provide needed amino acids for building and repairing muscle tissue to maximally stimulate muscle protein synthesis.[28,38,184-188] Although the exact timing of the postexercise window has not been determined, athletes interested in performance and skeletal muscle gain should consume protein as soon as possible after exercise.[189] Including fat during the recovery period may also be needed to replace intramyocellular lipid stores during periods of high-volume endurance training.[45,46] Chapter 3 provides more information on the timing of protein intake for athletes.

Current recommendations for postexercise fluid requirements are to consume up to 150% of the body mass loss (ie, fluid loss) during the exercise session or at least an amount greater than that lost to optimize recovery.[7,27,164,168] In general, a kilogram of body weight loss is approximately 1 L of fluid loss. Athletes participating in heavy, prolonged workouts should also include sodium and potassium in the recovery meal.[164,190] While vegetarians are likely to choose foods containing ample potassium (eg, fruits and vegetables), many may intentionally or unintentionally avoid sodium-containing foods. During heavy training, sodium intake can be of concern in athletes who avoid salt or processed foods (ie, the typical sweat loss is about 50 mEq/L or 1 g sodium per hour).[7,164] Thus, more liberal intakes of sodium are often appropriate among athletes. Counseling vegetarian athletes on sodium-containing foods to consume during the recovery period may be appropriate.

SPECIAL CONCERNS: RELATIVE ENERGY DEFICIENCY SYNDROME

Low energy availability—with or without eating disorders, reduced bone density, and altered menstrual function in women—provides a significant health risk for female and male athletes.[191] There is some indication that this condition, recently termed relative energy deficiency in sport (RED-S) and formerly identified as the female athlete triad, may be higher in vegetarians and vegetarian athletes, but the findings are not consistent.[192-194] In some cases, the apparent increased prevalence of RED-S or its components among vegetarians may be explained by study design or recruitment bias.[193]

For example, some studies have defined vegetarians as those having a low-meat diet and not necessarily a vegetarian diet and do not differentiate. Studies may also recruit a biased sample of vegetarians (ie, those with menstrual cycle disturbances may be more likely to volunteer for a study on menstrual cycle disturbances).[193] Furthermore, as will be reviewed later, proclaiming to be vegetarian may be perceived as a socially acceptable way to mask an eating disorder.[195-198] Professionals should certainly be cautioned to assess each athlete, including those following plant-based diets, and not make generalizations based on dietary preferences.[189]

The mechanism mediating the disruption of normal hypothalamic reproductive function is unknown, but evidence points to a favoring of energy availability (ie, the energy drain hypothesis), rather than stress or an overly lean body composition.[199] An earlier study, however, suggests that other factors may be linked to amenorrhea in women following a plant-based diet. In nonathletic women, Goldin and colleagues found that vegetarians had lower circulating estrogen concentrations—associated with higher fiber and lower fat intakes, higher fecal outputs, and two to three times more estrogen in their feces—compared with nonvegetarians.[200] Among athletes, retrospective recall studies have documented lower intakes of energy, protein, fat, and zinc, and higher intakes of vitamin A and fiber in athletes in those who are amenorrheic compared with those who are eumenorrheic.[201-204] Collectively, these findings suggest that the energy and nutrient composition of some vegetarian diets could predispose vegetarian athletes to amenorrhea and reduced bone density.

Because available research suggests that reproductive disruption typically occurs when energy availability (dietary energy intake minus exercise energy expenditure) is less than a threshold of 30 kcal/kg of lean body mass, vegetarian athletes who are amenorrheic should be counseled on how to meet energy needs on a vegetarian diet, which may include reducing fiber intake and increasing the frequency of meals and snacks.[191,199] For athletes in heavy training, a diet with excessive fiber may lower energy intake and potentially reduce enterohepatic circulation of sex steroid hormones.[200,205]

ASSESSING, COUNSELING, AND WORKING WITH VEGETARIAN ATHLETES

Assessment

The body size and composition of vegetarian athletes vary, as do their dietary practices, food choices, and reasons for being vegetarian. The sports dietitian should, therefore, first obtain and evaluate anthropometric measures, biochemical (laboratory) values, pertinent clinical information, and dietary and environmental factors, as discussed in Chapters 8 and 9. While laboratory and clinical data collected will vary, evaluation of mean corpuscular volume, hemoglobin, hematocrit, and 25(OH) vitamin D concentrations may be helpful. For female athletes, it is important to assess energy intake, menstrual function, training load, fatigue, history of injuries, and exercise performance to look for signs of the female athlete triad or RED-S.[191] Unintended weight or muscle loss, tiredness, fatigue, reduced strength gains, reduced performance, or loss of menstrual cycle function should be assessed, as these are signs that the diet may be lacking in total energy and possibly in certain macro- or micronutrients.

The dietary assessment should begin by determining which foods the athlete eliminates from the diet and which foods are acceptable. This will help assess nutrient adequacy and ensure that nutrients in omitted foods (such as dairy products) can be met with acceptable plant-based foods.

Although terms such as lacto-ovo-vegetarian, lacto-vegetarian, vegan, or strict vegetarian are commonly used to describe vegetarians, recent evidence-based analysis suggests that these very broad categories mask important variations within vegetarian diets and dietary practices.[2] For example, two lacto-ovo-vegetarian athletes may have different philosophies about dairy products that would require a different treatment plan. One may consume several servings of dairy products per day, while the other may eat only cheese and small amounts of dairy found in processed foods. Similarly, some vegans may be extremely strict, eliminating all commercially available foods that contain any ingredient that is animal derived or processed with an animal derivative (eg, commercial bread), while others will avoid only foods of obvious animal origin. Furthermore, some individuals claim to follow vegetarian diets when they mean that they avoid red meat but occasionally eat fish or poultry.

A thorough diet history followed by an analysis of energy and key nutrients, such as carbohydrate, protein, fat, fiber, calcium, vitamin D, iron, zinc, iodine, riboflavin, and vitamin B-12 is the best way to reliably assess the vegetarian athlete's diet. Computer nutrient databases may be helpful, but many do not contain an adequate selection of commercially available vegetarian food products. In many cases, it is useful to have the athlete keep food records and bring in food labels from vegetarian products that he or she consumes. The sports dietitian may find the recently developed 369-item vegan-specific questionnaire useful for some athletic populations and situations.[206]

Information collected about the environment should include discussion of the athlete's belief system (ie, why he or she has chosen to follow a vegetarian diet) and barriers to healthy eating. Although health, ecology, animal welfare, and religion are admirable reasons for following a vegetarian diet, desire to lose weight, lack of time, or creation of a certain social image may raise a red flag. Individuals who don't eat meat because it is the socially acceptable way to lose weight or because of limited time or food budgets have been labeled "new wave" vegetarians.[207] These individuals may be at health and nutritional risk due to their haphazard eating patterns and lack of a solid philosophy, which is what typically drives many vegetarians in their desire to eat well. The focus when working with new-wave vegetarians should be on improving the diet with more healthful plant-based but not necessarily vegetarian foods. A final concern is that vegetarianism may be used as a convenient and socially acceptable way for individuals with disordered eating tendencies to reduce energy and fat intake and thus mask their disordered eating behaviors.[195-198] Occasionally, vegetarianism may therefore be a red flag for disordered eating and increased risk for the female athlete triad and RED-S.[7,191]

Counseling and Nutrition Treatment

The role of the nutrition professional during counseling, nutrition education, and treatment is to work with the athlete to ensure adequate nutritional status given his or her lifestyle, income, and vegetarian belief system. Guidelines initially developed for counseling pregnant vegetarians are useful when working with the vegetarian population in general and include establishing rapport, reinforcing positive nutrition practices, prioritizing nutrition concerns, and providing individualized dietary recommendations.[208,209] It is also important to remember that nutritional requirements are for essential nutrients (eg, protein, calcium, and iron) rather than for specific foods (eg, meat or milk) or food groups (eg, meat group or dairy group). Given the position of the Academy of Nutrition and Dietetics on vegetarian diets, a vegetarian athlete should never be advised to consume meat or dairy to be healthy.[2] Box 16.4 contains tips for helping vegetarian athletes select a well-balanced vegetarian diet.

Box 16.4 Tips for Vegetarian Athletes

- Choose a variety of foods, including whole and enriched grains, fruits, vegetables, legumes, nuts, seeds, and, if desired, dairy products and eggs.
- Consume adequate energy to optimize performance and help meet other nutrient needs, including protein, iron, zinc, magnesium, and riboflavin. Decrease fiber and possibly increase energy intake by consuming one-third to one-half of cereal or grain servings from refined rather than whole-grain sources and by replacing some high-fiber fruit or vegetable servings with juice servings.
- To help meet energy needs, consume small, frequent meals and snacks and strive to obtain one-third to one-half of grains, fruits, and vegetables from more refined sources rather than whole-food sources, including enriched pasta, white rice, and fruit juice.
- Strive to consume a variety of protein-rich foods over the course of the day. Consumption of protein-rich foods along with carbohydrate foods in the 30 minutes after strenuous exercise may enhance recovery.
- Incorporate healthful fats in cooking and in dressing up foods, and limit foods that are high in saturated and *trans* fats.
- Include foods rich in n-3 fatty acids, such as flaxseeds; walnuts; and canola, flax, hemp, and walnut oils.
- If dairy products are not consumed, choose eight or more servings per day of calcium-rich foods (see Box 16.3 page 337).
- Obtain adequate vitamin D from regular sun exposure or through fortified foods or supplements. In the absence of adequate sun exposure, intake of vitamin D between 1,000 and 7,000 IU is needed daily to maintain optimal vitamin D status.
- To meet iron needs, consume a variety of iron-rich grains and legumes daily. Aim to consume a fruit or vegetable that contains vitamin C along with most meals to boost absorption.
- Incorporate legumes and a serving or two of nuts into the diet almost daily. These foods provide protein and an abundance of other nutrients, including iron, zinc, magnesium, and some calcium. Nuts also provide additional energy and healthful fats.
- Use iodized salt when cooking and in salting foods, particularly in areas where the concentration of iodine in the soil is low. Remember that the sodium needs of athletes are often increased due to sodium losses in sweat.
- Incorporate sources of vitamin B-12 in the diet each day. Vegan sources include 1 tablespoon of nutritional yeast, 1 cup (8 oz) of fortified soy milk, 1 oz (28 g) of fortified cereal, and 1.5 oz (42 g) of fortified meat analogue. Servings for vegetarians include ½ cup (4 oz) of cow's milk, 6 oz (172 g) yogurt, and one egg.
- Limit consumption of overly processed foods, which typically contain added sugars and unhealthful fats.

RESOURCES FOR IMPROVING THE DIET

Some athletes or active individuals—vegetarian or omnivore—may find it difficult to select a healthy well-balanced diet with adequate variety.[209] Factors such as lack of knowledge about food preparation, lack of time, and economic constraints may lead to a monotonous diet. Vegetarian cookbooks (particularly with pictures), videos, and credible websites can be used to provide ideas for increasing dietary variety and preparing simple meals. A tour of a supermarket or natural foods store may help identify products that are suitable for vegetarians. Vegetarian cooking classes for teams or individual athletes are also a great way to provide hands-on education and introduce new vegetarian foods and recipes.

SUMMARY

Athletes at all levels of performance can meet their energy and nutrient needs on a vegetarian diet that contains a variety of plant foods.[189] Depending on their food patterns, however, some athletes may have trouble meeting their dietary needs for certain key nutrients, including total energy, carbohydrate, protein, fat, calcium, vitamin D, iron, zinc, iodine, riboflavin, and vitamin B-12. Therefore, vegetarian athletes, like most athletes, may benefit from education on food choices that provide adequate energy and nutrients, thereby promoting optimal training, optimal performance, and good health.

Sports dietitians who work with vegetarian and vegan athletes and their trainers and coaches need to be sensitive to and knowledgeable about vegetarianism and exercise training. Athletes should be encouraged to eat a wide variety of plant foods; they should not be told that they need poultry, fish, or dairy products to obtain adequate nutrition. It is the position of the Academy of Nutrition and Dietetics that "appropriately planned vegetarian, including vegan, diets are healthful, nutritionally adequate, and may provide health benefits in the prevention and treatment of certain diseases" and can "meet the needs of competitive athletes."[2]

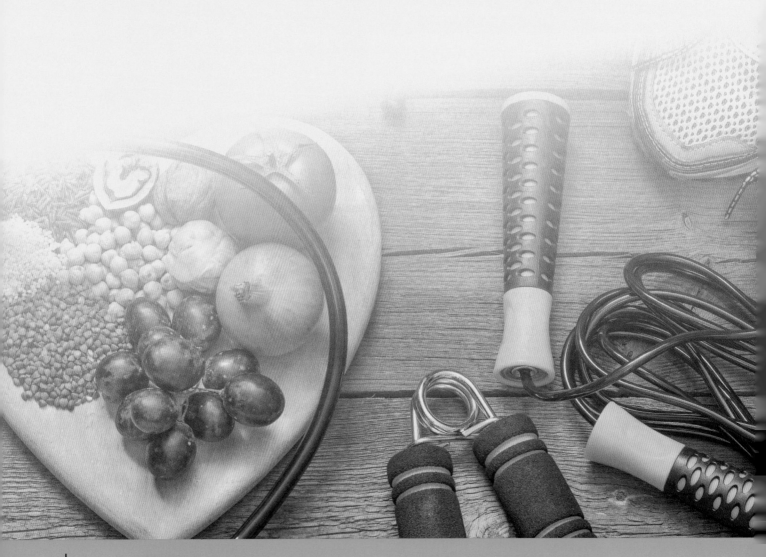

KEY TAKEAWAYS

A well-balanced vegetarian or vegan diet can support athletes at all levels of training and performance.

Meeting energy needs is a nutrition priority for all athletes, including vegetarian athletes.

A varied and well-balanced diet rich in whole grains, legumes, nuts, seeds, dried fruits, iron-fortified cereals, and green leafy vegetables can help ensure vegetarian athletes meet their needs for most nutrients.

Educating vegetarian athletes on food sources of carbohydrate, protein, fat, calcium, vitamin D, iron, zinc, iodine, riboflavin, and vitamin B-12 should help ensure adequate health and performance.

Consumer Publications

- Davis B, Melina V. *Becoming Vegan, Express Edition: The Everyday Guide to Plant-based Nutrition.* Summertown, TN: Book Publishing Co; 2013.
- Frazier M, Ruscigno M. *No Meat Athlete: Run on Plants and Discover Your Fittest, Fastest, Happiest Self.* Beverly, MA: Fair Winds Press; 2013.
- Larson-Meyer DE. *Vegetarian Sports Nutrition: Food Choices and Eating Plans for Fitness and Performance.* Champaign, IL: Human Kinetics; 2006.
- *USDA Choose MyPlate Tips for Vegetarians.* www.choosemyplate.gov/tips-vegetarians. Updated October 12, 2016.
- *Vegetarian Journal.* Bimonthly publication by the Vegetarian Resource Group, PO Box 1463, Baltimore, MD 21203. www.vrg.org/journal/.
- *Vegetarian Journal's Guide to Vegetarian and Vegan Restaurants in the US and Canada* (online version), Vegetarian Resource Group. Updates available at: www.vrg.org/restaurant/
- Yacoubou J. *Vegetarian Journal's Guide to Food Ingredients* (online version). Vegetarian Resource Group. www.vrg.org/ingredients/index.php.
- Wasserman D, Stahler C. *Meatless Meals for Working People: Quick and Easy Vegetarian Recipes.* 5th ed. Baltimore, MD: Vegetarian Resource Group; 2009.
- Wasserman D, Mangels R. *Simply Vegan: Quick Vegetarian Meals.* 5th ed. Baltimore, MD: Vegetarian Resource Group; 2013.

Professional Publications

- Carlson P, ed. *The Complete Vegetarian: The Essential Guide to Good Health.* Champaign, IL: University of Illinois Press; 2009.
- Mangels R, Messina V, Messina M. *The Dietitian's Guide to Vegetarian Diets: Issues and Applications.* 3rd ed. Sudbury, MA: Jones & Bartlett Learning; 2011.
- Mellina V, Craig W, Levin S. Position of the Academy of Nutrition and Dietetics: vegetarian diets. *J Acad Nutr Diet.* 2016;116(12):1970-1980.
- Sabaté J. *Vegetarian Nutrition.* Boca Raton, FL: CRC Press; 2001.

Quantity Recipes for Feeding Groups of Vegetarian Athletes

- Berkoff N. *Vegan in Volume: Vegan Quantity Recipes for Every Occasion.* Rev ed. Baltimore, MD: Vegetarian Resource Group; 2007.
- *Vegetarian Journal's Foodservice Update.* Periodic publication by the Vegetarian Resource Group, PO Box 1463, Baltimore, MD 21203. www.vrg.org/fsupdate/.

Resource Groups

- Vegetarian Nutrition Dietetic Practice Group of the Academy of Nutrition and Dietetics. www.vegetariannutrition.net.
- The Vegetarian Resource Group. www.vrg.org.

REFERENCES

1. Pelly FE, Burkhart SJ. Dietary regimens of athletes competing at the Delhi 2010 Commonwealth Games. *Int J Sport Nutr Exerc Metab.* 2014;24(1):28-36.

2. Mellina V, Craig W, Levin S. Position of the Academy of Nutrition and Dietetics: vegetarian diets. *J Acad Nutr Diet.* 2016;116(12):1970-1980.

3. Larson-Meyer DE. *Vegetarian Sports Nutrition. Food Choices and Eating Plans for Fitness and Performance.* Champaign, IL: Human Kinetics; 2006.

4. Leitzmann C. Vegetarian diets: what are the advantages? *Forum Nutr.* 2005;(57):147-156.

5. Reid MA, Marsh KA, Zeuschner CL, Saunders AV, Baines SK. Meeting the nutrient reference values on a vegetarian diet. *Med J Aust.* 2013;199(4):S33-40.

6. Goran MI. Variation in total energy expenditure in humans. *Obes Res.* 1995;3(S1):59-66.

7. Thomas DT, Erdman KA, Burke LM. Position of the Academy of Nutrition and Dietetics, Dietitians of Canada, and the American College of Sports Medicine: nutrition and athletic performance. *J Acad Nutr Diet.* 2016;116(3):501-528.

8. Otten JJ, Hellwig JP, Meyers LD, eds. Food and Nutrition Board, Institutes of Medicine. *The Dietary Reference Intakes: The Essential Guide to Nutrient Requirements.* Washington, DC: National Academies Press; 2006.

9. Institute of Medicine. *Dietary Reference Intakes for Energy, Carbohydrate, Fiber, Fat, Fatty Acids, Cholesterol, Protein, and Amino Acids.* Washington, DC: National Academies Press; 2005.

10. Cunningham JJ. A reanalysis fo the factors influencing basal metabolic rate in normal adults. *Am J Clin Nutr.* 1980;33(11):2372-2374.

11. US Department of Agriculture. MyPyramid. www.cnpp.usda.gov/mypyramid. Accessed November 8, 2016.

12. Messina V, Mangels AR, Messina M. *A Dietitian's Guide to Vegetarian Diets: Issues and Applications.* 2nd ed. Boston, MA: Jones & Bartlett Publishers; 2004.

13. Messina V, Melina V, Mangels AR. A new food guide for North American vegetarians. *J Am Diet Assoc.* 2003;103(6):771-775.

14. Casey A, Mann R, Banister K, et al. Effect of carbohydrate ingestion on glycogen resynthesis in human liver and skeletal muscle, measured by (13)C MRS. *Am J Physiol Endocrinol Metab.* 2000;278(1):E65-E75.

15. Bergstrom J, Hermansen L, Hultman E, Saltin B. Diet, muscle glycogen and physical performance. *Acta Physiol Scand.* 1967;71(2):140-150.

16. Goforth HW Jr, Laurent D, Prusaczyk WK, Schneider KE, Petersen KF, Shulman GI. Effects of depletion exercise and light training on muscle glycogen supercompensation in men. *Am J Physiol Endocrinol Metab.* 2003;285(6):E1304-E1311.

17. Nilsson L, Hultman E. Liver glycogen in man—the effect of total starvation or a carbohydrate-poor diet followed by carbohydrate refeeding. *Scand J Clin Lab Invest.* 1973;32(4):325-330.

18. Achten J, Halson SL, Moseley L, Rayson MP, Casey A, Jeukendrup AE. Higher dietary carbohydrate content during intensified running training results in better maintenance of performance and mood state. *J Appl Physiol (1985).* 2004;96(4):1331-1340.

19. Coggan AR, Swanson SC. Nutritional manipulations before and during endurance exercise: effects on performance. *Med Sci Sports Exerc.* 1992;24(suppl 9):331S-335S.

20. Spencer M, Yan Z, Katz A. Carbohydrate supplementation attenuates IMP accumulation in human muscle during prolonged exercise. *Am J Physiol.* 1991;261:C71-C76.

21. O'Keeffe K, Keith R, Wilson G, Blessing D. Dietary carbohydrate intake and endurance exercise performance of trained female cyclists. *Nutr Res.* 1989;9:819-830.

22. Brewer J, Williams C, Patton A. The influence of high carbohydrate diets on endurance running performance. *Eur J Appl Physiol Occup Physiol.* 1988;57(6):698-706.

23. Pizza F, Flynn M, Duscha B, Holden J, Kubitz E. A carbohydrate loading regimen improves high intensity, short duration exercise performance. *Int J Sport Nutr.* 1995;5:110-116.

24. Larson DE, Hesslink RL, Hrovat MI, Fishman RS, Systrom DM. Dietary effects on exercising muscle metabolism and performance by ^{31}P-MRS. *J Appl Physiol.* 1994;77:1108-1115.

25. Sugiura K, Kobayashi K. Effect of carbohydrate ingestion on sprint performance following continuous and intermittent exercise. *Med Sci Sports Exerc.* 1998;30(11):1624-1630.

26. Hargreaves M, Costill D, Coggan A, Fink W, Nishibata I. Effect of carbohydrate feedings on muscle glycogen utilization and exercise performance. *Med Sci Sports Exerc.* 1984;16(3):219-222.

27. Burke LM, Hawley JA, Wong SH, Jeukendrup AE. Carbohydrates for training and competition. *J Sports Sci.* 2011;29(suppl 1):17S-27S.

28. Phillips SM, Van Loon LJ. Dietary protein for athletes: from requirements to optimum adaptation. *J Sports Sci.* 2011;29(suppl 1):29S-38S.

29. Tipton KD, Witard OC. Protein requirements and recommendations for athletes: relevance of ivory tower arguments for practical recommendations. *Clin Sports Med.* 2007;26(1):17-36.

30. Lemon P, Mullin JP. Effect of initial muscle glycogen levels on protein catabolism during exercise. *J Appl Physiol Respir Environ Exerc Physiol.* 1980;48(4):624-629.

31. Babault N, Paizis C, Deley G, et al. Pea proteins oral supplementation promotes muscle thickness gains during resistance training: a double-blind, randomized, placebo-controlled clinical trial vs. whey protein. *J Int Soc Sports Nutr.* 2015;12:3.

32. Subcommittee on the Tenth Edition of the RDAs, Food and Nutrition Board, Commission on Life Sciences, National Research Council. *Recommended Dietary Allowances.* 10th ed. Washington, DC: National Academy Press; 1989.

33. Otten JJ, Hellwig JP, Meyers LD, eds, Institute of Medicine. *The Dietary Reference Intakes: The Essential Guide to Nutrient Requirements.* Washington, DC: National Academies Press; 2006.

34. Rand WM, Pellett PL, Young VR. Meta-analysis of nitrogen balance studies for estimating protein requirements in healthy adults. *Am J Clin Nutr.* 2003;77(1):109-127.

35. *Protein and Amino Acid Requirements in Human Nutrition: Report of a Joint FAO/WHO/UNU Expert Consultation.* WHO Technical Report Series No. 935. Geneva, Switzerland: WHO Press; 2002.

36. Young VR, Pellett PL. Plant proteins in relation to human protein and amino acid nutrition. *Am J Clin Nutr.* 1994;59(suppl 5):1203S-1212S.

37. Bergstrom J, Furst P, Vinnars E. Effect of a test meal, without and with protein, on muscle and plasma free amino acids. *Clin Sci (Lond).* 1990;79:331-337.

38. Tipton KD, Rasmussen BB, Miller SL, et al. Timing of amino acid-carbohydrate ingestion alters anabolic response of muscle to resistance exercise. *Am J Physiol Endocrinol Metab.* 2001;281(2):E197-206.

39. Mamerow MM, Mettler JA, English KL, et al. Dietary protein distribution positively influences 24-h muscle protein synthesis in healthy adults. *J Nutr.* 2014;144(6):876-880.

40. Tipton KD, Elliott TA, Cree MG, Aarsland AA, Sanford AP, Wolfe RR. Stimulation of net muscle protein synthesis by whey protein ingestion before and after exercise. *Am J Physiol Endocrinol Metab.* 2007;292(1):E71-E76.

41. Horvath PJ, Eagen CK, Fisher NM, Leddy JJ, Pendergast DR. The effects of varying dietary fat on performance and metabolism in trained male and female runners. *J Am Coll Nutr.* 2000;19(1):52-60.

42. Muoio DM, Leddy JJ, Horvath PJ, Awad AB, Pendergast DR. Effect of dietary fat on metabolic adjustments to maximal VO$_2$ and endurance in runners. *Med Sci Sports Exerc.* 1994;26(1):81-88.

43. Hoppeler H, Billeter R, Horvath PJ, Leddy JJ, Pendergast DR. Muscle structure with low- and high-fat diets in well trained male runners. *Int J Sports Med.* 1999;20(8):522-526.

44. Brown RC, Cox CM. Effects of high fat versus high carbohydrate diets on plasma lipids and lipoproteins in endurance athletes. *Med Sci Sports Exerc.* 1998;30(12):1677-1683.

45. Larson-Meyer DE, Newcomer BR, Hunter GR. Influence of endurance running and recovery diet on intramyocellular lipid content in women: a 1H NMR study. *Am J Physiol Endocrinol Metab.* 2002;282(1):E95-E106.

46. Larson-Meyer DE, Borkhsenious ON, Gullett JC, et al. Effect of dietary fat on serum and intramyocellular lipids and running performance. *Med Sci Sports Exerc.* 2008;40(5):892-902.

47. Thompson PD, Cullinane EM, Eshleman R, Kantor MA, Herbert PN. The effects of high-carbohydrate and high-fat diets on the serum lipid and lipoprotein concentrations of endurance athletes. *Metabolism.* 1984;33(11):1003-1010.

48. Laughlin GA, Yen SS. Nutritional and endocrine-metabolic aberrations in amenorrheic athletes. *J Clin Endocrinol Metab.* 1996;81(12):4301-4309.

49. Decombaz J, Schmitt B, Ith M, et al. Postexercise fat intake repletes intramyocellular lipids but no faster in trained than in sedentary subjects. *Am J Physiol Regul Integr Comp Physiol.* 2001;281:R760-R769.

50. Romijn J, Coyle EF, Sidossis LS, et al. Regulation of endogenous fat and carbohydrate metabolism in relation to exercise intensity and duration. *Am J Physiol.* 1993;265(3 pt 1):E380-E391.

51. Romijn JA, Coyle EF, Sidossis LS, Rosenblatt J, Wolfe RR. Substrate metabolism during different exercise intensities in endurance-trained women. *J Appl Physiol (1985).* 2000;88(5):1707-1714.

52. Ornish D, Brown S, Scherwitz L, et al. Can lifestyle changes reverse coronary heart disease? The Lifestyle Heart Trial. *Lancet.* 1990;336(8708):129-133.

53. Barnard ND, Katcher HI, Jenkins DJ, Cohen J, Turner-McGrievy G. Vegetarian and vegan diets in type 2 diabetes management. *Nutr Rev.* 2009;67(5):255-263.

54. Gould KL, Ornish D, Kirkeeide R, et al. Improved stenosis geometry by quantitative coronary arteriography after vigorous risk factor modification. *Am J Cardiol.* 1992;69:845-853.

55. Gould KL, Ornish D, Scherwitz L, et al. Changes in myocardial perfusion abnormalities by positron emission tomography after long-term, intense risk factor modification. *JAMA.* 1995;274(11):894-901.

56. Barnard ND, Cohen J, Jenkins DJ, et al. A low-fat vegan diet and a conventional diabetes diet in the treatment of type 2 diabetes: a randomized, controlled, 74-wk clinical trial. *Am J Clin Nutr.* 2009;89(5):1588S-1596S.

57. Lichtenstein AH, Appel LJ, Brands M, et al. Diet and lifestyle recommendations revision 2006: a scientific statement from the American Heart Association Nutrition Committee. *Circulation.* 2006;114:82-96.

58. Expert Panel on Detection, Evaluation, and Treatment of High Blood Cholesterol in Adults. Executive summary of the third report of the National Cholesterol Education Program (NCEP) Expert Panel on Detection, Evaluation, And Treatment of High Blood Cholesterol In Adults (Adult Treatment Panel III). *JAMA.* 2001;285(19):2486-2497.

59. US Departments of Health and Human Services, US Department of Agriculture. *Dietary Guidelines for Americans, 2005.* 6th ed. Washington, DC: US Government Printing Office; 2006.

60. US Department of Health and Human Services, US Department of Agriculture. *2015-2020 Dietary Guidelines for Americans.* https://health.gov/dietaryguidelines/2015/. Published December 2015. Accessed November 9, 2016.

61. Jeromson S, Gallagher IJ, Galloway SD, Hamilton DL. Omega-3 fatty acids and skeletal muscle health. *Mar Drugs.* 2015;13(11):6977-7004.

62. Williams CM, Burdge G. Long-chain n-3 PUFA: plant v. marine sources. *Proc Nutr Soc.* 2006;65(1):42-50.

63. Geppert J, Kraft V, Demmelmair H, Koletzko B. Docosahexaenoic acid supplementation in vegetarians effectively increases omega-3 index: a randomized trial. *Lipids.* 2005;40:807-814.

64. Conquer JA, Holub BJ. Supplementation with an algae source of docosahexaenoic acid increases (n-3) fatty acid status and alters selected risk factors for heart disease in vegetarian subjects. *J Nutr.* 1996;126(12):3032-3039.

65. Heaney RP, Recker RR, Saville P. Menopausal changes in calcium balance performance. *J Lab Clin Med.* 1978;92:953-963.

66. Myburgh KH, Hutchins J, Fataar AB, Hough SF, Noakes TD. Low bone density is an etiologic factor for stress fractures in athletes. *Ann Intern Med.* 1990;113(10):754-759.

67. Ruohola JP, Laaksi I, Ylikomi T, et al. Association between serum 25(OH)D concentrations and bone stress fractures in Finnish young men. *J Bone Miner Res.* 2006;21(9):1483-1488.

68. Wolman RL, Clark P, McNally E, Harries MG, Reeve J. Dietary calcium as a statistical determinant of trabecular bone density in amenorrhoeic and oestrogen-replete athletes. *Bone Miner.* 1992;17(3):415-423.

69. Lappe J, Cullen D, Haynatzki G, Recker R, Ahlf R, Thompson K. Calcium and vitamin D supplementation decreases incidence of stress fractures in female navy recruits. *J Bone Miner Res.* 2008;23(5):741-749.

70. Weaver CM, Plawecki KL. Dietary calcium: adequacy of a vegetarian diet. *Am J Clin Nutr.* 1994;59(suppl 5):1238S-1241S.

71. Weaver CM, Proulx WR, Heaney R. Choices for achieving adequate dietary calcium with a vegetarian diet. *Am J Clin Nutr.* 1999;70(suppl 3):543S-548S.

72. Heaney RP, Dowell MS, Rafferty K, Bierman J. Bioavailability of the calcium in fortified soy imitation milk, with some observations on method. *Am J Clin Nutr.* 2000;71(5):1166-1169.

73. Zhao Y, Martin BR, Weaver CM. Calcium bioavailability of calcium carbonate fortified soymilk is equivalent to cow's milk in young women. *J Nutr.* 2005;135(10):2379-2382.

74. Kohlenberg-Mueller K, Raschka L. Calcium balance in young adults on a vegan and lactovegetarian diet. *J Bone Miner Metab.* 2003;21(1):28-33.

75. Heaney RP, Dowell MS, Hale CA, Bendich A. Calcium absorption varies within the reference range for serum 25-hydroxyvitamin D. *J Am Coll Nutr.* 2003;22(2):142-146.

76. Holick MF. Sunlight and vitamin D for bone health and prevention of autoimmune diseases, cancers, and cardiovascular disease. *Am J Clin Nutr.* 2004;80(suppl 6):1678S-1688S.

77. Holick MF. The vitamin D epidemic and its health consequences. *J Nutr.* 2005;135(11):2739S-2748S.

78. Larson-Meyer DE, Willis KS. Vitamin D and athletes. *Curr SportsMed Rep.* 2010;9(4):220-226.

79. Larson-Meyer E. Vitamin D supplementation in athletes. *Nestle Nutr Inst Workshop Ser.* 2013;75:109-121.

80. Cannell JJ, Hollis BW, Sorenson MB, Taft TN, Anderson JJ. Athletic performance and vitamin D. *Med Sci Sports Exerc.* 2009;41(5):1102-1110.

81. Cannell JJ, Hollis BW. Use of vitamin D in clinical practice. *Altern Med Rev.* 2008;13(1):6-20.

82. Cannell JJ, Zasloff M, Garland CF, Scragg R, Giovannucci E. On the epidemiology of influenza. *Virol J.* 2008;5:29.

83. Willis KS, Smith DT, Broughton KS, Larson-Meyer DE. Vitamin D status and biomarkers of inflammation in runners. *Open Access J Sports Med.* 2012;3:35-42.

84. Hamilton B. Vitamin D and human skeletal muscle. *Scand J Med Sci Sports.* 2010;20(2):182-190.

85. Halliday TM, Peterson NJ, Thomas JJ, Kleppinger K, Hollis BW, Larson-Meyer DE. Vitamin D status relative to diet, lifestyle, injury, and illness in college athletes. *Med Sci Sports Exerc.* 2011;43(2):335-343.

86. Heller JE, Thomas JJ, Hollis BW, Larson-Meyer DE. Relation between vitamin D status and body composition in collegiate athletes. *Int J Sport Nutr Exerc Metab.* 2015;25:128-135.

87. Hamilton B, Grantham J, Racinais S, Chalabi H. Vitamin D deficiency is endemic in Middle Eastern sportsmen. *Public Health Nutr.* 2010;13(10):1528-1534.

88. Wang T, Bengtsson G, Karnefelt I, Bjorn LO. Provitamins and vitamins D_2 and D_3 in Cladina spp. over a latitudinal gradient: possible correlation with UV levels. *J Photochem Photobiol B.* 2001;62(1-2):118-122.

89. Holick MF, Biancuzzo RM, Chen TC, et al. Vitamin D2 is as effective as vitamin D3 in maintaining circulating concentrations of 25-hydroxyvitamin D. *J Clin Endocrinol Metab.* 2008;93(3):677-681.

90. Trang HM, Cole DE, Rubin LA, Pierratos A, Siu S, Vieth R. Evidence that vitamin D3 increases serum 25-hydroxyvitamin D more efficiently than does vitamin D2. *Am J Clin Nutr.* 1998;68(4):854-858.

91. Armas LA, Hollis BW, Heaney RP. Vitamin D2 is much less effective than vitamin D3 in humans. *J Clin Endocrinol Metab.* 2004;89(11):5387-5391.

92. Malczewska J, Raczynski G, Stupnicki R. Iron status in female endurance athletes and in non-athletes. *Int J Sport Nutr Exerc Metab.* 2000;10(3):260-276.

93. Malczewska J, Szczepanska B, Stupnicki R, Sendecki W. The assessment of frequency of iron deficiency in athletes from the transferrin receptor-ferritin index. *Int J Sport Nutr Exerc Metab.* 2001;11(1):42-52.

94. Woolf K, St Thomas MM, Hahn N, Vaughan LA, Carlson AG, Hinton P. Iron status in highly active and sedentary young women. *Int J Sport Nutr Exerc Metab.* 2009;19(5):519-535.

95. Zhu YI, Haas JD. Iron depletion without anemia and physical performance. *Am J Clin Nutr.* 1997;66(2):334-341.

96. Brownlie T, Utermohlen V, Hinton PS, Haas JD. Tissue iron deficiency without anemia impairs adaptation in endurance capacity after aerobic training in previously untrained women. *Am J Clin Nutr.* 2004;79(3):437-443.

97. Lamanca J, Haymes E. Effects of low ferritin concentrations on endurance performance. *Int J Sport Nutr.* 1992;2(4):376-385.

98. Peeling P, Dawson B, Goodman C, Landers G, Trinder D. Athletic induced iron deficiency: new insights into the role of inflammation, cytokines and hormones. *Eur J Appl Physiol.* 2008;103(4):381-391.

99. Robertson J, Maughan R, Davidson R. Faecal blood loss in response to exercise. *BMJ.* 1987;295:303-305.

100. Waller MF, Haymes EM. The effects of heat and exercise on sweat iron loss. *Med Sci Sports Exerc.* 1996;28(2):197-203.

101. Eichner E. Runner's macrocytosis: a clue to footstrike hemolysis. *Am J Med.* 1985;78:321-325.

102. Jones GR, Newhouse I. Sport-related hematuria: a review. *Clin J Sport Med.* 1997;7(2):119-125.

103. Craig WJ. Iron status of vegetarians. *Am J Clin Nutr.* 1994;59(suppl 5):1233S-1237S.

104. Coudray C, Bellanger J, Castiglia-Delavaud C, Remesy C, Vermorel M, Rayssignuier Y. Effect of soluble or partly soluble dietary fibres supplementation on absorption and balance of calcium, magnesium, iron and zinc in healthy young men. *Eur J Clin Nutr.* 1997;51(6):375-380.

105. Hallberg L, Hulthen L. Prediction of dietary iron absorption: an algorithm for calculating absorption and bioavailability of dietary iron. *Am J Clin Nutr.* 2000;71(5):1147-1160.

106. Saunders AV, Craig WJ, Baines SK, Posen JS. Iron and vegetarian diets. *Med J Aust.* 2013;199(suppl 4):11S-16S.

107. Platel K, Srinivasan K. Bioavailability of micronutrients from plant foods: an update. *Crit Rev Food Sci Nutr.* 2016;56(10):1608-1619.

108. Snyder AC, Dvorak LL, Roepke JB. Influence of dietary iron source on measures of iron status among female runners. *Med Sci Sports Exerc.* 1989;21(1):7-10.

109. Ball MJ, Bartlett MA. Dietary intake and iron status of Australian vegetarian women. *Am J Clin Nutr.* 1999;70(3):353-358.

110. Hinton PS, Giordano C, Brownlie T, Haas JD. Iron supplementation improves endurance after training in iron-depleted, nonanemic women. *J Appl Physiol (1985).* 2000;88(3):1103-1111.

111. Hinton PS, Sinclair LM. Iron supplementation maintains ventilatory threshold and improves energetic efficiency in iron-deficient nonanemic athletes. *Eur J Clin Nutr.* 2007;61(1):30-39.

112. Schumacher YO, Schmid A, Grathwohl D, Bultermann D, Berg A. Hematological indices and iron status in athletes of various sports and performances. *Med Sci Sports Exerc.* 2002;34(5):869-875.

113. Herbert V. Everyone should be tested for iron disorders. *J Am Diet Assoc.* 1992;92:1502-1509.

114. Micheletti A, Rossi R, Rufini S. Zinc status in athletes: relation to diet and exercise. *Sports Med.* 2001;31(8):577-582.

115. Lukaski HC. Micronutrients (magnesium, zinc, and copper): are mineral supplements needed for athletes? *Int J Sport Nutr.* 1995;5(suppl):74S-83S.

116. Hunt JR. Bioavailability of iron, zinc, and other trace minerals from vegetarian diets. *Am J Clin Nutr.* 2003;78(suppl 3):633S-639S.

117. Manore MM, Helleksen JM, Merkel J, Skinner JS. Longitudinal changes in zinc status in untrained men: effects of two different 12-week exercise training programs and zinc supplementation. *J Am Diet Assoc.* 1993;93:1165-1168.

118. Lukaski HC. Vitamin and mineral status: effects on physical performance. *Nutrition.* 2004;20(7-8):632-644.

119. Singh A, Moses FM, Deuster PA. Vitamin and mineral status in physically active men: effects of a high-potency supplement. *Am J Clin Nutr.* 1992;55:1-7.

120. Lonnerdal B. Dietary factors influencing zinc absorption. *J Nutr.* 2000;130(suppl 5S):1378S-1383S.

121. Hunt JR, Matthys LA, Johnson LK. Zinc absorption, mineral balance, and blood lipids in women consuming controlled lactoovovegetarian and omnivorous diets for 8 wk. *Am J Clin Nutr.* 1998;67(3):421-430.

122. Rosado JL, Diaz M, Gonzalez K, Griffin I, Abrams SA, Preciado R. The addition of milk or yogurt to a plant-based diet increases zinc bioavailability but does not affect iron bioavailability in women. *J Nutr.* 2005;135(3):465-468.

123. Krajcovicova-Kudlackova M, Buckova K, Klimes I, Sebokova E. Iodine deficiency in vegetarians and vegans. *Ann Nutr Metab.* 2003;47(5):183-185.

124. Lightowler HJ, Davies GJ. Iodine intake and iodine deficiency in vegans as assessed by the duplicate-portion technique and urinary iodine excretion. *Br J Nutr.* 1998;80(6):529-535.

125. Remer T, Neubert A, Manz F. Increased risk of iodine deficiency with vegetarian nutrition. *Br J Nutr.* 1999;81(1):45-49.

126. Waldmann A, Koschizke JW, Leitzmann C, Hahn A. Dietary intakes and lifestyle factors of a vegan population in Germany: results from the German Vegan Study. *Eur J Clin Nutr.* 2003;57(8):947-955.

127. Latham NK, Anderson CS, Reid IR. Effects of vitamin D supplementation on strength, physical performance, and falls in older persons: a systematic review. *J Am Geriatr Soc.* 2003;51(9):1219-1226.

128. Messina M, Redmond G. Effects of soy protein and soybean isoflavones on thyroid function in healthy adults and hypothyroid patients: a review of the relevant literature. *Thyroid.* 2006;16(3):249-258.

129. Rude RK, Singer FR, Gruber HE. Skeletal and hormonal effects of magnesium deficiency. *J Am Coll Nutr.* 2009;28(2):131-141.

130. Nielsen FH, Lukaski HC. Update on the relationship between magnesium and exercise. *Magnes Res.* 2006;19(3):180-189.

131. Woolf K, Manore MM. B-vitamins and exercise: does exercise alter requirements? *Int J Sport Nutr Exerc Metab.* 2006;16(5):453-484.

132. Herrmann W, Schorr H, Obeid R, Geisel J. Vitamin B-12 status, particularly holotranscobalamin II and methylmalonic acid concentrations, and hyperhomocysteinemia in vegetarians. *Am J Clin Nutr.* 2003;78(1):131-136.

133. Herrmann W, Geisel J. Vegetarian lifestyle and monitoring of vitamin B-12 status. *Clin Chim Acta.* 2002;326(1-2):47-59.

134. Watanabe F, Yabuta Y, Bito T, Teng F. Vitamin B_{12}-containing plant food sources for vegetarians. *Nutrients.* 2014;6(5):1861-1873.

135. Rauma A, Torronen R, Hanninen O, Mykkanen H. Vitamin B-12 status of long-term adherents of a strict uncooked vegan diet ("living food diet") is compromised. *J Nutr.* 1995;125:2511-2515.

136. Donaldson MS. Metabolic vitamin B12 status on a mostly raw vegan diet with follow-up using tablets, nutritional yeast, or probiotic supplements. *Ann Nutr Metab.* 2000;44(5-6):229-234.

137. Pawlak R, Parrott SJ, Raj S, Cullum-Dugan D, Lucus D. How prevalent is vitamin B(12) deficiency among vegetarians? *Nutr Rev.* 2013;71(2):110-117.

138. Belko AZ, Obarzanek E, Kalkwarf HJ, et al. Effects of exercise on riboflavin requirements of young women. *Am J Clin Nutr.* 1983;37(4):509-517.

139. Soares MJ, Satyanarayana K, Bamji MS, Jacob CM, Ramana YV, Rao SS. The effect of exercise on the riboflavin status of adult men. *Br J Nutr.* 1993;69(2):541-551.

140. Tang JE, Moore DR, Kujbida GW, Tarnopolsky MA, Phillips SM. Ingestion of whey hydrolysate, casein, or soy protein isolate: effects on mixed muscle protein synthesis at rest and following resistance exercise in young men. *J Appl Physiol (1985).* 2009;107(3):987-992.

141. Hartman JW, Tang JE, Wilkinson SB, et al. Consumption of fat-free fluid milk after resistance exercise promotes greater lean mass accretion than does consumption of soy or carbohydrate in young, novice, male weightlifters. *Am J Clin Nutr.* 2007;86(2):373-381.

142. Phillips SM, Hartman JW, Wilkinson SB. Dietary protein to support anabolism with resistance exercise in young men. *J Am Coll Nutr.* 2005;24(2):134S-139S.

143. Wilkinson SB, Tarnopolsky MA, Macdonald MJ, Macdonald JR, Armstrong D, Phillips SM. Consumption of fluid skim milk promotes greater muscle protein accretion after resistance exercise than does consumption of an isonitrogenous and isoenergetic soy-protein beverage. *Am J Clin Nutr.* 2007;85(4):1031-1040.

144. Balsom P, Soderlund E, Sjodin D, Hultman E. Creatine supplementation and dynamic high-intensity intermittent exercise. *Scand J Med Sci Sports.* 1993;3(3):143-149.

145. Delanghe J, De Slypere JP, De Buyzere M, Robbrecht J, Wieme R, Vermeulen A. Normal reference values for creatine, creatinine, and carnitine are lower in vegetarians. *Clin Chem.* 1989;35(8):1802-1803.

146. Shomrat A, Weinstein Y, Katz A. Effect of creatine feeding on maximal exercise performance in vegetarians. *Eur J Appl Physiol.* 2000;82(4):321-325.

147. Harris RC, Soderlund K, Hultman E. Elevation of creatine in resting and exercised muscle of normal subjects by creatine supplementation. *Clin Sci (Lond).* 1992;83(3):367-374.

148. Lukaszuk JM, Robertson RJ, Arch JE, et al. Effect of creatine supplementation and a lacto-ovo-vegetarian diet on muscle creatine concentration. *Int J Sport Nutr Exerc Metab.* 2002;12(3):336-348.

149. Burke DG, Chilibeck PD, Parise G, Candow DG, Mahoney D, Tarnopolsky M. Effect of creatine and weight training on muscle creatine and performance in vegetarians. *Med Sci Sports Exerc.* 2003;35(11):1946-1955.

150. Maughan RJ, Greenhaff PL, Hespel P. Dietary supplements for athletes: emerging trends and recurring themes. *J Sports Sci.* 2011;29(suppl 1):57S-66S.

151. Clarys P, Zinzen E, Hebbelinck M. The effect of oral creatine supplementation on torque production in a vegetarian and non-vegetarian population: a double blind study. *Veg Nutr.* 1997;1:100-105.

152. Baguet A, Everaert I, De Naeyer H, et al. Effects of sprint training combined with vegetarian or mixed diet on muscle carnosine content and buffering capacity. *Eur J Appl Physiol.* 2011;111(10):2571-2580.

153. Hobson RM, Saunders B, Ball G, Harris RC, Sale C. Effects of beta-alanine supplementation on exercise performance: a meta-analysis. *Amino Acids.* 2012;43(1):25-37.

154. Coyle E, Coggan A, Davis J, Sherman W. Current thoughts and practical considerations concerning substrate utilization during exercise. *Sports Sci Exch.* 1992;spring:1-4.

155. Sherman WM, Brodowicz G, Wright DA, Allen WK, Somonsen J, Dernbach A. Effects of 4 h preexercise carbohydrate feedings on cycling performance. *Med Sci Sports Exerc.* 1989;21(5):598-604.

156. Wright DA, Sherman WM, Dernbach AR. Carbohydrate feedings before, during, or in combination improve cycling endurance performance. *J Appl Physiol (1985).* 1991;71(3):1082-1088.

157. Wu CL, Williams C. A low glycemic index meal before exercise improves endurance running capacity in men. *Int J Sport Nutr Exerc Metab.* 2006;16(5):510-527.

158. Mondazzi L, Arcelli E. Glycemic index in sports nutrition. *J Am Coll Nutr.* 2009;28(suppl):455S-463S.

159. Below PR, Mora-Rodriguez R, Gonzalez-Alonso J, Coyle EF. Fluid and carbohydrate ingestion independently improve performance during 1 h of intense exercise. *Med Sci Sports Exerc.* 1995;27(2):200-210.

160. Ball TC, Headley SA, Vanderburgh PM, Smith JC. Periodic carbohydrate replacement during 50 min of high-intensity cycling improves subsequent sprint performance. *Int J Sport Nutr.* 1995;5(2):151-158.

161. Nicholas CW, Williams C, Lakomy HK, Phillips G, Nowitz A. Influence of ingesting a carbohydrate-electrolyte solution on endurance capacity during intermittent, high intensity shuttle running. *J Sports Sci.* 1995;13(4):283-290.

162. Currell K, Conway S, Jeukendrup AE. Carbohydrate ingestion improves performance of a new reliable test of soccer performance. *Int J Sport Nutr Exerc Metab.* 2009;19(1):34-46.

163. Hulston CJ, Jeukendrup AE. No placebo effect from carbohydrate intake during prolonged exercise. *Int J Sport Nutr Exerc Metab.* 2009;19(3):275-284.

164. American College of Sports Medicine, Sawka MN, Burke LM, Eichner ER, Maughan RJ, Montain SJ, Stachenfeld NS. American College of Sports Medicine position stand. Exercise and fluid replacement. *Med Sci Sports Exerc.* 2007;39(2):377-390.

165. Jeukendrup AE. Carbohydrate intake during exercise and performance. *Nutrition.* 2004;20(7-8):669-677.

166. Currell K, Jeukendrup AE. Superior endurance performance with ingestion of multiple transportable carbohydrates. *Med Sci Sports Exerc.* 2008;40(2):275-281.

167. Jeukendrup AE. Oral carbohydrate rinse: placebo or beneficial? *Curr Sports Med Rep.* 2013;12(4):222-227.

168. Shirreffs SM, Sawka MN. Fluid and electrolyte needs for training, competition, and recovery. *J Sports Sci.* 2011;29(suppl 1):39S-46S.

169. Pfeiffer B, Cotterill A, Grathwohl D, Stellingwerff T, Jeukendrup AE. The effect of carbohydrate gels on gastrointestinal tolerance during a 16-km run. *Int J Sport Nutr Exerc Metab.* 2009;19:485-503.

170. Neufer PD, Costill DL, Flynn MG, Kirwan JP, Mitchell JB, Houmard J. Improvements in exercise performance: effects of carbohydrate feedings and diet. *J App Physiol (1985).* 1987;62(3):983-988.

171. van der Brug GE, Peters HP, Hardeman MR, Schep G, Mosterd WL. Hemorheological response to prolonged exercise—no effects of different kinds of feedings. *Int J Sports Med.* 1995;16:231-237.

172. Lugo M, Sherman WM, Wimer GS, Garleb K. Metabolic responses when different forms of carbohydrate energy are consumed during cycling. *Int J Sport Nutr.* 1993;3:398-407.

173. Lancaster S, Kreider RB, Rasmussen C, et al. Effects of honey supplementation on glucose, insulin, and endurance cycling performance. *FASEB J.* 2001;15:LB315.

174. Gisolfi CV, Duchman SM. Guidelines for optimal replacement beverages for different athletic events. *Med Sci Sports Exerc.* 1992;24:679-687.

175. Saunders MJ, Kane MD, Todd MK. Effects of a carbohydrate-protein beverage on cycling endurance and muscle damage. *Med Sci Sports Exerc.* 2004;36(7):1233-1238.

176. Saunders MJ, Moore RW, Kies AK, Luden ND, Pratt CA. Carbohydrate and protein hydrolysate coingestions improvement of late-exercise time-trial performance. *Int J Sport Nutr Exerc Metab.* 2009;19(2):136-149.

177. Breen L, Tipton KD, Jeukendrup AE. No effect of carbohydrate-protein on cycling performance and indices of recovery. *Med Sci Sports Exerc.* 2009;42(6):1140-1148.

178. Jeukendrup AE, Tipton KD, Gibala MJ. Protein plus carbohydrate does not enhance 60-km time-trial performance. *Int J Sport Nutr Exerc Metab.* 2009;19:335-337; author reply 337-339.

179. van Essen M, Gibala MJ. Failure of protein to improve time trial performance when added to a sports drink. *Med Sci Sports Exerc.* 2006;38(8):1476-1483.

180. Why honey is not vegan. vegetus.org. www.vegetus.org/honey/honey.htm. Accessed November 10, 2016.

181. Burke LM, Collier GR, Hargreaves M. Muscle glycogen storage after prolonged exercise: effect of the glycemic index of carbohydrate feedings. *J Appl Physiol (1985).* 1993;75(2):1019-1023.

182. Jozsi AC, Trappe TA, Starling RD, et al. The influence of starch structure on glycogen resynthesis and subsequent cycling performance. *Int J Sports Med.* 1996;17(5):373-378.

183. Ivy JL, Goforth HW Jr, Damon BM, McCauley TR, Parsons EC, Price TB. Early postexercise muscle glycogen recovery is enhanced with a carbohydrate-protein supplement. *J Appl Physiol (1985).* 2002;93(4):1337-1344.

184. Rodriguez NR, Vislocky LM, Gaine PC. Dietary protein, endurance exercise, and human skeletal-muscle protein turnover. *Curr Opin Clin Nutr Metab Care.* 2007;10(1):40-45.

185. Roy B, Tarnopolsky M, MacDougall J, Fowles J, Yarasheski K. Effect of glucose supplement after resistance training on protein metabolism. *Clin J Sport Med.* 1997;8:70.

186. Roy BD, Luttmer K, Bosman MJ, Tarnopolsky MA. The influence of post-exercise macronutrient intake on energy balance and protein metabolism in active females participating in endurance training. *Int J Sport Nutr Exerc Metab.* 2002;12(2):172-188.

187. Levenhagen DK, Gresham JD, Carlson MG, Maron DJ, Borel MJ, Flakoll PJ. Postexercise nutrient intake timing in humans is critical to recovery of leg glucose and protein homeostasis. *Am J Physiol Endocrinol Metab.* 2001;280(6):E982-993.

188. Miller SL, Tipton KD, Chinkes DL, Wolf SE, Wolfe RR. Independent and combined effects of amino acids and glucose after resistance exercise. *Med Sci Sports Exerc.* 2003;35(3):449-455.

189. Thomas DT, Erdman KA, Burke LM. Position of the Academy of Nutrition and Dietetics, Dietitians of Canada, and the American College of Sports Medicine: nutrition and athletic performance. *J Acad Nutr Diet.* 2016;116(3):501-528.

190. Maughan RJ, Leiper JB, Shirreffs SM. Restoration of fluid balance after exercise-induced dehydration: effects of food and fluid intake. *Eur J Appl Physiol Occup Physiol.* 1996;73(3-4):317-325.

191. Nattiv A, Loucks AB, Manore MM, Sanborn CF, Sundgot-Borgen J, Warren MP, for the American College of Sports Medicine. American College of Sports Medicine position stand. The female athlete triad. *Med Sci Sports Exerc.* 2007;39(10):1867-1882.

192. Mountjoy M, Sundgot-Borgen J, Burke L, et al. The IOC consensus statement: beyond the Female Athlete Triad—Relative Energy Deficiency in Sport (RED-S). *Br J Sports Med.* 2014;48(7):491-497.

193. Barr SI. Vegetarianism and menstrual cycle disturbances: is there an association? *Am J Clin Nutr.* 1999;70(suppl 3):549S-554S.

194. Slavin J, Lutter J, Cushman S. Amenorrhea in vegetarian athletes [letter]. *Lancet.* 1984;1(8392):1474-1475.

195. O'Connor MA, Touyz SW, Dunn SM, Beumont JV. Vegetarianism in anorexia nervosa? A review of 116 consecutive cases. *Med J Aust.* 1987;147(11-12):540-542.

196. Huse DM, Lucas AR. Dietary patterns in anorexia nervosa. *Am J Clin Nutr.* 1984;40(2):251-254.

197. Robinson-O'Brien R, Perry CL, Wall MM, Story M, Neumark-Sztainer D. Adolescent and young adult vegetarianism: better dietary intake and weight outcomes but increased risk of disordered eating behaviors. *J Am Diet Assoc.* 2009;109(4):648-655.

198. Neumark-Sztainer D, Story M, Resnick MD, Blum RW. Adolescent vegetarians. A behavioral profile of a school-based population in Minnesota. *Arch Pediatr Adolesc Med.* 1997;151:833-838.

199. Loucks AB. Energy availability, not body fatness, regulates reproductive function in women. *Exerc Sport Sci Rev.* 2003;31(3):144-148.

200. Goldin BR, Adlercreutz H, Gorbach SL, et al. Estrogen excretion patterns and plasma levels in vegetarian and omnivorous women. *N Engl J Med.* 1982;307(25):1542-1547.

201. Kaiserauer S, Snyder AC, Sleeper M, Zierath J. Nutritional, physiological, and menstrual status of distance runners. *Med Sci Sports Exerc.* 1989;21(2):120-125.

202. Nelson ME, Fisher EC, Catsos PD, Meredith CN, Turksoy RN, Evans WJ. Diet and bone status in amenorrheic runners. *Am J Clin Nutr.* 1986;43(6):910-916.

203. Deuster PA, Kyle SB, Moser PB, Vigersky RA, Singh A, Schoomaker EB. Nutritional intakes and status of highly trained amenorrheic and eumenorrheic women runners. *Fertil Steril.* 1986;46(4):636-643.

204. Lloyd T, Buchanen JR, Bitzer S, Waldman CJ, Myers C, Ford BG. Interrelationship of diet, athletic activity, menstrual status, and bone density in collegiate women. *Am J Clin Nutr.* 1987;46(4):681-684.

205. Raben A, Kiens B, Richter EA, et al. Serum sex hormones and endurance performance after a lacto-ovo vegetarian and a mixed diet. *Med Sci Sports Exerc.* 1992;24(11):1290-1297.

206. Dyett P, Rajaram S, Haddad EH, Sabate J. Evaluation of a validated food frequency questionnaire for self-defined vegans in the United States. *Nutrients.* 2014;6(7):2523-2539.

207. Szabo L. The health risks of new-wave vegetarianism. *CMAJ.* 1997;156:1454-1455.

208. Johnston PK. Counseling the pregnant vegetarian. *Am J Clin Nutr.* 1988;48:901-905.

209. Mangels A. Working with vegetarian clients. *Issues Veg Diet.* 1995;5:1,4,5.

CHAPTER 17

NUTRITION AND EXERCISE GUIDANCE FOR THE PREGNANT ATHLETE

Kimberly Mueller, MS, RD, CSSD

INTRODUCTION

The changes during pregnancy from a fertilized egg to a fully formed newborn child are truly astounding. For the female athlete, these changes can also bring feelings of apprehension regarding their impact on training and successful return to sport. Concerns over how to properly fuel the child's development while maintaining a healthy weight gain, as well as what volume and intensity of exercise are appropriate and safe during each stage of pregnancy, are common and should be addressed. Some women also express concern that intensive training will impact their fertility. Therefore, registered dietitian nutritionists (RDNs), alongside a team of health professionals, play an integral role in helping the female athlete by providing menu planning and nutrition and fitness guidance in the prepreganancy period, through each stage of pregnancy, and during the postpartum period.

FERTILITY IN FEMALE ATHLETES

According to the Centers for Disease Control and Prevention, nearly 12.3% of women age 15 to 44 are unable to get pregnant or carry a child to term, a condition known as infecundity. Another 6.1% suffer from infertility, defined as the inability to get pregnant after 12 months of trying.[1] However, most women who present with fertility problems do not suffer from absolute infecundity and infertility—meaning there is no chance of conception. Rather, they suffer from subfecundity or subfertility, where likelihood of conception is good, especially when issues contributing to reproductive complication are remedied.

Subfertility and subfecundity are reported to be higher among athletic women. The combination of intense training routines and insufficient energy intake trigger unhealthy aberrations in the athlete's weight and body fat or imbalances in hormones essential to the regulation of their menstrual cycle may negatively influence fertility.[2-7] Even subtle menstrual disturbances, like luteal phase defects, characterized by poor endometrial maturation secondary to inadequate progesterone production and short luteal phases, have been linked to infertility and spontaneous abortions and are estimated to affect nearly half of all athletic women.[8] While other factors, such as age, affect infecundity and infertility, this section will focus on modifiable changes, including exercise routine, energy intake, weight status, and overall nutrition. Reducing infertility is a top priority of many health organizations, including Healthy People 2020.[9] RDNs and other health professionals have a unique opportunity to provide the guidance needed to help make significant headway in attaining this goal and to make a positive difference in the life of an athlete who aspires to be a mother.

Exercise and Reproductive Health

Exercise can reduce the risk of many adverse health outcomes, including infertility. Women who regularly exercise prepreganancy benefit from improvements in overall hormonal and metabolic profile, increased blood flow to the uterus and ovaries, enhanced insulin sensitivity and glucose homeostasis, reduced blood pressure, and decreased body fat or weight, especially in the abdominal region.[10,11] In addition, maternal gestational weight gain and odds of cesarean delivery are lower in women engaged in a prenatal exercise program, thereby helping to speed postpartum recovery.[12] Prenatal exercise can also reduce the odds of having a large newborn, defined as birth weight greater the 90th percentile for gestational age and sex, by 31% without altering the risk of having a small newborn, defined as birth weight less than the 10th percentile for gestational age and sex. Both high and low birth weights are typically associated with health risks for the newborn.[12] Even so, conflicted views remain regarding the optimal frequency, duration, and intensity of exercise during the prenatal period.[13]

Current evidence-based physical activity guidelines for adults, established by the US Department of Health and Human Services, recommend a minimum of 150 minutes per week of moderate-intensity activity, 75 minutes per week of vigorous intensity, or an equivalent combination of moderate- and vigorous-intensity aerobic activity in conjunction with moderate- to high-intensity muscle-strengthening exercises on two or more days of the week. Additional amounts are encouraged to extend health benefits. Vigorous intensity is defined in absolute terms as 6.0 metabolic equivalents or is defined in relative terms as 60% to 84% of aerobic capacity reserve (or heart rate reserve).[14] Many reproductive specialists, however, believe competitive sporting activity and exercise at an extreme (vigorous) level facilitates reproductive complications, elevating risk for infecundity and infertility and, thus, often recommend reductions in training volume and intensity to support conception.[13]

While research specific to the competitive athlete is lacking, early data evaluating exercise patterns and fertility have been equivocal; some studies show a lower risk of infecundity and infertility among vigorous exercisers,[15,16] and others showing increased risk at the highest levels of frequency or intensity.[17,18] There is evidence that the stress of exercise, coupled with insufficient nutrition to meet the metabolic demands of exercise, may result in conditions where conception is not possible (see Box 17.1.)[19-23] Exercise, especially energy-exhaustive endurance exercise, such as long-distance running, cycling, and triathlon, can impose significant stress on a women's homeostasis, lead to the release of excess cortisol into the bloodstream, and disturb reproductive function. Ensuring adequate energy intake to support baseline metabolic demands as well as the metabolic demands of exercise is critical to maintaining menstrual and reproductive integrity. Nutrition guidance from an RDN is important for the female athlete transitioning into pregnancy.

Box 17.1 Signs Exercise Stress May Be Too High[18-23]

Low energy availability

Menstrual dysfunction

Low bone mineral density

Substantial loss of weight

Body mass index <18.5 kg/m²

Body fat <12%

Elevated blood pressure

Nutrition and Reproductive Health

A woman's preconception nutrition and weight status help set the stage for a healthy pregnancy. Poor nutritional habits, especially when combined with aberrant weight status, are associated with compromised reproductive health and poor pregnancy outcomes for mother and child.[24,25]

Preconception Weight Status

The World Health Organization has defined what constitutes a healthy body mass index (BMI) in pregnant women (see Table 17.1, page 358).[26] According to the American Society for Reproductive Medicine, 12% of primary infertility results from deviations from a healthy weight status.[27]

Table 17.1 Weight Status According to Body Mass Index[26]	
Classification	**Body Mass Index, kg/m²**
Underweight	<18.5
Severe thinness	<16.00
Moderate thinness	16.00–16.99
Mild thinness	17.00–18.49
Healthy	18.50–24.99
Overweight	25.00–29.99
Obese	≥30.00
Moderate obesity	30.00–34.99
Severe obesity	35.00–39.99
Morbid obesity	≥40.00

Overweight or obesity is a condition exhibited by women over 18 years of age at a rate of 40% and 15% respectively.[28] Evidence demonstrates that this condition favors the development of ovulatory dysfunction and infertility, likely due to elevated insulin levels and insulin resistance.[28,29] One study revealed a decrease in the probability of natural conception of 4% per unit of BMI greater than 29 kg/m².[30] Furthermore, pre-partum obesity is associated with several adverse reproductive outcomes for mother and child, including gestational diabetes, hypertension, preeclampsia, miscarriage, caesarian delivery, preterm delivery, post-partum weight retention, and fetal growth disorders.[19,29,31]

Fortunately, ovulatory function and pregnancy rates, as well as pregnancy outcomes, have improved significantly after weight loss in women who are obese.[32] For example, a randomized controlled study of 49 obese women who are obese and undergoing fertility treatment demonstrated that a 12-week intervention consisting of a very-low-energy diet for the initial 6 weeks, followed by a hypocaloric diet combined with weekly group coaching sessions incorporating dietary, exercise, and behavioral guidance yielded greater anthropometric changes and significant improvements in pregnancy rate (48% vs 14%), as well as a marked increase in the number of live births (44% vs 14%). The number of fertility treatment cycles to achieve pregnancy also dropped by 50%.[33] Similarly, meaningful weight loss (≥ 10% of body weight) was shown to significantly improve conception (88% vs 54%) and live birth rates (71% vs 37%) in women who are overweight and struggling with infertility compared with those with minimal or no weight loss.[34] Thus, weight-loss counseling should be encouraged for women who are overweight and planning to conceive, with a focus on replacing nutrient-void and calorie-dense foods like soda and refined grains with lower-calorie, nutrient-rich alternatives like fruits, vegetables, whole grains, and legumes.

Underweight status (BMI < 18.5 kg/m²) contributes to an estimated 6% of infertility cases.[26] For the female athlete, a low body weight is often the result of chronic low energy availability (energy expenditure exceeds dietary energy intake) driven by strenuous exercise and conscious or subconscious restrictive eating patterns. This, in turn, can trigger hypothalamic dysfunction and suppress hormones, particularly gonadotropin-releasing factor, necessary for normal menstruation, ovulation, and conception.[35] Deficiencies in leptin, a hormone produced by fat cells in the body, may be a compounding factor in the development of reproductive dysfunction among female athletes. During periods of reduced or low energy availability, leptin concentration decreases independent of adiposity.[36]

Research has shown that negative effects on reproductive health resulte when energy availability falls below a threshold of 30 kcal/kg of fat-free mass daily.[37] Even a reduced energy availability of less than 45 kcal/kg of fat-free mass daily can lead to menstrual irregularities and can hurt bone mass, as well as slow metabolic rate, trigger hypoglycemia, and elevate blood cholesterol.[23,38] The combination of low energy availability (with or without an eating disorder), menstrual dysfunction, and diminished bone health is a condition known as the *female athlete triad*. This triad is estimated to affect up to 15% of female athletes, with a greater number experiencing any one of the conditions involved.[39] In 2014, the International Olympic Committee coined a new term, *relative energy deficiency in sport* (RED-S), to describe a syndrome of impaired physiological functioning caused by low energy availability. Like the female athlete triad, RED-S encompasses impairments in menstrual function and bone health and also includes detriments in metabolic rate, immunity, protein synthesis, and cardiovascular health.[40,41] Women who compete in sports where thinness is perceived to enhance performance, such as gymnastics, figure skating, ballet, and long-distance running, seem to be at greater risk for exhibiting symptoms of the female athlete triad and RED-S.[3,4,38,42-45]

Fortunately, more than 70% of women whose infertility stems from body weight disorders are likely to conceive spontaneously by restoring body weight to a healthy status.[27] RDNs, in conjunction with a behavior therapist or other mental health professional, can play a key role in helping women athletes establish and maintain a healthy relationship with food. Where necessary, this includes making corrections to energy balance for weight loss or gain as a means to facilitate a hormonal environment favorable for reproduction. For women who are overweight, especially those whose weight is greater than 120% of predicted ideal body weight, increased energy output through increases in physical activity or decreases in energy intake is warranted. For the athletes who are underweight, especially those with a body weight less than 95% of predicted ideal body weight, an increase in caloric load or a reduction in caloric expenditure through training are advised.

Optimizing energy availability (> 45 kcal/kg fat-free mass per day) through reductions in training or increases in energy intake is also crucial for female athletes of healthy weight who exhibit the symptoms of chronic anovulation, menstrual disorders, and secondary amenorrhea resulting from hypothalamic disorder. Screening tools such as the Low Energy Availability in Females Questionnaire and the Relative Energy Deficiency in Sport Clinical Assessment Tool can be helpful, especially when eating disorders are suspected.[41,46] When menses fails to return after 5 months, hormonal preparations may need to be incorporated into a therapeutic protocol as a means to protect against further reproductive complications and bone loss. Restoration of reproductive function may take as long as 6 months.

NUTRITION QUALITY

RDNs can assess and help implement positive diet and lifestyle changes to improve reproductive function and fertility results in female athletes.[47,48] Beyond sufficient energy consumption to support the metabolic demands of daily living, exercise, and the establishment of a healthy preconception weight status, evidence suggests that the quality of nutrition during the preconception period has implications for fertility and pregnancy outcomes. For example, a diet focused on plant-based rather than animal-based protein and fat has been shown to dramatically reduce the risk of impaired ovulation.[49,50] Impaired ovulation is estimated to contribute to 25% to 50% of infertility cases.[51] Furthermore, avoidance of *trans* fats is likely effective in protecting against infertility.[52] *Trans* fats are present in some industrially produced cakes and other sweets; potato chips, corn chips, and other snack foods; fast foods; powdered soups; and hard margarines containing hydrogenated vegetable oil.

For the female athlete undergoing in vitro fertilization and intracytoplasmic sperm injection, consumption of a Mediterranean-style diet rich in vegetables, fruits, fish, whole grains, and vegetable-based oils has been shown to increase blood folate and vitamin B-6, which correlates with successful fertility.[53] The benefits of healthy eating during the preconception period carry through pregnancy as well. Adherence to the alternate Mediterranean diet or the alternate Healthy Eating Index, both of which exclude wine, as well as the Dietary Approaches to Stop Hypertension diet, have been shown to lower the risk for developing gestational diabetes by 24%, 34%, and 46%, respectively, which, in turn, may help protect against obstetrical complications and birth defects associated with gestational diabetes.[54]

The use of a prenatal vitamin has been associated with a 73% lower incidence of infertility in women, likely due to improving ovarian function.[55-57] Inadequate folate intake can reduce ovarian response to internal gonadotropin, resulting in impaired ovulation and infertility. Higher intake of folate prepregnancy is also associated with reduced risk of miscarriage.[58] B vitamin supplements, especially folic acid, have been shown to reduce risk for fetal neural defects, such as spina bifida and anencephaly, congenital heart disease, and cleft lip and palate, by 70%.[59-61] Beyond eating foods rich in folic acid, all women of childbearing age should consume 400 mcg of folic acid daily from fortified foods or dietary supplements. For planned pregnancies, daily supplementation with prenatal vitamins for several months in advance of conception is often recommended to help achieve these goals.[55]

Frequent and excessive use of caffeine and alcohol are potentially detrimental to fertility. Intake of 300 mg or less of caffeine per day does not seem to affect risk of infertility or risk of adverse pregnancy outcomes, including miscarriage.[62] A daily intake above 500 mg of caffeine, however, has been shown to play a significant role in the development of subfecundity in a woman's first pregnancy.[63] Yet, a slightly lower dose of 455 mg/d (range: 3.71 to 3561 mg/d) did not significantly impact the success rate of pregnancy after in vitro fertilization. Even so, the authors of this study did note that the number of eggs decreased as the caffeine serum levels increased and that an increase in caffeine consumption was positively associated with the number of aborted pregnancies.[64] Consequently, the current American College of Obstetricians and Gynecologists recommends that all women attempting conception avoid exceeding 200 mg of caffeine per day or approximately one 12-ounce cup of coffee.[65]

Consumption of alcohol can trigger hypogonadism. This condition will worsen the more frequently a woman drinks and will interfere with hormonal homeostasis and fertility. Consumption of more than two drinks per day has been shown to increase relative risk of infertility by 60% in women.[66] For women undergoing in vitro fertilization, consumption of more than 25 g of ethyl alcohol (equivalent to approximately 18 ounces of beer, 7.5 ounces of wine, or 2.2 ounces 80-proof vodka) daily has been strongly associated with poorer-quality embryos.[67] As a result, abstinence from alcohol is recommended when attempting to conceive.[68]

A WOMAN ATHLETE'S PREGNANCY JOURNEY

Pregnancy triggers a cascade of hormonal aberrations that elicit physical and biomechanical changes in a woman athlete's metabolic, cardiovascular, and musculoskeletal makeup. These changes, which are essential for the optimal growth and development of a fetus, affect the nutritional demands and exercise capacity of the female athlete. As was true before pregnancy, maintaining fitness with an exercise program and making wise food choices during pregnancy are proven to provide a wealth of benefits for mother and child. Maternal benefits include enhanced cardiovascular fitness, prevention of urinary incontinence, gestational weight gain control, decreased musculoskeletal discomfort, reduced incidence of muscle cramps and edema, mood stability, and better management of blood sugars and blood pressure.[69-71] Fetal benefits include decreased fat mass, improved stress tolerance, and advanced neurobehavioral maturation.[69,72,73] On the flip side, failure to take certain precautions when exercising and being negligent of nutritional needs can be devastating to fetal growth and development and potentially dangerous to the athlete as well. This section will break down the key physiological challenges associated with each trimester of pregnancy and explore the recommended nutrient and exercise modifications that will help ensure a healthy pregnancy.

Key Physiological Challenges for Female Athletes

While most women discover the joy of pregnancy within a few days of missing their period early in the first trimester, some push through training sessions and competition for several weeks, even months, despite unusual fatigue, abnormal eating habits, dyspnea, nausea, bouts of dizziness, heartburn, and constipation before realizing that their symptoms are the result of pregnancy. As fetal growth accelerates in the second and third trimesters, increasing pressure on the bladder from the expanding uterus can lead to a frustrating and uncomfortable need to urinate multiple times during a workout as well as at rest. Furthermore, heartburn and reflux can escalate. Toward the end of pregnancy, fatigue returns, and musculoskeletal dysfunctions, such as lower back pain, pelvic pain, and leg cramps, can arise, making weight-bearing movement increasingly uncomfortable. Education on the causes of these common physiological challenges and guidance on remedies can help improve overall maternal well-being throughout the pregnancy and can improve pregnancy outcomes.[74]

FATIGUE

While fatigue can be caused by many things, including lack of sleep or poor nutrition, the unusual fatigue experienced by women early in pregnancy is generally the result of surging progesterone levels acting in concert with other hormonally driven changes within the cardiovascular system.[74] In the first few weeks of gestation, a notable rise in resting heart rate occurs.[75] From around week six to the end of the first trimester, blood volume expands approximately 10% to 15%, causing a 30% to 40% increase in cardiac output, as well as increases in pulse rate and stroke volume.[75,76] These cardiovascular changes can make a routine workout feel more difficult. Dyspnea driven by a 30% to 35% rise in tidal volume may also hinder workouts. Additionally, some women experience drops in blood pressure and consequent bouts of dizziness when getting up during the early weeks of pregnancy. These result from increased blood flow to the uterus and a substantial decrease in systemic vascular resistance.[77,78] Fortunately, as the body adapts to the hormonal and cardiovascular changes during early pregnancy, fatigue tapers. In fact, many women report surging energy levels and consequent increases in exercise patterns during the second trimester. Accelerating fetal growth patterns late in the second trimester and well into the third trimester place a greater energy demand on the body and, thus, fatigue often returns. Proper nutrition and hydration, continued exercise, and additional rest can be helpful in offsetting some of the fatigue experienced in late-stage pregnancy.[74,79]

MORNING SICKNESS

An estimated 70% of women worldwide are affected by nausea or vomiting, a condition known as morning sickness.[80,81] This can hamper a female athlete's ability to train, as well as her overall well-being during the first trimester and, in rare cases, throughout the pregnancy. Morning sickness and fatigue are common reasons why a pregnant athlete may consult a health professional. Severe nausea and vomiting, termed *hyperemesis gravidarum* (HG), is the number one cause of hospitalization in the first trimester, impacting 1.1% to 1.2% of pregnancies in the United States and worldwide.[80-82] Although the exact cause of morning sickness is unknown, changes in ovarian and placental hormones, including a surge in postconception estrogen levels, are likely responsible.[83]

The first 10 weeks of pregnancy are a delicate time for the developing embryo. Essential growth patterns occur that facilitate the development of every essential organ, including the brain, spinal cord, heart, lungs, and gastrointestinal tract. Failure to treat HG during the first trimester can have negative fetal consequences. For example, there is evidence that HG increases risk for low birth weight (< 2.5 kg) and restricts fetal growth throughout pregnancy, a condition called *intrauterine growth retardation*.[84-86] There is also preliminary evidence that HG may have long-term health ramifications for offspring, including childhood insulin resistance and psychological disorders in adulthood.[87]

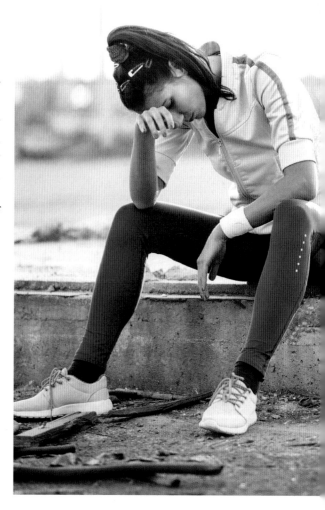

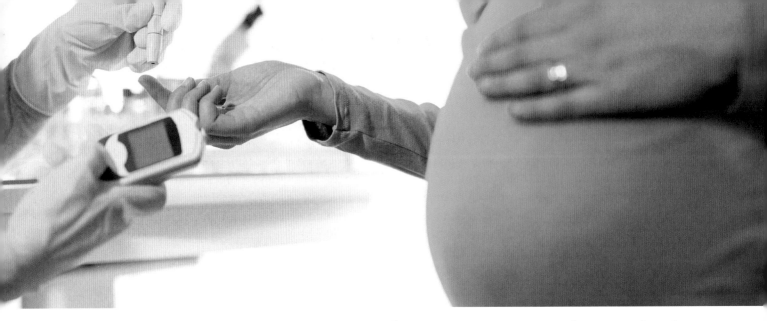

In cases of HG, hospitalization should be considered. Intravenous intervention is often required to address fluid and nutrition concerns, including dehydration, electrolyte imbalances, blood volume depletion, and nutrient deficiency and to ensure positive outcomes for the mother and child.[88,89] Nutrition treatment via nasogastric tube feedings is also an effective means to promote optimal maternal weight gain and favorable pregnancy outcomes.[90]

Of concern to some female athletes experiencing morning sickness, especially those with severe cases, are unnecessary or dramatic weight loss (> 5% of body weight), nutrient deficiency driven by an aversion to nutrient-dense foods, undernutrition, dehydration, electrolyte imbalances, and blood volume depletion.[82] In addition, a rare, dangerous complication of prolonged vomiting in pregnancy is Wernicke's encephalopathy. This condition is initiated by an acute deficiency of thiamine resulting from body stores being unable to meet increased metabolic demands and marked by confusion, ocular abnormalities, and ataxia. Thiamin replacement is indicated for women with Wernicke's encephalopathy.[91]

Treatment protocols for morning sickness should be tailored to the individual. Mild to moderate cases of morning sickness are most commonly addressed with diet and lifestyle changes, as well as nonpharmacologic supplements, such as vitamin B-6 and ginger.[88] Though there is a lack of science-based evidence to support these practices, common dietary recommendations based upon anecdotal reports of relief include the following[88,89]:

- Eat small, frequent meals to avoid an empty stomach or feelings of hunger.
- Eat dry, salty, and bland foods, such as crackers.
- Incorporate protein-rich foods, such as eggs, yogurt, nuts, and tuna at each feeding.
- Use an electrolyte-enhanced effervescent in water (eg, Nuun), homemade oral rehydration solution (6 teaspoon sugar, ½ teaspoon salt, 1 L water), or sports drink (eg, Gatorade) to aid rehydration in cases of vomiting.

Vitamin B-6 has over 50 years of evidence-based support from randomized, controlled studies and placebo-controlled clinical trials and can be safely taken during pregnancy at doses up to 200 mg/d.[92] The use of ginger products, which carry antiemetic qualities, has been supported in several studies at doses of up to 1,000 mg/d,[93,94] and some data suggest it is more effective than vitamin B-6 for relieving the severity of nausea, as well as decreasing the frequency of vomiting.[95]

CONSTIPATION

Constipation includes infrequent or painful bowel movements, at times leading to anorectal hemorrhoids. Approximately 13% of women experience these symptoms during pregnancy.[96] Surging levels of progesterone, which relax the smooth muscles of the digestive tract, and lower levels of the hormone motilin in early pregnancy cause food to travel much slower through the intestines, thus predisposing pregnant women to increased risk of constipation. In addition, increased water absorption from the intestines can make evacuation difficult due to dried-out stools. An elevated prepregnancy BMI greater than 24 and advanced maternal age (> 35 years) seem to increase this risk. Diet can also play a large role. Dietary supplementation with prenatal vitamins, which contain iron, a mineral that negatively impacts gut flora when consumed in excess, and calcium, a mineral that has a mild binding effect, can contribute to constipation. It is also not uncommon to see reduced fiber intake and less physical activity in women experiencing pronounced cases of fatigue and morning sickness, both factors that can exacerbate constipation.[96]

A simple explanation as to why constipation is occurring can provide comfort to the affected athlete. Easy resolutions include increasing fluid and dietary fiber intake, staying as active as possible throughout the day, and practicing postmeal defecation, when colonic activity is greatest.[96] Supplementation with fiber at meals, such as adding 4 to 6 tablespoons of bran or daily ingestion of bulk-forming agents like psyllium, methylcellulose, or polycarbophil with one or two glasses of water to help increase fecal water content, decrease colonic transit time, and increase stool weight may be necessary for women who struggle with diet and exercise modification for relief.[97] The use of probiotic supplements, especially *Bifidobacterium lactis*, has demonstrated improved whole gut transit time, stool frequency, and stool consistency.[98]

GASTROESOPHAGEAL REFLUX DISEASE

Heartburn and regurgitation are symptoms of gastroesophageal reflux disease (GERD), and they are estimated to affect upward of 80% of pregnant women. In early pregnancy, GERD symptoms are often associated with hormonal changes that initiate alterations in gastrointestinal transit time and decreases in lower esophageal sphincter pressure. Nausea and vomiting caused by GERD can occur later in pregnancy. Intragastric and intraabdominal pressure increasing secondary to the enlarged gravid uterus may exacerbate GERD symptoms.[99,100] The first line of defense should be implementing appropriate lifestyle and dietary adjustments. Using a food log to identify avoidable dietary triggers of GERD is helpful. The most common avoidable dietary triggers include acidic foods, like citrus and tomatoes, spicy foods, caffeine, carbonated beverages, peppermint, and chocolate. A high intake of animal fats has also been correlated with increased incidence of GERD symptoms, and, thus, plant-based diets are often encouraged as a dietary remedy.[101] In addition, eating smaller meals, not eating too close to bedtime, and wearing loose-fitting clothes have been explored as natural remedies.[101] When symptoms do not resolve with implementation of dietary and lifestyle changes, antacids, histamine-2 receptor antagonists, and proton pump inhibitors can be used safely under the guidance of a physician.[99]

FREQUENT URINATION

Early in pregnancy, human chorionic gonadotropin increases the rate of blood flow through the kidneys, thereby filling the bladder more rapidly and increasing urination frequency. Throughout the entirety of pregnancy, and especially late in the second and through the third trimester, the expanding uterus increases pressure on the bladder, thus enhancing the urge to urinate. Symptoms tend to crest when the baby drops to the pelvic area in preparation for delivery in the third trimester.[102] To alleviate some of the discomfort associated with frequent urination in pregnancy, the following strategies can be offered to pregnant women[103]:

- Reduce fluid intake before bedtime.
- Don't resist the need to urinate.
- Wear a sanitary pad to absorb leaks caused by coughing, sneezing, or physical activity.
- Incorporate Kegel exercises three to five times a day, in which the levator muscles are squeezed and held for 5 seconds, then released for 5 seconds, for 10 repetitions. These exercises help strengthen pelvic floor muscles and improve control over the urethra.

MUSCULOSKELETAL DYSFUNCTION

Musculoskeletal dysfunction is a common problem in pregnancy, especially during the second and third trimesters when a women's center of mass shifts anteriorly, causing an increase in lumbar lordosis and consequent low back and pelvic girdle pain. It is estimated that 33% to 85% of women experience lower back pain[104,105] while 20% to 37% experience pelvic girdle pain.[105,106] Other musculoskeletal issues common among pregnant women include calf muscle cramping, foot pain, and restless leg syndrome, impacting an estimated 47% to 64%, 37%, and 26% of women, respectively.[105,107] The exact mechanism for muscle cramping and pain is unknown, but they are thought to be triggered by muscle fatigue and nerve dysfunction rather than electrolyte deficiency or other abnormalities.[108] Fortunately, there does not seem to be a relationship between musculoskeletal dysfunction and complications during pregnancy or unfavorable fetal outcome. It can, however, make a pregnant athlete's comfort level decline, especially during the final few weeks of pregnancy.

When the athlete's body is experiencing pain, muscles tighten and compensate, which can cause asymmetry and misalignment of joints.[109,110] Continuing to train while exhibiting these misalignments can exacerbate them, prolong an athlete's postpartum recovery, and negatively influence their ability to safely return to competition.[110] Thus, education on proper body mechanics and safe, effective treatment options for pain management are important. Physical therapy is a proven effective and safe treatment option for musculoskeletal dysfunction in pregnancy and may include soft-tissue mobilization or massage, postural exercises, and strengthening and stabilization exercises to improve support of the pelvic girdle and pelvic floor.[111] Bracing or external supports can provide additional aid and help manage pain during exercise and daily life activities.[112,113] There is inconclusive evidence to support a wide range of marketed oral interventions for leg cramps, including magnesium, calcium, vitamin B, and vitamin C.[114] Support for passive stretching and deep tissue massage is equivocal, but both are harmless strategies that can be recommended to temporarily relieve cramps during pregnancy.[108]

Fueling During Pregnancy

Maintaining a good nutritional status throughout pregnancy is important for optimal fetal development and pregnancy outcome, as well as long-term health of the child. Evidence suggests that maternal dietary inadequacies early in pregnancy can impair placental development and function, which consequently can affect

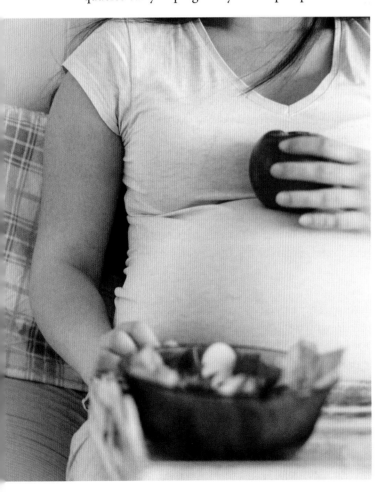

maternal-fetal transfer of nutrients and contribute to intrauterine growth restriction. Maternal dietary inadequacies that continue throughout pregnancy can also impact fetal growth and organ development through effects on the endocrine system or imprinted gene expression.[115] These developmental inadequacies increase risk for stillbirth; premature birth; low birth weight; perinatal mortality; infant neurologic, intestinal, respiratory, and circulatory disorders; birth defects; underdevelopment of some organs; cretinism; and brain damage.[116] Therefore, providing optimal nutrition and fueling guidance to pregnant athletes is important. Nutritional components leading to a healthy pregnancy include consumption of a wide variety of foods, prenatal vitamin and mineral supplementation, appropriate pregnancy weight gain, consistent moderate exercise unless contraindicated, adequate hydration, avoidance of alcohol and other harmful substances, and safe food handling.[117]

ENERGY REQUIREMENTS

Adequate calorie intake is required during pregnancy to accommodate energy deposition in maternal and fetal tissues, increases in basal metabolic rate (BMR), and changes in the energy cost of physical activity.[117-120] For athletes with a recent history of eating disorders, close monitoring by a team of health professionals, including an RDN, physician, and mental health specialist, may be warranted throughout pregnancy to protect against relapse and development of pregorexia, a term coined by the media to describe women who have an intense fear of gaining weight during pregnancy. Customized dietary guidance, including the possibility of reducing energy intake from targeted guidelines, and close physician monitoring is likely necessary for the a woman who is overweight or obese and who is gaining (or wishes to gain) less weight than recommended but has an appropriately growing fetus.[121-124]

First Trimester During early gestation, the energy demands of pregnancy are minimal, with BMR only increasing about 5% compared with the prepregnancy state in women with a healthy BMI. The increase in energy demands is slightly higher, 7%, in women with high BMIs.[118] As a result, significant adjustments to calorie intake are not required to accommodate the energy demands of pregnancy during the first trimester.[119] In fact, for many athletic women, especially those engaged in energy-exhaustive endurance exercise, overall daily calorie needs may actually decrease in pregnancy due to dramatic reductions in overall training load, nausea, and intense fatigue brought on by hormonal changes. A target energy intake of 45 kcal/kg prepregnancy fat-free mass per day plus the amount of energy exhausted during exercise should be encouraged during the first trimester of pregnancy.[117,125]

Second Trimester In the second trimester, most of the energy costs of pregnancy are attributed to maternal factors like expansion of blood volume, growth of the uterus and breasts, and fat storage. BMR gradually increases to a value that is approximately 11% greater than prepregnancy values in women with healthy BMIs. For women who are overweight or obese, BMR rises by approximately 16% from prepregnancy values.[118] Female athletes often report better energy levels and less nausea during the second trimester and thus often increase exercise patterns, further driving up daily calorie needs. To support the energy demands of pregnancy in the second trimester, a target energy intake of 45 kcal/kg prepregnancy fat-free mass per day plus an additional 340 kcal to accommodate increased pregnancy BMR plus the amount of energy exhausted during exercise should be encouraged.[117,125]

Third Trimester Fetal growth patterns peak during the third trimester, driving up BMR substantially from prepregnancy values. For women with BMR values in the healthy and overweight category, BMR increases by approximately 24% from prepregnancy values. For women with a BMR in the obese category, BMR increases by approximately 38% from prepregnancy values.[118] Pregnancy weight hits a peak in the third trimester, making some physical activities awkward. Additionally, fatigue returns for many women late in their pregnancy, and energy output from physical activity often decreases from second trimester norms. Thus total daily energy demands, for some, may not change much from second to third trimester. To support the energy demands of pregnancy in the third trimester, a target energy intake of 45 kcal/kg prepregnancy fat-free mass per day plus an additional 452 kcal to accommodate increased pregnancy BMR plus the amount of energy exhausted during exercise should be encouraged.[117,125]

Labor and Delivery The overall energy cost of reproduction, from conception through delivery, has been indicated at 75,000 to 85,000 kcal.[120] The actual energy cost of labor and delivery is dependent on duration, which may last between 13 and 17 hours for first-time pregnancies and substantially less time for each subsequent pregnancy. A meta-analysis of 385 studies published in 1990 or later examined the caloric needs of hospital births and revealed that the energy demands are similar to those of marathon runners.[126] The greatest rate of energy expenditure is experienced during the final transitional phase of labor when the mother is actively pushing. This phase typically lasts 30 minutes to 2 hours.

While there currently are no formal prelabor nutrition recommendations, it is prudent to consider that a carbohydrate-loading protocol in healthy women with noncomplicated pregnancies may be of possible benefit to performance because metabolically labor and delivery have been shown to be as demanding as continuous moderate exercise. Carbohydrate loading entails meeting a high intake of carbohydrate intake (9 to 12 g/kg body weight per day) for 24 to 48 hours while exercise is reduced to an easy taper as a means to enhance muscle glycogen stores and protect against premature muscle fatigue during exercise.[125,127] A more modest carbohydrate intake of 8 g/kg/d is likely to provide similar loading benefit provided energy intake is sufficient.[128] Prepregnancy weight should be used when calculating prelabor carbohydrate targets. Because it is hard to pinpoint the date of labor, unless an induction or cesarean section is scheduled, practitioners may simply encourage their patients to favor carbohydrate-rich foods as they near their due dates. Low-residue carbohydrate choices are preferable once labor begins to help minimize fecal matter and secretions in the intestines that may otherwise contribute to unpleasant gastrointestinal issues and other complications, such as pulmonary aspiration.[129]

Similar to prolonged exercise, a body in labor begins to use fat as an energy source when deprived of energy. This may cause an accumulation of fatty acids and ketones in both the mother and fetus. While this situation is well tolerated in the short term, left unmanaged during prolonged labor, ketosis can lead to ketoacidosis, which may reduce uterine contractions and lead to longer than typical labor, increased need for induction, increased need for forceps delivery, increased peripartum blood loss, and lower health scores in newborns.[126,130] Furthermore, energy deprivation is a form of maternal stress that may shunt blood away from the uterus and placenta and contribute to fetal distress.[126] Thus, traditional guidelines that advised against eating or drinking during labor due to concerns regarding aspiration, which can lead to pneumonia, have since been modified by the American College of Obstetricians and Gynecologists to allow low-risk women in the active phase of labor to ingest small quantities of clear fluids and foods, such as water, fruit juice without pulp, broth, gelatin products, carbonated beverages, tea, black coffee, sports drinks, and ice pops.[131] An isotonic sports drink, for instance, has been shown to lead to a statistically significant reduction in maternal ketone production compared with water and thus is a viable option for protecting against ketoacidosis and improving pregnancy outcome during prolonged labor.[132] Clear liquids also facilitate optimal hydration, which can be of concern in women who are not given intravenous fluids during labor.

There is skepticism as to whether a clear-liquid diet restriction is necessary, as improvements in anesthesia care make pain control during labor safer; risks related to aspiration indicate that fasting (nil per os) for healthy women is unnecesary. As a result, some obstetricians believe the extra energy associated with eating a light meal, including some solids, early in labor should be allowed because of the extra energy provided.[126] Studies defining the adequate nutritional diet and quantity to be ingested during labor as a means to optimize energy, comfort levels, and recovery are currently lacking, but, per tolerance and obstetrician and anesthesiologist approval, such easy-to-digest foods as bananas, applesauce, broth-based soups, toast, crackers, light sandwiches, yogurt, rice, quinoa, and cereal may be offered as fueling options. Contraindications for food intake during labor include eclampsia, preeclampsia, obesity, and the use of opioids to manage labor pain.[131]

Macronutrient Requirements

A balanced diet providing adequate carbohydrate, protein, fat, and essential fatty acids is important for healthy fetal development as well as protection against development of maternal health–compromising conditions, such as gestational diabetes and preeclampsia.

CARBOHYDRATE

Because the fetus uses glucose almost exclusively as its metabolic fuel, ensuring adequate maternal dietary intake of carbohydrate is a key factor in facilitating optimal fetal growth patterns throughout pregnancy. The current Recommended Dietary Allowance (RDA) for carbohydrate intake during pregnancy increases to 175 g/d, a slight increase from values of 130 g/d for nonpregnant women.[119] However, female athletes require 5 to 7 g carbohydrate per kilogram body weight to sustain muscle energy reserves and meet the metabolic demands of exercise.[125] Therefore, those women maintaining a moderate exercise program in pregnancy should be instructed to consume carbohydrate at a volume of 5 to 7 g/kg prepregnancy body weight plus an additional 45 g to support pregnancy.[119,125] Choosing nutrient-dense and fiber-rich carbohydrate sources, such as fruits, vegetables, beans, whole grains, seeds, and nuts, should be encouraged to help accommodate increased micronutrient demands and to reduce constipation, a common side effect early in pregnancy.

PROTEIN

The availability of adequate protein during pregnancy is essential to support fetal growth and development, (eg, via tissues such as the placenta and extraembryonic membranes) as well as accretion of maternal tissues like the heart, blood, and breast. While the majority of protein weight gain in the fetus occurs during the second and third trimesters of pregnancy, additional protein, above the prepregnancy recommendations of 0.8 g/kg body weight, is warranted during the first trimester to accommodate maternal adaptations involving protein and nitrogen metabolism that occur before there is a significant increase in fetal demand.[133] Current recommendations, however, do not support increasing intake until the second trimester

when 1.1 g/kg prepregnancy weight per day or an additional 25 g protein for singleton pregnancies and 1.4 g/kg prepregnancy weight per day or 50 g protein for twin pregnancies is advised.[119] Protein intake recommendations for strength and endurance-trained athletes are already 1.2 to 2.0 g/kg body weight per day, so it is prudent to advise pregnant athletes who will continue training routines during pregnancy to consume an additional 25 g daily (50 g for twins) during the second and third trimesters to accommodate increased protein turnover during exercise and pregnancy demands.[125,127] Also, encourage choosing high-quality sources of protein that include all essential amino acids, such as meat, eggs, poultry, dairy, and fish with a low mercury content (refer to section on Contraindicated Foods). Careful monitoring, including screening for protein deficiency, may be needed for female athletes engaged in vegan or vegetarian lifestyles to ensure that all essential amino acids are available for optimal fetal development and growth (see Chapter 16 for more about plant protein).

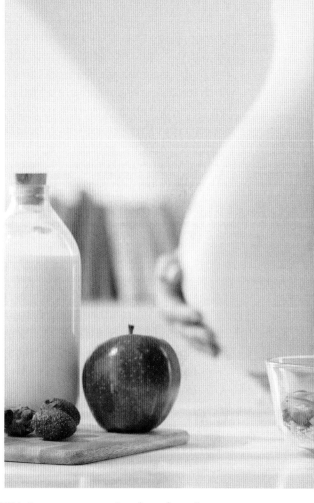

FAT

While recommendations for maternal fat intake during pregnancy remain the same as prepregnancy values (20% to 35% of total daily calorie intake), choosing healthy sources that are rich in essential fatty acids, such as n-3 and n-6 polyunsaturated fatty acids (PUFAs), can help support the rapid cellular growth and activity of the developing fetus early in pregnancy. The n-3 and n-6 PUFAs carry particular biological importance with docosahexaenoic acid (DHA), eicosapentaenoic acid (EPA), dihomo-γ-linolenic acid, and arachidonic acid playing metabolic, structural, and signaling roles.[134] Data have demonstrated that maternal dietary supplementation with DHA and EPA increases gestation length, enhances fetal growth, and reduces the risk of pregnancy complications.[135] Furthermore, enhanced maternal consumption of dietary n-3 long-chain PUFAs seems to exert long-term favorable effects on fetal immune function, especially as related to allergic and respiratory diseases.[136,137] Current intake recommendations for n-3 and n-6 fatty acids are indicated at 1.4 g/d and 13 g/d respectively, a 27% and 8% increase accordingly from prepregnancy values.[119] During pregnancy, women should eat 8 to 12 ounces of seafood low in methyl mercury a week, according to the Dietary Guidelines for Americans.[68] To accommodate these recommendations, pregnant women and those attempting to conceive should aim to consume one or two portions of fish per week, including oily fish.[138] Additional healthy sources of fat, such as avocados, nuts, seeds, and olives, should also be encouraged, while intake of *trans* fatty acids and animal-based saturated fats should be discouraged because they appear to promote deleterious metabolic effects on early stage fetal development.[139]

Micronutrient Requirements

Although deficiencies of any required nutrients during fetal development can result in health problems for the child during his or her lifetime, several nutrients are of particular importance because maternal inadequacies during pregnancy may contributing to devastating birth defects. Therefore, in addition to helping pregnant athletes achieve a balanced dietary intake, encouraging the use of multivitamins or prenatal vitamins is key to ensuring a healthy first trimester.

IRON

While hemoglobin mass does not significantly expand until the second and third trimesters of pregnancy, increased dietary intake of iron is recommended from the time of conception to accommodate normal iron losses, support fetal and placental growth, and build iron stores before demands become more pronounced.[140] The current RDA for iron during pregnancy is 27 mg/d, representing a 50% increase from prepregnancy values.[141] Female athletes may be at elevated risk for iron deficiency and iron-deficiency anemia due to heightened levels of hepcidin, a peptide hormone that inhibits iron absorption and sequesters iron in the macrophage. Research indicates that hepcidin concentrations increase in response to exercise, which makes early screening of added importance to this population.[142] Not only can iron deficiency and iron deficiency anemia exacerbate feelings of fatigue and compromise overall maternal health in the first trimester, but they can also contribute to poor pregnancy outcomes, including preterm delivery, prematurity, and small for gestational age birth weight.[140,143] In some cases, iron deficiency may escalate risk for pica, the act of craving substances (often non–food related) like ice, dirt, and clay, that contain little to no nutritional value. This behavior can be harmful for both mother and child, especially when the cravings include nonfood substances that increase the risk of exposure to toxic and parasitic ingredients. There also seems to be a correlation between iron deficiency and restless leg syndrome, making inclusion of questions regarding history of restless leg syndrome and pica of possible benefit when screening for deficiency.[144] In addition to incorporating iron-rich foods, such as lean meat, seafood, edamame, white beans, nuts, fortified grain products, and spinach, supplemental iron is recommended if ferritin levels drop below 70 μg/L. Suggested supplement guidelines are as follows[143]:

- Ferritin greater than 70 μg/L: no iron supplements
- Ferritin 31 to 70 μg/L: 30 to 40 mg ferrous iron per day
- Ferritin 30 to 15 μg/L: 60 to 80 mg ferrous iron per day
- Ferritin less than 15 μg/L and/or iron-deficiency anemia: therapeutic doses of 100 mg ferrous iron per day

FOLATE

Folate plays an integral role in the transformation of the neural tube into the brain and spinal cord during the first 28 days of pregnancy and provides consequent protection against neural tube defects like spina bifida and anencephaly. Folate requirements increase from preconception values of 200 mcg/d to 600 mcg/d during the first trimester.[145,146] Continued supplementation with 400 mcg/d in the second and third trimesters has been shown to increase maternal and cord blood folate status and prevent the increase in homocysteine concentration that otherwise occurs in late pregnancy; thus, supplementation may be of added benefit to pregnancy outcomes, and health in early childhood.[147] Ensuring adequate dietary consumption from such natural food sources as avocados, oranges, asparagus, green leafy vegetables, dried beans, and peas, as well as fortified grain products, should serve as the first line of defense. However, over-the-counter supplemental folate is often needed to achieve red blood cell folate levels associated with maximal protection against neural defect, especially when maternal nutrition is compromised secondary to morning sickness, a common first-trimester symptom.[146] Multivitamin tablets with folate are generally found in three formats:

- Regular over-the-counter multivitamins with 400 mcg to 600 mcg folate
- Prenatal over-the-counter multivitamins with 1,000 mcg folate
- Prescription multivitamins with 5,000 mcg folate

The higher doses of folate found in prenatal over-the-counter supplements are designed to protect against maternal folate deficiency as a result of fetal demand for the nutrient triumphing maternal demand. Prescription doses of folate are primarily reserved for women with a high risk for primary or recurrent neural tube or other folic acid–sensitive congenital anomalies To help mitigate possible concerns of high supplemental intakes of folate masking pernicious anemia, prescription doses of folate should be consumed in conjunction with 2.6 mcg/d of vitamin B-12.[146]

VITAMIN B-12

Because vitamin B-12 plays a fundamental role in neural myelination, brain development, and growth of the fetus, adequate intake during pregnancy is critical.[148] A dietary deficiency early in pregnancy is considered a risk factor for neural tube closure defects. Furthermore, maternal vitamin B-12 insufficiency (< 200 pmol/L) can lead to adverse pregnancy outcomes for mother and child, including preeclampsia, intrauterine growth retardation, impaired fetal brain function, preterm delivery, and low birth weight (< 2,500 g).[148] The RDA for vitamin B-12 increases by 8% from nonpregnancy values to 2.6 mcg/d to accommodate increased production of red blood cells, the manufacturing of genetic material, and healthy functioning of the nervous system. Some data suggest that doses as high as three times the RDA are of benefit to maternal and fetal health during pregnancy.[145,149] Including good dietary sources of vitamin B-12, such as eggs, cheese, milk products, meat, fish, shellfish, and poultry, as well as fortified grains and soy foods on a daily basis should be encouraged. Supplemental vitamin B-12 may be warranted for vegans and lacto-ovo-vegetarians, as well as women in resource-poor areas, to ensure optimal intake.[150,151]

ZINC

Zinc is a key micronutrient during pregnancy and particularly in the first trimester when organs begin to form and the immune system develops. To help accommodate fetal growth and development, the RDA for zinc increases from 8 mg/d to 11 mg/d during pregnancy.[141] Because suboptimal zinc status in pregnancy may elevate risk for numerous adverse pregnancy outcomes, including preeclampsia, gestational hypertension, low birth weight (< 2,500 g), premature delivery, labor and delivery complications, and congenital anomalies, supplemental zinc at doses up to 30 mg/d may be warranted in women who fail to fulfill the increased RDA for zinc through food intake.[152-154] Those women who follow plant-based diets often have difficulty acquiring sufficient zinc because the most abundant sources of zinc are animal based, and dietary phytates found in plant foods can interfere with zinc absorption.[155] In addition, women in low-income settings seem to be at greater risk for zinc deficiency and thus are likely to benefit from supplementation.[156]

CHOLINE

Choline helps support the structure and function of the brain and spinal cord during fetal development. It is also necessary for the synthesis of lecithin, an essential constituent of the human brain and nervous system, and acetylcholine, an important neurotransmitter. Results from both animal- and human-based studies suggest that maternal choline supplementation during pregnancy may help improve offspring cognitive function, stress response, and cerebral inhibition, thereby serving as a possible nutritional strategy to improve the lifelong health of a child.[157-159] Current Adequate Intake recommendation during all three trimesters of pregnancy is 450 mg/d, a 25 mg/d increase from prepregnancy values.[145] Good dietary sources of choline include cow's milk, egg yolk, liver, and peanuts.

VITAMIN D

Vitamin D is a key nutrient for establishing and maintaining optimal fetal and maternal bone health. It also aids in the uptake and metabolism of calcium and phosphorus and is consequently a critical component of bone mineralization and growth.[160-164] Poor maternal vitamin D status during pregnancy has been associated with fetal health complications, such as disordered skeletal homeostasis, congenital rickets, and fractures in newborns, with much of this damage being irreversible.[164-166]

Furthermore, there is mounting evidence that low maternal serum vitamin D levels may predispose the infant to lifelong chronic disease, including certain types of cancers, autoimmune disease, neurologic disease, insulin resistance, and cardiovascular disease.[167,168]

There is also some evidence that implies a tenuous link between suboptimal maternal vitamin D status and undesirable pregnancy outcomes, including infection, preeclampsia, gestational diabetes , preterm birth, and small for gestational age status.[168-173] It was estimated that anywhere from 5% to 84% of pregnant women across the globe either fail to consume the current RDA for vitamin D, which increased from 10 to 15 mcg/d (400 to 600 IU/d)or have inadequate serum vitamin D levels (< 20 ng/mL).[172,174] In the United States, the prevalence of vitamin D deficiency has been estimated to be 33% of the population.[175] Research among athletic populations suggests that maintaining a concentration of serum 25-hydroxyvitamin D— abbreviated 25(OH)D— ≥ 30 (preferrably ≥ 40) ng/mL range protects against common infectious illness, impaired muscle function, and stress fractures, all of which are important to the well-being of the female athlete during pregnancy, as well as to her return to sport after pregnancy.[176] Because vitamin D is found in very few foods and contribution of sun exposure to vitamin D status depends on many factors, including latitude, skin color, amount of skin exposed, duration of exposure, and use of sunscreens, vitamin D supplementation throughout pregnancy may be needed to achieve concentrations supportive of fetal and maternal health. Most prenatal vitamins contribute 10 mcg (400 IU) of vitamin D.

Some data suggest that supplementation with 25 to 50 mcg/d (1,000 to 2,000 IU vitamin D) throughout gestation may be warranted as a means to offer the infant substantial protection against vitamin D deficiency during the first 2 months of life.[177,178] However, it is important to note that excessive serum 25(OH)D concentration (> 50 ng/mL) can be equally dangerous because it can breach the placental barrier and adversely affect the total amount of calcium stored in fetal bones and ultimately lead to neonatal death.[179] Thus, supplementation with vitamin D is unnecessary in women with healthy serum 25(OH)D concentrations of 20 to 50 ng/mL, and supplementation at levels greater than 2,000 IU/d should be approached with caution.[179]

IODINE

Adequate intake of iodine throughout pregnancy is essential for fetal brain development and growth. It is also essential for maternal thyroid function. Dietary inadequacies have been shown to put a child at elevated risk for mental retardation, as well as growth, hearing, and speech problems, and put the mother at elevated risk for hypothyroidism.[180] Pregnancy hypothyroidism has been linked to several adverse pregnancy outcomes, including prematurity, low birth weight, miscarriage, preeclampsia, fetal death, and impaired fetal neurocognitive development.[180] Therefore, pregnant women should be advised to meet the current RDA of 220 mcg daily through dietary intake and supplementation.[181]

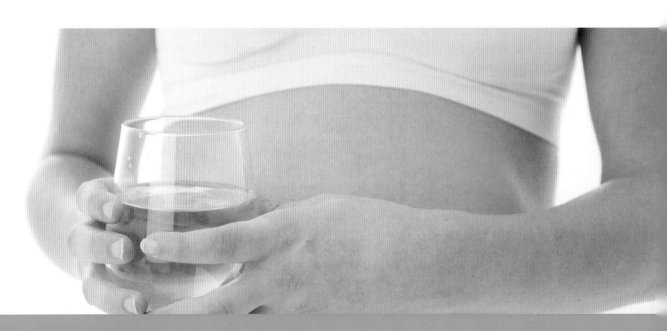

Hydration Needs

To accommodate substantial gestational blood water expansion, the adequate intake of fluid suggested to achieve a euhydrated state increases from 2.7 to 3 L/d during pregnancy.[182] However, because the amount of fluid needed to reach a euhydrated state can be highly variable, especially in athletes, urine color may be a valid alternative to mark urine concentration and overall hydration status in pregnant women. Current data suggest that pregnant women who present with a urine color ≥ 4 are likely to have a urine osmolality ≤ 500 mOsm/kg; thus, increased fluid intake is warranted to improve hydration status.[183] Female athletes should be advised to always carry fluids with them during workouts as well as during the day to avoid dehydration, which has been demonstrated to negatively affect amniotic fluid levels and initiate premature labor.

CONTRAINDICATED FOOD PRODUCTS, SUBSTANCES, AND SUPPLEMENTS IN PREGNANCY

Hormonal changes during pregnancy compromise the cell-mediated immune function of both pregnant women and their fetuses, making exposure to food-borne pathogens that can be passed to the fetus, like *Salmonella enterica* and *Listeria monocytogenes,* of particular concern during pregnancy. While maternal infection may be asymptomatic or present with mild flulike symptoms, including fever, muscle aches, and gastrointestinal symptoms, fetal or neonatal infection is often severe and potentially fatal.[184,185] In addition, substances like alcohol and caffeine and certain dietary supplements can penetrate the placenta and reach the fetus where they are only partially metabolized by the child's immature digestive system and thus may increase risk for adverse pregnancy outcomes, such as fetal alcohol spectrum disorder.[186-188] Therefore, pregnant women should be advised to take special precaution with intake of certain food and drink products, substances, and ingredients during pregnancy, including the following:

- raw fish and shellfish
- undercooked meat and poultry
- raw or soft-cooked eggs
- raw sprouts
- seafood with a high mercury content
- unpasteurized foods
- unwashed fruits and vegetables
- caffeine
- alcohol
- dietary supplements

Raw Fish and Shellfish

Raw fish, including oysters, clams, mussels, and scallops, and refrigerated, uncooked seafood, such as lox or Nova-style salmon or any kippered or smoked seafood, pose a greater threat of parasitic and bacterial infection than cooked fish and should be avoided during pregnancy. During preparation, fish should be cooked to an internal temperature of 145°F (63°C), at which point it will separate into flakes and appear opaque throughout. Shrimp, lobster, and scallops should be cooked until they are milky white. Clams, mussels, and oysters should be cooked until their shells open.[184,185]

Undercooked Meat and Poultry

Like raw seafood, undercooked meat and poultry are at greater risk of being contaminated with food-borne pathogens than their cooked counterparts, and thus special precautions need to be taken. A meat thermometer can be a helpful at-home tool to ensure that meats and poultry are cooked thoroughly. When dining out, meats should be requested well-done. Because hotdogs and lunch meat are carriers of the food-borne pathogen *L monocytogenes,* they should be cooked until steaming hot before consumption.[184,185]

Raw or Soft-Cooked Eggs

A carrier of *S enterica,* eggs are among the most common causes of salmonella infection. Therefore, consumption of raw or undercooked eggs is discouraged during pregnancy. Food products containing raw or partially cooked eggs, such as eggnog, custard, cookie dough, cake batter, and any hollandaise, mayonnaise, or caesar salad dressing made with raw eggs should also be avoided during pregnancy.[114,115] Eggs that have been pasteurized to reduce the risk of food-borne illness in dishes that are not cooked or are only lightly cooked, such as liquid egg products or eggs pasteurized in the shell, are safe for consumption.

Raw Sprouts

Raw sprouts, like alfalfa, clover, radish, and mung bean, are vulnerable to bacteria entering through cracks in their seeds before sprouting. Thus, consumption is risky and discouraged during pregnancy.[184,185]

Seafood High in Mercury

Because high levels of the organometallic compound methylmercury can be toxic to the nervous system of a fetus, certain fish, like tilefish from the Gulf of Mexico, king mackerel, shark, and swordfish, should be avoided during pregnancy. As a safe alternative, consuming up to 12 ounces of fish and shellfish with lower counts of methylmercury, such as shrimp, canned light tuna, salmon, catfish, pollock, anchovies, and trout, is recommended.[184,185]

Unpasteurized Foods

While many grocery store chains do not carry unpasteurized foods, such as milk, soft cheeses (eg, queso blanco, queso fresco, queso panela, Camembert, Brie, feta, and blue), and juice, due to heightened risk that they carry food-borne pathogens, some stores do sell them. Pregnant women should read labels while food shopping, especially when at a nonchain or farmers market, and should buy and consume only pasteurized products. When dining out, pregnant women are advised to check with the kitchen before ordering certain types of cheeses and juices.[184,185]

Caffeine

Caffeine crosses over the placenta, and the developing fetus is ill-equipped to fully metabolize the stimulant, which creates the potential adverse pregnancy outcomes of miscarriage, preterm labor, and low-birth-weight babies. Therefore, caffeine intake of less than 200 mg/d during pregnancy is recommended, with abstinence indicated for women with known caffeine sensitivities before pregnancy.[187] Education on common caffeine-containing products and their caffeine doses, including coffee, tea, energy drinks, and some soft drinks, should be provided early in pregnancy. It is important to also educate clients on the lesser-known contributors to dietary caffeine intake, including such dietary supplement ingredients as guarana, yerba mate, kola or kola nut, cocoa, citrus aurantium (bitter orange), and various sports foods that contain caffeinated gels and blocks.

Alcohol

Because alcohol passes freely through the placenta to the fetus, no level of consumption is verified safe during pregnancy. Abuse of alcohol during pregnancy is linked to fetal alcohol syndrome, which is characterized by malformations of the skeletal system, heart, and brain; growth problems; central nervous system problems; poor motor skills; increased mortality; and problems with learning, memory, social interaction, attention span, problem solving, speech, and hearing. Even moderate intake of alcohol, which, for women, is a 5-ounce glass of wine or a 12-ounce beer, can elicit fetal alcohol effects marked by mental and behavioral impairments.[186] Thus, pregnant women should be advised to avoid alcohol throughout pregnancy.

Dietary Supplements

Dietary ingredients in dietary supplements, including vitamins, minerals, herbs or other botanicals, and amino acids, are not subject to the premarket safety evaluations required of food ingredients and medications. Because of this, the efficacy and safety of these products during pregnancy is questionable, and, thus, their use is discouraged unless specifically recommended by a health care provider for pregnancy health. Ingredients found in dietary supplements reach the fetus primarily by crossing the placenta. Exposure during pregnancy to some ingredients and substances in dietary supplements can indirectly impact the fetus by initiating uterine contractions and premature labor or by lowering maternal blood pressure, which, in turn, may reduce blood flow to the placenta and the consequent supply of oxygen and nutrients to the fetus, increasing the risk of the child being born at a low birth weight.[187] Exposure during pregnancy to some ingredients found in dietary supplements may also directly cause damage, abnormal development, and death of the fetus.[188]

WEIGHT GAIN RECOMMENDATIONS

Over the years, there has been considerable discussion regarding the optimal quantity of weight gain in pregnancy for both maternal and fetal health. Currently, the Institute of Medicine (IOM) and the American College of Obstetricians and Gynecologists recommend a total weight gain of 25 to 35 lb for singleton pregnancies in women with a healthy BMI (18.5 to 24.9).[121,122] A slightly greater weight gain of 28 to 40 lb for singleton pregnancies is recommended for female athletes who enter pregnancy underweight (BMI < 18.5).[119,120] Women who are overweight (BMI = 25 to 29.9) are encouraged to minimize pregnancy weight gain to 15 to 25 lb for singleton pregnancies.[121,122] Women who are obese (BMI > 30) should minimize pregnancy weight gain to 11 to 20 lbs for singleton pregnancies.[120,121] For twin pregnancies, the IOM recommends a total gestational weight gain of 37 to 54 lb for women of normal weight, 31 to 50 lbs for women who are overweight, and 25 to 42 lb for women who are obese.[121]

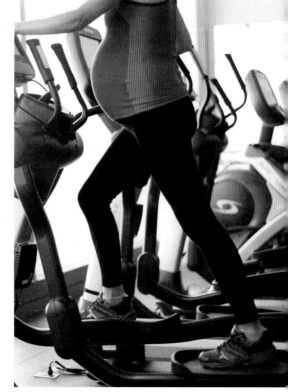

Singleton pregnancy-associated weight gain during the first trimester of 1.1 to 4.4 lb can be attributed to the expanding uterus, growing breasts, and increased blood volume. It makes up only a small percentage of total recommended pregnancy weight gain. Slightly more weight gain is attributed to the same causes for twin pregnancies. During the second and third trimesters, when fetal growth increases dramatically, a weekly weight gain of approximately 1 lb for singleton pregnancies and 1.5 lb for twin pregnancies is recommended for women with underweight and healthy prepregnancy BMIs. The recommended weekly weight gain for women who are overweight and obese during the second and third trimester is 0.6 and 0.5 lb, respectively, for singleton pregnancies and slightly higher for twin pregnancies.[121] Some experts speculate that if adequate fetal growth is occurring, even lower rates of pregnancy weight gain in women who are overweight and obese may be warranted to help optimize the long-term health of the child.[123,124] Maintaining a healthy rate of weight gain in pregnancy has been shown to decrease risk for several adverse maternal and neonatal outcomes, including gestational diabetes, hypertension, cesarean birth, fetal macrosomia, preterm birth, stillbirth, small or large for gestational age, and low birth weight.[121-124,189,190]

Especially relevant for female athletes interested in making a postpartum athletic comeback is the finding that staying within IOM weight-gain guidelines during pregnancy helps reduce the risk of retaining more than 2 kg pregnancy weight at 18 months postpartum and beyond, regardless of prepregnancy weight status.[191] Therefore, it is important for RDNs and other health professionals working with pregnant athletes to discuss the IOM pregnancy weight-gain guidelines and to provide appropriate diet and exercise guidance to help achieve these goals.

EXERCISE IN PREGNANCY

Some female athletes fear that their training may trigger miscarriage or cause harm to their child, so they stop exercise completely upon discovery of their pregnancy. Current evidence does not substantiate these concerns. In fact, the evidence demonstrates that moderate resistance and cardiovascular exercise during pregnancy is not a direct cause of miscarriage and instead may offset some of the discomforts associated with nurturing fetal growth and support a healthy pregnancy.[4,192-194]

For a competitive athlete, the excitement of pregnancy can be overshadowed by concern for how pregnancy weight gain will affect her body, sport performance, and ability to return to competition. Helping the athlete transition from a "train to win" or "train to perform" to a "train for health" mind-set is not always easy. Education on exercise tolerance and countraindications and benefits from a maternal, fetal, and athletic standpoint can go a long way in providing comfort to the athlete and establishing the framework for a healthy pregnancy (see Box 17.2).

Box 17.2 Exercise During Pregnancy

For pregnant women who want to exercise throughout pregnancy, the American College of Sports Medicine provides the following recommendations[127]:

Safety: As changes in weight distribution occur, balance and coordination may be affected. Exercise programs should be modified if they pose a significant risk of abdominal injury or fatigue as opposed to relaxation and an enhanced sense of well-being. Until more information is available, exercising in the supine or prone positions should be avoided after the first trimester.

Environment: Temperature regulation is highly dependent on hydration and environmental conditions. Exercising pregnant women should ensure adequate fluid intake before, during, and after exercise; wear loose-fitting clothing; and avoid high heat and humidity to protect against heat stress, especially in the first trimester.

Growth and Development: The pregnant woman should monitor her level of exercise and adjust her dietary intake to ensure proper weight gain. If pregnancy is not progressing normally or if vaginal bleeding, membrane rupture, persistent pain, or chronic fatigue is noted, exercise should be stopped until medical evaluation can be completed. Also, if regular contractions occur more than 30 minutes after exercise, medical evaluation should be sought. This may signify preterm labor.

Mode: Weight-bearing and non–weight-bearing exercise are thought to be safe during pregnancy. Improved maternal fitness is a well-known benefit of non–weight-bearing exercise, such as swimming and cycling. Weight-bearing exercises are similarly beneficial as long as they are comfortable. Swimming and stationary cycling are excellent non–weight-bearing exercises and may be recommended. Walking, jogging, and low-impact aerobic programs are good choices when weight-bearing exercise is to be considered.

Heavy weight lifting or similar activities that require straining are to be discouraged. Bicycle riding, especially during the second and third trimesters, should be avoided because of changes in balance and the risk of falling. Exposure to the extremes of air pressure, such as scuba diving and high-altitude exercise in nonacclimatized women, should be avoided.

Intensity: Pregnancy is probably not a time for serious competition. For women who are continuing their regular exercise during pregnancy, exercise intensity should not exceed prepregnancy levels. The intensity of exercise should be regulated by how hard a woman believes she is working. Moderate to hard is quite safe for a woman who is accustomed to this level of exercise.

Exercise: A healthy woman with a normal pregnancy may either continue her regular exercise regimen or begin a new exercise program during pregnancy. For your particular exercise prescription and its duration, check with your physician.

Reprinted with permission of the American College of Sports Medicine, ACSM Current Comment Exercise During Pregnancy.

POSTPARTUM RECOMMENDATIONS

After welcoming a new baby, many mothers are eager to resume exercise activities and are motivated to eat healthfully as a means to help shed their pregnancy weight and facilitate a strong return to competition. There is some anecdotal evidence to suggest that athletic performance may improve postpartum. A complete disregard for the physiological changes that occur in the body after childbirth, however, is unwise. The transition into becoming a new mother presents unique challenges an athlete must consider, such as the high energy cost of breastfeeding. Disregarding these new obstacles can place an athlete who is a new mother at heightened risk for injury, compromise her overall health, and hinder her ability to successfully return to sport. Health practitioners working with athletes who are new mothers can play an integral role facilitating a successful return to sport by providing education and guidance on proper nutrition during breastfeeding, nutrition and fitness strategies to promote healthful weight loss, and appropriate precautions to take when returning to sport activity.

Nutrition and Breastfeeding

It is the position of the Academy of Nutrition and Dietetics that exclusive breastfeeding provides optimal nutrition and health protection for the first 6 months of life and that breastfeeding with complementary foods from 6 months until at least 12 months of age is the ideal feeding pattern for infants.[195]

Many female athletes express concern about their milk production and composition being negatively affected by exercise training and consequently choose to supplement with formula or delay their return to fitness activity until after weaning. However, there is currently no evidence to support the notion that exercise training, even at moderate-to-high intensity hurts the production or composition of breast milk, including important immune factors (secretory immunoglobulin A , lactoferrin, and lysozyme).[196,197]

Ensuring adequate nutrition to support the metabolic demands of lactation is critical. For an athlete, the combined energetic costs of breastfeeding and physical training can be extremely demanding. Failure to consume adequate calories can exacerbate postpartum fatigue and interfere with both nursing and fitness performance. Mean milk production of 749 g/d (~26 oz/d) requires an additional 453 kcal/d or approximately 17 kcal/oz of milk produced to support the metabolic demands of lactation.[198] With women's daily milk production being variable, a range of 300 to 500 kcal is often recommended. Thus, a target energy intake of 45 kcal/kg fat-free massper day plus an additional 300 to 500 kcal to accommodate lactation plus the amount of energy needed for physical activity should be encouraged.[125,198]

Because breastfeeding may reduce bone density by as much as 5% due to osteoclastic activity, it is prudent to encourage nursing women to regularly consume foods rich in calcium to ensure that they acquire the RDA of 1,000 mg of calcium.[199] While bone mass is generally recovered once the child is weaned, the rate and extent of recovery can be influenced by the duration of lactation and postpartum amenorrhea and may differ by skeletal site.[200]

Healthy Weight-Loss Strategies

Body composition and body weight are two of many factors that contribute to optimal exercise performance and overall health. Returning to prepregnancy form is a goal that most athletes strive to achieve postpartum. Practitioners can play a key role in providing the tools needed to promote healthy fat loss, optimized health, and enhanced performance. Research has shown that average weight retention at 1 year postpartum falls to around 2.0 kg, with the greatest rate of weight loss occurring in the first 3 months postpartum and then continuing at a slow and steady rate until about 6 months postpartum.[201] Women who exclusively breastfeed for at least 3 months have been shown to exhibit significantly less weight retention than those who supplement or discontinue breastfeeding before 3 months.[202] Recent data have shown exercise programs with objectively defined goals, such as heart rate or total steps, and those with intensive dietary intervention, including self-monitoring through the use of food journals, to be highly effective in aiding sustained postpartum weight loss.[203,204] For women who began their pregnancy at a healthy weight and gained the recommended amount of weight during pregnancy, a gradual weight loss not to exceed 4.5 lb/mo should be encouraged after the first month postpartum and until prepregnancy weight is achieved.[205]

Return to Sport

While obstetricians often recommend waiting to exercise until after the first postpartum checkup, generally scheduled 4 to 6 weeks after delivery, an earlier return to physical training is usually safe, provided the absence of medical or surgical complications during labor and delivery, according to the American College of Obstetricians and Gynecologists.[206] However, there are hormonal and physiological changes to the postpartum body that can increase risk for injury when too much activity is taken on too soon. One of the biggest challenges results from a hormone called relaxin. For up to 6 months after childbirth, and even longer for nursing mothers, the body produces relaxin, which, in turn, relaxes the muscles, joints, and ligaments, contributing to instability. These changes can make high-impact exercise, such as running, lifting heavy weights, and quick changes of direction, potentially dangerous to an athlete postpartum. This is especially true for women with pelvic floor weakness because constant and excessive downward pressure on the pelvic floor can increase postpartum risk for hemorrhage, prolapse, and urine leakage.[207] Daily pelvic floor exercises should be encouraged immediately after childbirth to strengthen these muscles. Due to these concerns, lower-impact activities, such as swimming, elliptical, and body weight exercises, should be the focal point of any conditioning program during the early postpartum stages or until pelvic floor stability is established. See Box 17.3 for information on postpartum recovery.

Box 17.3 The Pregnancy-Performance Connection[16]

Overcoming performance roadblocks is not an easy feat, but with perseverance, there are key physiological benefits that can facilitate a women's successful return to sporting competition.

According to James Clapp III, MD, a renowned researcher in the area of exercise and pregnancy, women who regularly train at a moderately hard level of perceived effort about an hour a day throughout pregnancy and are able to resume a similar pattern soon after delivery will experience significant improvements in exercise economy, meaning the cost of oxygen to perform a specific workload is lower, and maximum aerobic capacity will increase about 10%, even if overall training load is lighter compared with prepregnancy.

These benefits are thought to last about a year postpartum, possibly more. While scientific evidence supporting the translation to athletic performance in high-performing endurance athletes is lacking, it is thought to be one reason why so many women athletes come back stronger after giving birth.

Before Pregnancy:

Female athletes who have struggled to maintain a normal menstrual cycle, defined as experiencing menstruation every 28 to 30 days, at any point during training or competition may need to reduce overall training load or increase energy intake.

Body weight and fat gain may be necessary for female athletes carrying very low body weights, as defined by a BMI less than 18.5.

Developing healthy weight-loss strategies, including exercise, for women with a BMI greater than 25 will help boost fertility by enhancing insulin function and improving the body's overall hormone profile.

Consuming a balanced plant-focused diet and supplementing with prenatal vitamins, which provide key fertility nutrients, such as folate and iron, are nutrition strategies shown to boost fertility.

Limiting caffeine intake to no more than 200 mg/d and abstaining from alcohol preconception is recommended to improve fertility.

During Pregnancy:

Advising the pregnant athlete on how to achieve a balanced dietary intake, adhere to food safety recommendations, and take multivitamins or prenatal vitamins is key to ensuring a healthy pregnancy.

A target energy intake of 45 kcal/kg prepregnancy fat-free mass per day plus the amount of energy burned during exercise should be encouraged during the first trimester of pregnancy with an additional 340 kcal and 452 kcal being warranted in the form of carbohydrate and protein during the second and third trimesters to support increased fetal growth patterns.

Adequate intake of fluid suggested for maintaining a euhydrated state increases from 2.7 to 3 L/d during pregnancy to accommodate substantial gestational blood volume expansion.

For a healthy woman with a normal pregnancy, a regular exercise regimen should be encouraged under the supervision of her physician.

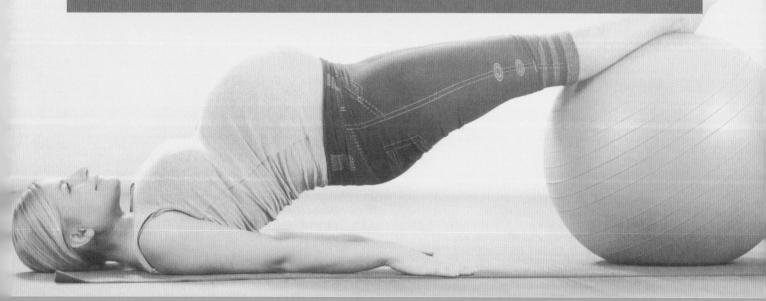

After Pregnancy:

It is the position of the Academy of Nutrition and Dietetics that exclusive breastfeeding provides optimal nutrition and health protection for the first 6 months of life and that breastfeeding with complementary foods from 6 months until at least 12 months of age is the ideal feeding pattern for infants.

A target energy intake of 45 kcal/kg fat-free mass per day plus an additional 300 to 500 kcal to accommodate lactation plus the amount of energy needed for physical activity should be encouraged.

For women who began their pregnancy at a healthy weight and gained the recommended amount of weight during pregnancy, a gradual weight loss not to exceed 4.5 lb/mo should be encouraged after the first month postpartum and until prepregnancy weight is achieved.

While obstetricians often recommend waiting to exercise until after the first postpartum checkup, generally scheduled 4 to 6 weeks after delivery, an earlier return to more physical training is generally safe, provided there were no medical or surgical complications during labor and delivery, according to the American College of Obstetricians and Gynecologists.

REFERENCES

1. Key statistics from the National Survey of Family Growth (data are for 2011-20130). Centers for Disease Control and Prevention website. www.cdc.gov/nchs/fastats/infertility.htm. Updated February 15, 2016. Accessed December 14, 2016.

2. Marquez S, Molinero O. Energy availability, menstrual dysfunction, and bone health in sports; an overview of the female athlete triad. *Nutr Hosp.* 2013;28(4):1010-1017.

3. De Souza MJ, Toombs RJ, Scheid JL, O'Donnell E, West SL, Williams NI. High prevalence of subtle and severe menstrual disturbances in exercising women: confirmation using daily hormone measures. *Hum Reprod.* 2010;25(2):491-503.

4. Weinstein Y, Weinstein A. Energy balance, body composition and the female athlete triad syndrome. *Harefuah.* 2012;151(2):97-101, 127, 126.

5. Ahrens KA, Vladutiu CJ, Mumford SL, et al. The effect of physical activity across the menstrual cycle on reproductive function. *Ann Epidemiol.* 2014;24(2):127-134.

6. Orio F, Muscogiuri G, Ascione A, et al. Effects of physical exercise on the female reproductive system. *Minerva Endocrinol.* 2013;38(3):305-319.

7. Gibbs JC, Williams NI, Mallinson RJ, Reed JL, Rickard AD, De Souza MJ. Effect of high dietary restraint on energy availability and menstrual status. *Med Sci Sports Exerc.* 2013;45(9):1790-1797.

8. De Souza MJ. Menstrual disturbances in athletes: a focus on luteal phase defects. *Med Sci Sports Exerc.* 2003;35(9):1553-1563.

9. Centers for Disease Control and Prevention. Healthy People 2020. National Center for Health Statistics, US Department of Health and Human Services. www.cdc.gov/nchs/healthy_people/hp2020.htm. Updated October 14, 2011. Accessed October 3, 2016.

10. Surehka T, Himabindu Y, Sriharibabu M, Pandey AK. Impact of physical activity on ovarian reserve markers in normal, overweight, and obese reproductive age women. *Indian J Physiol Pharmacol.* 2014;58(2):162-165.

11. Orio F, Muscogiuri G, Ascione A, et al. Effects of physical exercise on the female reproductive system. *Minerva Endocrinol.* 2013;38(3):305-319.

12. Wiebe HW, Boule NG, Chari R, Davenport MH. The effect of supervised prenatal exercise on fetal growth: a meta-analysis. *Obstet Gynecol.* 2015;125(5):1185-1194.

13. Kehler AK, Heinrich KM. A selective review of prenatal exercise guidelines since the 1950s until present: written for women, health care professionals, and female athletes. *Women Birth.* 2015;28(4):e93-e98.

14. US Department of Health and Human Services. 2008 physical activity guidelines for Americans. https://health.gov/PAGUIDELINES/pdf/paguide.pdf. Published October 2008. Accessed October 3, 2016.

15. Chavarro JE, Rich-Edwards JW, Rosner BA, Willett WC. Diet and lifestyle in the prevention of ovulatory disorder infertility. *Obstet Gynecol.* 2007;110(5):1050-1058.

16. Rich-Edwards JW, Spiegelman D, Garland M, et al. Physical activity, body mass index, and ovulatory disorder infertility. *Epidemiology.* 2002;13(2):184-190.

17. Gudmundsdottir SL, Flanders WD, Augestad LB. Physical activity and fertility in women: the North-Trøndelag Health Study. *Hum Reprod.* 2009;24(12):3196-3204.

18. Wise LA, Rothman KJ, Mikkelsen EM, Sorensen HT, Riis AH, Hatch EE. A prospective cohort study of physical activity and time to pregnancy. *Fertil Steril.* 2012;97(5):1136-1142.

19. Maimoun L, Georgopoulos NA, Sultan C. Endocrine disorders in adolescent and young female athletes: impact on growth, menstrual cycles, and bone mass acquisition. *J Clin Endocrin Metab.* 2014;99(11):4037-4050.

20. Brooks KA, Carter JG. Overtraining, exercise, and adrenal insufficiency. *J Nov Physiother.* 2013;3(125):pii:11717.

21. Kreher JB, Scwartz JB. Overtraining syndrome: a practical guide. *Sports Health.* 2012;4(2):128-138.

22. Meczekalski B, Katulski K, Czyzyk A, Podfigurna-Stopa A, Maciejewska-Jeske M. Functional hypothalamic amenorrhea and its influence on women's health. *J Endocrinol Invest.* 2014;37(11):1049-1056.

23. Melin A, Tornberg AB, Skouby S, et al. Energy availability and the female athlete triad in elite endurance athletes. *Scand J Med Sci Sports.* 2015;25(5):610-622.

24. Sharma R, Biedenharn KR, Fedor JM, Agarwal A. Lifestyle factors and reproductive health: taking control of your fertility. *Reprod Biol Endocrinol.* 2013;11:66.

25. Provost MP, Acharya KS, Acharya CR, et al. Pregnancy outcomes decline with increasing recipient body mass index: an analysis of 22,317 fresh donor/recipient cycles from the 2008-2010 Society for Assisted Reproductive Technology Clinic Outcome Reporting System registry. *Fertil Steril.* 2015;105(2):364-368.

26. World Health Organization. *Obesity: Preventing and Managing the Global Epidemic.* Report of a WHO Consultation. WHO Technical Report Series 894. Geneva, Switzerland: World Health Organization; 2000.

27. Bates WG for the Prevention of Infertility Committee of the American Society for Reproductive Medicine. Abnormal body weight: a preventable cause of infertility. http://www.reproductivefacts.org/globalassets/asrm/asrm-content/learning--resources/patient-resources/protect-your-fertility3/bodyweight_infertility.pdf. Accessed July 24, 2017.

28. Obesity and overweight. World Health Organization website. www.who.int/mediacentre/factsheets/fs311/en/. Updated January 2015. Accessed October 4, 2016.

29. Marsh CA, Hecker E. Maternal obesity and adverse reproductive outcomes: reducing the risk. *Obestet Gynecol Surv.* 2014;69(10):622-628.

30. Jungheim ES, Travieso JL, Carson KR, Moley KH. Obesity and reproductive function. *Obstet Gynecol Clin North Am.* 2012;39(4):479-493.

31. van der Steeg JW, Steures P, Eijkemans MJ, et al. Obesity affects spontaneous pregnancy chances in subfertile, ovulatory women. *Hum Reprod.* 2008;23(2):324-328.

32. Sim KA, Partridge SR, Sainsbury A. Does weight loss in overweight or obese women improve fertility treatment outcomes? A systematic review. *Obes Rev.* 2014;15(1):839-850.

33. Sim KA, Dezarnaulds GM, Denyer GS, Skilton MR, Caterson ID. Weight loss improves reproductive outcomes in obese women undergoing fertility treatment: a randomized controlled trial. *Clin Obes.* 2014;4(2):61-68.

34. Kort JD, Winget C, Kim SH, Lathi RB. A retrospective cohort study to evaluate the impact of meaningful weight loss on fertility outcomes in an overweight population with infertility. *Fertil Steril.* 2014;101(5):1400-1403.

35. Sowińska-Przepiera E, Andrysiak-Mamos E, Jarząbek-Bielecka G, et al. Functional hypothalamic amenorrhoea—diagnostic challenges, monitoring, and treatment. *Endokrynol Pol.* 2015;66(3):252-260.

36. Niedźwiedzka B1, Jagielska G, Bartoszewicz Z, Kondracka A, Brzozowska A, Karowicz-Bilińska A. [Assessment of neuropeptide Y, leptin and leptin-receptor concentrations in teenagers suffering from anorexia nervosa]. *Ginekol Pol.* 2013;84(4):268-276.

37. Loucks AB. Energy availability, not body fatness, regulates reproductive function in women. *Exerc Sport Sci Rev.* 2003;31(3):144-148.

38. Melin A, Tornberg AB, Skouby S, et al. Low-energy density and high fiber intake are dietary concerns in female endurance athletes. *Scand J Med Sci Sports.* 2016;26(9):1060-1071.

39. Gibbs JC, Williams NI, De Souza MJ. Prevalence of individual and combined components of the female athlete triad. *Med Sci Sports Exerc.* 2013;45(5):985-996.

40. Mountjoy M, Sundgot-Borgen J, Burke L, et al. The IOC consensus statement: beyond the Female Athlete Triad—Relative Energy Deficiency in Sport (RED-S). *Br J Sport Med.* 2014;48(7):491-497.

41. Mountjoy M, Sundgot-Borgen J, Burke L, et al. RED-S CAT. Relative Energy Deficiency in Sport (RED-S) Clinical Assessment Tool (CAT). *Br J Sport Med.* 2015;49(7):421-423.

42. Folscher LL, Grant CC, Fletcher L, Janse van Rensberg DC. Ultra-marathon athletes at risk for the female athlete triad. *Sports Med Open.* 2015;1(1):29.

43. Bacchi E1, Spiazzi G, Zendrini G, Bonin C, Moghetti P. Low body weight and menstrual dysfunction are common findings in both elite and amateur ballet dancers. *J Endocrinol Invest.* 2013;36(5):343-346.

44. Gibbs JC, Williams NI, Scheid JL, Toombs RJ, De Souza MJ. The association of a high drive for thinness with energy deficiency and severe menstrual disturbances: confirmation in a large population of exercising women. *Int J Sport Nutr Exerc Metab.* 2011;21(4):280-290.

45. Doyle-Lucas AF, Akers JD, Davy BM. Energetic efficiency, menstrual irregularity, and bone mineral density in elite professional female ballet dancers. *J Dance Med Sci.* 2010;14(4):146-154.

46. Melin A, Tornberg AB, Skouby S, et al. The LEAF questionnaire: a screening tool for the identification of female athletes at risk for the female athlete triad. *Br J Sports Med.* 2014;48(7):540-545.

47. Hammiche F, Laven JS, van Mil N, et al. Tailored preconceptional dietary and lifestyle counseling in a tertiary outpatient clinic in The Netherlands. *Hum Reprod.* 2011;26(9):2432-2441.

48. Walfisch A, Koren G. Preconception counseling: rational, practice and challenges. *Minerva Ginecol.* 2011;63(5):411-419.

49. Sinska B, Kucharska A, Dmoch-Gajzlerska E. The diet in improving fertility in women. *Pol Merkur Lekarski.* 2014;36(216):400-402.

50. Chavarro JE, Rich-Edwards JW, Rosner BA, Willet WC. Protein intake and ovulatory infertility. *Am J Obstet Gynecol.* 2008;198(2):210.e1-e7.

51. Weiss RV, Clapauch R. Female infertility of endocrine origin. *Arq Bras Endocrinol Metabol.* 2014;58(2):144-152.

52. Szostak-Wegierek D. Nutrition and fertility. *Med Wieku Rozwoj.* 2011;15(4):431-436.

53. Vujkovic M, de Vries JH, Lindemans J, et al. The preconception Mediterranean dietary pattern in couples undergoing in vitro fertilization/intracytoplasmic sperm injection treatment increases the chance of pregnancy. *Fertil Steril.* 2010;94(6):2096-2101.

54. Tobias DK, Zhang C, Chavarro J, et al. Adherence to dietary patterns and lower risk of gestational diabetes mellitus. *Am J Clin Nutr.* 2012;96(2):289-295.

55. Wilson RD, Audibert F, Brock JA, et al. Pre-conception folic acid and multivitamin supplementation for the primary and secondary prevention of neural tube defects and other folic acid-sensitive congenital anomalies. *J Obstet Gynaecol Can.* 2015;37(6):534-552.

56. Chavarro JE, Rich-Edwards JW, Rosner BA, Willett WC. Use of multivitamins, intake of B vitamins, and risk of ovulatory infertility. *Fertil Steril.* 2008;89(3):667-676.

57. Chavarro JE, Rich-Edwards JW, Rosner BA, Willett WC. Iron intake and risk of ovulatory infertility. *Obstet Gynecol.* 2006;108(5):1145-1152.

58. Gaskins AJ, Rich-Edwards JW, Hauser R, et al. Maternal prepregnancy folate intake and risk of spontaneous abortion and stillbirth. *Obstet Gynecol.* 2014;124(1):23-31.

59. Gardiner PM, Nelson L, Shellhaas CS, et al. The clinical content of preconception care: nutrition and dietary supplements. *Am J Obstet Gynecol.* 2008;199(6):345S-356S.

60. De-Regil LM, Fernández-Gaxiola AC, Dowswell T, Peña-Rosas JP. Effects and safety of periconceptional folate supplementation for preventing birth defects. *Cochrane Database Syst Rev.* 2010;(10):CD007950. doi:10.1002/14651858.CD007950.pub2.

61. Buhling KJ, Grajecki D. The effect of micronutrient supplements on female fertility. *Curr Opin Obstet Gynecol.* 2013;25(3):173-180.

62. Morgan S, Koren G, Bozzo P. Is caffeine consumption safe during pregnancy? *Can Fam Physician.* 2013;59(4):361-362.

63. Bolumar F, Olsen J, Rebagliato M, Bisanti L, and the European Study Group on Infertility Subfecundity. Caffeine and delayed conception: a European multicenter study on infertility and subfecundity. *Am J Epidemiol.* 1997;145(4):324-334.

64. Al-Saleh I, El-Doush I, Grisellhi B. Coskun S. The effect of caffeine consumption on the success rate of pregnancy as well as various performance parameters of in-vitro fertilization treatment. *Med Sci Monit.* 2010;16(12):CR598-CR605.

65. American College of Obstetrics and Gynecology, Committee on Obstetric Practice. Committee opinion no. 462. Moderate caffeine consumption during pregnancy. *Obstet Gynecol.* 2010;116:467-468. (Position reaffirmed 2015.)

66. Eggert J, Theobald H, Engfeldt P. Effects of alcohol consumption on female fertility during an 18-year period. *Fertil Steril.* 2004;81(2):379-383.

67. Wdowiak A, Sulima M, Sadowska M, Grzegorz B, Bojar I. Alcohol consumption and quality of embryos obtained in programmes of in vitro fertilization. *Ann Agric Environ Med.* 2014;21(2):450-453.

68. US Department of Agriculture. *Dietary Guidelines for Americans, 2015.* https://health.gov/dietaryguidelines/2015/guidelines/

69. Symons Downs D, Chasan-Taber L, Evenson KR, Leiferman J, Yeo S. Physical activity and pregnancy: past and present evidence and future recommendations. *Res Q Exerc Sport.* 2012;83(4):485-502.

70. Sanabria-Martinez G, Garcia-Hermosa A, Poyatos-León R, Álvarez-Bueno C, Sánchez-López M, Martinez-Vizcaino V. Effectiveness of physical activity interventions on preventing gestational diabetes mellitus and excessive maternal weight gain: a meta-analysis. *BJOG.* 2015;122(9):1167-1174.

71. Hinman SK, Smith KB, Quillen DM, Smith MS. Exercise in pregnancy: a clinical review. *Sports Health.* 2015;7(6):527-531.

72. Sanabria-Martinez G, Garcia-Hermoso A, Poyatos-León R, González-Garcia A, Sánchez-López M, Martinez-Vizaino V. Effects of exercise-based interventions on neonatal outcomes: a meta-analysis of randomized controlled trials [published online May 14, 2015]. *Am J Health Promot.*

73. Szymanski LM, Satin AJ. Exercise during pregnancy: fetal responses to current public health guidelines. *Obstet Gynecol.* 2012;119(3):603-610.

74. Nasik E, Eryilmaz G. Incidence of pregnancy-related discomforts and management approaches to relieve them among pregnant women. *J Clin Nurs.* 2014;23(11-12):1736-1750.

75. Tan EK, Tan EL. Alterations in physiology and anatomy during pregnancy. *Best Pract Res Clin Obstet Gyenacol.* 2013;27(6):791-802.

76. Bernstein IM, Ziegler W, Badger GJ. Plasma volume expansion in early pregnancy. *Obstet Gynecol.* 2001;97(5 pt 1):669-672.

77. Hegewald MJ, Crapo RO. Respiratory physiology in pregnancy. *Clin Chest Med.* 2011;32(1):1-13.

78. Berry MJ, McMurray RG, Katz VL. Pulmonary and ventilator responses to pregnancy, immersion, and exercise. *J Appl Physiol (1985).*1989;66(2):857-862.

79. Gaston A1, Prapavessis H. Tired, moody, and pregnant? Exercise may be the answer. *Psychol Health.* 2013;28(12):1353-1369.

80. Einarson TR, Piwko C, Koren G. Prevalence of nausea and vomiting of pregnancy in the USA: a meta analysis. *J Popul Ther Clin Pharmacol.* 2013;20(2):e163-e170.

81. Einarson TR, Piwko C, Koren G. Quantifying the global rates of nausea and vomiting of pregnancy: a meta analysis. *J Popul Ther Clin Pharmacol.* 2013;20(2):e171-e183.

82. Decarme G, Dochez V. [*Hyperemesis gravidarum*: A review]. *Presse Med.* 2015;44(12 pt 1):1226-1234.

83. Sanu O, Lamont RF. *Hyperemesis gravidarum*: pathogenesis and the use of antiemetic agents. *Expert Opin Pharmacother.* 2011;12(5):737-748.

84. Veenendaal MV, van Abeelen AF, Painter RC, van der Post JA, Rosebloom TJ. Consequences of *hyperemesis gravidarum* for offspring: a systematic review and meta-analysis. *BJOG.* 2011;118(11):1302-1313.

85. Fejzo MS, Poursharif B, Korst LM, et al. Symptoms and pregnancy outcomes associated with extreme weight loss among women with *hyperemesis gravidarum.* J Womens Health (Larchmt). 2009;18(12):1981-1987.

86. Hastoy A, Lien Tran P, Lakestani O, Barau G, Gerardin P, Boukerrou M. [*Hyperemesis gravidarum* and pregnancy outcomes]. *J Gynecol Obstet Biol Reprod (Paris).* 2015;44(2):154-163.

87. Ayyavoo A, Derraik JG, Hofman PL, Cutfield WS. *Hyperemesis gravidarum* and long-term health of the offspring. *Am J Obstet Gynecol.* 2014;210(6):521-525.

88. Maltepe C, Koren G. The management of nausea and vomiting of pregnancy and hyperemesis gravidarum—a 2013 update. *J Popul Ther Clin Pharmacol.* 2013;20(2):e184-e192.

89. Herrell HE. Nausea and vomiting of pregnancy. *Am Fam Physician.* 2014;89(12):965-970.

90. Stokke G, Gjelsvik BL, Flaatten KT, Birkeland E, Flaatten H, Trovik J. *Hyperemesis gravidarum*, nutritional treatment by nasogastric tube feeding: a 10-year retrospective cohort study. *Acta Obstet Gynecol Scand.* 2015;94(4):359-367.

91. Kotha VK, De Souza A. Wernicke's encephalopathy following *Hyperemesis gravidarum*. A report of three cases. *Neuroradiol J.* 2013;26(1):35-40.

92. Association of Professors of Gynecology and Obstetrics. APGO Educational Series on women's health issues. *Nausea and Vomiting of Pregnancy.* Boston, MA: Jespersen & Associates, LLC; 2011:1-26.

93. Viljoen E, Visser J, Koen N, Musekiwa A. A systematic review and meta-analysis of the effect and safety of ginger in the treatment of pregnancy-associated nausea and vomiting. *Nutr J.* 2014;13:20.

94. Saberi F, Sadat Z, Abedzadeh-Kalahroudi M, Taebi M. Effect of ginger on relieving nausea and vomiting in pregnancy: a randomized, placebo-controlled trial. *Nurs Midwifery Stud*. 2014;3(1):e11841.

95. Ensiyeh J, Sakineh MA. Comparing ginger and vitamin B-6 for the treatment of nausea and vomiting: a randomized controlled trial. *Midwifery*. 2009;25(6):649-653.

96. Shi W, Xu X, Zhang Y, Guo S, Wang J, Wang J. Epidemiology and risk factors of functional constipation in pregnant women. *PLoS One*. 2015;10(7):e0133521.

97. Longo SA, Moore RC, Canzoneri BJ, Robichaux A. Gastrointestinal conditions during pregnancy. *Clin Colon Rectal Surg*. 2010;23(2):80-89.

98. Dimidi E, Christodoulides S, Fragkos KC, Scott SM, Whelan K. The effect of probiotics on functional constipation in adults: a systematic review and meta-analysis of randomized controlled trials. *Am J Clin Nutr*. 2014;100(4):1075-1084.

99. Law R, Maltepe C, Bozzo P, Einarson A. Treatment of heartburn and acid reflux associated with nausea and vomiting of pregnancy. *Can Fam Physician*. 2010;56(2):143-144.

100. Ramu B, Mohan P, Rajasekaran MS, Jayanthi V. Prevalence and risk factors for gastroesophageal reflux in pregnancy. *Trop Gastroenterol*. 2011;30(3):144-147.

101. Vazquez JC. Heartburn in pregnancy. *BMJ Clin Evid*. 2015;2015.pii:1411.

102. Liang CC, Chang SD, Lin SJ, Lin YJ. Lower urinary tract symptoms in primiparous women before and during pregnancy. *Arch Gynecol Obstet*. 2012;285(5):1205-1210.

103. Boyle R, Hay-Smith EJ, Cody JD, Mørkved S. Pelvic floor muscle training for prevention and treatment of urinary and fecal incontinence in antenatal and postnatal women: a short version Cochrane review. *Neurourol Urodyn*. 2014;33(3):269-276.

104. Stuber KJ, Wynd S, Weiss CA. Adverse events from spinal manipulation in the pregnant and postpartum periods: a critical review of the literature. *Chiropr Man Therap*. 2012;20:8.

105. Ramachandra P, Maiya AG, Kumar P, Kamath A. Prevalence of musculoskeletal dysfunctions among Indian pregnant women. *J Pregnancy*. 2015;2015:437105.

106. Aldabe D, Ribeiro DC, Milosavljevic S, Dawn Bussey M. Pregnancy-related pelvic girdle pain and its relationship with relaxin levels during pregnancy: a systematic review. *Eur Spine J*. 2012;21(9):1769-1776.

107. Hensley JG. Leg cramps and restless legs syndrome during pregnancy. *J Midwifery Womens Health*. 2009;54(3):211-218.

108. Allen RE, Kirby KA. Nocturnal leg cramps. *Am Fam Physician*. 2012;86(4):350-355.

109. Bhardwaj A, Nagandla K. Musculoskeletal symptoms and orthopaedic complications in pregnancy: pathophysiology, diagnostic approaches and modern management. *Postgrad Med J*. 2014;90(1066):450-460.

110. Noon ML, Hoch AZ. Challenges of the pregnant athlete and low back pain. *Curr Sports Med Rep*. 2012;11(1):43-48.

111. Tseng PC, Puthussery S, Pappas Y, Gau ML. A systematic review of randomised controlled trials on the effectiveness of exercise programs on Lumbo Pelvic Pain among postnatal women. *BMC Pregnancy Childbirth*. 2015;15:316.

112. Flack NA, Hay-Smith EJ, Stringer MD, Gray AR, Woodley SJ. Adherence, tolerance and effectiveness of two different pelvic support belts as a treatment for pregnancy-related symphyseal pain—a pilot randomized trial. *BMC Pregnancy Childbirth*. 2015;15:36.

113. Cakmak B, Inanir A, Nacar MC, Filiz B. The effect of maternity support belts on postural balance in pregnancy. *PM R*. 2014;6(7):624-628.

114. Zhou K, West HM, Zhang J, Xu L, Li W. Interventions for leg cramps in pregnancy. *Cochrane Database Syst Rev*. 2015;8:CD010655.

115. Belkacemi L, Nelson DM, Desai M, Ross MG. Maternal undernutrition influences placental-fetal development. *Biol Reprod*. 2010;83(3):325-331.

116. Ramakrishnan U, Grant F, Goldenberg T, Zongrone A, Martorell R. Effect of women's nutrition before and during early pregnancy on maternal and infant outcomes: a systematic review. *Paediatr Perinat Epidemiol*. 2012;26(suppl 1):285-301.

117. Kaiser LL, Campbell CG, Academy Positions Committee Workgroup. Practice paper of the Academy of Nutrition and Dietetics abstract: nutrition and lifestyle for a healthy pregnancy outcome. *J Acad Nutr Diet*. 2014;114(9):1447.

118. Butte NF, Wong WW, Treuth MS, Elis KJ, O'Brian Smith E. Energy requirements during pregnancy based on total energy expenditure and energy deposition. *Am J Clin Nutr*. 2004;79(6):1078-1087.

119. Panel on Macronutrients, Panel on Macronutrients, Panel on the Definition of Dietary Fiber, Subcommittee on Upper Reference Levels of Nutrients, Subcommittee on Interpretation and Uses of Dietary Reference Intakes, and the Standing Committee on the Scientific Evaluation of Dietary Reference Intakes, Food and Nutrition Board, Institute of Medicine. *Dietary Reference Intakes for Energy, Carbohydrate, Fiber, Fat, Fatty Acids, Cholesterol, Protein, and Amino Acids*. Washington, DC: The National Academies Press; 2002.

120. Butte NF, King JC. Energy requirements during pregnancy and lactation. *Public Health Nutr.* 2005;8(7A):1010-1027.

121. Rasmussen KM, Yaktine AL, eds; Committee to Reexamine IOM Pregnancy Weight Guidelines; Food and Nutrition Board; Board on Children, Youth, and Families; Institute of Medicine; National Research Council. *Weight Gain During Pregnancy: Reexamining the Guidelines.* Washington, DC: The National Academies Press; 2009.

122. American College of Obstetrics and Gynecology, Committee on Obstetric Practice. Committee opinion no. 548. Weight gain during pregnancy. *Obstet Gynecol.* 2013;121:210-212. (Reaffirmed 2015.)

123. Mehta SH, Kruger M, Sokol RJ. Institute of Medicine guidelines for appropriate pregnancy weight gain for obese women may be too high. *J Reprod Med.* 2015;60(7-8):324-328.

124. Truong YN, Yee LM, Caughey AB, Cheng YW. Weight gain in pregnancy: does the Institute of Medicine have it right? *Am J Obstet Gynecol.* 2015;212(3):362.e1-e8.

125. Maughan R, Burke L, and the Nutrition Working Group of the International Olympic Nutrition for Athletes. A practical guide to eating for health and performance. www.olympic.org/documents/reports/en/en_report_833.pdf. 2012. Accessed December 1, 2015.

126. Most healthy women would benefit from light meal during labor. American Society of Anesthesiologists. www.asahq.org/about-asa/newsroom/news-releases/2015/10/eating-a-light-meal-during-labor. Published November 6, 2015. Accessed December 1, 2015.

127. Thomas DT, Erdman KA, Burke LM. Position of the Academy of Nutrition and Dietetics, Dietitians of Canada, and the American College of Sports Medicine: Nutrition and athletic performance. *J Acad Nutr Diet.* 2016;116(3):501-528.

128. Delidicque L, Francaux M. Recommendations for healthy nutrition in female endurance runners: an update. *Front Nutr.* 2015;2:17.

129. Vanhauwaert E, Matthys C, Verdonck L, De Preter V. Low-residue and low-fiber diets in gastrointestinal disease management. *Adv Nutr.* 2015;6(6):820-827.

130. Maharaj D. Eating and drinking in labor: should it be allowed? *Eur J Obstet Gynecol Reprod Biol.* 2009;146(1):3-7.

131. American College of Obstetricians and Gynecologists, Committee on Obstetric Practice opinion no. 441. Oral intake during labor. *Obstet Gynecol.* 2009;114:714.

132. Kubli M, Scrutton MJ, Seed PT, O'Sullivan G. An evaluation of isotonic "sports drinks" during labor. *Anesth Analg.* 2002;94:404-408.

133. Kalhan SC. Protein metabolism in pregnancy. *Am J Clin Nutr.* 2000;71(suppl 5):1249S-1255S.

134. Haggarty P. Fatty acid supply to the human fetus. *Annu Rev Nutr.* 2010;30:237-255.

135. Jones ML, Mark PJ, Waddell BJ. Maternal dietary omega-3 fatty acids and placental function. *Reproduction.* 2014;147(5):R143-152.

136. Rogers LK, Valentine CJ, Keim SA. DHA supplementation: current implications in pregnancy and childhood. *Pharmacol Res.* 2013;70(1):13-19.

137. Shek LP, Foong-Fong Chong M, Yi Lim J, Soh SE, Chong YS. Role of dietary long-chain polyunsaturated fatty acids in infant allergic and respiratory diseases. *Clin Dev Immunol.* 2012; 2012:730568.

138. Koletzko B, Boey CC, Campoy C, et al. Current information and Asian perspectives on long-chain polyunsaturated fatty acids in pregnancy, lactation, and infancy: systematic review and practice recommendations from an early nutrition academy workshop. *Ann Nutr Metab.* 2014;65(1):49-80.

139. Mennitti LV, Oliveira JL, Morais CA, et al. Type of fatty acids in maternal diets during pregnancy and/or lactation and metabolic consequences of the offspring. *J Nutr Biochem.* 2015;26(2):99-111.

140. Milman N. Iron in pregnancy. How do we secure an appropriate iron status in the mother and child? *Ann Nutr Metab.* 2011;59(1):50-54.

141. Panel on Micronutrients, Subcommittees on Upper Reference Levels of Nutrients and of Interpretation and Use of Dietary Reference Intakes, Standing Committee on the Scientific Evaluation of Dietary Reference Intakes, Food and Nutrition Board, Institute of Medicine. *Dietary Reference Intakes for Vitamin A, Vitamin K, Arsenic, Boron, Chromium, Copper, Iodine, Iron, Manganese, Molybdenum, Nickel, Silicon, Vanadium, and Zinc.* Washington, DC: National Academy Press; 2001.

142. McClung JP. Iron status and the female athlete. *J Trace Elem Med Biol.* 2012;26(2-3):124-126.

143. Alwan NA, Cade JE, McArdle HJ, Greenwood DC, Hayes HE, Simpson NA. Maternal iron status in early pregnancy and birth outcomes: insights from the child's vascular health and iron in pregnancy study. *Br J Nutr.* 2015;113(12):1985-1992.

144. Singh A, Chaudhary R, Sonker A, Pandey HC. Importance of donor history of restless leg syndrome and pica to access iron deficiency. *Transfus Apher Sci.* 2016;54(2):259-261.

145. Institute of Medicine (US) Standing Committee on the Scientific Evaluation of Dietary Reference Intakes and its Panel on Folate, Other B Vitamins, and Choline. *Dietary Reference Intakes for Thiamin, Riboflavin, Niacin, Vitamin B-6, Folate, Vitamin B-12, Pantothenic Acid, Biotin, and Choline.* Washington, DC: National Academy Press; 1998.

146. Wilson RD, Genetics Committee, Audibert F, et al. Pre-conception folic acid and multivitamin supplementation for the primary and secondary prevention of neural tube defects and other folic acid sensitive congenital anomalies. *J Obstet Gynaecol Can.* 2015;37(6):534-552.

147. McNulty B, McNulty H, Marshall B, et al. Impact of continuing folic acid after the first trimester of pregnancy: findings of a randomized trial of folic acid supplementation in the second and third trimesters. *Am J Clin Nutr.* 2013;98:92-98.

148. Finkelstein JL, Layden AL, Stover PJ. Vitamin B-12 and perinatal health. *Adv Nutr.* 2015;6(5):552-563.

149. Bae S, West AA, Yan J, et al. Vitamin B-12 status differs among pregnant, lactating and control women with equivalent nutrient intakes. *J Nutr.* 2015;145(7):1507-1514.

150. Duggan C, Srinivasan K, Thomas T, et al. Vitamin B-12 supplementation during pregnancy and early lactation increases maternal, breast milk, and infant measures of vitamin B-12 status. *J Nutr.* 2014;144(5):758-764.

151. Kaiser L, Allen LH. Position of the American Dietetic Association: nutrition and lifestyle for a healthy pregnancy outcome. *J Am Diet Assoc.* 2008;108(3):553-561.

152. Ma Y, Shen X, Zhang D. The relationship between serum zinc level and preeclampsia: a meta-analysis. *Nutrients.* 2015;7(9):7806-7820.

153. Tande DL, Ralph JL, Johnson LK, Scheett AJ, Hoverson BS, Anderson CM. First trimester dietary intake, biochemical measures, and subsequent gestational hypertension among nulliparous women. *J Midwifery Women's Health.* 2013;58(4):423-430.

154. Nossier SA, Naeim NE, El-Sayed NA, Abu Zeid AA. The effect of zinc supplementation on pregnancy outcomes: a double blind, randomized controlled trial, Egypt. *Br J Nutr.* 2015;114(2):274-285.

155. Foster M, Herulah UN, Prasad A, Petocz P, Samman S. Zinc status of vegetarians during pregnancy: a systematic review of observational studies and meta-analysis of zinc intake. *Nutrients.* 2015;7(6):4512-4525.

156. Ota E, Mori R, Middleton P, et al. Zinc supplementation for improving pregnancy and infant outcomes. *Cochrane Database Syst Rev.* 2015;2:CD000230.

157. Jiang X, West AA, Caudill MA. Maternal choline supplementation: a nutritional approach for improving offspring health. *Trends Endocrinol Metab.* 2014;25(5):263-273.

158. Blusztajn JK, Mellott TJ. Neuroprotective actions of perinatal choline nutrition. *Clin Chem Lab Med.* 2013;51(3):591-599.

159. Blusztajn JK, Mellott TJ. Choline nutrition programs brain development via DNA and histone methylation. *Cent Nerv Syst Agents Med Chem.* 2012;12(2):82-94.

160. Shin JS, Choi MY, Longtine MS, Nelson DM. Vitamin D effects on pregnancy and the placenta. *Placenta.* 2010;31(12):1027-1034.

161. Shaw NJ, Mughal MZ. Vitamin D and child health part 1 (skeletal aspects). *Arch Dis Child.* 2013;98(5):363-367.

162. Pettifor JM, Prentice A. The role of vitamin D in paediatric bone health. *Best Pract Res Clin Endocrinol Metab.* 2011;25(4):573-584.

163. Marshall I, Mehta R, Petrova A. Vitamin D in the maternal-fetal-neonatal interface: clinical implications and requirements for supplementation. *J Matern Fetal Neonatal Med.* 2013;26(7):633-638.

164. Moon RJ, Harvey NC, Cooper C. Endocrinology in pregnancy: influence of maternal vitamin D status on obstetric outcomes and the fetal skeleton. *Eur J Endocrinol.* 2015;173(2):R69-83.

165. Zhu K, Whitehouse AJ, Hart PH, et al. Maternal vitamin D status during pregnancy and bone mass in offspring at 20 years of age: a prospective cohort study. *J Bone Miner Res.* 2104;29(5):1088-1095.

166. Specker BL. Does vitamin D during pregnancy impact offspring growth and bone? *Proc Nutr Soc.* 2012;71(1):38-45.

167. Shaw NJ, Mughai MZ. Vitamin and child health: part 2 (extraskeletal and other aspects). *Arch Dis Child.* 2013;98(5):368-372.

168. Olmos-Ortiz A, Avila E, Durand-Carbajal M, Diaz L. Regulation of calcitriol biosynthesis and activity: focus on gestational vitamin D deficiency and adverse pregnancy outcomes. *Nutrients.* 2015;7(1):443-480.

169. Wagner CL, Baggerly C, McDonnell S, et al. Post-hoc analysis of vitamin D status and reduced risk of preterm birth in two vitamin D pregnancy cohorts compared with South Carolina March of Dimes 2009-2011 rates. *J Steroid Biochem Mol Biol.* 2016;155(pt B):245-251.

170. Wei SQ. Vitamin D and pregnancy outcomes. *Curr Opin Obstet Gynecol.* 2014;26(6):438-447.

171. Schneuer FJ, Roberts CL, Guilbert C, et al. Effects of maternal serum 25-hydroxyvitamin D concentrations in the first trimester on subsequent pregnancy outcomes in an Australian population. *Am J Clin Nutr.* 2014;99(2):287-295.

172. Brannon PM. Vitamin D and adverse pregnancy outcomes: beyond bone health and growth. *Proc Nutr Soc.* 2012;71(2):205-212.

173. Achkar M, Dodds L, Giguere Y, et al. Vitamin D status in early pregnancy and risk of preeclampsia. *Am J Obstet Gynecol.* 2015;212(4):511.e1.

174. Ross AC, Taylor CL, Yaktine AL, Del Valle HB, eds, for the Committee to Review Dietary Reference Intakes for Vitamin D and Calcium, Institute of Medicine (US). *Dietary Reference Intakes for Calcium and Vitamin D.* Washington, DC: The National Academies Press, 2011.

175. Ginde AA, Sullivan AF, Mansbach JM, Camargo CA Jr. Vitamin D insufficiency in pregnant and nonpregnant women of childbearing age in the United States. *Am J Obstet Gynecol.* 2010;202(5):436.e1-8.

176. Larson-Meyer E. Vitamin D supplementation in athletes. *Nestle Nutr Inst Workshop Ser.* 2013;75:109-121.

177. March KM, Chen NN, Karakochuk CD, et al. Maternal vitamin D3 supplementation at 50 ug/d protects against low serum 25-hydroxyvitamin D in infants at 8-wk of age: a randomized controlled trial of 3 doses of vitamin D beginning in gestation and continued in lactation. *Am J Clin Nutr.* 2015;102(2):402-410.

178. Grant CC, Stewart AW, Scragg R, et al Vitamin D during pregnancy and infancy and infant serum 25-hydroxyvitamin D concentration. *Pediatrics.* 2014;133(1):3143-3153.

179. Lieben L, Stockmans I, Moermans K, Carmeliet G. Maternal hypervitaminosis D reduces fetal bone mass and mineral acquisition and leads to neonatal lethality. *Bone.* 2013;57(1):123-131.

180. Obican SG, Jahnke GD, Soldin OP, Scialli AR. Teratology public affairs committee position paper: Iodine deficiency in pregnancy. *Birth Defects Res.* 2012;94(part A):677-682.

181. Swanson C, Zimmerman M, Seaff S, et al. Summary of an NIH workshop to identify research needs to improve the monitoring of iodine status in the United States and to inform the DRI. *J Nutr.* 2012;142(6):1175S-1185S.

182. Panel on Dietary Reference Intakes for Electrolytes and Water, Standing Committee on the Scientific Evaluation of Dietary Reference Intakes, Food and Nutrition Board, Institute of Medicine of the National Academies. *Dietary Reference Intakes for Water, Potassium, Sodium, Chloride, and Sulfate.* Washington, DC: The National Academies Press; 2005.

183. McKenzie AL, Muñoz CX, Ellis LA, et al. Urine color as an indicator of urine concentration in pregnant and lactating women [published online November 16, 2015]. *Eur J Nutr.*

184. Tam C, Erebara A, Einarson A. Food-borne illness during pregnancy. *Can Fam Physician.* 56(4):341-343.

185. US Department of Agriculture, Food and Drug Administration. Food safety for pregnant women. www.fda.gov/downloads/Food/FoodborneIllnessContaminants/UCM312787.pdf. Published 2006 (revised 2011). Accessed December 1, 2015.

186. American Academy of Pediatrics. AAP says no amount of alcohol should be considered safe during pregnancy. www.aap.org/en-us/about-the-aap/aap-press-room/pages/AAP-Says-No-Amount-of-Alcohol-Should-be-Considered-Safe-During-Pregnancy.aspx. Published October 19, 2015. Accessed December 1, 2015.

187. The American College of Obstetricians and Gynecologists, Committee on Obstetric Practice. Committee opinion no. 462. Moderate caffeine consumption during pregnancy. www.acog.org/Resources-And-Publications/Committee-Opinions/Committee-on-Obstetric-Practice/Moderate-Caffeine-Consumption-During-Pregnancy. Published August 2010. Accessed December 1, 2015.

188. Schweitzer AS. Dietary supplements during pregnancy. *J Perinat Educ.* 2006;15(4):44-45.

189. Hung TH, Chen SF, Hsu JJ, Hsieh TT. Gestational weight gain and risks for adverse perinatal outcomes: a retrospective cohort study based on the 2009 Institute of Medicine guidelines. *Taiwan J Obstet Gynecol.* 2015;54(4):421-425.

190. Asvanarunat E. Outcomes of gestational weight gain outside the Institute of Medicine guidelines. *J Med Assoc Thai.* 2014;97(11):1119-1125.

191. Haugen M, Brantsaeter AL, Winkvist A, et al. Associations of pre-pregnancy body mass index and gestational weight gain with pregnancy outcome and postpartum weight retention: a prospective observational cohort study. *BMC Pregnancy Childbirth.* 2014;14:201.

192. Thorell E, Goldsmith L, Weiss G, Kristiansson P. Physical fitness, serum relaxin and duration of gestation. *BMC Pregnancy Childbirth.* 2015;15:168.

193. Petrov Fieril K, Glantz A, Fagevik Olsen M. The efficacy of moderate-to-vigorous resistance exercise during pregnancy: a randomized controlled trial. *Acta Obstet Gynecol Scand.* 2015;94(1):35-42.

194. American College of Sports Medicine. ACSM Current Comment. Exercise during pregnancy. www.acsm.org/docs/current-comments/exerciseduringpregnancy.pdf?sfvrsn=4. Accessed December 1, 2015.

195. Lessen R, Kavanaugh K. Position of nutrition and dietetics: promoting and supporting breastfeeding. *J Acad Nutr Diet.* 2015;115(3):444-449.

196. Dewey KG, Lovelady CA, Nommsen-Rivers LA, McCrory MA, Lonnerdal B. A randomized study of the effects of aerobic exercise by lactating women on breast-milk volume and composition. *N Engl J Med.* 1994;330(7):449-453.

197. Lovelady CA, Hunter CP, Geigerman C. Effect of exercise on immunologic factors in breast milk. *Pediatrics.* 2003;111(2):E148-152.

198. Butte NF, King JC. Energy requirements during pregnancy and lactation. *Public Health Nutr.* 2005;8(7A):1010-1027.

199. Oliveri B, Parisi MS, Zeni S, Maultalen C. Mineral and bone mass changes during pregnancy and lactation. *Nutrition.* 2004;20(2):235-240.

200. Kim HJ, Kwon H, Oh SW, et al. Breast feeding is associated with postmenopausal bone loss: findings from the Korea National Health and Nutrition Examination Survey. *Korean J Fam Med.* 2015;36(5):216-220.

201. Ferrari RM, Siega-Riz AM, Evernson KR, Moos MK, Melvin CL, Herring AH. Provider advice about weight loss and physical activity in the postpartum period. *J Womens Health.* 2010;19(3):397-406.

202. López-Olmedo N, Hernández-Cordero S, Neufeld LM, Garcia-Guerra A, Mejia-Rodriguez F, Gómez-Humaran M. The associations of maternal weight change with breastfeeding, diet and physical activity during the postpartum period *Matern Child Health J.* 2016;20(2):270-280.

203. Nascimento SL, Pudwell J, Surita FG, Adamo KB, Smith GN. The effect of physical exercise strategies on weight loss in postpartum women: a systematic review and meta-analysis. *Int J Obes (Lond).* 2014;38(5):626-635.

204. Lim S, O'Reilly S, Behrens H, Skinner T, Ellis I, Dunbar JA. Effective strategies for weight loss in post-partum women: a systematic review and meta-analysis. *Obes Rev.* 2015;16(11):972-987.

205. Subcommittee for a Clinical Application Guide, Committee on Nutritional Status During Pregnancy and Lactation, Food and Nutrition Board, Institute of Medicine. *Nutrition During Pregnancy and Lactation: An Implementation Guide.* Washington, DC: National Academy Press; 1992.

206. American College of Obstetricians and Gynecologists, Committee on Obstetric Practice. Committee opinion no. 650. Physical activity and exercise during pregnancy and the postpartum period. *Obstet Gynecol.* 2015;126:e135-142.

207. Kahyoglu SH, Balkanli KP. Effect of pelvic floor muscle exercise on pelvic floor muscle activity and voiding functions during pregnancy and the postpartum period *Neurourol Urodyn.* 2016;35(3):417-422.

208. Yan-na Z, Qing-kai W, Hul C, Yin-cheng T. Relationship between serum relaxin levels and female pelvic floor prolapse. *J Shanghai Jiotong University.* 2012;32(4):393-395.

CHAPTER 18

DISORDERED EATING IN ATHLETES

Christina Scribner, MS, RDN, CSSD, CEDRD, and Katherine A. Beals, PhD, RDN, CSSD, FACSM

INTRODUCTION

The purpose of this chapter is to provide an overview of theoretical and applied science related to the provision of nutrition therapy in the treatment of eating disorders (EDs) and disordered eating (DE) among athletes. To successfully provide treatment, the caregiver must first understand, and the recipient must *feel* understood and safe. This chapter will provide background to aid in development of a greater understanding of afflicted individuals, as well as an overall view of the spectrum of DE and EDs within the athletic population.

The chapter offers a variety of potential strategies to consider based upon the individual needs of the patient or client and resources of the provider for achieving nutritional rehabilitation as identified through maintenance of weight within a healthy range, determined by a combination of body mass index or growth trajectory, reproductive health, and predominantly healthful thoughts and behaviors related to food and body that result in an overall state of health.

This chapter offers insight regarding the variety of factors that play into development of these disorders, prevalence data, issues in identification and diagnosis, and treatment. The registered dietitian nutritionist (RDN) is an integral member of a multidisciplinary treatment team. A review of therapeutic modalities and treatment models, qualifications and therapeutic qualities of effective dietitians, and best-practice strategies in the provision of medical nutrition therapy as part of a multidisciplinary approach is provided. The knowledge and experience of veteran sports dietitians in treating athletes with EDs is offered as practical clinical suggestions and a case example. Finally, suggestions for preventing EDs and DE among athletes are shared.

Importance of Subject to Sports Nutrition

One's self-identity is socially and culturally constructed; social group attitudes, practices, and a sense of belonging influence ideals and behaviors. The culture of the athlete's sport is one social group subject to a host of influences. Elite athletes are commonly held in high esteem because they achieve goals that relatively few others do. Athletes are recognized for their performance, as well as their physical appearance, leading to real or perceived pressure from the general population, as well as from within the sport, to conform to expectations regarding physique. Psychological traits of the athlete may also contribute to the development of an ED (eg, mental toughness, commitment to training, pursuit of excellence, coachability, selfless commitment, perfectionism, performance despite pain).[1] Furthermore, the age of onset for EDs seems to parallel the age for elite athletic participation. Byrne and McLean suggest that the developmental changes of puberty increase vulnerability for athletes, particularly for women, in terms of their attitudes about weight, shape, and their athletic performance.[2] Western culture's obsession over and objectification of the physical form may put athletes at even greater risk for the development of a negative body image and EDs related to the stresses of performance and internalization of a sociocultural preference for thinness.

With the increasing visibility of EDs in athletes has come the need to recruit personnel for programs that will identify, treat, and prevent EDs. Sports dietitians are often among the first to come into contact with an athlete with DE or an EDs and are almost always an integral member of a treatment team. It is essential that the sports dietitian has a firm understanding of EDs and is prepared to provide appropriate nutrition-based care.

EATING DISORDER CLASSIFICATIONS

EDs are diagnosed and classified according to criteria published by the American Psychiatric Association (APA). The APA has published the *Diagnostic and Statistical Manual* (*DSM*) since the mid-20th century, with numerous updates and revisions since then. At the time of this writing, the most current revision of the *DSM* is the fifth edition, known as *DSM-5*. EDs are covered in the chapter titled "Feeding and Eating Disorders." It describes "persistent disturbances of eating or eating-related behavior that results in the altered consumption or absorption of food and that significantly impairs physical health or psychosocial functioning."[3] Detailed and updated descriptions for each of the EDs is available online from the APA.[4]

Table 18.1 Summary of *Diagnostic and Statistical Manual-V* Feeding and Eating Disorders[3]

Disorder	Characteristics	Specificity
Anorexia nervosa (AN)	Dietary restriction of energy intake relative to requirements, leading to significantly low (less than minimally normal or for youth less than minimally expected) body weight in the context of age, sex, developmental trajectory, and physical health. Intense fear of gaining weight or becoming fat leads to behaviors that interfere with weight gain. Disturbance in the way one's body weight or shape is experienced, undue influence of body weight or shape on self-evaluation or persistent lack of recognition of the seriousness of low body weight. Subtypes include: • Restricting type (ICD-10: F50.01) • Binge-eating/purging type (ICD-10: F50.02)	Current Severity Mild: Body mass index (BMI) ≥17 Moderate: BMI 16–16.99 Severe: BMI 15–15.99 Extreme: BMI <15 Remission types: Partial: After full criteria for AN were met, the patient no longer meets low body weight but continues to experience intense fear of gaining weight/becoming fat or has behaviors that interfere with weight gain, or has disturbance in self-perception of weight and shape. Full: After full criteria for AN were met, none of the criteria have been met for a sustained period.
Bulimia nervosa (BN)	Recurrent episodes of binge-eating (eating in a discrete period of time an amount of food that is definitely larger than what most people would eat in a similar time period and under similar circumstances with a feeling that one cannot stop or control what or how much is eaten). Recurrent inappropriate compensatory behaviors/purging intended to prevent weight gain (eg, self-induced vomiting; misuse of laxatives, diuretics, or other medications; fasting; excessive exercise). Self-evaluation is unduly influenced by body shape and weight. Behaviors occur on average once a week for 3 months. Disturbance does not occur exclusively during episodes of AN.	Current Severity Mild: Average 1–3 episodes of inappropriate compensatory behaviors per week. Moderate: Average 4–7 episodes of inappropriate compensatory behaviors per week. Severe: Average 8–13 episodes of inappropriate compensatory behaviors per week. Extreme: Average 14 or more episodes of inappropriate compensatory behaviors per week. Remission types: Partial: After full criteria for BN were met, the patient no longer meets all of the criteria for a sustained period. Full: After full criteria for BN were met, none of the criteria have been met for a sustained period.

Continued on next page

Disorder	Characteristics	Specificity
Binge-eating disorder (BED)	Recurrent binge eating (as described for BN) episodes are present. Binge-eating episodes are associated with 3 or more of the following: • Eating much more rapidly than normal. • Eating until feel uncomfortably full. • Eating large amounts of food in the absence of physical hunger. Eating alone and feeling embarrassed by how much one is eating. Feeling disgusted with oneself, depressed, or very guilty afterward. Marked distress regarding binge eating. Binge eating occurs, on average, at least once a week for 3 months. Binge eating is not associated with recurrent use of inappropriate compensatory behavior and does not occur exclusively during the course of AN or BN. (ICD-10: F50.8)	Current Severity Mild: 1–3 binge eating episodes per week. Moderate: 4–7 binge eating episodes per week. Severe: 8–13 binge eating episodes per week. Extreme: 14 or more binge eating episodes per week. Remission types: Partial: After full criteria for BED were met, the patient engages in binge eating at an average frequency of less than once per week. Full: After full criteria for BED were met, none of the criteria have been met for a sustained period.
Avoidant/restrictive food intake disorder (ARFID)	An eating or feeding disturbance that manifests by persistent failure to meet appropriate nutritional and/or energy needs resulting in (1) significant weight loss or failure to achieve expected weight gain or faltering growth in children, (2) significant nutritional deficiency, (3) dependence on enteral feeding or oral nutritional supplements, (4) marked interference with psychosocial functioning. Disturbance is not better explained by a lack of available food or by a cultural practice. ARFID does not entail disturbance in body weight or shape, nor is it attributable to another eating disorder or mental disorder. The eating disturbance is not attributable to a concurrent medical condition and is not better explained by another mental disorder. When it co-occurs with another condition or disorder, the severity of the eating disturbance exceeds that routinely associated with the condition or disorder and warrants additional clinical attention. (ICD-10: F50.8)	Full remission: When after criteria for ARFID have been met, the criteria have not been met for a sustained period.
Pica	Persistent eating of nonnutritive, nonfood substances that are not part of a culturally supported or socially normative practice over a period of at least 1 month. The eating behavior is inappropriate for the developmental level of the individual. When the eating behavior occurs in the context of another mental disorder (eg, intellectual disability, autism, schizophrenia) or medical condition (eg, pregnancy), it is sufficiently severe to warrant additional clinical attention. (ICD-10: F98.3 [in children]) (ICD-10: F50.8 [in adults])	Full remission: When after criteria for pica have been met, the criteria have not been met for a sustained period.

Continued on next page

Disorder	Characteristics	Specificity
Rumination disorder	Repeated regurgitation of food (rechewed, reswallowed, or spit out) that is not related to another gastrointestinal or medical condition, nor does it occur exclusively during the course of AN, BN, BED, or ARFID, for at least 1 month. If the symptoms occur in the context of another mental disorder (eg, intellectual disability or another neurological disorder), they are sufficiently severe to warrant additional clinical attention. (ICD-10: F98.21)	Full remission: When after criteria for rumination disorder have been met, the criteria have not been met for a sustained period.
Other specified feeding or eating disorder	Applies to symptoms characteristic of a feeding and eating disorder that cause clinically significant distress or impairment in social, occupational, or other important areas of functioning, but do not meet the full criteria for any of the other diagnostic classes. (ICD-10: F 50.8)	Atypical AN (eg, lacks the significant weight criteria for AN). BN (of low frequency and/or limited duration). BED (of low frequency and/or limited duration). Purging disorder: Recurrent purging behavior to influence weight or shape in the absence of binge eating. Night eating syndrome: Recurrent episodes of night eating manifested by awakening from sleep or by excessive food consumption after the evening meal that causes significant distress and/or impairment of functioning. Disorder is not explained by other mental or binge eating disorder, including substance use or effect of medication.
Unspecified feeding or eating disorder	Applies to presentation of symptoms characteristic of a feeding and eating disorder that cause clinically significant distress or impairment in social, occupational, or other important areas of functioning but do not meet the full diagnostic criteria for any of the other disorders in feeding and eating disorders. This category may also apply in situations when the provider does not specify why criteria do not meet a more specific diagnosis or has insufficient information to make another specific feeding and eating disorder diagnosis (eg, urgent care settings). (ICD-10: F50.8)	

The Spectrum of Disordered Eating and Eating Disorders

When one is suffering from DE, there are changes in thoughts and behaviors, which may be transient. For example, someone may engage in DE in an attempt to lose weight in response to grief over the loss of a loved one or relationship, in answer to the stress related to athletic events, or in reaction to an injury or illness. The food-related behaviors that result reflect a *temporary* change in eating patterns and critical self-evaluation. DE may also reflect long-term attitudes and behaviors and is sometimes described simply as "an unhealthy relationship with food" or subclinical ED. When DE occurs for prolonged periods, it may result in significant physical and psychological damage and may progress into a clinical ED. While less extreme forms of DE are much more prevalent than clinical EDs, both DE and EDs are worthy of serious attention and have potential for medical instability or even death. At the time of publication, the term *disordered eating* has not been specifically defined by the authoritative organizations (eg, the Academy for Eating Disorders, National Eating Disorders Association, or International Association of Eating Disorder Professionals).

To be diagnosed with a clinical ED, an individual must meet a standard set of criteria as outlined in the *DSM-5*.[3,5] An eating disorder refers to a potentially life-threatening mental illness that can have long-standing adverse consequences on the individual's psychosocial and physical health and reduces quality of life.[5,6] When someone has an ED, thoughts and behaviors related to food and body consume much of his or her life. An ED involves complex thought processes and typically affects numerous body systems leading to multiple, serious physical and psychosocial problems.

The DSM identifies clinical disorders based upon useful criteria that define problematic behavioral disorders across the life span. The updated diagnostic criteria of *DSM-5* for anorexia nervosa (AN) and bulimia nervosa (BN) differ from diagnostic criteria in the previous edition by not requiring the overvaluation of weight, shape, or other body image disturbance.[3,7] Binge eating disorder (BED) is considered the most common ED in the United States.[8] It was first included in *DSM-5* as its own category of ED.

Similarly, avoidant-restrictive food intake disorder (ARFID) was introduced as an ED in *DSM-5*. Yet, ARFID, like BED, is not new but was previously captured under umbrella category of ED not otherwise specified (EDNOS) in the fourth edition of the *DSM*. EDNOS has been renamed and divided into two categories: other specified feeding and eating disorders (OSFED) and unspecified feeding or eating disorder. ARFID describes individuals who experience clinically significant struggles with food and eating, but whose symptoms do not better match the criteria for another feeding or eating disorder.

It is not always immediately clear when an individual's decision to limit or avoid food is disordered because many public health problems of our time are related to food. Von Essen and Mårtensson reported on young adults in Sweden who attempt to utilize food choice as a means toward a healthy lifestyle. Their findings revealed that the preferred diet was typically organic and that their food practices included both "looking inward" for direction on food choice and using food as an "outward bound" strategy toward making the world more understandable and friendly.[9] It is common to see food choice reflecting an individual's knowledge or belief about how food affects physical, mental, or social health, as well as planet health. However, there is a point at which trends in eating do not support optimal health, as with EDs.

Steven Bratman, MD, author of *Health Food Junkies*, coined the term *orthorexia* in a 1977 issue of *Yoga Journal*.[10] Diagnostic criteria for orthorexia nervosa (ON) have been proposed to identify the pathological eating pattern characterized by an extreme and unhealthy obsession to eat right.[11] The criteria included consumption of a nutritionally unbalanced diet related to preoccupation with food purity or the effect of food on physical or emotional health; rigid avoidance of foods deemed unhealthy; a sense of worry and guilt related to transgressions; intolerance of others' food beliefs; and spending excessive amounts on food relative to one's income. Additional criteria identify impaired physical health (eg, malnutrition) resulting from nutritional imbalance and severe distress. Lastly, the obsessive preoccupation with food is not an exacerbation of another disorder. People with ON avoid foods that they perceive as being unhealthy, that contain ingredients they feel are undesirable, or were prepared in a manner that violates their value system. Case reports among individuals with such preoccupations reveal similar severe medical findings as found with malnutrition secondary to AN.[11]

It is important to recognize that ED symptoms rarely exist in isolation and that afflicted individuals often cross over between and among various EDs, presenting with changing symptoms over the course of the illness. Crossover is more common in the initial years of illness. For example, individuals with AN-restrictive subtype, may develop symptoms of binge eating or purging AN, and then *cross over* to BN. Transition between specific ED categories and unspecified EDs is common, with the movement to an unspecified ED often representing movement toward recovery.[12]

Anna, a 15-year-old girl with a 10-lb weight loss over the last 3 years, is currently at less than the first percentile for height and weight. Her growth chart has not shown normal progress in weight since age 12. Anna has changed primary care providers in the past year, and little transitional information was shared between them. While Anna's parents have noticed that she has gotten thinner, it has not raised alarm. It was not until Anna failed to heal after surgery related to a sports injury that her state of malnutrition was noted. Anna was initially diagnosed with anorexia nervosa (AN) based on her low body weight and osteopenia. However, as treatment progressed, it was clear that Anna was enthused about her nutrition prescription to eat more, especially of some foods, as well as to gain weight. Yet, she faced various obstacles in her effort. Her parents were concerned about the future possibility of obesity that could result from unscrupulous teenage eating. Snack foods were severely limited at home in an attempt to persuade Anna to "eat like an athlete." Anna's sister was diagnosed with celiac disease, and Anna took on some concern that she too should limit her intake of carbohydrate-rich foods to "be her best." Concern about carbohydrates was reinforced by her high school team trainer who advised the team to avoid all white foods to reduce body fat. Furthermore, Anna had begun to refer to sweets (carbohydrate- and fat-rich foods) that she previously enjoyed as "gross and disgusting." Anna and her parents participated in several psychotherapy appointments. They responded extremely well to family nutrition psychoeducation and a parent-focused nutrition therapy approach provided by the registered dietitian nutritionist.

In this example, the diagnosis was changed from AN to avoidant/restrictive food intake disorder because Anna did not exhibit the fear of weight gain or body image concerns typical of AN. Anna's primary obstacle to consumption of adequate food was familial food rules, learned disgust of certain foods related to fear of becoming obese, and the familial history of celiac disease. Anna received two 400-kcal supplemental formulas daily, in addition to meals and snacks to reach her minimum healthy weight before transitioning to a full solid diet with expanded food choices. Anna was monitored for refeeding syndrome during the early stages of nutritional rehabilitation.

Excessive Exercise in Disordered Eating and Eating Disorders

Issues with physical activity often coexist with eating problems; some people avoid activity and others depend on it. While less than 20% of American adults and youth reach the guidelines for aerobic physical activity, a subset of people engage in excessive exercise, which can lead to a host of negative physical and mental effects, including musculoskeletal injuries, metabolic derangements, cardiovascular stress, nutrient deficiencies, anxiety, and depression.[13,14] The term *exercise* falls under the umbrella of physical activity. Physical activity refers to a variety of types of bodily movement; exercise is undertaken with a purpose and a structure that includes repetition. Avoidance of exercise or excessive exercise alone do not qualify as an ED, yet, exercise may be a method of purging unwanted caloric intake or may present as a behavior related to another disorder that includes compulsive or obsessive behavior concomitant to diagnosis of an ED. Excessive exercise is commonly explained by patients as their means of managing uncomfortable thoughts or emotions.

Excessive exercise has often been referred to in the literature as exercise addiction. Landolfi distinguished between healthy (committed) levels of exercise and exercise addiction.[15] Criteria for exercise addiction included continued exercise regardless of physical injury, psychological, or social consequences (eg, personal inconvenience or disruption to other areas of life, including marriage, employment, and lack of time for other activities that interfere with exercise). Exercise addiction is related to intrinsic rewards, as well as the experience of disturbing sensations of deprivation when unable to exercise. Committed exercisers are motivated by extrinsic rewards and do not suffer severe withdrawal symptoms (as identified by Cook and Hausenblas in their characterization of exercise dependence) when they cannot exercise.[16] Excessive exercisers lack life-balance and engage in a level of exercise that is not sustainable in terms of long-term physical, psychological, and social health outcomes.[15]

Prevalence of Disordered Eating and Eating Disorders Among Athletes

The estimated prevalence of DE among athletes ranges from 6% to 45% in female athletes and 0% to 19% in male athletes.[17] Prevalence estimates for the clinically recognized EDs among competitive athletes tend to be somewhat lower for female athletes. Estimates are as follows: AN (0% to 6.7%), BN (0% to 12.1%), and EDNOS (2% to 13.4%); for male athletes: AN (0%), BN (0% to 7.5%), and EDNOS (0% to 9.7%).[18] The range of prevalence estimates is likely explained by discrepancies in one or more of the following: the screening instruments/assessment tools used; definitions of ED employed; and the athlete populations, including ages, studied.

Most studies examining the prevalence of EDs among athletes have utilized one or more of the currently available self-report instruments, such as the Eating Attitudes Test (EAT), Eating Disorder Inventory (EDI), Three-Factor-Eating Questionnaire, and the Bulimia Test Revised (BULIT-R). Not only do self-report instruments likely underestimate true ED prevalence because athletes may be reluctant to disclose this information on a questionnaire, but most have not been validated in an athletic population.[19] Moreover, the variety of measures used in these studies makes inconsistencies in prevalence estimates more likely and comparisons of studies more difficult. Studies have also varied widely in how they have defined *eating disorder*. While some studies adhered to the strict *DSM-5* criteria and required rigorous interviews to diagnose EDs, others used self-report questionnaires, symptom checklists, and risk factor identifiers that are more likely indicative of DE. Of course, using stricter criteria will result in lower prevalence estimates, while using more liberal criteria will result in higher prevalence estimates. Finally, studies have varied greatly in the sample populations studied, including the ages of athletes, types of athletes (eg, recreational, high school, collegiate and elite athletes, as well as physically active individuals), and types of sports. It is not surprising that the prevalence of EDs would be higher in a homogenous sample of athletes representing thin-build sports, characterized by low body weight and low body fat, such as in running, gymnastics, and figure-skating, compared with a heterogeneous sample of athletes from a wide range of sports.

To obtain an accurate, unbiased estimate of prevalence, it is important to use a sufficiently large sample size ($N \geq 100$) and a variety of sports to ensure adequate heterogeneity. Table 18.2 presents the most recent (post-1990) prevalence studies that meet the aforementioned criteria. From the data contained within the table, it is possible to make some general conclusions regarding the prevalence of DE and EDs among athletes. First, the prevalence of DE is significantly greater than the prevalence of the clinical EDs (AN, BN, and EDNOS) among athletes. Second, with a few exceptions, the majority of studies suggest that the prevalence of DE is greater among athletes compared with nonathletic control subjects, while the prevalence of clinical ED is similar. The exceptions to this seem to be found among high school athletes, which could be explained by the shorter exposure to sport-specific DE triggers, as well as the use of self-reported questionnaires, which may not be appropriate for adolescents.[17] Among athletes, the prevalence of DE has consistently been shown to be higher in those that participate in thin-build or weight-dependent sports.[17] These sports can be categorized into three groups: (1) aesthetic sports, such as diving, figure skating, gymnastics, and synchronized swimming; (2) sports in which low body mass and body-fat levels are considered a physical or biomechanical advantage, such as distance running, road cycling, and triathlon; and (3) sports that require weight categories for competition, such as lightweight rowing, weight lifting, and wrestling.[19] Finally, the prevalence of EDs and DE is higher among female athletes compared with male athletes.[17] Interestingly, research suggests that there is an interaction between sex and sport in terms of DE prevalence. For example, Schaal and colleagues reported that the prevalence of DE was highest in endurance sports among female athletes, while in males it was most prevalent in the weight-dependent sports.[20]

Table 18.2 Summary of Recent (Post-1990) Studies Examining the Prevalence of Disordered Eating in Athletes[20-49]

Study/ Country	Sample	Instrument	Prevalence
Thiemann et al (2015) Germany[21]	108 German professional athletes (46 in aesthetic and 62 in ball-game sports) and 108 nonathletic control subjects	Self-report questionnaire and clinical interview	17% of athletes from aesthetic sports, 3% of athletes from ball-game sports, and 2% of nonathletes were classified as having an ED.[a]

Continued on next page

Study/ Country	Sample	Instrument	Prevalence
Fortes et al (2014) Portugal[22]	580 male and female high school athletes and 362 age-matched nonathletes	EAT-26[b]	18% of female athletes and 14% of male athletes showed ED symptoms based on EAT-26 scores compared with 26% and 15% of female and male nonathletes, respectively.
Chatterton and Petrie (2013) United States[23]	732 male collegiate athletes	Q-EDD[c]; 7 items from the BULIT-R[d]	16% reported DE[e] symptoms; 1% were classified as ED (EDNOS[f]).
Goltz et al (2013) Brazil[24]	150 male athletes in aesthetic and weight-dependent sports	EAT-26, BITE[g], BSQ[h]	DE behaviors and body image dissatisfaction were found in 43 athletes (28%) in aesthetic sports and 23 (15%) athletes in weight-dependent sports.
Martinsen and Sundgot-Borgen (2013) Norway[25]	611 elite adolescent male and female athletes and 355 adolescent male and female control subjects	A two-stage screening process consisting of a questionnaire developed by the authors, including subscales of the EDI-2[i], weight history, and self-reported history of EDs (stage 1), followed by a clinical interview using the EDE[j] and EDE-Q[k] (stage 2)	After the initial screening, 51% of the control subjects and 25% of the athletes were classified as "at risk" for an ED. In stage 2, the prevalence of EDs among the total population of athletes and control subjects was estimated to be 7% vs 2%, with the ED prevalence higher for female athletes than male athletes (14% vs 3%, $P < .001$) and female and male control subjects (5% vs 0%, $P < 0.001$).
Schaal et al (2011) France[20]	2,067 male and female elite athletes	Psychological evaluation using *DSM-IV*[l] criteria for clinical EDs	6% of female athletes and 4% of male athletes indicated a current/ongoing ED; 11% of female athletes and 5.5% of male athletes reported a history of EDs.
Thein-Nissenbaum et al (2011) United States[26]	311 female high school athletes	EDE-Q	35% of female athletes presented with symptoms of DE.
Martinsen et al (2010) Norway[27]	606 elite male and female high school athletes and 355 male and female control subjects	Questionnaire developed by the authors, including dieting, use of pathogenic weight control methods, and the drive for thinness and body dissatisfaction subscales from the EDI[m]	45% of female athletes and 13% of male athletes reported symptoms of DE compared with 71% and 30% of female and male control subjects, respectively.
Greenleaf et al (2009) United States[28]	204 female collegiate athletes	Q-EDD and BULIT-R	2% of athletes were classified as having an ED; 26% had symptoms consistent with DE.

Continued on next page

Study/ Country	Sample	Instrument	Prevalence
Rosendahl et al (2009) Germany[29]	576 male and female high school athletes and 291 adolescent male and female control subjects	EAT-26	27% of female athletes and 10% of male athletes met the criteria for DE based on EAT-26 scores compared with 36% of female and 12% of male controls.
Petrie et al (2008) United States[30]	203 collegiate male athletes	Q-EDD and BULIT-R	None of the athletes presented with a clinical ED; 19% showed symptoms of EDs based on the two self-report instruments.
Torstveit et al (2008) Norway[31]	186 adolescent and adult female elite athletes and 145 nonathletic femal control subjects	EDE-Q and clinical interview	33% of athletes and 21% of nonathletic control subjects were classified with an ED based on the clinical interview.
Nichols et al (2007) United States[32]	423 female high school athletes	EDE-Q	20% of athletes met the EDE-Q criteria for DE.
Nichols et al (2006) United States[33]	170 female high school athletes	In-depth interview developed by the author using the EDE	18% met the criteria for DE.
Beals and Hill (2006) United States[34]	112 female collegiate athletes	Questionnaire developed by the authors, including the EDE-Q and Eating Disorder Inventory Symptom Checklist	3% of athletes self-reported a clinical ED; 23% of athletes met the criteria for DE.
Toro et al (2005) United Kingdom[35]	283 elite female athletes competing in 20 sports	EAT and CETCA[n] (based on *DSM-III-R*[o] criteria)	11% of the athletes exceeded the EAT cutoff score; 2.5% and 20% of the athletes met the CETCA criteria for AN[p] and BN,[q] respectively.
Sundgot-Borgen and Torstveit (2004) Norway[36]	660 Norwegian elite female athletes	A two-stage screening process consisting of a questionnaire developed by the authors, including subscales of the EDI, weight history, and self-reported history of EDs (stage 1) followed by a clinical interview using the EDE (stage 2)	21% (n = 121) of the female athletes were classified "at risk" after the initial screening; results of the clinical interview indicated that 2% met the criteria for AN, 6% for BN, 8% for EDNOS, and 4% for anorexia athletica.
Byrne and McClean (2002) Australia[37]	263 elite male and female athletes and 263 nonathletic male and female control subjects	CIDI[r] and number of self-report questionnaires.	22% of female athletes and 4% of male athletes were classified with an ED compared with 5.5% of female control subjects and no male control subjects.

Continued on next page

Table 18.2 Summary of Recent (Post-1990) Studies Examining the Prevalence of Disordered Eating in Athletes[20-49] (Continued)

Study/ Country	Sample	Instrument	Prevalence
Beals and Manore (2002) United States[38]	425 female collegiate athletes	EAT-26 and EDI-BD[s]	3% and 2% of the athletes self-reported a diagnosis of clinical AN and BN, respectively; 15% and 32% of the athletes scored above the designated cutoff scores on the EAT-26 and EDI-BD, respectively.
Johnson et al (1999) United States[39]	562 female collegiate athletes	EDI-2 and questionnaire developed by the authors using *DSM-IV* criteria	None of the athletes met the *DSM-IV* criteria for AN, while 1% met the criteria for BN. 2% and 6% of the athletes believed they might have AN and BN, respectively. Subclinical AN and BN were identified in 3% and 9% of the women, respectively. 35% to 38% demonstrated DE behaviors (eg, binge eating, vomiting, laxatives, diuretics, diet pills, elevated drive for thinness subscale score, elevated body dissatisfaction score).
Sundgot-Borgen (1993) Norway[40]	522 Norwegian elite female athletes	EDI and in-depth interview developed by the author based on *DSM-III* criteria	1%, 8.0%, and 8% were diagnosed with AN, BN, and anorexia athletica, respectively.

a ED, eating disorder

b EAT-26, Eating Attitudes Test (see source 45)

c BULIT-R, Bulimia Test Revised (see source 43)

d Q-EDD, Questionnaire for Eating Disorder Diagnosis (see source 49)

e DE, disordered eating

f EDNOS, eating disorder not otherwise specified

g BITE, Bulimic Investigatory Test, Edinburgh (see source 41)

h BSQ, Body Shape Questionnaire (see source 42)

i EDI-2, Eating Disorder Inventory-2 (see source 48)

j EDE, Eating Disorder Examination (see source 46)

k EDE-Q, Eating Disorder Examination Questionnaire

l *DSM-IV, Diagnostic and Statistical Manual of Psychiatric Disorders, Fourth Edition* (see source 44)

m EDI, Eating Disorder Inventory (see source 47)

n CETCA, Eating Disorders Assessment Questionnaire

o *DSM-III, Diagnostic and Statistical Manual of Psychiatric Disorders, Third Edition*

p AN, anorexia nervosa

q BN, bulimia nervosa

r CIDI, Composite International Diagnostic Interview

p EDI-BD, Eating Disorder Inventory, Body Dissatisfaction subscale (see source 47)

HEALTH RISKS ACROSS THE SPECTRUM OF DISORDERED EATING AND EATING DISORDERS

All individuals suspected of having an ED need to have a thorough medical assessment. Not only can an ED be misdiagnosed, but EDs affect multiple organ systems and lead to acute and potentially chronic complications throughout the body. While one may be normal and healthy with a body weight that is on the lower or higher end of the weight spectrum, the two extremes of disordered energy balance are represented by undernutrition characterized as semistarvation or starvation on one end of the spectrum and overnutrition leading to obesity on the other end. Significant and lasting health issues with weight loss or weight gain occur only when energy intake is consistently mismatched with energy needs; individual responses to under- or overnutrition vary, and some individuals lose weight or gain weight more or less than others. Although the energy-related responses to severe dietary restriction are not well understood, the body seems to strive to maintain consistency in terms of body composition as evidenced by the maintenance of percent body fat during weight cycling and after weight regain following semistarvation. Dual-energy x-ray absorptiometry (DEXA) and magnetic resonance imaging (MRI) are tools currently used to determine changes in body composition.[50]

Undernutrition

Undernutrition commonly refers to deficiency of energy or a deficit of one or more essential nutrients, including low energy availability (LEA). Inadequate energy intake relative to nutritional needs may be acute or chronic, resulting from physical or psychological constraints. For example, athletes may experience a reduction in appetite, rather than the expected drive for more food to meet energy needs. There may be environmental factors that reduce the availability of food, such as travel, scheduling, or time. Furthermore, lack of understanding regarding nutritional needs, poor time management, and poor food preparation or shopping skills, as well as the pressure of achieving a body ideal associated with a sport, increase susceptibility to developing DE or an ED among those seeking to alter their body through fad or extreme diets.

Athletes who restrict their dietary intake to control calories or otherwise limit the types of food they will eat (eg, vegetarian) are at greater risk for LEA. Similarly, athletes who engage in prolonged physical activity are also at risk.[6] LEA due to dietary restraint or exercise without sufficient food intake appears to be the start of the DE continuum, so it may be the common mechanistic factor underlying the ED onset. The reason some athletes cross the line from dieting and use of extreme weight-loss methods to clinical ED is not yet known, but it seems that a genetic predisposition combined with vulnerability in terms of the athlete's age, the type of sport practiced, and mental health status and history are involved. Recent research hypothesizes that thoughts and emotions originating from fear of fatness or intense drive for thinness may lead to goal-oriented behaviors that lead to changes in brain signaling that are similar to those seen with drug addiction and result in automatic, habit-like disordered behaviors.[51] The difficulty in effectively treating EDs may be related to these neural changes that result in people engaging in behaviors unconsciously, commonly referred to as being in autopilot.

Although decreased adipose appears to constitute the majority of body mass lost under severe dietary restriction, protein is also mobilized from organs and skeletal muscle, and, under the stress of acute or chronic infection, protein mobilization for gluconeogenesis predominates.[52] Utilization of DEXA and MRI methodologies in the eating disordered population would provide greater insight regarding the effects of dietary restriction on energy expenditure and protein mobilization from low metabolic rate tissue (fat mass and skeletal muscle) vs high metabolic rate organs, such as the heart, liver, and kidneys.[50] The proportion of weight lost from adipose tissue and lean tissue depends in large part on the amount of stored adipose tissue available, such that a leaner person will lose a greater proportion from lean tissue during dietary restriction. Degenerative changes in lean tissue include compromise of the heart, reduced erythropoiesis, immune system depression, and impaired capacity of the liver to metabolize drugs or toxic substances in the diet.[52]

The depletion of fatty tissues and liver glycogen stores result in liver transaminase abnormalities (elevated aspartate transaminase and alanine transaminase). Severe caloric restriction may result in fatal hypoglycemia due to depletion of substrate to maintain safe blood glucose levels.[53] Depletion of substrates needed for hormone production—estrogen deficiency in females and testosterone deficiency in males—also occurs as a result of an energy-deficient diet.[54] Substrate depletion due to inadequate energy availability affects nerve conduction and results in muscle fiber atrophy and weakness. Thus, the neuromuscular system, which includes the brain, spinal cord, nerves, and all of the muscles in the body (including organ tissue), is often regarded as the most significantly affected system in severe AN.[55]

Overnutrition

Overeating that leads to excessive food intake or overweight may affect health and performance. Some people restrict their intake early in the day and then find themselves overeating later. This behavior is commonly referred to as *back-loading* and may involve binge eating, which is eating more than a normal person would during a discrete period, accompanied by a sense of guilt or shame. The physical health risks of ED that include binge eating include digestive and menstrual problems, joint and muscle pains, and headache. In addition, when eating leads to overweight, as in BED, the health risks include type 2 diabetes, hypertension, heart disease and strokes, certain types of cancer, sleep apnea, osteoarthritis, fatty liver disease, kidney disease, and, among women, irregular menstruation, infertility, and pregnancy problems. The health risks also include psychosocial problems, such as missing school, work, or social activities.[56]

Cardiovascular

Special attention is given to abnormalities in cardiovascular function. Cardiovascular abnormalities include abnormal heart rhythm (arrhythmia), abnormally rapid heart rate (tachycardia), abnormally slow resting heart rate (bradycardia), hypotension, and mitral valve prolapse, among others. Cardiovascular abnormalities warrant referral to a specialist for evaluation with an electrocardiogram.

Generally accepted norms for resting pulse are 60 to 100 beats per minute (bpm). However, a review of the literature did not reveal an authoritative source for defining heart rate limits for the application of these clinical terms. Spodick suggests a lower threshold of 50 bpm and an upper threshold of 90 bpm as a red flag, alerting providers to potential cardiac abnormality.[57] Similarly, an adolescent with a heart rate of less than 50 bpm will be identified as being bradycardic.[58] Monitoring heart rate does not require specialized instrumentation. RDNs may routinely monitor heart rate as an indicator of changes in health and dietary adequacy. Bradycardia is the most common cardiovascular complication of AN and should not be confused with the long-term sinus node sickness that athletes often consider a confirmation of their cardiovascular fitness, the bradycardia commonly known as athlete's pulse.[54] While neither type of bradycardia is well understood, among those who are calorically restricted and underweight, bradycardia is thought to be a physiological downregulation of metabolism to conserve energy. The mechanism of bradycardia in a person with AN may be different from that in a well-nourished, endurance athlete. It is thought that the increased vagal tone, decreased glycogen content of myocardial cells, and atrophy result from inadequate caloric intake.[59] The difference may be explained to the patient or client by checking the pulse at rest and then with minimal exertion. According to Jennifer Gaudiani, MD (oral communication, June 2015), tachycardia upon standing and walking across the room is a result of cardiac deconditioning and the weakness of malnutrition; the heart of a well-nourished athlete would have little response (less than 20 bpm increase) to the energy demands of standing and walking a short distance.

Hypoglycemia and concomitant depletion of liver glycogen necessary to maintain blood glucose have been associated with sudden death in persons with severe AN.[60] Congestive heart failure and mitral valve prolapse may also result from malnutrition.[61] Even though the cardiac complications of AN may result in death, overall they are largely considered, at least in the early stages, reversible and likely to result in full recovery.[55]

Changes in cardiovascular function among those suffering from EDs, as well as seemingly well-nourished, endurance-trained athletes, are not well understood. While reduction of resting heart rate among athletes engaged in long-term training for ultraendurance events is typically considered a benign adaptation to maintain normal cardiac output and blood pressure concomitant to conditioning that increases stroke volume and vagal tone, recent evidence suggests that it too may be pathological and indicative of remodeling of the heart and not due to changes in resting autonomic tone.[62]

The vulnerable years of adolescence pose a special concern for those with DE and EDs, both from the standpoint of acute and chronic effects and the challenge of recognition. Young athletes may not present with the typical signs and symptoms and may be overlooked. Be on the alert for growth stunting, failure to maintain growth trajectory, or pubertal delay.[63] Inadequate energy intake negatively affects growth and development, interfering with accrual of bone density and the formation of organ systems. When LEA leads to underdevelopment or wasting of skeletal, smooth, or cardiac muscle, numerous acute and chronic complications, including sudden death in severe cases, may result.[64]

Gastrointestinal System

Patients with EDs frequently complain of gastrointestinal (GI) distress and bloating. These complaints may precede or accompany diagnosis of ED. GI issues, such as bloating, are common among all medical disciplines, and this is perhaps why they are generally not specifically addressed in many ED treatment programs. While the pathophysiology behind these gut complaints is complicated, is incompletely understood, and may warrant a differential diagnosis, some health providers simply explain to the patient that GI issues are a result of restrictive food choices. As elucidated by Lacy and colleagues, the gut microbiome (also called microflora) is influenced by food choice, including the method of feeding as an infant and habitual diet.[65] Changes in microflora can result in changes in intestinal function, such as producing excess gas. These changes may be due to a host of factors, including immune function, alterations in the mucosal barrier, and production of short-chain fatty acids and vitamins. GI distress has also been related to psychosocial distress with perceived severity of bloating related to anxiety and depression. Thus, it comes as no surprise that the approximately 500 species of gut microbiota have recently gained recognition as a potential factor in ED development, maintenance, and recovery because of their impact on energy metabolism and body weight, as well as anxiety and depression.[65,66] This area is still largely unexplored, but preliminary evidence suggests that the intestinal microbiota may have biological and psychological effects.

Superior mesenteric artery syndrome is a partial blockage of the upper bowel caused by loss of the fatty tissue that normally serves as a pad between the gut and the superior mesenteric artery and aorta. Loss of the fat pad results in compression of the upper bowel. Nutritional deficiencies in energy intake, protein, and minerals resulting from dietary restriction or purging may affect the muscles and tendons, disturbing contraction and reflexes, which may trigger muscle spasms.[62] Individuals with this syndrome need medical supervision until the condition corrects with renourishment.

Reproductive Function

Reproductive function may be affected by an ED. It is common for menstruation to be interrupted, especially among those suffering from AN. Leptin is secreted from adipocytes; a deficiency in leptin triggers an adaptive metabolic response to energy distribution, including disruption of the hypothalamic-gonadal axis. Dysregulation of the hypothalamic-gonadal axis leads to suppression of reproductive hormones and menstrual disturbance among females. Use of oral contraceptives or other estrogen replacements have not been shown to benefit individuals who suffer menstrual disturbance resulting from chronic insufficient energy intake to meet caloric needs.[54] Restoring nutrition and maintaining body weight within a healthy range is the necessary treatment, although in clinical practice, resumption of menses frequently lags restoration of weight. To resume normal function, it may be necessary to nudge body weight slightly above (eg, 5 lb) the weight at which menstruation ceased.

Menstrual dysfunction, hypercortisolemia, and reduced levels of androgens, leptin, and insulin-like growth factor 1 are associated with low-bone mineral density. While it is common to associate the essential nutrients calcium and vitamin D with bone growth and development, once bone loss has occurred, supplementation with these nutrients is insufficient to treat or prevent low bone density. Unfortunately, research fails to show that full recovery from an ED will completely reverse damage to bone or the reproductive system. Long-term fracture risk and future problems with fertility may persist.[54,67] The best medicine at this time is treatment of the ED and nutritional restoration.

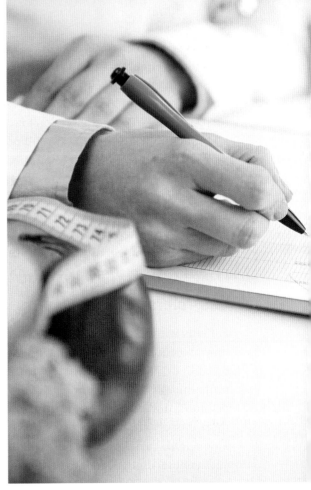

Comorbidities

By and large, EDs do not exist in isolation. Both psychological and physical comorbidities are found with EDs. The vast majority of people suffering from an ED also suffer from another concurrent mental disorder, and it is of extreme importance that a comprehensive assessment for comorbidities is included in the evaluation of anyone presenting to the practitioner showing symptoms of an ED.

Many people with an ED display a co-occurring personality disorders, such as obsessive-compulsive disorder, dependent personality disorder, or bipolar disorder. It is worthwhile to note that body dysmorphic disorder, characterized by preoccupation with perceived defects in physical appearance, is described as an obsessive-compulsive disorder in *DSM-5*, not as an eating disorder.[4] These personality disorders may predispose development of an ED, or a personality disorder may be a consequence of malnutrition. The famous Keys semistarvation study of conscientious objectors during World War II demonstrated not only the physical effects of dietary restriction to achieve a 25% weight reduction but also psychological distress, including development of anxiety, depression, rigidity, obsessions, and irritability.[68] Nutritional rehabilitation improves many of these personality traits, although some linger.[6]

ED behaviors may limit availability of vitamins and minerals, but clinical micronutrient deficiency does not occur as frequently as expected in the ED population.[69] Overnutrition (obesity) is a problem for some people. While most people who are obese do not have BED, up to two-thirds of people with BED are obese and are at risk of the medical complications of obesity.[8]

Special Considerations for Athletic Performance

Surprisingly, anecdotal evidence (eg, reports from coaches and personal accounts by athletes with DE) suggests that athletes practicing DE behaviors often experience an initial, albeit transient, increase in performance. The reasons for this temporary increase in performance are not completely understood but are thought to be related to the initial physiological and psychological effects of starvation and purging.[70] Starvation and purging are physiological stressors and, as such, produce an upregulation of the hypothalamic-pituitary-adrenal axis (eg, the fight-or-flight response) and an increase in the adrenal hormones: cortisol, epinephrine, and norepinephrine. These hormones have a stimulatory effect on the central nervous system that can mask fatigue and evoke feelings of euphoria in an athlete with an ED. In addition, the initial decrease in body weight (particularly before there is a significant decrease in muscle mass) may induce a transient increase in relative maximal oxygen uptake per kilogram of body weight (VO_2 max).[71] Moreover, with weight loss, athletes may feel lighter, which may afford them a psychological boost, particularly if they believe that lighter is better in terms of performance.

It should be emphasized that the increase in performance sometimes seen with DE is only temporary. Eventually, the body will break down and performance will suffer. The decrement in performance seen with chronic or severe energy restriction is likely due to one or more of the following factors: nutrient deficiencies, anemia, fatigue, reduced cardiovascular function, frequent infection, illness, or injuries.[19] As previously described, individuals with BN may purge or attempt to compensate for their bingeing episodes by using diuretics, laxatives, or enemas; self-induced vomiting; or excessive exercise. If the purging or compensatory behaviors place the athlete in a state of negative energy balance, then the potential effects on performance are similar to those seen with chronic or severe energy restriction. Also, the GI blood losses that often result from chronic vomiting can contribute to iron losses and increase the risk of iron-deficiency anemia. Excessive exercise, especially given inadequate energy and nutrient intakes, invariably leads to overuse injuries, such as stress fractures. In addition to the resulting energy and nutrient deficiencies, purging poses some unique problems regarding athletic performance, most notably dehydration and electrolyte abnormalities.[70]

The effects of DE on athletic performance are a function of the severity and duration of the DE behaviors as well as the physiological demands of the sport.[19] Thus, an individual who engages in severe energy restriction or who has been bingeing and purging for a long time will likely experience a greater decrement in performance than one who has engaged in milder weight-control behaviors for a shorter time. Likewise, those who participate in endurance sports and other physical activities with high energy demands (eg, distance running, swimming, cycling, basketball, and field and ice hockey) are likely to be more negatively affected than are those in sports with lower energy demands (eg, diving, gymnastics, weight lifting). Finally, athletes who train at a high intensity (eg, elite athletes) are likely to have greater performance decrements than those who engage in lower-intensity exercise (eg, recreational athletes).

ETIOLOGY AND RISK FACTORS FOR THE DEVELOPMENT OF DISORDERED EATING AND EATING DISORDERS

Why do some people develop EDs while others do not? An understanding of why one develops an ED is important in reducing stigma, providing effective treatment, and preventing the ED. Among the most prevalent reasons individuals engage in behaviors that they know are harmful and costly to them psychologically, socially, or in terms of performance and do not seek treatment are shame and fear of being misunderstood or blamed for their ED. Risk factors include biological characteristics (eg, genetic differences in the allele) and environmental events (eg, teasing or bullying) or experiences (eg, cultural ideal of thinness) that precede and are associated with an increase in the probability that one will develop an outcome or illness, in this case an ED.[72]

Sex and Age

Sex and age are the two characteristics that are most indicative of risk for an ED. In every study of the prevalence of ED, females outnumber males. However, gender appears to be less of a factor for BED and EDNOS than for AN or BN. Males and females with EDs often engage in similar behaviors but with different goals. For example, females are more likely to focus on weight-control behaviors while males often focus on loss of fat and increasing muscularity. Estimates of male athletes with an ED or DE varies among studies, but prevalence rates are higher than among the general population. The age of adolescence has long been recognized as the period of greatest vulnerability in terms of developing AN or BN; BED, on the other hand, has an onset well into adulthood.[72]

ENVIRONMENTAL

A variety of environmental factors may influence the development of an ED. Examples include the family environment, the sociocultural environment, and environmental experiences of stress and trauma.

FAMILY OF ORIGIN

Thinking about how the family contributes to the development of an ED has changed over time. While early research focused on family dysfunction, more recently the family has been considered to be part of the larger sociocultural environment. The following types of family dysfunction play a relatively small role in the etiology of eating disturbance and development of ED: (1) high-conflict home environment, (2) lack of familial cohesion, (3) poor communication, (4) deficient problem-solving skills, (5) high levels of emotional expression (general criticism, hostility) or low levels of emotional expression, and (6) modeling of dieting or negative body comments.[73]

CULTURE

Eating plays an important role in the lives of people in most cultures around the globe, and habits that are considered acceptable vary widely among groups. Thus, EDs have been conceptualized as culture-bound syndromes, implying that they occur uniquely in certain cultures or that they represent a culturally shaped expression of an underlying disease.[12,72] Prevalence and risk of ED suggests that variation, both within and among groups, is largely determined by socioeconomic status; religious affiliation; cultural ideals for body weight, shape, or size; media exposure; local environment (suburban vs urban settings); and the influence of other people who play a significant role.[74] Socioeconomic status has long been held to be a factor in the development of an ED based on the observation that higher-status individuals are thinner than those of lower status. However, research does not support a direct association between socioeconomic status and onset of an ED.[72]

According to Striegel-Moore and Bulik, epidemiologic studies on demographics, such as race, ethnicity, or sexual orientation (including homosexuality) are lacking, and thus we cannot draw valid conclusions and offer reliable insight regarding risk associated with cross-cultural differences.[72] EDs occur around the world and may reflect changes in body ideals. Media messages parallel the sociocultural ideal. Levine and Murnen report that the mass media sends many types of messages, in both form and content, that "present, elaborate, and reinforce, in a salient fashion, the schematic ingredients, that is, the 'nervosa,' of severely disordered eating…" and that those messages include "unattainable for most…to dichotomous, contradictory, and mystifying messages about passion, abandon, and indulgence versus control of hunger, sexuality, and other desires."[75] Evidence suggests that media exposure increases body-image concerns at least in the short run.[72]

SUBCULTURE OF THE ATHLETE

Evidence shows that people live and associate with specific cultures and subcultures. Culturally based value for a specific body weight, shape, or size, and exposure or social pressure to conform to the norm play a significant role in body-image concerns, such as overvaluation of thinness, weight, shape, or body composition.[72] Both aesthetic (appearance) sports and nonaesthetic sports often involve revealing attire, focusing attention on the body and body consciousness.[1] Excessive exercise to control body shape and weight has been observed among 40.3% to 54.5% of persons with an ED.[55] While athletic participation may play a role in appreciation of one's body, thereby serving as a protective factor, traditionally, sports participation has been stereotyped as more masculine than feminine.[76,77]

Although attention on the body and sexualization of athletes may adversely affect both males and females, females have been targeted, from both subtle suggestions to revealing attire on the cover of mainstream magazines.[77] On a more positive note, a recent analysis of female athlete coverage on mainstream media revealed an increase in both the

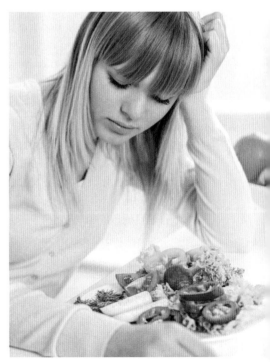

frequency and serious tone of coverage. Focus on females as serious competitors has grown, emphasizing their psychological and emotional strengths and athletic performance rather than their physical appearance and personal relationships.[78] More widespread representation of females may prompt others to value their physical abilities over how their bodies look and serve as a point of reference for athletic girls and women in the development of their own self-concept.[77]

While all athletes should be considered at risk for development of an ED, those who seem to have the highest prevalence of EDs are athletes involved in sports that emphasize a low body weight and low body fat, combined with regulations in some weight-sensitive sports.[79]

Higher levels of performance (eg, elite vs collegiate) generally predict more EDs; however, the evidence is inconsistent. Based upon questionnaire results from German high school students, Rosendahl and colleagues reported higher risk of EDs among nonathlete females (36.1%) and nonathlete males (12.3%) vs female athletes (12.3%) and male athletes 10.4%.[29] In contrast, Martinsen and Sundgot-Borgen used a two-stage approach (survey followed by a clinical interview) among male and female Norwegian adolescents and found the rates of EDs higher among elite athletes than among age-matched nonathlete controls.[25]

TRAUMA

An association between trauma, both emotional (eg, feelings of failure, loss) and physical (eg, sexual abuse, injury) and development of an ED is well established. Many people with EDs reveal a history of trauma during the course of treatment and may be diagnosed with posttraumatic stress disorder. Although the specific mechanism that leads to ED development is not understood, psychobiological dysregulation may put some people at greater risk than others.[6]

IDENTIFICATION, DIAGNOSIS, AND TREATMENT

Identification

People with ED are typically identified through the use of questionnaires to screen for ED. Ideally, a two-stage approach, as recommended by Jacobi and colleagues[80], that utilizes a broad screen for those at risk, followed by a more specific assessment, such as the clinical interview employed by Martinsen and Sundgot-Borgen would more accurately identify individuals with an ED.[25,]In research, there seems to be a preference for questionnaires, perhaps because self-reporting questionnaires are easy to administer, efficient, and economical. Furthermore, anonymity likely enhances ease or honesty in response, compared with a face-to-face interview.

The EAT in either the original 40-item version or the shorter 26-item version, the EDI, and the Eating Disorder Examination Questionnaire (EDE-Q) are among the most widely used screening tools for EDs. The EDE-Q is the self-report version of the Eating Disorder Examination Interview (EDE), recognized as one of the gold standard instruments used in the validation of screening tools.[81] The EDE is reportedly the most commonly used interview tool in clinical studies but may not be practical in many situations due to the time and training required for the interviewers.[6]

Be cautious in the use of these tools among populations where they have not been validated, such as the athletic population, in which individuals are thought to be two to three times more at risk compared with nonathletes.[6,81] Knapp and others describe a variety of tools used to identify ED among female athletes, including the Survey of Eating Disorders among Athletes (SEDA), the Female Athlete Screening Tool (FAST), the BUILT-R, the Brief Eating Disorder in Athletes Questionnaire (BEDA-Q), and the Athletic Milieu Direct Questionnaire (AMDQ), which may be better choices for identifying EDs.[82] Lease and Bond compare tools designed to identify maladaptive exercise—Obligatory Exercise Questionnaire (OEQ), Exercise Dependence Scale (EDS), and Frequency, Intensity, Time Index Scale (FIT)—and their associations with DE symptomology.[83]

Overall, the fields needs better identification of athletes at risk. The 2008 National Athletic Trainers' Association position statement recommends that more people involved in the health and performance of athletes, including certified athletic trainers, health care providers, and coaches, become more skilled in observing the behaviors of athletes as a means of detecting DE.[84]

Diagnosis

The very people who serve as first responders in terms of ED recognition and referral for treatment (coaches, primary care doctors, RDNs) have relatively little formal preparation according to "A National Survey of Eating Disorder Training."[85] It is not uncommon for professionals to miss the symptoms of EDs in a culture that idolizes the thin and fit and, in fact, even inadvertently promote DE and EDs through comments or body measurements. The diagnosis of an ED is based on specific criteria and may include physical, behavioral, and cognitive domains. Although the RDN may be among the first to recognize the signs and symptoms of an ED, it is considered outside the scope of the RDN's role to make the conclusive diagnosis. It is essential that patients be referred to a physician who is familiar with EDs for thorough physical and psychological examination to rule out other diseases.

The Treatment Team

EDs are being recognized more commonly, yet, statistically speaking, EDs remain relatively rare conditions in the general population and need to be addressed by people who are experienced in them. Professional ED organizations maintain the view that effective treatment usually involves clinicians from various health disciplines, including mental health professionals, physicians, RDNs, and nurses knowledgeable about EDs. Inclusion of a physical therapist experienced with EDs is gaining support. Although not all treatment teams include all members for the duration of treatment, thorough assessment and treatment are warranted. Clinical decisions will be deferred to the individual who holds the highest level of responsibility and liability (eg, the physician).

Levels of Care

A fundamental goal of ED treatment is to work with the patient at the lowest effective level of care. The outpatient setting is less disruptive and less costly than higher levels of care, which are not necessary for the treatment of most people.[86] However, a subset of people with an ED will require the safety, structure, and support offered by inpatient or day treatment programs.[87] The APA publishes guidelines for the care of individuals with EDs. Overall physical condition, psychologal state, behaviors, and social circumstances all play roles in the decision making regarding the appropriate level of care. Adults who weigh less than approximately 85% of individually estimated healthy body weight are known to have difficulty gaining weight outside of a highly structured, supervised program.[88] Even those who have weights 85% or more above expected body weight may also require higher levels of care due to medical or psychiatric necessity. Levels of care include 24-hour inpatient programs; partial hospital programs, which entail being at the hospital part of every day; intensive outpatient programs, in which patients attend part of most days of the week; variable setting, practitioner, support, and schedule programs, known as outpatient programs; and support groups.

At all levels of care, transition planning is important. When an individual is served by a hospital program, it is recommended that they stay until consistency in food intake and a healthy body weight is achieved and maintained to reduce the chances of relapse. The APA recommends that a specific clinician be identified as the primary care coordinator to ensure continuity and attention to important aspects of treatment.[88] The Disordered Eating and Eating Disorders (DEED) subunit of the Sports, Cardiovascular, and Wellness Nutrition (SCAN) group of the Academy of Nutrition and Dietetics provides informational matieral, such as a fact sheet for transitional care for use by RDNs.[89]

Nutrition therapists participate in the transition of care between levels of care and between providers. DEED provides an evidence-based advanced practice guide titled "Transitioning Care Effectively," specifically for the RDN to assist in the matriculation from one level of care to another.[89]

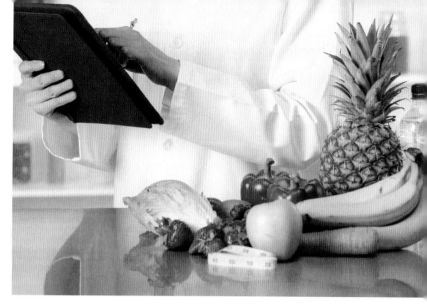

NUTRITION COUNSELING

Each patient with an ED brings his or her unique circumstances to the treatment team; athletes are no exception. Remember that athletes with an ED are people first. As such, they can be expected to hold the same thoughts, beliefs, hopes, and fears that other people with EDs do. We have observed EDs as diseases wherein doubt frequently surfaces: doubt about the seriousness of the ED behaviors, doubt about what recovery will look like, and doubt in both their ability to recover and their treatment team. Thus, it is imperative that providers who treat people with EDs are specifically prepared to work with this population. The sports dietitian who has an existing relationship with an athlete who has an ED may be well positioned to help him or her but may also benefit from networking or coordinating care with another RDN who has expertise in the treatment of EDs. Recognize and respect your limits. Inadequate or harmful care puts individuals with EDs at even greater risk for abandoning or avoiding treatment and for loss of faith in the medical system.[53]

RDNs who work with people who have EDs have chosen to work in a field where there is substantial disagreement and debate about many aspects of the disorders, including etiology, labels and diagnoses, therapeutic modalities, and what constitutes recovery. However, those who work with the athletic population encounter people regularly, if not daily or hourly, who hold some degree of body dissatisfaction and concern about eating. These concerns, sometimes referred to as normative dissatisfaction, are important predictors of the possible onset of an ED.

It is important that all members of the treatment team recognize that the patient or client is the one who determines if or when he or she ultimately chooses to recover, partially or fully. It is our responsibility to bring our best effort forward and support our patients based on where they are, recognizing what they are willing and able to do with regard to keeping themselves safe and avoiding further harm. At times this may result in involuntary treatment. In the world of sports nutrition, we often practice harm reduction, recognizing the limits of our ability to effect change in another person. However, when treating a person with a life-threatening ED, harm reduction rarely applies.

Work with people who have these dysfunctions is demanding, and those who serve their patient or client best will be equally committed to self-care. To that end, we recommend regular collaboration among treatment team members as a source of support and for setting therapeutic boundaries. Recognize the patient or client, coach, training staff, family, and significant others as potential resources (see Box 18.2 on page 406 for professional resources).

Role of the Registered Dietitian Nutritionist

RDNs who work with patients with DE or EDs work as medical nutrition therapists. RDNs who work with athletes *will* encounter individuals suffering from DE and EDs; thus, it is imperative that one develops the skills and qualifications to treat these serious disorders. One must demonstrate proficiency in the delivery of medical nutrition therapy (MNT) for individuals with EDs, contributing both technical and collaborative expertise within the treatment team.[90] While MNT is widely endorsed by professional organizations in the treatment of EDs, no standard exists for the delivery of nutrition therapy among the DE or ED population.[91] Mittnacht and Bulik assessed for best nutrition counseling practices for AN among a select group of 21 RDNs identified as recognized experts in the treatment of ED.[92] Interestingly, consensus (>85% agreement) regarding nutritional treatment among these experts was reached on only 35% (47 of 133) of questions and statements delivered via the Delphi method.

Box 18.2 Professional Organizations as Resources

Professional Organization	Resources Available
Academy for Eating Disorders website: www.aedweb.org	Brochure: Eating Disorders: Critical Points for Early Recognition and Medical Risk Management in the Care of Individuals With Eating Disorders
	Professional listserv
	International conferences and meetings
	Webinars for members
	Continuing education
Academy of Nutrition and Dietetics website: www.eatright.org	Position paper: Nutrition Intervention in the Treatment of Eating Disorders
	Position paper: Nutrition and Athletic Performance
	Standards of Practice and Standards of Professional Performance in Disordered Eating and Eating Disorders
	Standards of Practice and Standards of Professional Performance for Registered Dietitian Nutritionists in Sports Nutrition and Dietetics
	Disordered Eating and Eating Disorders (DEED) subunit of the Sports, Cardiovascular, and Wellness Nutrition (SCAN) dietetic practice group (www.scandpg.org):
	DEED Advance Practice Guidelines and Fact Sheets
	SCAN conferences
Binge Eating Disorder Association website: www.bedaonline.com	Conferences
International Association of Eating Disorders Professionals Foundation website: www.iaedp.com	Conferences and local chapters
	Certification as an expert in eating disorders
National Eating Disorder Association website: www.nationaleatingdisorders.org	Conferences
	Hotline
	Workshops and symposiums

Mittnacht and Bulik stated that the following are integral parts of the RDN role[92]:

- Set patient goals (including goal weights for children and adolescents, but not for adults).
- Address weight-related issues, while emphasizing healthy state over a healthy weight.
- Develop meal plans based upon current food intake and moving toward improvement.
- Address body image and psychological issues.
- Apply psychological therapy techniques as part of nutrition counseling.
- Involve parents in the treatment of children and adolescents.
- Engage patients in recovery based upon the patient's values and goals.
- Educate patients about scientific evidence related to the genetic components and medical consequences of EDs.
- Adjust treatment approach based on the individual and their circumstances.

The therapeutic delivery of nutrition care demands that the RDN possess the aptitude to combine technical skill with the development and delivery of nutrition care plans. It is imperative that the RDN is able to empathetically listen to the patient's story, reflect back to the patient what has been heard, understand the patient's values, and creatively assist in identifying goals and strategies that will restore the patient's health. The sports dietitian plays a central role in helping individuals who overexercise recognize the adverse effects of their actions on sports performance, as well as on physical, emotional, and social health.

The effective RDN working with people who have DE or EDs will possess relational skills to engage and appropriately challenge patients or clients to do the work required for recovery. Additional counseling skills include inquiry and the modeling of mindfulness, empathy, authenticity, affirmation, courage, calm, warmth, appropriate humor, and playfulness. The RDN may work with family members and guide them in taking a supervisory role during mealtimes that demonstrates a caring and compassionate attitude, as well as consistency in expectations about meals in terms of amount eaten, time to completion, and acceptable behaviors. Taken together, these skills enable RDNs to build and sustain a close therapeutic relationship with the patient or client and a strong partnership with the treatment team, including family members, coaches, and trainers.

RDNs who treat athletes with EDs will best serve this population by having a solid foundation in both sports nutrition and EDs. The certified specialist in sports dietetics (CSSD) certification, offered through the Commission on Dietetic Registration, and the certified eating disorders registered dietitian (CEDRD) certification, offered through the International Association of Eating Disorders Professionals, verify foundational knowledge in these areas. RDNs versed in the details of the nutrition care process and who have an aptitude for health and wellness coaching, if not a certificate, are well positioned to work

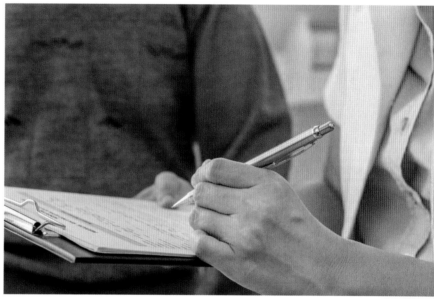

with the athlete with an ED. RDNs coming from this background will support the patient or client in the provision of safe and effective nutritional recovery and then will utilize counseling and coaching skills to support the patient through full nutrition rehabilitation and return to sport when appropriate.

It is imperative that providers recognize the unpredictability of ED and maintain vigilance in treatment. For example, it is important to check vitals and laboratory tests, as well as proceed with the awareness that individuals with EDs seem to wear a mask, frequently reporting that they are fine, based on an obscured view of their condition. Clients frequently do not feel that they are sick enough or that they deserve care. Furthermore, they are ambivalent about the desire for change in their food selection or body weight. Stereotypes abound regarding EDs, and individuals who do not fit the image of having an ED may either disregard the symptoms or feel unworthy of medical attention. Thompson and Sherman describe the phenomenon of "presumption of health," in which people often automatically associate competition in sport as a reflection of health.[1] Lack of awareness, training, or the desire to recognize DE and EDs may result in coaches, family members, and medical providers missing clues that there is a serious problem.

Expanded Role of the Registered Dietitian Nutritionist in Medical Monitoring and Coordination

When properly trained, the RDN may further contribute to the treatment of people with EDs by monitoring vital signs, along with providing psychoeducation around the signs of malnutrition and nutritional recovery. RDNs also assess hydration status through urine color, urine frequency, and urine specific gravity. Some people with EDs restrict fluid intake and others may fluid load, typically in an attempt to either misguide the treatment team regarding their body weight or in an attempt to quiet hunger signals. Related to fluid intake, some people consume caffeine in hopes of suppressing appetite, stimulating metabolism, or both.

Phases of Nutrition Therapy

Graves and Scribner describe three phases of nutrition therapy with which an athlete familiar with recovery from physical injury may be likely to identify.[91] The phases move from high levels of structure that keep the athlete safe from further injury to eating with flexibility and for optimal performance. Phase 1 is described as providing a foundation for healing, similar to casting a broken bone; phase 2 is the rehabilitation phase, which may involve painful change likened to having a cast removed and progressing to physical therapy to regain flexibility and strength; and phase 3 is described as striving to achieve one's full potential or synergy, with the RDN serving as an ally to patient-driven progress. The role of the RDN shifts from expert mode in prescribing specific meal plans and nutritional supplements to a nutrition coach role. This model supports the athlete in holding a vision of recovery as an injured athlete returning to his or her sport based upon readiness as determined by progress in healing.

Therapeutic Approaches

The nutrition therapist working with people with DE may draw from a variety of domains, including compassionate communication (also known as nonviolent communication), motivational interviewing, and appreciative inquiry, as well as well as a number of psychological therapy practices. In the content that follows, we present some of the more common therapeutic approaches and modalities that RDNs may utilize in providing MNT to those who have an ED.

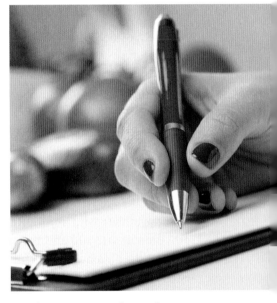

COGNITIVE BEHAVIORAL THERAPY

Cognitive behavioral therapy (CBT) is often regarded as the leading evidence-based treatment for adults with EDs, although it is generally considered to be more effective for treating BN and BED than AN.[93,94] CBT is based on the premise that thoughts (cognition) and emotions lead to eating disordered actions and behaviors.[87] CBT begins with education about the disease, and patients learn to recognize thought patterns and the power of those patterns and triggers that lead to symptomatic behavior. Recovery is focused on managing self-defeating thought patterns and engaging in planned strategies through the phases of CBT that lead to healthful, recovery-oriented behavioral patterns. There are various forms of CBT, but the basics of CBT provide the foundation for other therapies.[87]

DIALECTICAL BEHAVIOR THERAPY

Dialectical behavior therapy (DBT), originally developed by Marsha Linehan, utilizes elements from CBT, with the additions of mindfulness, distress tolerance, and acceptance, which now permeate behavioral approaches.[95] DBT has been modified for the treatment of patients with complex, multidiagnostic EDs.[96,97] When DBT is applied in the treatment of EDs, individuals learn rational thinking and decision-making skills that allow them to move beyond black-and-white thinking to develop coping strategies for perceived crises. Examples of skills include walking the middle path, regulating emotions, and improving interpersonal effectiveness.[95]

ACCEPTANCE AND COMMITMENT THERAPY

Like DBT, acceptance and commitment therapy (ACT) moves the focus of treatment from changing cognition to accepting thoughts.[98] ACT, developed by Steven Hayes, Kelly Wilson, and Kirk Strosahl, is increasingly recognized as a viable ED treatment intervention.[99] ACT differs from CBT in that rather than striving to change or control the way they think, people learn that thoughts may be uncontrollable. ACT teaches recognition and tolerance of negative thoughts and feelings in an effort to live a better life in the face of distress, accepting pain as a normal part of living.[98]

ACT is founded on these principles: accept your thoughts and feelings and be present; choose a valued direction; and take action. Thus, the primary goal of ACT is to create a rich and meaningful life while accepting the pain that accompanies it. ACT embodies the belief that we will have pain and suffering. ED patients are viewed as attempting to avoid the pain of life.[100]

FAMILY-BASED TREATMENT

The role of the family in the treatment and etiology of EDs has changed dramatically; parents, who were once veiwed negatively, are now an integral part of the recovery. The term *family-based treatment* (FBT) emerged from the family-based, home-based treatment practiced at Maudsley Hospital in London. The treatment model is fairly brief (15 to 20 outpatient sessions over 6 to 12 months) and includes three phases: (1) uniting parents to take temporary control of all food-related decisions and restore a healthful weight range; (2) transitioning control back to the adolescent; and (3) establishing normal adolescent development and identity. FBT is a manualized approach with guides for treatment of AN and BN among adolescents. Practitioners, programs, and institutions, depending on circumstances, frequently adapt the FBT approach. Adaptation may result in loss of treatment fidelity as the empirical support for FBT is based on its clear structure. Some of the difficulties in adhering to FBT include the consistent time commitment required of family members and the sibling involvement in therapy.[100] Although FBT does not specifically use the expertise of the RDN, training on FBT is offered to professionals through the Training Institute at Stanford University.[101]

Many of the strategies used in FBT have long been utilized by RDNs treating other illness of childhood (eg, diabetes, food allergy), such as educating parents regarding food, nutrition, and metabolism, including dispelling misinformation and myths, and effectively training parents to support their children in eating. The principles of FBT may also be utilized with older patients or clients by enlisting the support of those who play the supportive roles of the family.

MOTIVATIONAL INTERVIEWING

Motivational interviewing (MI) emphasizes four general principles: expressing empathy, developing discrepancy, rolling with resistance, and supporting self-efficacy. RDNs who are trained in MI utilize these principles to help patients and clients become increasingly aware of thoughts and feelings that lead to behaviors. Awareness of precipitating thoughts and feelings facilitate the resolution of resistance to change.[102]

EXPOSURE TREATMENT

Exposure treatment with response prevention is considered an adjunct therapeutic technique.[103] RDNs frequently engage in therapeutic meals and snacks with patients, as well as help parents and others support providers expose patients to foods that are fearful to them in order to gain familiarity and confidence in adding those foods back into the diet. A progressive twist on the concept of exposure therapy is to change one's relationship with food through involvement in growing and cooking food. The act of nurturing a seed or small plant, harvesting, and then sharing a meal are recognized as pleasures, reflections of identity, and connection. These same strategies are being used among athletes and RDNs in pursuit of a diet that brings some structure and assurance that needs are being met, while at the same time are used to heal or promote one's relationship with food.

Psychoeducation and Dietary Manipulation

There is no clear protocol for manipulating macronutrients (carbohydrates, proteins, or fats) or micronutrients (vitamins and minerals) among the ED population. The RDN explores and addresses beliefs held about benefits and risks of energy-producing nutrients, vitamins, and minerals and about the use of supplements, including ergogenic agents. While it is beyond the scope of this chapter to describe the details of dietary manipulation, meal plans generally progress from specific (referring to dosing of food as medicine based on amount and timing) to more general, with the end goal of establishing an adequate nutrient intake and balance among food groups and variety of foods. The type of eating plan depends on the type and severity of the disorder as well as the individual patient needs. Most patients express a desire to return to normal eating, characterized by mindfulness and intuition. Retraining the patient to eat in response to internal cues, utilizing mindfulness or an approach termed *intuitive eating,* would generally follow weight restoration and requires that the patient be at a place where she or he can integrate interoceptive awareness (ability to perceive physical, bodily sensations) with emotional regulation and respond to her or his own needs in a timely manner. One principle of intuitive eating is unconditional permission to eat. Keeping in mind food addiction theory, implementation of all the principles of mindful or intuitive eating may need to be delayed or may never be effective or appropriate.[104] As previously described, the RDN may apply an assortment of psychological therapy techniques as part of MNT. We find that athletes generally understand, at least cognitively, the need for carbohydrate-rich foods as fuel for the brain, power for muscles, and a vehicle for fiber and phytochemicals. They also relate to the necessity of adequate protein as a bridge supporting satiety signals, as well as a connector for building muscle and producing neurotransmitters.[91] While the fears of eating may apply to any of the macronutrients, fear of body fat often translates into fear of food fat.

Athletes are not immune to nutrition myths, and they are aware that weight loss may result in an initial performance improvement. What they have a difficult time understanding is the transience of this benefit. The first impression is lasting, and even after continued efforts to lose weight through dietary restriction that result in nutritional deficits, fatigue, loss of strength, impaired immunity, and illness, the initial success may propel the athlete and, through contagion, teammates or others watching to move along the same path toward developing a clinical ED, including purging by vomiting, use of diuretics or laxatives, or excessive exercise.[6] The devastation of a poor performance due to injury or illness pales in comparison to the potential for a life-threatening cardiac event due to hypoglycemia, dehydration, or electrolyte imbalance. RDNs are uniquely qualified to educate athletes and coaches on the critical role of nutrition to health and performance.

When a semistarved person is identified (eg, an athlete identified with LEA), a thorough nutritional and medical assessment, with ongoing monitoring, is warranted. Rapid restoration of nutrition, especially among adults, can be life threatening when it results in a rapid shift of phosphorus from the serum into the cells. Low serum phosphorus can cause muscle breakdown (eg, rhabdomyolysis), blood cell dysfunction, respiratory failure, seizure, and cardiac arrest.[53]

The term *refeeding* may refer to either (1) the process of restoring nutrition or (2) the potentially life-threatening condition that results from improved energy intake (especially from carbohydrate), known as refeeding syndrome. It is important to know that theoretically any patient could experience refeeding syndrome in the process of increasing nutritional intake. While no single indicator exists to precisely identify who will develop refeeding syndrome, the National Institute for Health and Care Excellence guideline 32 provides criteria for identifying those at higher risk (Table 18.3).[105]

Traditionally, the strategy toward restoring nutrition has been to "start low, go slow" in terms of caloric intake. However, recent research suggests that refeeding risk varies depending on the degree of malnutrition, the age of the patient or client, and the ratio of carbohydrate to fat and protein.[54] Initially, carbohydrate intake may be less than 50% of calories in an attempt to reduce risk of refeeding syndrome. This lower percentage of carbohydrate goes against conventional wisdom of sports nutrition and is met with resistance among some athletes and sometimes their family members and coaching or training staff. The restoration of energy intake is incrementally increased, by 100 to 200 kcal daily or by up to 400 kcal every 3 days with close medical supervision. Caloric needs for a person who is severely energy restricted defy typical calculations and may be upward of 3,000 to 4,000 kcals/d, even at low physical activity and concurrent with indicators of downregulation of metabolism. Research suggests that the thermic effect of food may be elevated from between 14% and 30% among those with AN by psychological state (eg, anxiety and depression related to eating) and hormonal response to stress.[106,107] More research is needed to

Table 18.3 Criteria for Determining People at High Risk of Developing Refeeding Problems[105]

Patient has one or more of the following:	OR	Patient has two or more of the following:
Body mass index (BMI) <16		BMI <18.5
Unintentional weight loss greater than 15% within the previous 3–6 months		Unintentional weight loss greater than 10% within the previous 3–6 months
Little or no nutritional intake for more than 10 days		Little or no nutritional intake for more than 5 days
Low levels of potassium, phosphate, or magnesium prior to feeding		A history of alcohol drug or abuse including insulin, chemotherapy, antacids, or diuretics

understand the metabolic changes and needs of patients with EDs. The RDN provides psychoeducation regarding nutritional needs, develops and modifies meal plans, supervises food and beverage intake, and provides overall accountability for meeting nutritional needs.

RETURNING TO COMPETITION

Progression in Physical Activity

Determining appropriate levels of physical activity based on both nutritional status and emotional readiness can be a responsibility of the RDN, especially if the athlete does not have a multidisciplinary sports medicine team. When a patient or client wishes to increase physical activity, it is important to explore his or her intention, as well as potential benefits and risks. In general, gradual return to physical activity is recommended. However, because some athletes have an addictive nature regarding physical activity, they may never be able to safely return to physical activity at the competitive level.

Return-to-Play Guidelines

Athletes who present with an ED or otherwise have signs or symptoms of dysfunction (energy deficiency relative to energy intake or exercise dependence) should undergo a thorough medical examination for safe participation. The International Olympic Committee introduced the syndrome called relative energy deficiency in sport (RED-S) to extend and emphasize the risks described in the female athlete triad to include males and persons from various ethnic groups.[108,109] People seem to relate to the simple red-yellow-green categorization of participation in activity used in the RED-S return-to-play scorecard. The simple stoplight metaphor speaks to the varying levels of risk that guide return to play. Following medical history and examination, an athlete would be classified into one of the following: red light = high risk; yellow light = moderate risk; and green light = low risk. For example, a red light is assigned to an athlete with any of the following: diagnosis of an ED, serious psychological or physiological condition, engagement in extreme dieting, or bradycardia. Yellow light is assigned to an athlete based on the following: maintaining an abnormally low body fat for an extended time; experiencing a 5% to 10% loss of body weight within a month; having interrupted growth or development (adolescent athletes); or having LEA, low bone density, abnormal menstruation, or stress fractures associated with hormonal abnormality or LEA. Furthermore, athletes who are deemed to put other athletes at risk or are not making the expected progress in treatment of DE will be labeled as yellow light. Those athletes who engage in health-promoting eating habits, maintain a healthy physique while consuming adequate caloric intake, and are psychologically and physiologically healthy are assigned the green light for full participation. Moderate-risk (yellow light) athletes may continue to train if a treatment plan is followed; return to competition requires medical clearance. High-risk (red light) athletes are not permitted to practice or compete and are under a written health contract governing return-to-play.[110] Many athletic training programs employ their own specific return to play protocol, and protocols may vary from program to program.

PREVENTING DISORDERED EATING AND EATING DISORDERS AMONG ATHLETES

RDNs are increasingly recognized for their therapeutic role. RDNs trained in therapeutic modalities play a parallel role with other therapists on the treatment team by aligning the language and goals addressed in nutrition therapy with psychotherapy. For clients, this facilitates recognition of the supportive therapeutic role the RDN plays beyond the imposing intake of unwanted food or setting activity limits for the patient who is overexercising. Those who work in this field are called upon to be cognizant of the many ways in which we may unwittingly find ourselves promulgating the very thing we seek to prevent, identify, and treat. In all that we do, we need to be wary of the words we use and the messages we send regarding the physical and emotional environment we provide. Be cautious about associating any body weight, shape, or size with disease or disorder. The most recent edition of the *DSM-5* recognizes that AN can occur at any weight; therefore, it is imperative to not provide admiration, praise, and encouragement for current body weight when first meeting a person with AN.

Prevention programs are generally divided into three categories as defined by the Caplan model: primary, secondary, and tertiary. Primary (also known as universal) prevention aims to reduce the number of cases in a population by targeting people who do not have signs or symptoms. Secondary prevention seeks to reduce the prevalence by selectively targeting high-risk individuals and those who may be showing early signs or symptoms. Tertiary prevention is directed toward minimizing the damaging effects among those who have been diagnosed with a disorder.[5] It is often difficult to discriminate between populations that are targets for primary or secondary interventions because differentiation between healthy individuals and those with a subclinical condition may be difficult. Reactive prevention efforts are directed at creating resistance to potential risk factors, whereas proactive prevention seeks to reduce or eliminate exposure to known risk factors.[5] Little empirical evidence exists regarding prevention of DE and EDs among athletes. Peer-led and professionally led programs have been modified to address some of the unique needs and circumstances of the culture of the athlete.[6]

At any level, prevention begins with awareness of risks, signs, and symptoms. Often, dietary restriction, which results in relative energy deficiency, is the first sign of an ED.[6] Unfortunately, relatively little is actually known about the diets of athletes. This calls for greater attention to the dietary and weight management practices of athletes.[111]

Some additional factors that place an athlete at risk for RED-S include: injuries and illness (injured athletes fear unwanted weight gain during recovery); decline in quality of performance due to loss of lean body mass and strength; sharing of nutrition myths or pressure to lose weight by misinformed training staff; fear of eating when traveling, perhaps especially in fast-food restaurants; lack of nutrition knowledge or skills to choose or prepare nutritious food; and personality traits of a good athlete (eg, perfectionism, competitiveness, willingness to train through pain).[1,6,79]

Additional efforts toward prevention include the following:

- Develop mandatory educational programs for coaches, trainers, and athletes across all sports regarding the risk factors, signs, and symptoms of DE and EDs.[6]
- Educate male and female athletes about the female athlete triad and RED-S so they recognize the nutrition and health requirements necessary for safe participation in sport.[108]
- Adopt a protocol to identify EDs and appropropriate actions to take. Consider the International Olympic Committee RED-S Clinical Assessment Tool, the Female Athlete Triad Cumulative Risk Assessment Tool, and a sample athlete contract for clearance and ready-to-play decisions .[110,111]

- Monitor modeling beliefs and behaviors in an effort to reduce contagion between athletes and influential others.
- Deemphasize body weight and composition.
- Promote healthful eating behaviors.
- Destigmatize ED.
- Fosterindividuality among and within athletes.

FUTURE NEEDS

Formal ED curricula include various programs, in brief training workshops, specialized ED conferences, web-based courses; techniquest include collaborative learning, teaching, and supervision.[86] Despite these programs, more training is needed, specifically for RDNs on therapeutic modalities for the ED population. While education does not directly translate to changes in attitude or behavior, education does contribute to awareness. Educational programs for athletes and coaches that emphasize the central role of nutrition in both physical and mental health, in addition to weight as a factor in performance, increase awareness of the potential detriment of critical comments about body size, weight, or shape and create safe and trusting relationship to encourage open communication about eating problems.[112] Although the determinants of mental health are complex, the emerging and compelling evidence for nutrition as a crucial factor in the high prevalence and incidence of mental disorders suggests that diet is as important to psychiatry as it is to cardiology, endocrinology, and gastroenterology. Evidence is steadily growing for the relationship between dietary quality (and potential nutritional deficiencies) and mental health and for the select use of nutrient-based supplements to address deficiencies or for use as monotherapies or augmentation therapies.

SUMMARY

This chapter summarizes EDs, especially among the athletic population. While there are data that suggest individual risk factors, it is important to view every athlete as at risk. If we address the entire culture of sport, we are more likely to make strides toward the prevention of EDs on a large scale, affecting countless at-risk athletes. It is also important that we dispel the commonly held belief that those with DE or other specified feeding and eating disorders are not as at risk as those diagnosed with other EDs. Similarly, it is a mistake to presume health based on performance or simple observation. It is imperative that those who work with athletic populations recognize their own attitudes and gaps in knowledge and seek to improve skills. RDNs should seek out opportunities to increase their knowledge of EDs by seeking out formal education opportunities.

KEY TAKEAWAYS

EDs are much more than diets gone too far.

View every athlete as at risk for an ED.

RDNs who treat those with EDs require specialized training and experience.

Utilize a multidisciplinary treatment team in collaboration and support.

Be aware of your own biases and commit to model good self care.

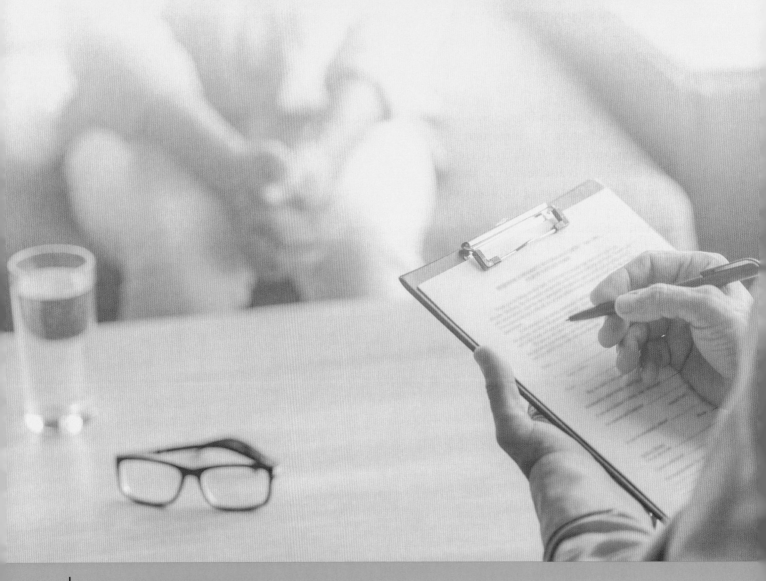

REFERENCES

1. Thompson RA, Sherman RT. *Eating Disorders in Sport.* New York, NY: Routledge; 2010.

2. Byrne S, McLean N. Eating disorders in athletes: a review of the literature. *J Sci Med Sport.* 2001;4(2):145-159.

3. American Psychiatric Association, ed. *Diagnostic and Statistical Manual of Mental Disorders, Fifth Edition (DSM-5).* Arlington VA: American Psychiatric Association; 2013.

4. American Psychiatric Association, ed. *Diagnostic and Statistical Manual of Mental Disorders, Fifth Edition (DSM-5).* American Psychiatric Association Publishing. http://psychiatryonline.org/doi/book/10.1176/appi.books.9780890425596. Published 2013. Accessed January 3, 2016.

5. Filion AJ, Haines J. Why prevention? The case for upstream strategies. In: Smolak L, Levine MP, eds. *The Wiley Handbook of Eating Disorders.* Chichester, UK: John Wiley & Sons, Ltd; 2015: 557-568.

6. Coelho GM de O, Gomes AI da S, Ribeiro BG, Soares E de A. Prevention of eating disorders in female athletes. *Open Access J Sports Med.* 2014;5:105-113.

7. Hay P, Girosi F, Mond J. Prevalence and sociodemographic correlates of DSM- eating disorders in the Australian population. *J Eat Disord.* 2015;3(19).

8. National Eating Disorders Association website. www.nationaleatingdisorders.org/. Accessed December 10, 2015.

9. Von Essen E, Martensson F. Young adults' use of food as a self-therapeutic intervention. *Int J Qual Stud Health Well-being.* 2014;9. doi:http://dx.doi.org/10.3402/qhw.v9.23000.

10. Bratman S, Knight D. *Health Food Junkies: Orthorexia Nervosa: Overcoming the Obsession with Healthful Eating.* New York, NY: Broadway Books; 2000.

11. Moroze RM, Dunn TM, Holland CJ, Yager J, Weintraub P. Microthinking about micronutrients: a case of transition from obsessions about healthy eating to near-fatal "orthorexia nervosa" and proposed diagnostic criteria. *Psychosomatics.* 2015;56(4):397-403.

12. Uher R, Rutter M. Classification of feeding and eating disorders: review of evidence and proposals for ICD-11. *World Psychiatry.* 2012;11(2):80-92.

13. Healthy People 2020. HealthyPeople.gov website. www.healthypeople.gov/2020/default.aspx. Accessed October 23, 2015.

14. O'Keefe JO, Patil HR, Lavie CJ, Magalski A, Vogel RA, McCullough PA. Potential adverse cardiovascular effects from excessive endurance exercise. *Mayo Clin Proc.* 2012;87(6):587-595.

15. Landolfi E. Exercise addiction. *Sports Med.* 2013;43(2):111-119.

16. Cook BJ, Hausenblas HA. The role of exercise dependence for the relationship between exercise behavior and eating pathology: mediator or moderator? *J Health Psychol.* 2008;13(4):495-502.

17. Bratland-Sanda S, Sundgot-Borgen J. Eating disorders in athletes: overview of prevalence, risk factors and recommendations for prevention and treatment. *Eur J Sport Sci.* 2013;13(5):499-508.

18. Petrie T, Greenleaf C. Athletes, physical activity, dancers, and eating disorders. In: Smolak L, Levine MP, eds. *The Wiley Handbook of Eating Disorders.* Chichester, UK: John Wiley & Sons; 2015:463-478.

19. Beals K. *Disordered Eating Among Athletes: A Comprehensive Guide for Health Professionals.* Champaign, IL: Human Kinetics; 2004.

20. Schaal K, Tafflet M, Nassif H, et al. Psychological balance in high level athletes: gender-based differences and sport-specific patterns. *PLoS One.* 2011;6(5):e19007.

21. Thiemann P, Legenbauer T, Vocks S, Platen P, Auyeung B, Herpertz S. Eating disorders and their putative risk factors among female German professional athletes. *Eur Eat Disord Rev.* 2015;23:269-276.

22. Fortes LS, Kakeshita I, Almeida S, Gomes A, Ferreira M. Eating behaviours in youths: a comparison between female and male athletes and non-athletes. *Scand J Med Sci Sports.* 2014;24:e62-e68.

23. Chatterton J, Petrie TA. Prevalence of disordered eating and pathogenic weight control behaviors among male collegiate athletes. *Eat Disord.* 2013;21:328-341.

24. Goltz F, Stenzel L, Schneider C. Disordered eating behaviors and body image in male athletes. *Rev Bras Psiquiatr.* 2013;35:237-242.

25. Martinsen M, Sundgot-Borgen J. Higher prevalence of eating disorders among adolescent elite athletes than controls. *Med Sci Sports Exerc.* 2013;45(6):1188-1197.

26. Thein-Nissenbaum J, Rauh M, Carr K, Loud K, McGuine T. Associations between disordered eating, menstrual dysfunction, and musculoskeletal injury among high school athletes. *J Orthop Sports Phys Ther.* 2011;41:60-69.

27. Martinsen M, Bratland-Sanda S, Eriksson AK, Sundgot-Borgen J. Dieting to win or to be thin? A study of dieting and disordered eating among adolescent elite athletes and non-athlete controls. *Br J Sports Med.* 2010;44:70-76.

28. Greenleaf C, Petrie T, Carter J, Reel J. Female collegiate athletes: prevalence of eating disorders and disordered eating behaviors. *J Amer Coll Health.* 2009;57:489-495.

29. Rosendahl J, Bormann B, Aschenbrenner K, Aschenbrenner F, Strauss B. Dieting and disordered eating in German high school athletes and non-athletes. *Scand J Med Sci Sports.* 2009;19(5):731-739.

30. Petrie TA, Greenleaf C, Reel J, Carter J. Prevalence of eating disorders and disordered eating behaviors among male collegiate athletes. *Psych Men Masc.* 2008;9:267-277.

31. Torstveit M, Rosenvinge J, Sundgot-Borgen J. Prevalence of ED and the predictive power of risk models in female elite athletes: a controlled study. *Scand J Med Sci Sports.* 2008;18(1):108-118.

32. Nichols J, Rauh M, Barrack M, Barkai H, Pernick Y. Disordered eating and menstrual irregularity in high school athletes in lean-build and nonlean-build sports. *Int J Sport Nutr Exerc Metab.* 2007;17:364-377.

33. Nichols J, Rauh M, Lawson M, Ji M, Barkai H. Prevalence of the female athlete triad syndrome among high school athletes. *Arch Pediatr Adolesc Med.* 2006;160:137-142.

34. Beals K, Hill A. The prevalence of disordered eating, menstrual dysfunction, and low bone mineral density among US collegiate athletes. *Int J Sport Nutr Exerc Metab.* 2006;16:1-23.

35. Toro J, Gailiea B, Martinez-Mallén E, et al. Eating disorders in Spanish female athle. *Int J Sports Med.* 2005;26(8):679-700.

36. Sundgot-Borgen J, Torstveit MK. Prevalence of eating disorders in elite athletes is higher than in the general population. *Clin J Sport Med.* 2004;14(1):25-32.

37. Byrne S, McLean N. Elite athletes: effects of the pressure to be thin. *J Sci Med Spor.* 2002;5:80-94.

38. Beals K, Manore M. Disorders of the female athlete triad among collegiate athletes. *Int J Sport Nutr Exerc Metab.* 2002;12:281-293.

39. Johnson C, Powers P, Dick R. Athletes and eating disorders: the National Collegiate Athletic Association study. *Int J Eat Disord.* 1999;26:179-188.

40. Sundgot-Borgen J. Prevalence of eating disorders in elite female athletes. *Int J Sport Nutr.* 1993;3:29-40.

41. Fairburn C, Beglin S. Assessment of eating disorders: interview or self-report questionnaire? *Int J Eat Disord.* 1994;16:363-370.

42. Cooper P, Taylor M, Cooper Z, Fairburn C. The development and validation of the body shape questionnaire. *Int J Eat Disord.* 1987;6:485-494.

43. Thelen M, Farmer J, Wonderlich S, Smith M. A revision of the bulimia test: the BULIT-R. *J Consult Clin Psychol.* 1991;3:119-124.

44. *Diagnostic and Statistical Manual of Mental Disorders.* 4th ed. Washington, DC: American Psychiatric Association; 1994.

45. Garner D, Olmstead M, Bohr Y, Garfinkel P. The Eating Attitudes Test: psychometric features and clinical correlates. *Psychol Med.* 1982;12:871-878.

46. Cooper Z, Fairburn C. The eating disorder examination: a semi-structured interview for the assessment of the specific psychopathlology of eating disorders. *Int J Eat Disord.* 1987;6:1-8.

47. Garner D, Olmsted M, Polivy J. Development and validation of a multidimensional eating disorder inventory for anorexia nervosa and bulimia. *Int J Eat Disord.* 1983;2:15-34.

48. Garner D. *Eating Disorder Inventory-2 Manual.* Odessa, Fl: Psychological Assessment Resources; 1991.

49. Mintz L, O'Halloran M, Mulholland A, Schneider P. Questionnaire for eating disorder diagnosis: reliability and validity of operationalizing DSM-IV criteria into a self-report format. *J Couns Psychol.* 1997;6:485-494.

50. Kosmiski L, Schmiege S, Mascolo M, Gaudiani J, Mehler P. Chronic starvation secondary to anorexia nervosa is associated with an adaptive suppression of resting energy expenditure. *J Clin Endocrinol Metab.* 2014;99(3):908-914.

51. O'Hara CB, Keyes A, Renwick B, Leyton M, Campbell IC, Schmidt U. The effects of acute dopamine precursor depletion on the reinforcing value of exercise in anorexia nervosa. *PLoS One.* 2016;11(1):e0145894.

52. Physical status: the use and interpretation of anthropometry. Report of a WHO expert committee. Technical Report Series No. 854. 1995. World Health Organization website. www.who.int/childgrowth/publications/physical_status/en/. Accessed May 5, 2016.

53. Gaudiani JL, Mehler PS. Rare medical manifestations of severe restricting and purging: "Zebras," missed diagnoses, and best practices. *Int J Eat Disord.* 2016;49(3):331-344.

54. Mehler PS, Krantz MJ, Sachs KV. Treatments of medical complications of anorexia nervosa and bulimia nervosa. *J Eat Disord.* 2015;3:15.

55. Fisher B, Schenkman M. Functional recovery of a patient with anorexia nervosa: physical therapist management in the acute care hospital setting. *Phys Ther.* 2012;92(4):595-604.

56. Binge eating disorder. National Institute of Diabetes and Digestive and Kidney Diseases website. www.niddk.nih.gov/health-information/health-topics/weight-control/binge_eating/Pages/binge-eating-disorder.aspx. Accessed January 1, 2016.

57. Spodick DH. Normal sinus heart rate; appropriate rate thresholds for sinus tachycardia and bradycardia. *South Med J.* 1996;89(7):666-667.

58. Chiu SN, Lin LY, Wang JK, et al. Long-term outcomes of pediatric sinus bradycardia. *J Pediatr.* 2013;163(3):885-889.

59. Yahalom M, Spitz M, Sandler L, Heno N, Roguin N, Turgeman Y. The significance of bradycardia in anorexia nervosa. *Int J Angiol.* 2013;22(2):83-94.

60. Mehler PS, Brown C. Anorexia nervosa–medical complications. *J Eat Disord.* 2015;3:11.

61. Birmingham CL. Medical complications and diagnosing eating disorders. In: Smolak L, Levine MP, eds. *The Wiley Handbook of Eating Disorders*. Chichester, UK: John Wiley & Sons, Ltd; 2015:170-182.

62. D'Souza AD, Bucchi A, Johnsen AB, et al. Exercise training reduces resting heart rate via downregulation of the funny channel HCN4. *Nat Commun.* 2014;5:3775. doi:10.1038/ncomms4775.

63. Campbell K, Peebles R. Eating disorders in children and adolescents: state of the art review. *Pediatrics.* 2014;134(3):582-592.

64. Sidiropoulos M. Anorexia nervosa: the physiological consequences of starvation and the need for primary prevention efforts. *McGill J Med.* 2007;10(1):20-25.

65. Lacy BE, Gabbard SL, Crowell MD. Pathophysiology, evaluation, and treatment of bloating: hope, hype, or hot air? *Gastroenterol Hepatol (NY).* 2011;7(11):729-739.

66. Kleiman SC, Carroll IM, Tarantino LM, Bulik CM. Gut feelings: a role for the intestinal microbiota in anorexia nervosa? *Int J Eat Disord.* 2015;48(5):449-451.

67. Faje AT, Fazeli PK, Miller KK, et al. Fracture risk and areal bone mineral density in adolescent females with anorexia nervosa. *Int J Eat Disord.* 2014;47(5):458-466.

68. Kalm LM, Semba RD. They starved so that others be better fed: remembering Ancel Keys and the Minnesota Experiment. *J Nutr.* 2005;135(6):1347-1352.

69. Hadigan CM, Anderson EJ, Miller KK, et al. Assessment of macronutrient and micronutrient intake in women with anorexia nervosa. *Int J Eat Disord.* 2000;28(3):284-292.

70. Otis CL, Goldingay R. *The Athletic Woman's Survival Guide: How to Win the Battle Against Eating Disorders, Amenorrhea, and Osteoporosis.* Champaign, IL: Human Kinetics Publishers; 2000.

71. Ingjer F, Sundgot-Borgen J. Influence of body weight reduction on maximal oxygen uptake in female elite athletes. *Scand J Med Sci Sports.* 1991;1(3):141-146.

72. Striegel-Moore RH, Bulik CM. Risk factors for eating disorders. *Am Psychol.* 2007;62(3):181-98.

73. Crowther J, Smith KE, Williams GA. Familial risk factors and eating disorders. In: Smolak L, Levine MP, eds. *The Wiley Handbook of Eating Disorders*. Chichester, UK: John Wiley & Sons, Ltd; 2015:338-351.

74. Wildes JE, Forbush KT. Ethnicity as a risk factor for eating disorders. In: Smolak L, Levine MP, eds. *The Wiley Handbook of Eating Disorders*. Chichester, UK: John Wiley & Sons, Ltd; 2015:chap 25.

75. Levine MP, Murnen SK. Media and eating disorders In: Smolak L, Levine MP, eds. *The Wiley Handbook of Eating Disorders*. Chichester, UK: John Wiley & Sons, Ltd; 2015:324-337.

76. Smolak L, Murnen SK, Ruble AE. Female athletes and eating problems: a meta-analysis. *Int J Eat Disord.* 2000;27(4):371-380.

77. Daniels EA. Sex objects, athletes, and sexy athletes: how media representations of women athletes can impact adolescent girls and college women. *J Adolesc Res.* 2009;24(4):399-422.

78. Wolter S. A quantitative analysis of photographs and articles on espnW: positive progress for female athletes. *Commun Sport.* 2015;3(2):168-195.

79. Sundgot-Borgen J, Meyer NL, Lohman TG, et al. How to minimise the health risks to athletes who compete in weight-sensitive sports review and position statement on behalf of the Ad Hoc Research Working Group on Body Composition, Health and Performance, under the auspices of the IOC Medical Commission. *Br J Sports Med.* 2013;47(16):1012-1022.

80. Jacobi C, Abascal L, Taylor CB. Screening for eating disorders and high-risk behavior: caution. *Int J Eat Disord.* 2004;36(3):280-295.

81. Rodgers RF, Franko DL. Screening for eating disorders. In: Smolak L, Levine MP, eds. *The Wiley Handbook of Eating Disorders*. Chichester, UK: John Wiley & Sons, Ltd; 2015:509-523.

82. Knapp J, Aerni G, Anderson J. Eating disorders in female athletes: use of screening tools. *Curr Sports Med Rep.* 2014;13(4):214-218.

83. Lease H, Bond M. Correspondence between alternate measures of maladaptive exercise, and their associations with disordered eating symptomatology. *J Behav Addict.* 2013;2(3):153-159.

84. Bonci CM, Bonci LJ, Granger LR, et al. National athletic trainers' association position statement: preventing, detecting, and managing disordered eating in athletes. *J Athl Train.* 2008;43(1):80-108.

85. Mahr F, Farahmand P, Bixler E, et al. A national survey of eating disorder training *Int J Eat Disord.* 2015;48(4):443-445.

86. National Institute for Health and Care Excellence. Core interventions in the treatment and management of anorexia nervosa, bulimia nervosa and related eating disorders. Clinical Guideline 9. www.nice.org.uk/guidance/cg9. Published 2004. Accessed October 12, 2015.

87. Dalle Grave R, Calugi S, Conti M, Doll H, Fairburn CG. Inpatient cognitive behaviour therapy for anorexia nervosa: a randomized controlled trial. *Psychother Psychosom*. 2013;82(6):390-398.

88. Yager J, Devlin MJ, Halmi KA, et al. American Psychiatric Association. Practice guideline for the treatment of patients with eating disorders. 3rd ed. http://psychiatryonline.org/pb/assets/raw/sitewide/practice_guidelines/guidelines/eatingdisorders.pdf. Published 2006. Accessed October 30, 2015.

89. American Dietetic Association, Dietitians of Canada, American College of Sports Medicine, Rodriguez NR, Di Marco NM, Langley S. American College of Sports Medicine position stand. Nutrition and athletic performance. *Med Sci Sports Exerc*. 2009;41(3):709-731.

90. Tholking MM, Mellowspring AC, Eberle SG, et al. American Dietetic Association: standards of practice and standards of professional performance for registered dietitians (competent, proficient, and expert) in disordered eating and eating disorders (DE and ED). *J Am Diet Assoc*. 2011;111(8):1242-1249.

91. Graves LL, Scribner C. Medical nutrition therapy for eating disorders. In: Smolak L, Levine MP, eds. *The Wiley Handbook of Eating Disorders*. Chichester, UK: John Wiley & Sons, Ltd; 2015:843-858.

92. Mittnacht AM, Bulik C. Best nutrition counseling practices for the treatment of anorexia nervosa: a Delphi study. *Int J Eat Disord*. 2015;48(1):111-122.

93. Beck AT. The past and future of cognitive therapy. *J Psychother Pract Res* 1997;6(4):276-284.

94. Anderson AE, Yager J. Eating disorders. In: Sadock BJ, Sadock VA, Ruiz P, eds. *Kaplan and Sadock's Comprehensive Textbook of Psychiatry*. vol 1. 9th ed. Philadelphia, PA: Lippincott Williams and Wilkins; 2009:2128-2149.

95. Rathaus JH, Miller AL. *DBT Skills Manual for Adolescents*. New York, NY: Guilford Press; 2014.

96. Federici A, Wisniewski L. An intensive DBT program for patients with multidiagnostic eating disorder presentations: a case series analysis. *Int J Eat Disord*. 2013;46:322-331.

97. Federici A, Wisniewski L, Ben-Porath DD. Development and feasibility of an intensive DBT outpatient program for multi-diagnostic clients with eating disorders. *J Couns Dev*. 2012;90:330-338.

98. Gorham E. The use of acceptance and commitment therapy (ACT) in the treatment of eating disorders. Paper presented at: 3rd annual Rocky Mountain Eating Disorders Conference; 2011; Denver, CO.

99. Juarascio A, Shaw J, Forman E, et al. Acceptance and commitment therapy as a novel treatment for eating disorders: an initial test of efficacy and mediation. *Behav Modif*. 2013;37(4):459-489.

100. Ciao AC, Anderson K, Le Grange D. Family approaches to treatment. In: Smolak L, Levine MP, eds. *The Wiley Handbook of Eating Disorders*. Chichester, UK: John Wiley & Sons, Ltd; 2015:828-842.

101. Mettler S, Mitchell N, Tipton KD. Increased protein intake reduces lean body mass loss during weight loss in athletes. *Med Sci Sports Exerc*. 2010;42(2):326-337.

102. Miller WR, Rollnick S. *Motivational Interviewing: Preparing People for Change*. New York, NY: Guilford; 2002.

103. Brauhardt A, de Zwaan M, Hilbert A. The therapeutic process in psychological treatments for eating disorders: a systematic review. *Int J Eat Disord*. 2014;47:565-584.

104. Schulte EM, Joyner MA, Potenza MN, Grilo CM, Gearhardt AN. Current considerations regarding food addiction. *Curr Psychiatry Rep*. 2015;17(4):563.

105. National Institute for Health and Care Excellence. Nutrition support for adults: oral nutrition support, enteral tube feeding and parenteral nutrition. *Clinical Guideline 32*. www.nice.org.uk/guidance/cg32/chapter/1-Guidance. Published February 2006. Accessed August 28, 2016.

106. Rigaud D, Verges B, Colas-Linhart N, et al. Hormonal and psychological factors linked to the increased thermic effect of food in malnourished fasting anorexia nervosa. *J Clin Endocrinol Metab*. 2007;92(5):1623-1629.

107. Castellini G, Castellani W, Lelli L, et al. Association between resting energy expenditure, psychopathology and HPA-axis in eating disorders. *World J Clin Cases*. 2014;2(7):257-264.

108. Mountjoy M, Sundgot-Borgen J, Burke L, et al. The IOC consensus statement: beyond the Female Athlete Triad—Relative Energy Deficiency in Sport (RED-S). *Br J Sports Med*. 2014;48(7):491-497.

109. Nattiv A, Loucks AB, Manore MM, Sanborn CF, Sundgot-Borgen J, Warren MP; American College of Sports Medicine. American College of Sports Medicine position stand. The female athlete triad. *Med Sci Sports Exerc*. 2007;39(10):1867-1882.

110. Mountjoy M, Sundgot-Borgen J, Burke L, et al. RED-S CAT. Relative Energy Deficiency in Sport (RED-S) Clinical Assessment Tool (CAT). *Br J Sports Med*. 2015;49(7):421-423.

111. De Souza MJ, Nattiv A, Joy E, et al. 2014 Female Athlete Triad Coalition consensus statement on treatment and return to play of the female athlete triad: 1st International Conference held in San Francisco, California, May 2012 and 2nd International Conference held in Indianapolis, Indiana, May 2013. *Br J Sports Med.* 2014;48(4):289.

112. Sarris J, Logan AC, Akbaraly TN, et al. Nutritional medicine as mainstream in psychiatry. *Lancet Psychiatry.* 2015;2(3):271-274.

CHAPTER 19

NUTRITION FOR ATHLETES WITH DIABETES
Sally Hara, MS, RDN, CSSD, CDE

INTRODUCTION

The scientific understanding of the interplay between diabetes and physical exercise is rapidly increasing. Our expanding knowledge of the biochemical regulation of muscle metabolism, exercise endocrinology, pathophysiology of diabetes, and exercise prescription allows for better decision making for athletes with diabetes. Likewise, recent research and developments have contributed to many improvements in the treatment of diabetes, including new types of oral and injectable medications, designer insulins, insulin pumps, and continuous glucose monitors, to name a few. As this book goes to print, many new medications and devices are in human trials or are awaiting approval by the US Food and Drug Administration. The many advances in diabetes management have made it possible for people with diabetes to safely partic-

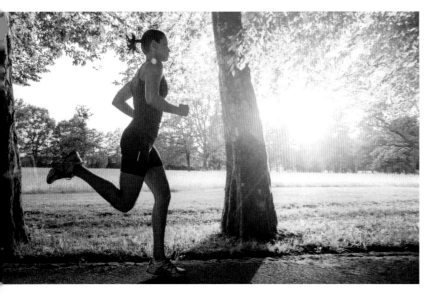

ipate in nearly all levels and types of sports.[1] Consequently, the number of athletes who have diabetes continues to increase. They range from youth and recreational athletes to elite professional, collegiate, and Olympic athletes.[1-4] These athletes are involved in a wide variety of sports and training regimens, each presenting its own unique set of challenges.[1, 5-7] Balancing blood sugar management and athletic performance is challenging. Athletes with diabetes often feel as if they are walking a tightrope, or as one person with type 1 diabetes (T1D) expressed it, "balancing on the edge of a razor blade." Today, athletes with diabetes have opportunities and resources that did not exist even a decade ago, and having the support of knowledgeable professionals can be a significant benefit. A sports dietitian who understands the needs of athletes with diabetes can be a valuable part of the athlete's support team, which typically includes a certified diabetes educator (CDE) and an endocrinologist.

Physical activity affects glucose metabolism and thus has a significant impact on blood glucose control in people with diabetes. Much has been written about the role of exercise as a key component to diabetes management for people with type 2 or gestational diabetes.[8-10] Barring any contraindication, the US government's physical activity recommendation for pregnant women, including those with gestational diabetes, is 150 minutes of moderate exercise per week, unless they were more physically active before pregnancy.[10,11] Similarly, the American College of Sports Medicine and the American Diabetes Association recommend that people with type 2 diabetes (T2D) aim for at least 150 minutes of moderate exercise each week to help improve glucose control. They suggest aerobic exercise intensity of 40% to 70% of VO_2 max and anaerobic exercise for a minimum of one set of 10 to 15 repetitions using 8 to 10 resistance exercises for most people with T2D.[3,9] Such recommendations are intentionally designed to be moderate in intensity to encourage activity sustainable for 20 to 60 minutes to assist with weight loss.

However, managing diabetes in athletes is a complex endeavor that goes beyond simply encouraging physical activity for the purpose of improving blood glucose control.[1,3,5] Athletes with diabetes have two important goals: optimize sports performance and control blood glucose. Professionals working with this population must be aware of both of these goals and must place maintaining the athlete's overall health as a third, equally important, goal. It is common for athletes with diabetes and health professionals to become so focused on blood glucose management that they lose sight of the need to fuel for performance. And, as with many athletes, there is a tendency to become so focused on meeting performance goals that they lose sight of general nutritional needs for good health. When developing a quality sports nutrition plan for athletes with diabetes, it is necessary to consider all three of the aforementioned goals. To do so, the sports dietitian or nutritionist must have a good understanding of sports nutrition, energy metabolism, exercise physiology, exercise endocrinology, and the pathophysiology of the various types of diabetes.

Though there are some general guidelines for exercise and diabetes, most have been developed with sedentary or mildly active individuals in mind and do not allow for many of the variables that competitive athletes need to consider. This chapter will attempt to provide an overview of topics relevant to registered dietitian nutritionists (RDNs) who work with athletes with diabetes and to other professionals involved in such athletes' training, coaching, and medical care.

As with all athletes, the nutritional needs of athletes with diabetes are unique for each person. Factors to consider include the type of diabetes; the progression of the disease; the presence of complications; the type, intensity, and duration of training; the athlete's level of fitness; the type of diabetes medications and their mode of delivery; the individual blood glucose patterns; and the habits of each individual athlete. There is no one-size-fits-all protocol for designing a sports nutrition plan for athletes with diabetes. However, having an understanding of the variables that need to be assessed and how they affect each other will enable RDNs to design nutrition plans that address the needs of athletes with diabetes.

TYPES OF DIABETES

It is estimated that 86 million Americans have prediabetes and 29.1 million have diabetes (about 9.3% of the general population). Of these 29.1 million, 8.1 million are undiagnosed, and 1.25 million have T1D. There are nearly 1.4 million new diagnoses of diabetes in the United States each year, including an estimated 40,000 diagnoses of T1D.[12-14] Professionals working with athletes with diabetes should be aware that the term *diabetes* is used to refer to several diseases, each of which has unique implications for successful management. While it is commonly taught that there are three types of diabetes—type 1, type 2, and gestational—in reality there are at least five major types and numerous rare variations. Understanding the pathophysiology of each of these diseases helps us to accurately anticipate the potential impact of physical activity.

Type 1 Diabetes

Approximately 5% to 10% of people with diabetes have T1D.[13-15] T1D is an autoimmune disease in which the body's immune system produces antibodies that attack the β-cells of the pancreas. Destruction of the β-cells results in an inability to produce insulin and subsequent reliance on exogenous insulin for survival.[15]

Type 2 Diabetes

T2D is a progressive metabolic disease characterized by insulin resistance and decreased insulin secretion.[15] In early stages, blood glucose may be normal due to increased insulin secretion in response to food. This is the body's attempt to compensate for insulin resistance in hepatic and muscle cells, but this reaction is not an effective long-term fix. Over time, insulin resistance in peripheral cells continues to increase, or the pancreas cannot continue to overproduce insulin at the level necessary to maintain normal glucose levels. Consequently, blood glucose levels begin to rise despite normal or high levels of circulating insulin. In this early scenario, people may have metabolic syndrome or prediabetes. As the metabolic disorder progresses, blood glucose continues to climb due to increases in insulin resistance or pancreatic β-cell failure. Genetic predisposition is associated with T2D, but lifestyle can also have a significant influence on its development and the extent and rate of disease progression. Approximately 90% of people with diabetes in the United States have T2D and, of these, about 50% of men and 70% of women are obese when diagnosed.[15] The observed correlation between obesity and T2D is likely due to the confluence of genetic predisposition and unhealthy lifestyle habits.[15] Likely due to the positive effects of physical exercise on insulin sensitivity, T2D is relatively rare in competitive athletes but not unheard of.[3,5]

Gestational Diabetes

Gestational diabetes is also characterized by insulin resistance. It is associated with insulin resistance due to pregnancy and is possibly related to obesity and genetic predisposition.[15] If a woman is diagnosed at her initial prenatal visit, it is assumed the diabetes was a preexisting condition and is classified as overt rather than gestational diabetes. In gestational diabetes, there is a failure to increase β-cell insulin production in response to the increased insulin resistance that typically occurs secondary to hormonal changes associated with pregnancy.

Latent Autoimmune Diabetes in Adults

Latent autoimmune diabetes (LADA) in adults is sometimes referred to as type 1.5 diabetes. It accounts for about 10% of T1D. LADA is classified as a slowly progressing variation of T1D and is often misdiagnosed as T2D. People with LADA may go for many years without the need for exogenous insulin, even though there is a progressive autoimmune deterioration of the pancreatic β-cells.[15] Because LADA has associated insulin resistance, symptoms of diabetes manifest earlier in regards to degree of β-cell failure than in other forms of T1D. LADA is initially controlled with diet but eventually requires a basal-bolus insulin regimen similar to that of classic T1D. As the disease progresses, the pancreas may produce inconsistent quantities of insulin in a manner similar to a prolonged honeymoon phase of newly diagnosed classic T1D. People with LADA are typically over 35 years old and are not obese.

Mature-Onset Diabetes of the Young

Mature-onset diabetes of the young (MODY) accounts for less than 5% of all diabetes cases and usually has its onset during adolescence or young adulthood.[14] It is caused by any number of monogenetic gene mutations that limit the body's ability to produce insulin but do not completely destroy the β-cells. People with MODY generally are not overweight and do not have symptoms associated with metabolic syndrome. Typically, they can be successfully treated with oral agents and do not require exogenous insulin.[16]

Polycystic Ovary Syndrome

Though not a form of diabetes, polycystic ovary syndrome (PCOS) deserves a mention in this chapter because of its shared pathophysiology with T2D and its prevalence among athletes. PCOS is a metabolic disorder characterized by peripheral insulin resistance, menstrual dysfunction, hirsutism, and infertility. It is believed to be a manifestation of metabolic syndrome in women of childbearing age. Thus, women with PCOS are at an increased risk for T2D, dyslipidemia, and chronic low-grade inflammation.[5] There is an associated hormonal imbalance such that women with PCOS typically have abnormally high levels of androgen hormones, including testosterone. The surplus testosterone predisposes these women to increased muscle mass compared with their peers, and it is not uncommon for women with PCOS to be athletic due to their disposition. It is thought that most women with this condition remain undiagnosed.[17-19] The compensatory hyperinsulinemia associated with insulin resistance also predisposes these women to maintain a higher body fat percentage than their peers, which may result in increased pressure from coaches and trainers to lose weight.[17,18] This is often an unrealistic goal that can lead to disordered eating or underfueling. Focus should instead be placed on training and conditioning to improve skill and performance. Irregular menses and reproductive dysfunction are also hallmarks of PCOS and are often mistaken for overtraining or underfueling.[20] Identifying PCOS can be a boon for athletes because it can help explain existing physical symptoms and set them on the right path to treatment. Due to the common occurence of insulin resistance, the management of PCOS is often similar to that of T2D with regards to nutrition therapy and medications.

PHYSIOLOGICAL RESPONSE TO EXERCISE

Energy Metabolism

Understanding how to best fuel athletes with diabetes is a unique challenge. As described in Chapter 1, the amount and type of fuel consumed during exercise is dependent on the type, intensity, and duration of the activity, as well as the available fuel mix and the athlete's degree of physical fitness.

Anaerobic exercise depends almost exclusively on glucose as a fuel source.[1,5,21] To help meet the high demand for glucose during anaerobic exercise, the body augments the glucose supply via glycolysis and gluconeogenesis. Thus, anaerobic activities can potentially increase blood glucose in athletes with diabetes. This rise in blood glucose may be sustained for prolonged periods in some athletes and may be short-lived in others. When glycogen stores begin to deplete, however, there may be a rapid drop in blood glucose, resulting in hypoglycemia.

Aerobic exercise is highly dependent on glucose in the early stages but shifts to a greater dependence on fat as a fuel source as duration increases beyond about 20 minutes. Aerobic exercise is less likely to cause sustained elevated blood glucose because the need for glucose as a fuel source is significantly lower; thus, the liver is not inclined to supplement the glucose supply. A typical blood glucose pattern for endurance athletes who do not have diabetes includes a short initial spike in blood glucose followed by a steady state, then a gradual decline as glycogen stores are depleted, if they are not supplemented with exogenous sources of carbohydrates during exercise. Though most endurance athletes with diabetes also experience the initial rise in blood glucose with the onset of exercise, the pattern that follows will vary depending on the type of diabetes, medications on board, and individual differences unique to each athlete.[1,5,6,21]

Exercise Endocrinology

The energy pathways used during exercise are mediated by hormonal responses to exercise. An understanding of exercise endocrinology and hormonal control of carbohydrate metabolism is essential to accurately predict blood glucose patterns in athletes with diabetes. At the onset of exercise, the catecholamines epinephrine and norepinephrine are released. These, in turn, trigger the secretion of other metabolic hormones including glucagon, growth hormone, and cortisol.[1,6] A summary of these counterregulatory or stress hormones, their actions, and adaptations to exercise can be found in Table 19.1 (page 424). In general, these hormones facilitate the mobilization of metabolic fuels from storage to working muscles. Insulin, by contrast, is a storage hormone that facilitates the transport of fuels into cells. A primary function of insulin is facilitating the transport of glucose into cells where it is either used as an immediate fuel source or stored

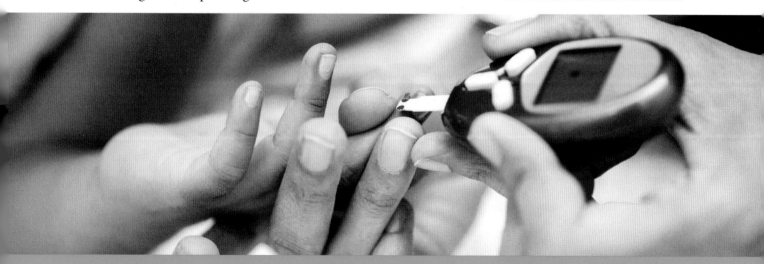

as glycogen (in liver and muscle cells). Insulin also facilitates the uptake of circulating amino acids and free fatty acids into cells and stimulates glycogen synthesis, protein synthesis, and lipogenesis, thus promoting fuel storage. Insulin inhibits the actions of counterregulatory hormones that promote mobilization of fuels out of storage, via lipolysis, proteolysis, and gluconeogenesis processes. Conversely, counterregulatory hormones inhibit insulin production, thus allowing for the mobilization of glucose, amino acids, and free fatty acids to be available to fuel the muscles and brain.[6,22]

Table 19.1 Endocrine Response to Exercise[22]

Hormone	Hormone Effects	Onset of Exercise	Recovery	Adaptation to Exercise
Glucagon	Stimulates hepatic glucose production via glycolysis and gluconeogenesis Stimulates lipolysis Facilitates uptake of free fatty acids (FFAs) Inhibits insulin	Increase	Increase	Smaller increase in glucose levels during exercise at both absolute and relative workloads
Epinephrine	Stimulates muscle and some hepatic glycolysis Mobilizes FFAs from adipose tissue Stimulates hepatic gluconeogenesis Inhibits insulin production	Increase	Increase	Decreased secretion at rest Same exercise intensity
Norepinephrine	Directly stimulates lipolysis Indirectly suppresses glucose utilization Stimulates amino acids(AA) storage	Increase	Nominal	Nominal
Growth hormone	Stimulates hepatic glucose production via glycolysis and gluconeogenesis Stimulates lipolysis Facilitates uptake of FFAs Inhibits insulin	Increase	Nominal	Less dramatic rise during exercise
Cortisol	Mobilizes AAs and glycerol as substrate for hepatic gluconeogenesis Mobilizes FFAs as fuel source for muscles Blocks glucose uptake into adipocytes and muscles	Increase in heavy exercise only	Nominal	Slight elevations during exercise
Insulin	Increases glycogen synthesis Increases lipogenesis Increases AA uptake Increases potassium uptake Decreases proteolysis Decreases gluconeogenesis Decreases renal sodium excretion	Decrease	Dramatic increase	Increased sensitivity to insulin Decrease in insulin during exercise

It is important to understand that insulin production is inhibited at the onset of exercise. While a primary function of insulin is to facilitate the transport of glucose into cells, the mechanism by which this occurs is often oversimplified by educators, who imply that when insulin binds to insulin receptors, it escorts blood glucose into cells. More accurately, when insulin binds to receptors on the surface of cells, the glucose transporter type 4 (GLUT4) within the cell is activated and migrates to the interior surface of the cell membrane. The GLUT4 that actually moves glucose into the cell.

Physical exercise, independent of insulin, also activates GLUT4. Thus, during exercise, insulin is not needed to transport glucose into cells of working muscles, and insulin production is necessarily inhibited to allow the cells to switch from a fuel storage mode to a fuel utilization mode. Additionally, exercising muscles have increased insulin sensitivity, making them more responsive to any insulin that is present.[6] A useful mnemonic analogy is: *Insulin opens the cell doors, and exercise opens the cell windows—both allow glucose into cells.*

During recovery from exercise, glucagon remains high for approximately an hour after exercise. At the cessation of exercise, high concentrations of glucagon and catecholamine are retained, insulin sensitivity of muscles increases, intestinal absorption of glucose increases, and insulin production rebounds. During the hour following exercise, the body is primed to store glycogen. Insulin sensitivity and insulin production remain high for several hours, allowing the body to transport glucose into muscles three to five times faster than normal. The elevated glucagon encourages hepatic glucose production, which is used to replenish muscle glycogen. While fuel storage is most efficient during this phase, completely replenishing glycogen stores can take up to 48 hours postexercise.[6,22]

For athletes with T1D, all insulin is exogenously supplied, so the body does not have the ability to downregulate insulin during exercise. These athletes are, therefore, at greater risk of hypoglycemia secondary to exercise than those who produce their own insulin because some amount of baseline circulating insulin (from injection of long-acting insulin or an insulin pump's basal rate) remains present even after exercise has activated GLUT4 receptors independent of insulin. Using the previously mentioned analogy, this means the cell doors and cell windows are open simultaneously, and insulin sensitivity is high due to exercise, allowing for rapid depletion of blood glucose.[1,6,9,23] Postexercise, athletes with T1D often experience an initial rise in blood glucose, followed by a decrease in blood glucose. The rise is a result of continued hepatic glucose output without the compensatory insulin response that people without diabetes experience. The eventual decrease in blood glucose corresponds with the decreased concentration of stress hormones, in conjunction with increased insulin sensitivity. It is essential to realize that each athlete with T1D has a unique pattern of postexercise glucose response.[1,5,24]

This pattern varies in regards to timing and magnitude of the glucose response. Some athletes with T1D will experience a dramatic spike in blood glucose immediately after exercise, while others may have a delayed rise in blood glucose that could occur up to several hours later. The timing and extent of the post-exercise rise in blood sugar is also dependent on the type of exercise and can vary for different types or intensities of activities for a single athlete.[24] Knowing an athlete's patterns helps to determine how to tailor insulin recommendations and the ideal timing of recovery nutrition. Determining this pattern is most easily performed using a continuous glucose monitor (CGM), though it can be roughly estimated by multiple finger-stick glucose checks postexercise.[25]

In athletes with T2D, insulin sensitivity and insulin secretion will typically be elevated postexercise, as with athletes who do not have diabetes. These athletes typically have a net decrease in blood glucose postexercise. Athletes who have T2D and take insulin will benefit from additional monitoring around exercise and may need to consider reducing their insulin dose if blood glucose is consistently low postexercise.[24]

Training Adaptations

In addition to the acute responses to exercise, training adaptations occur that affect energy metabolism. As an athlete's level of fitness improves, insulin sensitivity increases and exercise-induced insulin secretion declines. There is a decreased secretion of epinephrine and growth hormone response to exercise that subsequently decreases exercise-induced hepatic glucose production.[22]

These adaptations in a person with T2D may result in decreased insulin secretion in response to ingested carbohydrate, decreased levels of circulating insulin between feedings, and a subsequent decreased tendency to store fat. Since hallmarks of T2D are insulin resistance and increased hepatic glucose production, regular exercise, especially exercise that involves large muscle groups, can be an effective tool to manage blood glucose. As training intensity increases and fitness improves, monitoring blood glucose trends and adjusting doses of diabetes medications as appropriate are highly recommended.[1] This is especially important for athletes with T2D who take insulin or oral hypoglycemic agents, such as sulfonylureas, which put them at an increased risk of hypoglycemia. However, even those taking medications such as glucophage may be able to successfully decrease their dose or discontinue their diabetes medications as their fitness improves. This may require negotiating with the prescribing medical provider to decrease the dose in a stepwise progression, bearing in mind that most diabetes specialists lack experience with athletes.

For athletes with T1D, the primary implications of adaptations to exercise include an increased risk of hypoglycemia secondary to increased insulin sensitivity and decreased hepatic glucose production.

DIABETES MANAGEMENT PLAN

Assessment

The initial assessment of an athlete with diabetes should include a number of parameters. Assessing the athlete's understanding of diabetes and readiness to manage it are top priorities. Inquire about the following:

- How often does the athlete check his or her blood glucose?
- What challenges does the athlete encounter in checking blood glucose?
- Can the athlete feel if his or her blood glucose is too high or too low?
- Does the athlete know how to effectively treat hyperglycemia and hypoglycemia?
- Does the athlete understand how diet affects blood glucose and know how to appropriately adjust diet or insulin as dictated by pattern management of blood glucose readings?
- Does the athlete understand how stress (psychological or physiological) can affect blood glucose?
- Does the athlete understand how various types of exercise can affect blood glucose patterns?

Commitment to a diabetes management plan that maintains adequate glycemic control is necessary for safe athletic participation.[1] The preparticipation medical exam should ensure that the athlete is up to date on recommended routine diabetes screenings for cardiovascular disease, renal function, retinopathy, and

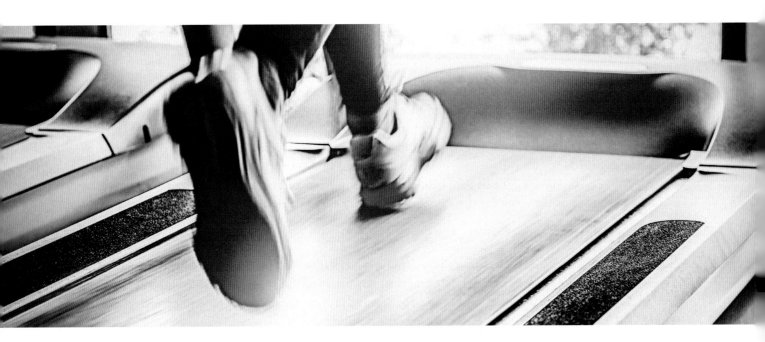

neuropathy (including a diabetic foot exam). Laboratory tests should include fasting blood glucose, hemoglobin A1c, blood lipids, and glomerular filtration rate. Athletes who take metformin should also be screened for vitamin B-12 deficiency.

Glucose Monitoring

The management plan for athletes with diabetes needs to anticipate blood glucose response to training and competition. Thus, self-monitoring of blood glucose (SMBG) is essential. The data from SMBG can be used to determine how to adjust food, medication, and other parameters that may be affecting blood glucose. SMBG and pattern management are critical skills for all athletes with diabetes. Athletes should understand how insulin, exercise, and carbohydrate intake affect their blood glucose values and performance. Frequent monitoring helps identify asymptomatic hypoglycemia or hyperglycemia and allows the individual to treat each situation. Ideally, blood glucose should be between 70 and 150 mg/dL, but realistically, most athletes with T1D maintain a range of 120 to 180 mg/dL. Frequency of monitoring depends on type of diabetes, type of medication, and individual needs. While most athletes with diabetes who are in need of tight control of blood glucose check their blood glucose before each meal and at bedtime, recommendations can vary based on individual needs. Blood glucose goals provided by CDEs or endocrinologists are typically appropriate for the general population of people with diabetes; however, athletes also need to check blood glucose around exercise for safety's sake. With exercise, an athlete with diabetes will benefit from knowing their initial blood glucose concentration as well as its direction and rate of change before exercise. This can be determined by taking at least three blood glucose readings at 20- to 30-minute intervals. The slope of the line created by these blood glucose data points will indicate the rate and direction the blood glucose is trending. This information allows the athlete to make preemptive adjustments to prevent hypoglycemia and hyperglycemia. If possible, it is also advisable to check blood glucose every 30 to 60 minutes during prolonged exercise, within 30 minutes postexercise, and then every 2 to 4 hours after exercise. If preexercise blood glucose is between 100 and 250, it is generally safe to begin training. Athletes who take insulin should check for ketones when blood glucose is greater than 250 mg/dL. If ketones are present, the athlete should avoid exercise and drink water or other noncarbohydrate fluids. If blood glucose is greater than 300 mg/dL and no ketones are present, the athlete may proceed with caution.[5,6] Blood glucose can be measured with finger sticks using a glucometer or with a CGM. For convenience's sake, most serious athletes use a CGM if they are able to safely position a CGM sensor and monitor to accommodate the demands of their sports.

BLOOD GLUCOSE MONITORING WITH A CONTINUOUS GLUCOSE MONITOR

Recently, CGMs have become commonly used by individuals on insulin therapy. The CGM is a small medical device that utilizes a subcutaneous sensor to measure the glucose in interstitial fluid. It collects information every 5 minutes and transmits the sensor glucose value to a receiver. Because the interstitial fluid glucose levels differ slightly from blood glucose, the CGM uses an algorithm to project a blood glucose value from sensor glucose measured values. CGM receivers can be programmed individually for target ranges and will sound an alarm if sensor glucose is too high or too low. To prevent alarm fatigue, it is common for these ranges to be set outside of target blood glucose goals; thus, when the CGM alarm sounds, the individual is more responsive to his or her needs. The receiver provides both a predicted blood glucose value and the blood glucose trend. A standard blood glucose meter gives a single blood glucose value but no predicted direction.[25] Manufacturers suggest that a CGM sensor can be worn for up to 7 days, though this varies among individuals. The use of a CGM does not negate the use of a blood glucose monitor (glucometer). At the time of this printing, CGM technology is less precise than blood glucose monitors. To maximize the accuracy of approximations to blood glucose, CGMs must be calibrated to a blood glucose value every 12 hours (using a glucometer). Additionally, there is a lag time between the equilibration of interstitial glucose and blood glucose of 5 to 15 minutes that a CGM cannot accurately predict. Thus, quickly fluctuating blood glucose values in an athlete may present a significant obstacle to accurate readings.[26] As such, glucose values measured on a CGM should be verified by a glucometer and should not be used for estimating insulin needs. The value of a CGM is its usefulness in tracking instantaneous blood glucose trends. It gives the user the ability to identify the direction and rate that their blood glucose is trending, which is extremely helpful for adjusting insulin and carbohydrate intake before blood glucose is out of control. However, a glucose meter and standard SMBG practices should be used to accurately quantify CGM data.[27] The most useful information provided by CGMs is the direction and rate of change in blood glucose and the blood glucose alarm—especially when it may prevent a potentially fatal overnight low.

Noninsulin Diabetes Medications

Noninsulin pharmacologic diabetes therapies are used primarily to treat T2D, though some are also used to treat PCOS, gestational diabetes, and other types of diabetes. The majority of these are oral medications, but there are also a few noninsulin injectables. A list of these medications can be found in Table 19.2, along with a brief description of the functions, alternative names, and considerations for athletes with diabetes.

Table 19.2 Diabetes Medications and Considerations for Athletes[28]

Drug Class and Uses	Generic and Brand Names	Delivery	Considerations for Athletes
Biguanides 　Decrease hepatic glucose output 　Formerly a T2D[a] medication; now used in T1D[b], gestational diabetes mellitus, and polycystic ovary syndrome	Metformin (Glucophage, Glumetza, Fortamet)	Oral pill	May contribute to vitamin B-12 deficiency
Sulfonylureas 　Stimulate β-cell insulin release over sustained time 　T2D medication	Glyburide (Micronase, Diabeta, Glynase) Glipizide (Glucotrol) Glimepiride (Amaryl)	Oral pill	Significant contribution to hypoglycemia, especially in conjunction with exercise
DPP-4 inhibitors[c] 　Prolong action of native glucagon-like peptide action in which gastric emptying is delayed and insulin secretion is stimulated	Sitagliptin (Januvia) Saxagliptin (Onglyza) Linagliptin (Tradjenta) Alogliptin (Nesina)	Oral pill	No hypoglycemia
SGLT2[d] inhibitors 　"Glucoretic" 　Increase glucose excretion in urine 　T2D medication	Canagliflozin (Invokana) Empagliflozin (Jardiance) Dapagliflozin (Farxiga) Ipragliflozin (Suglat)	Oral pill	Hypotension
Thiazolidinediones 　Increase insulin sensitivity at muscle 　T2D medication	Pioglitazone (Actos) Rosiglitazone (Avandia)	Oral pill	May increase peripheral fracture risk
Meglitinides 　Stimulate rapid insulin burst	Repaglinide (Prandin) Nateglinide (Starlix)	Oral pill	Hypoglycemia
Dopamine receptor agonists 　Reset circadian rhythm 　T2D medication	Bromocriptine mesylate (Cycloset)	Oral pill	Hypotension

Continued on next page

Table 19.2 Diabetes Medications and Considerations for Athletes[28] (Continued)

Drug Class and Uses	Generic and Brand Names	Delivery	Considerations for Athletes
Glucosidase inhibitors Delay carbohydrate absorption	Acarbose (Precose) Miglitol (Glyset)	Oral pill	Does not cause hypoglycemia, but if hypoglycemia occurs, treatment is with dextrose or pure glucose; also reconsider carbohydrate sources for fueling
Incretin mimetics Stimulate glucose-dependent insulin release, slow gastric emptying, suppress glucagon release, promote satiety T2D medication; used "off label" for T1D	Exenatide (Byetta) Exenatide XR (Bydureon) Liraglutide (Victoza) Dulaglutide (Trulicity) Albiglutide (Tanzeum)	Injectable, twice a day, once a day, or once a week	Does not cause hypoglycemia, but the athlete's fuel plan for event may need to be altered due to decreased appetite and suppressed glucagon release
Amylins Mimetic Slows gastric emptying, suppresses glucagon release, promotes satiety T1D medication or T2D with insulin use	Pramlintide (Symlin)	Injectable before meals	Does not cause hypoglycemia; may occur concomitantly with insulin Insulin dose must be reduced when using pramlintide and reduced further with exercise and pramlintide

[a] T1D = type 1 diabetes
[b] T2D = type 2 diabetes
[c] DPP-4 = dipeptidyl peptidase 4
[d] SGLT2 = sodium-glucose cotransporter 2

Insulin Supplementation

The principles of obtaining euglycemia are the same for athletes with T1D and athletes with T2D: adjusting carbohydrates, insulin, and exercise.[29] The RDN or sports nutritionist is often adept at adjusting carbohydrates for exercise, but it is beyond the scope of practice for most RDNs to prescribe insulin adjustments. Thus, consulting with a CDE for insulin adjustment recommendations is suggested. There are several types of insulin available for diabetes management. The onset, peak, and duration of the types of insulin being used by an athlete are important considerations when assessing factors contributing to blood glucose fluctuations. It is appropriate to consult with the athlete's diabetes treatment team before making recommendations for insulin adjustments. Be mindful that health care providers often assume that individuals who take insulin know how to properly adjust their insulin doses. Unfortunately, this is not always true, especially for those who have not had access to a CDE. Trial and error alone is generally inadequate education for diabetes self-management.

Insulin can be divided into three general categories: basal, bolus, and mixed. Basal insulin is a long-acting insulin designed to mimic the glycogenic response of the liver, providing a relatively steady baseline amount of insulin. It is commonly provided via a once-daily injection or insulin pump. Bolus insulin is a fast-acting insulin taken specifically to keep blood glucose levels under control when food is consumed or to correct hyperglycemia. Mixed insulin is a combination of fast-acting and long-acting insulin that is taken by an injection one or two times daily. It is primarily used by people with T2D who require supplemental insulin. It lacks the dosing flexibility required by most people with T1D. Basal-bolus therapy describes regimens utilizing both basal (long-acting) and bolus (fast-acting) insulins that are designed to closely mimic physiologic secretion.[30] Table 19.3 (page 430) provides a description of common types of insulin.

Table 19.3 Types of Insulin[a,30,31]

Action of Insulin	Insulin Name	Onset	Peak	Duration
Bolus: Rapid acting	Aspart (NovoLog) Lispro (Humalog) Glulisine (Apidra)	5–15 min	30–90 min	<5 h
Bolus: Ultra rapid acting; inhaled human insulin	Afrezza	12–15 min	30 min	2.5 h
Bolus: Short acting	Regular	30–60 min	2–3 h	5–8 h
Basal: Intermediate	Isophane insulin (NPH)	2–4 h	4–10 h	10–16 h
Basal: Long acting	Detemir (Levemir)	3–8 h	No peak	6–24 h
Basal: Long acting	Glargine (Lantus) Glargine (Toujeo)	2–4 h 6 h	No peak No peak	20–24 h 24–32 h
Basal: Long acting	Degludec (Tresiba)	30–90 min	No peak	42 h
Bolus + basal: Intermediate + rapid acting	NovoLog Mix 70/30 Humalog mix 75/25	5–15 min	Dual peaks	10–16 h
Bolus + basal: Intermediate + short acting	NPH plus regular combination 70/30 50/50	30–60 min	Dual peaks	10–16 h

[a] Because insulin action times can vary with each injection, time periods listed are general guidelines only.

MULTIPLE DAILY INJECTIONS

Multiple daily injections (MDIs), a type of basal-bolus therapy, attempts to mimic normal pancreatic insulin secretion. As the name implies, the therapy requires several insulin injections or inhaled insulin doses per day. These insulin doses are timed to approximate normal insulin patterns, with a sustained basal level in the background and supplemental insulin boluses to accommodate carbohydrate consumption and to correct hyperglycemia. Injections are given via an insulin pen or a vial and syringe. An insulin pen is a discrete unit that has a self-contained insulin cartridge and a dial for adjustable dosing.[31]

INSULIN PUMP

An insulin pump is a small computerized device that infuses insulin subcutaneously through a tiny catheter, allowing for more precise management of insulin dosing than MDIs and tighter control of blood glucose. Insulin pumps are primarily used for managing T1D and for insulin-dependent T2D. To maximize blood glucose control, insulin pumps must be properly programmed and adjusted for individual needs. An athlete's physiological insulin requirements may be altered as demands of training, level of conditioning, and body weight change. Female athletes may also find variations in insulin needs relative to menstrual cycle phases, especially during the premenstrual phase when there is often increased insulin resistance and subsequent hyperglycemia. Insulin pumps allow for more tailored basal insulin coverage than injections of long-acting insulin.[32] Insulin pumps use only rapid-acting insulins and are programmed to deliver a small continuous infusion of basal insulin. This basal rate is calculated based on the amount of long-acting insulin that would otherwise be used as basal insulin, distributed over 24 hours. For example, if an individual were switching from MDIs to a pump and taking 24 units of Lantus (long-acting insulin) daily, the basal rate for a pump might start at 1.0 unit/h, giving a total of 24 units in 24 hours. However, infused rapid-acting insulin is absorbed more efficiently in hourly increments than single-dose, injected, long-acting insulin, so a CDE may recommend that the pump be programmed with 75% of the current long-acting insulin amount; thus, the hourly infusion rate of rapid-acting insulin for this individual would be (24 units × 0.75)/24 hours = 0.75 unit/h. One useful, and often underutilized, feature of insulin pumps is their ability to be programmed with multiple basal rates within a single day to accommodate variations in insulin sensitivity. For example, people who are consistently more insulin resistant in the early morning (the dawn phenomenon) are able to program a higher than usual basal insulin rate for the early morning hours to prevent elevated blood glucose. Athletes are able to set temporary basal rates to accommodate the physiological changes that occur around training. This allows for improved diabetes management and improved athletic performance due to more stable blood glucose. Athletes with T1D will often decrease their basal rate during training or competition, especially for endurance sports. However it is not advised for athletes with insulin pumps to disconnect from pump therapy for greater than 1 hour. Disconnecting for longer than 1 hour puts the athlete at increased risk for hyperglycemia and ketones due to the missed basal insulin dose. In addition to basal rates, insulin pumps are programmed to accommodate the wearer's unique response to food and insulin by setting an insulin-to-carbohydrate ratio (ICR) and an insulin sensitivity factor (ISF). These are highly individualized calculations that are agreed upon by the CDE and prescribing physician. The ICR estimates how many units of insulin per gram of carbohydrate ingested are required for glycemic control. The ISF estimates how much 1 unit of insulin will decrease blood glucose independent of eating. (ISF is sometimes calculated for 0.5 units if the individual has high insulin sensitivity.) It is important to note that both of these variables can be dynamic for athletes because insulin sensitivity and insulin-independent absorption of blood glucose are affected by exercise and stress (short term) and by adaptation of training. See Table 19.4 for an example of insulin pump settings.

Table 19.4 Example of Insulin Pump Settings[27]

Basal Rates[a]	Insulin:Carbohydrate Ratio[b]		Sensitivity[c]		Insulin Action[d]
12 AM: 0.50 u/h	12 AM	1:12	12 am	1:40	4 h
4 AM: 0.55 u/h	12 PM	1:14			
8 AM: 0.40 u/h	5 PM	1:10			
4 PM: 0.45 u/h					
10 PM: 0.50 u/h					

[a] Units delivered per hour.
[b] One unit of insulin covers (x) grams of carbohydrates.
[c] One unit of insulin not assigned to carbohydrates lowers blood sugar by (x) mg/dL.
[d] Time assumed one bolus of insulin is active once infused.

ACTIVE INSULIN

Active insulin is defined as the calculated amount of insulin remaining for a period of time post bolus or injection. It is also commonly referred to as insulin on board. Duration of insulin action refers to how long a bolus of insulin will lower blood glucose. It typically takes at least 4 to 6 hours for all of the insulin action from a bolus of insulin to stop decreasing blood glucose. Taking more insulin while there is still active insulin on board has an additive effect referred to as *stacking insulin doses*. It is one of the most common causes of hypoglycemia.[23] When programming insulin pumps, CDEs take into consideration peak insulin action and duration of insulin action to minimize low blood glucose caused by stacking. Other factors considered when programming insulin pumps are individual differences in insulin sensitivity, insulin clearance, and gastric emptying. A CDE may program an insulin pump to accommodate for such differences by decreasing the dosage interval for an athlete who has high insulin sensitivity or by increasing it for individuals with gastroparesis or renal insufficiency, who are less efficient at clearing blood glucose and/or insulin from their system. It is more difficult to estimate active insulin of individuals on MDI insulin therapy than for those using insulin pumps.

TRAVEL AND STORAGE

Many types of insulin are stable at room temperature for up to 28 days, after which they must be discarded. It is best to refrigerate insulin until needed (36°F to 46°F). Do not freeze insulin; this will decrease its effectiveness.[23,33] Athletes in cold-weather sports who carry insulin with them should keep it in an inside pocket to insulate it from potentially freezing temperatures. In general, insulin exposed to extreme temperatures may lose its effectiveness. A diabetes management plan should include specific strategies for storing insulin at appropriate temperatures.[34] This can be done by storing it in an insulated bag, special insulin storage containers with freezer packs, or a convenient type of light-weight carrying case, which, when soaked in water, keeps insulin cool for up to 48 hours.[35] To avoid exposure to extreme temperatures, insulin and other medications should be kept with the person they are prescribed for and not in a cargo hold when traveling.[5] It is also advisable that these athletes carry a written copy of all prescriptions, extra diabetes supplies, and food that can be used to treat hypoglycemia or used as a small meal should the need arise.[36]

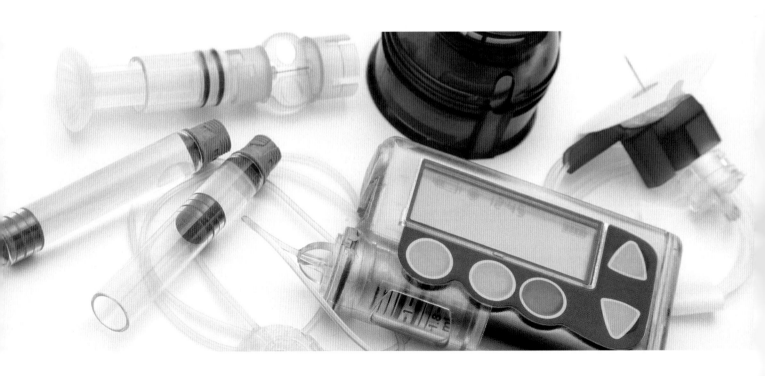

GLYCEMIC CONTROL AND SPORT PERFORMANCE

A primary concern for managing athletes with diabetes is preventing acute complications of hypoglycemia and hyperglycemia.[1] There is no singe means to do this. The type of diabetes, duration, intensity and type of exercise, and various medications can each affect glycemic control.

Preventing and Managing Hypoglycemia

Exercise may increase risk of hypoglycemia in individuals who take insulin or insulin secretagogues (which enhance insulin production) if the medication dose or carbohydrate ingestion are not carefully adjusted. This is due to the insulin-independent ability of exercise to lower blood glucose. Consumption of carbohydrate is advised around exercise if blood glucose value is below 120 mg/dL. Some endurance athletes may find that drinking whole milk before exercise can effectively stabilize their blood glucose, presumably because of the mix of macronutrients it contains. Some athletes who have a known pattern of significant blood glucose declines during exercise often find it necessary to start exercise with a blood glucose that is above their normally recommended blood glucose range, especially if they are participating in sports during which they will be unable to ingest carbohydrate. For athletes who take insulin, knowing how much active insulin is on board helps to accurately predict additional carbohydrate needs.[23]

However, when there is a consistent pattern of hypoglycemia in response to exercise, it is preferable, and often possible, to prevent this by adjusting insulin or other medications. If an athlete has a clear pattern of hypoglycemic tendencies during or after exercise, it is prudent to decrease insulin to proactively prevent hypoglycemic events. For athletes who use insulin pumps, this is often achieved by temporarily decreasing the basal insulin. The extent and timing of the temporary adjustment will depend on the individual athlete's typical blood glucose patterns, which give an indication of changes in the ISF around exercise. The degree to which athletes need to decrease basal insulin varies greatly. Some will reduce by 10%; others may reduce by 70%. Individual insulin sensitivity and endocrine response to types of exercise are significant variables affecting insulin needs around exercise. Many athletes find it helpful to decrease basal insulin 30 to 60 minutes before exercise to effectively limit active insulin on board and to increase back to a normal basal rate near the cessation of exercise, based on their historical blood glucose trends around exercise.[3] Data from a CGM can be useful in identifying blood glucose patterns for individual athletes and subsequently adjusting insulin dosing accordingly.

Following exercise, athletes on insulin therapy often experience late-onset hypoglycemia.[1,5] This can occur within a few hours of exercise but often manifests as decreased overnight blood glucose and is typically most pronounced following prolonged or particularly intense exercise. Determining each athlete's blood glucose pattern around exercise is key to preventing delayed hypoglycemic events. If an athlete has a known pattern of low overnight blood sugars following intense workouts, it may be prudent to decrease the overnight basal rate on an insulin pump or decrease the long-acting bedtime insulin dose for those using MDIs. It is also common for athletes to experience lower blood glucose the following day. This pattern is common in T1D endurance athletes after an event such as a triathlon, marathon, century cycle, or mountain climb. CGM can be extremely useful for detecting delayed hypoglycemia and alerting the wearer in time to treat it.

MILD AND MODERATE HYPOGLYCEMIA

Hypoglycemia is defined as a blood glucose value less than 70 mg/dL. Symptoms of mild hypoglycemia may include an urgency to eat, nervousness, shakiness, or excessive perspiration.[37] If blood glucose continues to decline, neurologic symptoms of moderate hypoglycemia will arise. These symptoms typically correspond to blood glucose less than 55 mg/dL and may include changes in mood, such as irritability, anxiety, restlessness, or anger; confusion; difficulty concentrating; blurred vision; dizziness; headache; low energy; poor coordination; slurred speech; or decreased communication.[5,23,38,39] Because not all individuals have the same signs and symptoms, it is advisable to ask athletes with diabetes how they personally react when their blood glucose is low and how they would like teammates and coaching staff to respond when symptoms are noticed.

This is an important part of the diabetes care plan because it is possible for individuals with diabetes to have hypoglycemia unawareness, in which case they do not experience the physical symptoms of hypoglycemia and may not recognize it. Mood, behavior, and judgment are still typically impaired, making recognition of such signs by colleagues a valuable asset. Factors that contribute to hypoglycemia unawareness include having diabetes for many years, a recent history of frequent low blood glucose, a rapid decline in blood glucose, a hypoglycemic event within the previous 24 to 48 hours, stress or depression, alcohol consumption within the previous 12 hours, or use of β-blockers.[23] Conversely, individuals may sometimes experience symptoms of hypoglycemia when blood glucose is within normal range. This can happen if their body is used to chronically high blood glucose or if blood glucose is dropping rapidly. If an athlete has blood glucose within normal range but is experiencing symptoms of hypoglycemia due to a rapid drop in blood glucose, it may be prudent to take action to prevent further decline in blood glucose.

Suspected hypoglycemia should be confirmed with measured blood glucose values before treatment. Blood glucose data obtained via a finger stick and glucometer or current CGM data can be used to verify true hypoglycemia or a significant downward trend, which warrant treating. In most cases of mild and moderate hypoglycemia, individuals are able to self-treat hypoglycemic events using the 15:15 rule. This simple protocol suggests consuming 15 g of a quick-acting carbohydrate source, such as glucose tablets, gel, or juice, then rechecking blood glucose after 15 minutes. If blood glucose has not responded to treatment, the protocol is repeated until blood glucose is within acceptable limits.[28,40] The physiological effects of hypoglycemia lag behind the treated blood glucose as it is on the rise. The 15-minute checks verify that blood glucose is indeed returning to acceptable limits. The second check helps ensure that the individual did not overcorrect and end up with rebounded high blood glucose. In anticipation of such events, an athlete's diabetes management plan should stipulate having a source of quick-acting carbohydrate readily available at all times.

If an athlete is experiencing low blood glucose and is responsive but has no rapid uptake carbohydrate source available, performing a quick bout of intense exercise (eg, 10 jumping jacks) may cause the body to release its own glucagon to stimulate hepatic glucose production and result in a temporary increase in blood glucose. This alternative method will not be effective if glycogen stores are depleted, but in many instances it does have the desired effect.

SEVERE HYPOGLYCEMIA

Severe hypoglycemia typically occurs when blood glucose falls below 35 to 40 mg/dL and the individual is nonresponsive or too debilitated to self-treat with oral carbohydrate.[39] Symptoms of severe hypoglycemia may include an altered state of consciousness, coma, seizure, or hypothermia.[5,37,39] Severe hypoglycemia is a medical emergency demanding immediate attention. In some cases it may be treated orally with assistance from others, but if the patient cannot safely swallow or is unable to cooperate, a glucagon injection may be necessary.[28] Athletes with diabetes who take insulin should have a glucagon kit readily available during training and competition, and their diabetes plan should have designated individuals who are trained to prepare and administer it if needed. The glucagon kit is available by prescription and consists of a syringe of saline that must be freshly mixed into a small vial of dry glucagon powder before injection.[23] It is injected into the buttocks, thigh, or deltoid and works immediately to increase blood glucose by stimulating production and release of glucose from the liver.[23,28,39] Effectiveness may be impaired if liver function is compromised by recent consumption of alcohol or by hepatic disease.[39]

Preventing and Managing Hyperglycemia

Hyperglycemia is simply defined as blood glucose above normal. The normal blood glucose range may vary between athletes but is generally defined as blood glucose of 70 to 120 mg/dL. While transient hyperglycemia is not uncommon, prolonged or extreme hyperglycemia is a cause for concern. Chronic high blood glucose (ie, blood glucose >250 mg/dL) can result in long-term complications, including damage to nerves, eyes, kidneys, and blood vessels. Common symptoms of chronic hyperglycemia are fatigue, thirst, frequent urination, and possible urinary tract or genital yeast infections. People with chronic hyperglycemia may not feel well but can continue usual daily activities. By contrast, episodes of acute hyperglycemia can be life threatening. Signs and symptoms of progressing hyperglycemia may include nausea, dehydration, reduced cognition, slowed visual reaction time, and fatigue. Severe hyperglycemia may result in diabetic ketoacidosis (DKA), with possible additional symptoms that include rapid breathing, fruity odor to the breath, extreme fatigue/sleepiness, inattentiveness, decreased appetite, increased thirst, and frequent urination.[28,41] Most commonly associated with T1D, though possible with other types, DKA is due to insufficient insulin to transport glucose into cells and results in metabolic acidosis, severe dehydration, and electrolyte imbalance. Any action that increases blood glucose and decreases insulin action can contribute to the development of DKA.[28] Athletes with T1D are advised to have urine ketone strips or a ketone meter available to test for ketoacidosis when blood glucose is excessively high.[41] In athletes with T2D, hyperosmolar hyperglycemic state (HHS) is the most common form of acute hyperglycemic illness. HHS is the result of high blood glucose (>600 mg/dL) compounded by profound dehydration (plasma osmo-

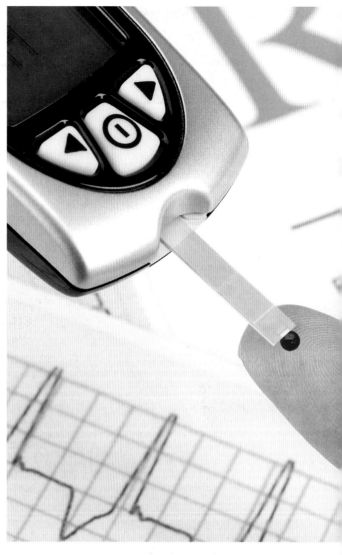

lality >320 mOsm/kg). There may be associated loss of 12% or more of body weight. Symptoms of HHS are similar to those of DKA but with the notable absence of ketones.[28] Both DKA and HHS are life threatening and require immediate treatment. The goals of treatment include rehydrating, restoring electrolyte balance, and providing insulin to normalize blood glucose. Prevention of severe hyperglycemia includes attention to hydration. Exercising with ketones is dangerous and can lead to DKA. Athletes with blood glucose levels greater than 250 mg/dL without ketones should hydrate to help bring blood glucose into a desired range. If athletes have glucose levels greater than 250 mg/dL with ketones, they should treat with insulin and hydration and not exercise until ketones are cleared.

Exercise-induced hyperglycemia is most often associated with short-duration, high-intensity exercise that stimulates endogenous production of glucose in the liver. Any type of physiological or psychological stress can also contribute to elevated blood glucose due to the action of stress hormones. Thus, an illness, injury, inflammation, pain, or even pre-event jitters can influence blood glucose. In most such cases, blood glucose will decline without intervention after the cessation of exercise, so caution should be used when considering treating hyperglycemia with insulin because this may result in subsequent hypoglycemia.[5,6,41,42] Hyperglycemia can also occur if an insulin pump fails, if the insulin is expired or spoiled from extreme temperature exposure, or if the injection site is bad due to excessive scar tissue. In these instances, it is entirely appropriate to provide the missing insulin to correct the hyperglycemia. The diabetes management plan should include protocols for treating hyperglycemia using a sliding scale for insulin based on the insulin sensitivity of the individual athletes. Bear in mind that insulin sensitivity may increase around exercise, decreasing the amount of insulin needed to correct elevated blood glucose.

Nutrition Prescription for Athletes with Diabetes

Sports nutrition plans for athletes with diabetes, as for any athletes, must be tailored to meet individual needs. Athletes with diabetes have the same basic nutritional needs as nonathletes with diabetes, which means their carbohydrate and energy requirements are higher than those of nonathletes who have diabetes. Nutrition strategies differ depending on the type of diabetes. Unfortunately, many diabetes educators do not understand exercise endocrinology or the unique nutritional needs of athletes. The most common mistake made by athletes with diabetes is to restrict carbohydrates as a means to control blood glucose. By doing so, they often compromise athletic performance in favor of well-controlled blood glucose. This is not a necessary compromise.

NUTRITION PRESCRIPTION

Athletes with T2D, PCOS, and MODY will need to adjust carbohydrate intake to manage blood sugar. However, carbohydrate recommendations should be kept as close to those of nonathletes with diabetes as possible to help meet performance needs. Strategies that maximize carbohydrate intake and control blood glucose focus on distributing carbohydrates throughout the day. Often this means timing larger carbohydrate intake at the times of day when insulin sensitivity is highest, such as evening and postexercise. Because there may be a need to limit, but not overrestrict, carbohydrate in T2D, there is often more emphasis on "just-in-time fueling" for these athletes. This simply means that they may need to intentionally fuel just before and during exercise to provide fuel for optimal performance. This is suggested because they are not able to efficiently process relatively large doses of carbohydrate, so their glycogen stores are likely to be smaller than those of athletes who do not have diabetes.

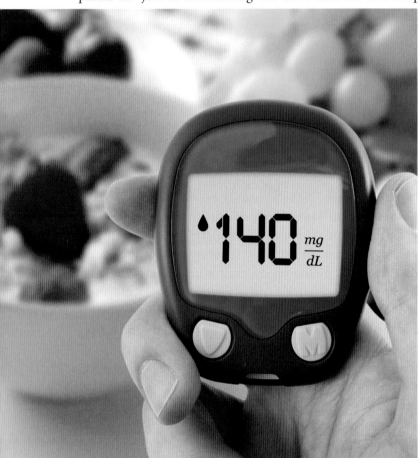

TYPE I DIABETES NUTRITION PRESCRIPTION

For athletes with T1D, insulin is adjusted to fit the recommended sports nutrition plan. It is important to realize that insulin is a prescription medication, and only providers who are qualified to prescribe it can legally make adjustments to an athlete's insulin prescription. It is advisable to consult with a CDE or endocrinologist when insulin adjustments are deemed necessary. That said, most CDEs and endocrinologists are not well acquainted with exercise endocrinology and the nutritional needs of athletes, so they will likely benefit from the expertise and guidance of a professional who is skilled in sports nutrition prescriptions.

When working with athletes with T1D, the sports dietitian must first consider the sports nutritional needs of the athlete and design a nutrition plan appropriate for the athlete's sport, preferences, and training. One must be mindful that athletes with diabetes do not have the option of carbohydrate loading in the traditional sense. If an athlete with T1D attempted to significantly increase carbohydrate intake in the days preceding a sporting event (ie, carbohydrate loading), the athlete would have to significantly alter his or her insulin dosing to accommodate this. Doing so would risk compromising blood glucose control and training. The better approach for athletes with diabetes is to find a macronutrient balance and energy level that meets their training needs and focus more on keeping their glycogen stores topped off rather than maximized. This will mean just-in-time fueling strategies must be built into their nutrition plans, and timing and distribution of foods—especially carbohydrate food sources—may be more important than for nonathletes with diabetes. The most common mistake made by athletes with diabetes is excessive restriction of carbohydrates. Many have been taught that limiting carbohydrate is necessary for managing blood sugars. In athletes with T1D, it is often necessary to titrate carbohydrate up to the estimated amount needed for optimizing performance, making corresponding incremental adjustments in insulin in the process.

ADJUSTING INSULIN

Adjusting insulin is not in the scope of practice of the RDN; however, an RDN or CDE may be able to make minor adjustments that are protected by protocol. Regardless, understanding how and when adjustments are made can help when coordinating care and communicating with the diabetes management team. Adjustments for exercise are usually focused around a reduction of insulin delivery. There are many published sources for guidelines.[1,3,43-49] The guidelines suggest a reduction in basal rates in pumps by 25% to 50% before exercise, during exercise, and for a period after exercise. Basal injections can be reduced as well. It is also recommended that mealtime boluses before exercise be reduced in anticipation of the insulin-independent reduction of blood glucose associated with many types of exercise. This may result in a slightly elevated pre-exercise blood glucose but will help ensure that adequate glucose is available to fuel active muscles during exercise and will help prevent exercise-induced hypoglycemia.

While it is common for athletes and those helping to manage their diabetes to adjust food intake to prevent or treat exercise-related hypoglycemia, this is not typically the best approach for optimizing athletic performance. Athletes with T1D have the same general sports nutritional needs as athletes without diabetes.[3] Thus, their nutrition plan needs to be set to support their training and competition goals. Recommendations for macronutrients and nutrient timing before and during exercise are similar to those for their peers without diabetes. Once the training diet is constructed, the insulin can be adjusted accordingly. Athletes with T1D are often in the habit of adjusting their diet to manage blood glucose around exercise, but restricting intake can lead to compromised athletic performance or recovery. Many athletes with T1D habitually begin exercise with blood glucose in the range of 200 to 350 mg/dL, with the intent of avoiding exercise-induced hypoglycemia. If this is a consistent practice, it is usually more appropriate to decrease basal or long-acting insulin than to eat to keep up with the medication. Athletes who use an insulin pump can set a temporary basal rate that is decreased about 20 to 60 minutes before exercise and during exercise. For those prone to blood glucose spikes immediately after exercise, turning the basal rate back up about 30 minutes before the end of exercise can help normalize postexercise blood glucose. For those who have a delayed postexercise blood glucose spike, the timing and duration of the temporary basal rate may necessarily differ to accommodate individual blood glucose patterns around exercise. There is no one-size-fits-all recommendation for insulin adjustments.[1,3,5] The size, duration, and timing of insulin adjustments must be tailored to individual athletes. As mentioned previously, the type, duration, and intensity of exercise will influence blood glucose levels around exercise, as will the amount of stored glycogen, nutrient timing, stress factors surrounding exercise, and individual differences. Athletes with T1D are often heard saying, "This is what I do, but your mileage may vary." Athletes with T1D on MDIs sometimes benefit from decreasing their long-acting insulin and adjusting their mealtime insulin as needed to manage blood glucose on exercise days. Recreational athletes on MDIs sometimes choose to take their long-acting insulin in the morning rather than at bedtime so they can be more spontaneous about outdoor activities that may be weather dependent. Optimizing both blood glucose and athletic performance, including fueling to make exercise easier and more enjoyable, requires an understanding of the blood glucose patterns around exercise of individual athletes so that nutrient timing and insulin dosing and timing can be adjusted to best support the unique needs of each athlete.

T1D is a complex autoimmune disease that has many associated risks and complications. Professionals who work with athletes with T1D benefit from being informed about adjunct concerns that may affect these athletes. Knowing about special considerations helps professional recognize and be prepared to address these issues if needed.

Autoimmune Disorders

Professionals working with athletes with T1D should be aware that these individuals are at an increased risk for other autoimmune diseases. Because of common genetic predisposition and the interplay between environmental and immunologic factors, individuals with T1D are at a higher risk for developing other autoimmune disorders than the general population.[50,51]

CELIAC DISEASE

Celiac disease is one of the most common coexisting autoimmune diseases for people with T1D. The reported incidence varies between 3% and 16%, with a mean of 8%.[50-53] People with celiac disease cannot tolerate gluten. The immune response to gluten damages the inner lining of the small intestine, resulting

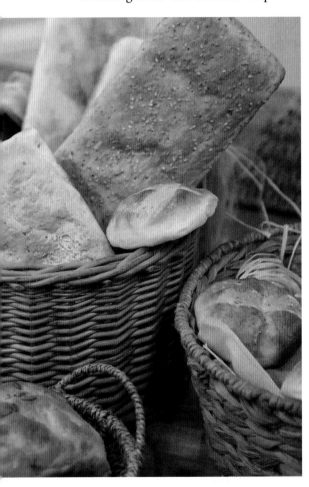

in malabsorption of nutrients and often gastrointestinal (GI) distress.[54] Most cases of celiac disease among people with T1D are diagnosed within 5 years of the initial diagnosis of T1D, but onset of celiac disease is not limited to this time frame. It is recommended that people with T1D be screened for celiac disease at initial diagnosis and within the next 2 to 5 years.[53] Cohn and colleagues from the University of Chicago Department of Medicine recommend screening annually for the first 4 years after initial T1D diagnosis, then every 2 years for the next 6 years.[50] Thereafter, screening for celiac disease is not generally part of standard protocols unless an individual presents with suspicious signs or symptoms.[50,53] Classic symptoms of celiac disease include diarrhea, GI bloating, possible weight loss, and failure to thrive and delayed puberty in children. Nonclassic symptoms may include constipation, neuropathy, ataxia, and heartburn. Not everyone with celiac disease experiences GI symptoms. In fact, the majority of people with T1D who have celiac disease do *not* present with classic symptoms or may have only very mild GI symptoms, which can be overlooked. Other possible indicators of celiac disease are iron-deficiency anemia and low bone density.[50] These clinical signs are a result of poor micronutrient absorption secondary to inflamed and damaged intestinal villa. Because anemia and low bone density (often identified as a result of stress fractures) are not uncommon in athletes, it is very important for sports dietitians to be aware of this possible non–sports-related etiology of these conditions, especially in populations at high risk for celiac disease. Iron-deficiency anemia that does not respond to iron supplementation may warrant screening for celiac disease. Screening for celiac disease involves a relatively easy and common set of serologic tests. The most sensitive and specific tests currently include serum transglutaminase immunoglobulin A (IgA), endomydial IgA and deaminated gliadin peptide IgA, and immunoglobulin G antibodies. Screening for native gliadin antibodies is no longer recommended due to reported wide variability in diagnostic accuracy.[50] It is important to be aware that these tests are only valid if the patient is currently consuming the gluten that the antibodies would be reacting to. If the person has been following a gluten-free diet, the antibodies will not be present, even if they have celiac disease. Because of this, and because screening for celiac disease is typically a test covered by most medical insurance in the United States, it is recommended that individuals who may have celiac disease be screened before starting a gluten-free diet. The gold standard for diagnosing celiac disease is the intestinal biopsy. Celiac disease is characterized by damaged intestinal villi that appear flattened and atrophied.[50]

Treatment of celiac disease in athletes with T1D is the same as for those without T1D: adherence to a gluten-free diet (no wheat, barley, or rye). It is highly advised that athletes with celiac disease work with an RDN to learn appropriate diet modifications to avoid gluten while still meeting nutritional needs for sport performance. Without guidance, deciphering the correct types and balance of foods can overwhelm and frustrate busy athletes. Fortunately, there are now numerous gluten-free options that did not exist even 10 years ago. The athlete with celiac disease should be counseled on how to avoid cross-contamination from facilities that prepare both gluten-free and non-gluten-free foods, tips for traveling, easy gluten-free meal options, and recovery snacks. Perhaps the easiest approach is to start by assessing what sources of carbohydrate the athlete already consumes that do not contain gluten (potatoes, milk, rice, rice noodles, yams, corn tortillas, legumes, fruit, etc), then start to introduce and experiment with gluten-free specialty foods. There are some wonderful resources available to RDNs and consumers, including those by the Gluten Intolerance Group, the Celiac Disease Foundation, and the National Institutes of Health.[54-56]

AUTOIMMUNE THYROID DISEASES

Autoimmune thyroid diseases constitute 30% of all the autoimmune diseases. They are qualified as organ-specific, attacking only the thyroid gland. The most crucial of these are Hashimoto's disease and Graves' disease.[57]

Hashimoto's Disease Hashimoto's disease, also known as Hashimoto's thyroiditis, autoimmune thyroiditis, and chronic lymphocytic thyroiditis, is characterized by chronic inflammation of the thyroid gland caused by antibodies attacking and damaging thyroid cells. It is a progressive disease that damages the thyroid, resulting in hypothyroidism. It can eventually destroy the thyroid.[58] People with T1D are at a higher risk for Hashimoto's disease than the general population because of some genetic overlap between these two endocrine autoimmune disorders. Individuals who have both T1D and celiac disease appear to have an even greater risk than those who only have T1D.[51] Hashimoto's disease can present with various combinations of symptoms, which may make diagnosis difficult.[58] Symptoms can include constipation, difficulty concentrating or thinking, dry skin, enlarged neck or presence of goiter, fatigue, hair loss, heavy and irregular menses, intolerance to cold, mild weight gain, and, in the progressed disease state, a small or shrunken thyroid gland.[59] Because each of these symptoms can be indicative of other disorders, it is good for the sports dietitian to be aware of them and be able to recognize that they may be indicative of thyroid disease when seen clustered together. Treatment of Hashimoto's disease consists of hormone replacement therapy to compensate for the decreased production of thyroxin.

Graves' Disease People with T1D also have an increased risk for Graves' disease, an autoimmune disease that results in hyperthyroidism. Symptoms of Graves' disease include nervousness or irritability, fatigue or muscle weakness, heat intolerance, trouble sleeping, hand tremors, rapid and irregular heartbeat, frequent bowel movements or diarrhea, weight loss, or goiter. In rare instances, Graves' disease can present with symptoms of thickening and reddening of the skin on the shins. This condition, known as pretibial myxedema or Graves' dermopathy, is typically painless. Occasionally, people with Graves' disease may have eyes that appear enlarged due to their eyelids being retracted back into the eye sockets, causing their eyes to seemingly bulge from the eye sockets. This condition is called Graves' ophthalmopathy. Graves' disease does not have any stand-alone nutrition therapy. Though antithyroid medications are sometimes used, Graves' disease is most commonly treated by destroying or removing all or part of the overactive thyroid with radioiodine therapy or surgery, followed by hormone replacement therapy if necessary. Of course, nutrition support can be beneficial during recovery, especially if nutrition deficiencies developed as a result of the hyperactive thyroid.[60]

If a thyroid disorder is suspected in an athlete with T1D, it is generally wise to screen for autoimmune thyroid diseases by requesting the appropriate serum thyroid antibody tests along with a thyroid panel (thyroid-stimulating hormone, free T4, T3).[59]

RHEUMATOID ARTHRITIS

Lastly, it is good for professionals working with athletes who have T1D to be aware that this population has a higher than typical risk of rheumatoid arthritis, another autoimmune disorder. It is typical for serious athletes to experience inflammation in association with training, and inflammation is even believed to be a necessary part of the recovery process. However, if an athlete with T1D experiences chronic inflammation that cannot be attributed to overtraining, poor technique, inadequate nutrition, or poor recovery habits, it may be prudent to screen for rheumatoid arthritis. As with the aforementioned autoimmune disorders, screening for rheumatoid arthritis also involves a specific serum antibody test.[61]

It is always best not to make assumptions about the etiology of symptoms, whether those assumptions may be based on the fact that someone is an athlete or that they are in a higher risk category for an autoimmune disorder. However, it is good for professionals working with athletes to be aware of increased risks that individuals may have based on personal medical history.

Disordered Eating

Because disordered eating is prevalent in many sports, it is always wise to screen for this in athletes. It is particularly important to do so with athletes who have T1D, because they have an additional and dangerous component to add to their weight-loss arsenal. Withholding insulin can be a very effective means of inducing weight loss, but it is extremely dangerous for athletes with T1D because it results in hyperglycemia and often results in ketosis.[3,62,63] See Chapter 18 for information on eating disorders in athletes.

OTHER FACTORS AFFECTING GLYCEMIC CONTROL

Circadian Rhythms

Circadian rhythms refer to naturally occurring biological rhythms that follow a daily pattern. Of particular relevance to people with diabetes are the diurnal variations in glucose metabolism. These are primarily mediated via direct autonomic innervations that target organs from the hypothalamus and are independent of insulin or glucagon levels

Secretion of glucocorticoid typically increases before dawn and targets the liver to stimulate hepatic glucose production. Other actions tied to our circadian rhythms in anticipation of a need for energy in the day include reduction in skeletal muscle blood flow and increased insulin resistance.[64-66] This is often referred to as the dawn phenomenon and helps explain why blood glucose is often highest in the morning, despite coming off of an overnight fast. This is important to keep in mind for athletes who may train and compete at different times of day.

Sleep

College athletes may sacrifice sleep to studying to meet academic demands. Professional athletes frequently lose sleep when they travel between time zones. And endurance athletes and outdoor adventurers often begin the day before dawn. What effect does sleep deprivation have on glycemic control? In one study, subjects who went without sleep for 1 to 5 days developed insulin resistance and β-cell dysfunction, resulting in increased fasting and postprandial glucose levels.[64] In another study, subjects who restricted sleep to 4 to 5 hours per night exhibited a decline in glucose tolerance, decreased muscle glucose uptake, increased hepatic glucose output, and pancreatic β-cell dysfunction.[64,67]

Altitude and Ambient Temperature

Athletes often perform in extraordinary conditions that include high altitude and extreme temperatures. While obvious examples include mountain climbers, skiers, rock climbers, or endurance trail runners, teams who travel from sea level destinations several thousand feet higher also experience radical climate changes. Altitude exposure can increase levels of epinephrine, norepinephrine, and cortisol, causing a subsequent rise in blood glucose.[68] Temperature extremes (heat and cold), humidity, and high altitude can cause physiological stress that results in elevated counterregulatory hormones and subsequent hyperglycemia despite exercise.[34] Frequent glucose monitoring is warranted, but the glucometer readings may be inaccurate at high altitude and in extreme heat or cold.[2] Additionally, heat and cold can destroy insulin, so efforts must be made to insulate it from the elements. Dehydration is also common under such extreme conditions and contributes to increased blood glucose. Refer to Box 19.1 (page 442).[6,24,34,68,69]

WHEN IS EXERCISE CONTRAINDICATED?

- **Retinopathy**: Exercise is contraindicated for individuals with T1D or T2D who have proliferative diabetic retinopathy.[38] In this particular complication of diabetes, vigorous-intensity aerobic or resistance exercise can increase risk of vitreous hemorrhage or retinal detachment.[70]
- **Peripheral neuropathy**: Individuals with peripheral neuropathy may have decreased pain sensation that can alter kinesthetic or proprioceptive sensation during physical activity. Peripheral neuropathy can increase the risk of skin breakdown, infection, and Charcot joint destruction. Proper footwear and daily self-examination of feet can detect skin breakdown early.[38]
- **Autonomic neuropathy**: Individuals with autonomic neuropathy can be at an increased risk of exercise-induced injury through a lowered cardiac responsiveness, postural hypotension, impaired thermoregulation, impaired night vision due to decreased papillary reaction, and greater risk of hypoglycemia.[38] These individuals should be monitored by a cardiologist prior to training.
- **Albuminuria and nephropathy**: Exercise can increase urinary protein excretion. There is no evidence that vigorous-intensity exercise increases the rate of progression of diabetic kidney disease.[70]

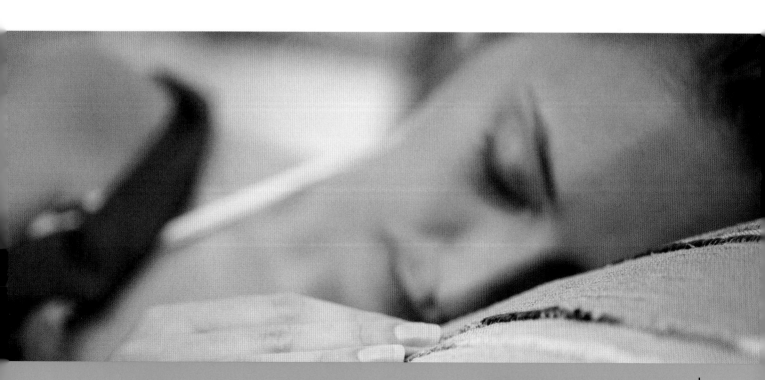

Exercise Type	Blood Glucose Response
High-intensity and anaerobic exercise Example: High-intensity interval training, strength training, sprints, calisthenics	Increases blood glucose May stay elevated for duration of training May decrease over time, especially if glycogen stores are low and athlete is not fueling while training
Steady-state aerobic exercise Example: Endurance running, hiking, Nordic skiing, endurance cycling	Initial increase in blood glucose followed by gradual decrease Risk of hypoglycemia with prolonged exercise, especially if glycogen stores are low or insulin on board is excessive
Stress	Increases blood glucose Competition-day stress often raises blood glucose
Illness	Increases blood glucose Anything from catching a cold to breaking a bone can cause physiological stress that will raise blood glucose
Sleep	Inadequate sleep can cause enough stress to increase blood glucose
Time of day (circadian rhythms)	Blood glucose is often highest in the early morning hours due to higher insulin resistance at that time Some athletes with diabetes who take insulin do well to have different basal rates and/or carbohydrate-to-insulin ratios for different times of day An important consideration if competition is at a different time of day than usual practice
Altitude	Can vary between athletes; the stress and/or increased risk of dehydration may cause increased blood glucose Cold conditions may rerquire more energy expenditure to keep warm, resulting in decreased blood glucose Glucometers, insulin pumps, and continuous glucose monitors may not work as accurately at higher altitudes
Ambient temperature	Heat and humidity may enhance absorption rate of insulin, which decreases blood glucose Cold environments require more glucose to keep warm, which decreases blood glucose If the body is too stressed, there could result in increased blood glucose
Hydration	Dehydration causes physiological stress and more concentrated blood, which means increased blood glucose

Athletes with diabetes present with challenges that need to be addressed.

If there is a determined athlete and a solid plan for training and diabetes management, there is no reason diabetes needs to prevent these athletes from achieving great feats.

Athletes with diabetes are often more prepared than other athletes on the course or field. By necessity, they have to think through variables and anticipate potential needs more carefully than others.

Preparation and planning are key to the success of athletes with diabetes. Each athlete should have an individual diabetes management plan for training and competition that includes prevention and treatment strategies. It is also advisable to have a diabetes management kit that includes emergency plans, medications, and items to treat hypoglycemia if needed.

Managing an athlete with diabetes demands a team approach and necessitates excellent communication between members of the team. The team includes medical professionals (endocrinologist, CDEs, and others) who are involved in the athlete's diabetes care, pertinent members of the coaching and training staff, the sports dietitian, and, most importantly, the athlete. The better the communication, the better the outcome.

Every athlete with diabetes has unique needs. Understanding the underlying science will provide valuable insights, but for best results, there must also be an understanding of each athlete's individual blood glucose response to exercise. Flexible treatment is key to success!

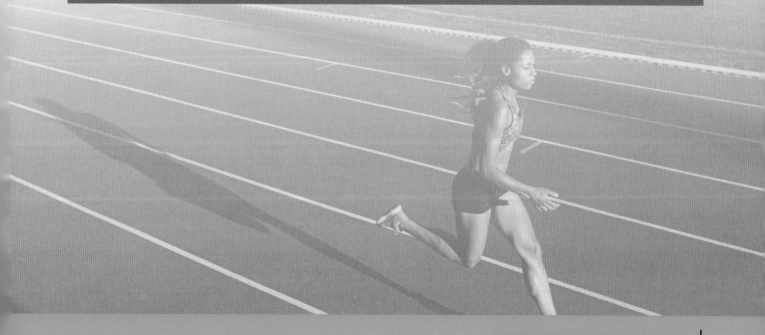

REFERENCES

1. Lisle D, Trojian T. Managing the athlete with type 1 diabetes. *Curr Sports Med Rep.* 2006;5(2):93-98.

2. Nathan DM. Diabetes: advances in diagnosis and treatment. *JAMA.* 2015;314(10):1052-1062.

3. Hornsby WG Jr, Chetlin RD. Management of competitive athletes with diabetes. *Diabetes Spectr.* 2005;18(2):102-107.

4. Diabetes fame–athletes. dLife website. www.dlife.com/diabetes/famous_people/sports. Published November 2015. Accessed January 20, 2016.

5. Harris GD, White RD. Diabetes in the competitive athlete. *Curr Sports Med Rep.* 2012;11(6):309-315.

6. Colberg SR. *Diabetic Athlete's Handbook.* Champaign, IL: Human Kenetics; 2009.

7. Ratjen I, Weber KS, Roden M, Herrmann ME, Müssig K. Type 1 diabetes mellitus and exercise in competitive athletes. *Exp Clin Endocrinol Diabetes.* 2015;123(7):419-422.

8. 2014 National diabetes statistics report. Centers for Disease Control and Prevention website. www.cdc.gov/diabetes/data/statistics/2014statisticsreport.html. Updated May 14, 2015. Accessed September 29, 2015.

9. Dugan J. Exercise recommendations for patients with type 2 diabetes. *JAAPA.* 2016;29(1):13-18.

10. Mottola MF, Ruchat SM. Exercise guidelines for women with gestational diabetes. In: Radenkovic M, ed. *Gestational Diabetes.* London, Canada: Intech; 2011:339-361.

11. US Department of Health and Human Services. Physical activity guidelines for Americans. Health.gove website. www.health.gov/paguidelines. 2008. Accessed October 8, 2016.

12. Statistics about diabetes. American Diabetes Association website. www.diabetes.org/diabetes-basics/statistics. Updated April 1, 2016. Accessed January 14, 2016.

13. Centers for Disease Control and Prevention. *National Diabetes Statistics Report: Estimates of Diabetes and Its Burden in the United States, 2014.* Atlanta, GA: U.S. Department of Health and Human Services; 2014.

14. Type 1 diabetes facts. JDRF website. www.jdrf.org/about/fact-sheets/type-1-diabetes-facts/. Accessed July 29, 2016.

15. Bardsley J, Magee M. Pathophysiology of the metabolic disorder. In: Mensing C, McLaughlin S, Halstenson C, eds. *The Art and Science of Diabetes Self-Management Education Desk Reference.* 2nd ed. Chicago, IL: American Association of Diabetes Educators; 2011:285-308.

16. National Institute of Diabetes and Digestive and Kidney Diseases, National Institutes of Health. *Monogenic Forms of Diabetes: Neonatal Diabetes Mellitus and Maturity-onset Diabetes of the Young.* Bethesda, MD: National Diabetes Information Clearinghouse; 2007. NIH Publication No. 07–6141. www.niddk.nih.gov/health-information/health-topics/Diabetes/monogenic-forms-diabetes-neonatal-diabetes-mellitus-maturity-onset-diabetes-young/Documents/Monogenic_Diabetes_508.pdf. Accessed January 20, 2016.

17. Barber TM, Dimitriadis GK, Andreou A, Franks S. Polycystic ovary syndrome: insight into pathogenesis and a common association with insulin resistance. *Clin Med (Lond).* 2015;15(suppl 6):72S-76S.

18. Domecq JP, Prutsky G, Mullan RJ, et al. Lifestyle modification programs in polycystic ovary syndrome: systematic review and meta-analysis. *J Clin Endocrinol Metab.* 2013;98(12):4655-4664.

19. Højlund K, Metabolism and insulin signaling in common metabolic disorders and inherited insulin resistance. *Dan Med J.* 2014;61(7):B4890.

20. Hagmar M, Berglund B, Brismar K, Hirschberg AL. Hyperandrogenism may explain reproductive dysfunction in Olympic athletes. *Med Sci Sports Exerc.* 2009;41(6):1241-1248. doi: 10.1249/MSS.0b013e318195a21a.

21. McArdle WD, Katch FI, Katch VL. *Exercise Physiology: Energy, Nutrition, and Human Performance.* 3rd ed. Malvern, PA: Lea & Febiger; 1991.

22. Borer K. *Exercise Endocrinology.* Champaign, IL: Human Kinetics; 2003.

23. Walsh J, Roberts R. *Pumping Insulin.* San Diego, CA: Torrey Pines Press; 2006.

24. Colberg S, Sigal RJ, Fernhall B, et al. Exercise and type 2 diabetes. The American College of Sports Medicine and the American Diabetes Association: joint position statement. *Diabetes Care.* 2010;33:e147-e167

25. Continuous glucose monitoring. National Institute of Diabetes and Digestive and Kidney Diseases website. www.niddk.nih.gov/health-information/health-topics/Diabetes/continuous-glucose-monitoring/Pages/index.aspx. Published 2008. Accessed January 12, 2016.

26. Iscoe KE, Campbell JE, Jamnik V, Perkins BA, Ridell MC. Efficacy of continuous real-time blood glucose monitoring during and after prolonged high-intensity cycling exercise: spinning with a continuous glucose monitoring system. *Diabetes Technol Ther.* 2006;8:627-635.

27. Vettoretti M, Facchinetti A, Sparacino G, Cobelli C. Patient decision-making of CGM sensor driven insulin therapies in type 1 diabetes: in silico assessment. *Conf Proc IEEE Eng Med Biol Soc 2015.* 2015:2363-2366.

28. Sisson E, Cornell S. Pharmacotherapy for glucose management. In: Mensing C, McLaughlin S, Halstenson C, eds. *The Art and Science of Diabetes Self-Management Education Desk Reference.* 2nd ed. Chicago, IL: American Association of Diabetes Educators; 2011:329-330.

29. Waserman D, Davis S, Sinman B. Fuel metabolism during exercise in health and diabetes. In: Ruderman N, Devlin J, Schneider S, eds. *Handbook of Exercise in Diabetes.* Alexandria, VA: American Diabetes Association; 2002:63-99.

30. Elliott J, Reece S. Insulin therapy: new options. *Pract Diabetology.* 2015;34(4):15-17.

31. Spollett G. Basal-bolus insulin therapy. *Pract Diabetology.* 2002;21(1):33-36.

32. Millstein R, Becerra N, Shubrook J. Insulin pumps: beyond basal-bolus. *Clev Clin J Med.* 2015;82(12):835-841.

33. Insulin storage and syringe safety. American Diabetes Association website. www.diabetes.org/living-with-diabetes/treatment-and-care/medication/insulin/insulin-storage-and-syringe-safety.html. Edited April 7, 2014. Accessed May 24, 2016.

34. de Mol P, de Vries ST, de Koning EG, Gans RO, Bilo HJ, Tack CJ. Physical activity at altitude: challenges for people with diabetes. *Diabetes Care.* 2014;37:2404-2413.

35. Keeping insulin cool. Diabetes.co.uk website. www.diabetes.co.uk/travel/keeping-insulin-cool.html. Accessed December 20, 2016.

36. Handelsman Y, Bloomgarden ZT, Grunberger G, et al. American Association of Clinical Endocrinologists and American College of Endocrinology clinical practice guidelines for developing a diabetes mellitus commprehensive care plan. *Endocr Pract.* 2015;21(suppl 1):1-87. www.aace.com/files/dm-guidelines-ccp.pdf. Accessed March 1, 2016.

37. Davis S, Lastra-Gonzalez G, eds. Diabetes and low blood sugar (hypoglycemia). The Hormone Foundation website. http://press.endocrine.org/doi/pdf/10.1210/jcem.93.8.9993. Published September 2008. Accessed May 23, 2016.

38. American Diabetes Association. Standards of medical care for patients with diabetes mellitus. *Diabetes Care.* 2016;39(suppl 1):13S-28S.

39. Clayton D, Woo V, Yale J-F, Canadian Diabetes Association Clinical Practice Guidelines Expert Committee. Canadian Diabetes Association 2013 Clinical Practice Guidelines for the Prevention and Management of Diabetes in Canada: hypoglycemia. http://guidelines.diabetes.ca/browse/chapter14. Published 2013. Accessed May 24, 2016.

40. Treating hypoglycemia. Diabetes Self-Management website. www.diabetesselfmanagement.com/managing-diabetes/treatment-approaches/understanding-insulin/treating-hypoglycemia/. Published July 25, 2006. Accessed May 24, 2016.

41. Jimenez C, Corcoran M, Crawley J, et al. National Athletic Trainers' Association position statement: management of the athlete with type 1 diabetes mellitus. *J Athl Train.* 2007;42(4):536-545.

42. Jensen TE, Richter EA. Regulation of glucose and glycogen metabolism during and after exercise. *J Physiol.* 2012;590(5):1069-1076.

43. American Association of Clinical Endocrinologists and American College of Endocrinology. Comprehensive diabetes management algorithm. *Endocr Pract.* 2015;21(4)e7.

44. Exercise and sport in diabetes, 2nd ed, part 7: adjusting insulin dosing for physical activity. DiabetesInControl website. www.diabetesincontrol.com/exercise-and-sport-in-diabetes-2nd-ed-part-7-adjusting-insulin-dosing-for-physical-activity/. Published June 18, 2012. Accessed February 29, 2016.

45. Kinshuck D. Insulin dose adjustment for physical exercise. Diabeticretinopathy.org.uk. www.diabeticretinopathy.org.uk/prevention/insulindoseexercise.htm. Accessed October 8, 2016.

46. Gulve EA. Exercise and glycemic control in diabetes: benefits, challenges, and adjustments to pharmacotherapy. *Phys Ther* .2008;88(11):1297-1321. doi: 10.2522/ptj.20080114.

47. Rabasa-Lhoret R, Bourque J, Ducros F, Chiasson JL. Guidelines for premeal insulin dose reduction for postprandial exercise of different intensities and durations in type 1 diabetic subjects treated intensively with a basal-bolus insulin regimen (ultralente-lispro). *Diabetes Care.* 2001;24(4):625-630.

48. Adjusting insulin doses. DiabetesMotion website. www.diabetesmotion.com/#!adjusting-insulin-doses/cs1r. Accessed February 29, 2016

49. Campbell MD, Walker M, Bracken RM, et al. Insulin therapy and dietary adjustments to normalize glycemia and prevent nocturnal hypoglycemia after evening exercise in type 1 diabetes: a randomized controlled trial. *BMJ Open Diabetes Res Care.* 2015;3(1):e000085.

50. Cohn A, Sofia AM, Kupfer SS. Type 1 diabetes and celiac disease: clinical overlap and new insights into disease pathogenesis. *Curr Diabetes Rep.* 2014;14(8):517.

51. Kurien M, Mollazadegan K, Sanders DS, Ludvigsson JF. Celiac disease increases risk of thyroid disease in patients with type 1 diabetes: a nationwide cohort study. *Diabetes Care.* 2016;39(3):371-375.

52. Madvariya M, Joshi R. Prevalence and clinical profile of celiac disease in children with type 1 diabetes mellitus. *Indian J Endocrinol Metab.* 2015;19(6):797-803.

53. Pham-Short A, Donaghue KC, Ambler G, Phelan H, Twigg S, Craig ME. Screening for celiac disease in type 1 diabetes: a systematic review. *Pediatrics.* 2015;136(1):e170-e176.

54. The National Institute of Diabetes and Digestive and Kidney Diseases, National Institutes of Health. Celiac disease. www.niddk.nih.gov/health-information/health-topics/digestive-diseases/celiac-disease/Pages/facts.aspx. June 2015. Accessed January, 20, 2016.

55. Gluten Intolerance Group. www.gluten.org. 2015. Accessed January 20, 2016.

56. Celiac Disease Foundation. https://celiac.org/. Accessed January 20, 2016.

57. Pyzik A, Grywalska E, Matyjaszek-Matuszek B, Roliński J. Immune disorders in Hashimoto's thyroiditis: what do we know so far? *J Immunol Res.* 2015;2015:979167. Epub April 27, 2015.

58. Genetic and Rare Diseases Information Center. Hashimoto's Syndrome. National Institutes of Health website. https://rarediseases.info.nih.gov/diseases/6570/hashimotos-syndrome. Accessed December 20, 2016.

59. US National Library of Medicine. Chronic thyroiditis (Hashimoto disease). Medline Plus website. www.nlm.nih.gov/medlineplus/ency/article/000371.htm. Reviewed February 3, 2016. Accessed January 20, 2016.

60. Graves disease. The National Institute of Diabetes and Digestive and Kidney Diseases website. www.niddk.nih.gov/health-information/health-topics/endocrine/graves-disease/Pages/fact-sheet.aspx. Published August 2012. Accessed January 20, 1016.

61. US National Library of Medicine. Rheumatoid arthritis. Medline Plus website. www.nlm.nih.gov/medlineplus/rheumatoidarthritis.html. January 2014. Accessed January 2016.

62. Bermudez O, Sommer J. T1D Intel: Learning about the dual diagnosis of an eating disorder and type 1 diabetes. T1D Intel. JDRF website. www.jdrf.org/blog/2012/10/15/t1d-intel-learning-about-the-dual-diagnosis-of-an-eating-disorder-and-type-1-diabetes/. Published October 15, 2012. Accessed July 15, 2016.

63. Eating Disorders/"Diabulimia" in Type 1 Diabetes. Joslin Diabetes Center website www.joslin.org/info/Eating_Disorders_Diabulimia_in_Type_1_Diabetes.html. Published 2016. .

64. Accessed July 15, 2016.

65. Briançon-Marjollet A, Weiszenstein M, Henri M, Thomas A, Godin-Ribuot D, Polak J. The impact of sleep disorders on glucose metabolism: endocrine and molecular mechanisms. *Diabetol Metab Syndr.* 2015:24;7:25.

66. Challet E. Keeping circadian time with hormones. *Diabetes Obes Metab.* 2015;17(suppl 1):76-83.

67. Armstrong MJ, Sigal RJ. Physical activity clinical practice guidelines: what's new in 2013? *Can J Diabetes.* 2013;37(6):363-366.

68. Halson SL. Sleep in elite athletes and nutritional interventions to enhance sleep. *Sports Med.* 2014;44(suppl 1):13S-23S.

69. Richards P, Hillebrandt D. The practical aspects of insulin at high altitude. *High Alt Med Biol.* 2013;14(3):197-204.

70. Valletta JJ, Chipperfield AJ, Clough GF, Byrne CD. Metabolic regulation during constant moderate physical exertion in extreme conditions in type 1 diabetes. *Diabetes Med.* 2012;29(6):822-826.

71. Colberg SR. *Exercise and Diabetes: A Clinician's Guide to Prescribing Physical Activity.* Alexandria, VA: American Diabetes Association; 2013.

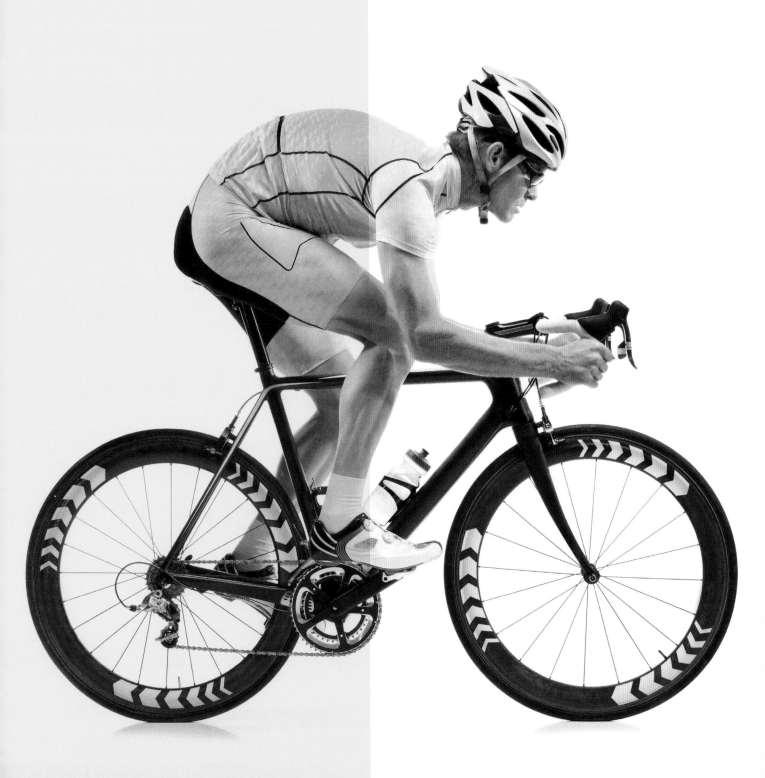

SECTION 4

SPORTS-SPECIFIC NUTRITION GUIDELINES

The practice of sports nutrition has come a long way. The chapters in this section synthesize the science of sports nutrition and exercise to provide guidelines for athletes participating in sports ranging from the very-high-intensity but short all-out effort (like the 100-m sprint that crowns the "fastest" athlete in the world) to the ultraendurance events (like the Run Around Australia, which covers 9,053 miles in 191 days of competition). Athletes have very different nutritional needs depending on exercise intensity and duration. These chapters pinpoint the nutritional requirements for training and competition for athletes competing in very-high-intensity, high-intensity short-duration, high-intensity intermittent exercise, endurance, and ultraendurance events. The science, as well as practical tips for fueling athletes, is provided to help sports dietitians establish food and fluid tips to help athletes achieve their dreams. The section ends with a brand-new chapter that explores emerging areas of opportunities for sports registered dietitian nutritionists, such as CrossFit, obstacle course races, motorsports, performance artists (eg, dancers, marching band), first responders, and more.

CHAPTER 20

NUTRITION FOR SHORT-DURATION VERY-HIGH- AND HIGH-INTENSITY SPORTS

Christine A. Karpinski, PhD, RD, CSSD, LDN, and Janet Walberg Rankin, PhD, FACSM

INTRODUCTION

Limited research focuses on high-intensity sports compared with endurance or intermittent sports, and even less focuses on what is referred to as short-duration, very-high-intensity and high-intensity sports. Events typically included in the very-high-intensity category are sports or training that requires all-out effort or near maximal effort ($>90\%$ VO_2 max or 1 repition maximum) and lasts less than 30 seconds. Short-duration, high-intensity sports require near maximal effort that can last several minutes.

These sports are often referred to as power sports or explosive sports and can include single sprints (eg, run, cycle, swim, skate), middle-distance events (eg, running, rowing), jumping or throwing events (field), or a single move or play during the course of a game or match (eg, football, baseball, basketball, soccer). Olympic and power weightlifting and certain strength-training protocols can also fall into this category. Table 20.1 lists examples of events that involve short-duration, very-high-intensity and high-intensity, exercise.

Bodybuilding and physique competitions (eg, bikini, figure, fitness) are not included in this chapter because their strength-training programs are typically higher volume, use higher repetition ranges (10 to 12 repetitions), include more muscle groups, and incorporate little rest between sets, compared with most power athletes.[1] Another unique aspect of bodybuilding and other aesthetic sports is that the competition is not intended to generate power or speed, as the athlete holds an isometric pose for up to 20 seconds. Lastly, the diet of bodybuilders and physique competitors drastically varies during different phases of training, with the ultimate goal being to achieve a body-fat level below guidelines recommended for most performance athletes. Although common among coaches and competitors, these practices are not supported by scientific literature. Refer to the At a Glance section for more information on physique sports.

Because these events are extremely short duration, the importance of nutritional implications can be minimized by athletes and coaches; however, for these sports, hundredths of seconds can be the difference between first and second place, and nutrition can play an important role in the outcome. These athletes face unique nutritional challenges due to the nature of their sport, including demanding training schedules, multiple-event days, travel, and a high level of focus. For example, an elite swim sprinter can train up to 3 or 4 hours per day, yet his or her event lasts less than 2 minutes. It is common for track and field athletes and gymnasts to have several events in one day with limited recovery time between events. This chapter will review the energy systems and substrate utilization involved in these types of sports; typical dietary intake; energy, macronutrient, and micronutrient needs; nutritional guidelines; and nutritional strategies that address training and competition for athletes involved in short-duration, very-high-intensity and high-intensity sports.

ENERGY SYSTEM AND SUBSTRATE UTILIZATION

The performance of high-intensity and very-high-intensity efforts in sport depends on many factors, including reaction time, muscle power, skill, muscle fiber type, and psychological issues. From a metabolic standpoint, adenosine triphosphate (ATP) availability, rate of breakdown, and rate of ATP resynthesis are critical. The rate of ATP production needed to perform these events is high. For example, the power output during a 30-second sprint is approximately twice that achieved at maximum oxygen consumption (VO_2 max), and the energy need for a 1,500-m running race may be approximately 115% of maximal oxygen consumption.[2] A substantial amount of the ATP to fuel these events is produced anaerobically. The shorter the duration of maximal effort, the higher the percentage of ATP generated from anaerobic sources. For example, ATP used in a 30-second sprint is approximately 80% anaerobically generated, whereas a 10-second sprint is approximately 97% anaerobically fueled.[3] Although the specific crossover point varies by individual, in general, events of effort longer than 2 minutes obtain a majority of ATP from the aerobic system, and the contribution from anaerobic pathways diminishes.

The briefest, highest intensity efforts are fueled by ATP produced anaerobically by the breakdown of creatine phosphate (PCr) within the muscle. The maximal rate of ATP production (μmol/s/kg) is estamated at 6.0 for PCr but only 1.5 for anaerobic glycolysis, and 0.24 and 0.5 for aerobic generation via fat and carbohydrate, respectively.[4] This means that efforts that require very rapid ATP use will rely heavily on PCr breakdown. Because PCr stores are limited and the use of these stores is rapid with high-intensity work, it is possible to substantially reduce them during a brief exercise bout. For example, research shows that a 30-second sprint decreased PCr by 75%, a 20-second sprint (eg, 200-m run, 50-m swim) decreased it by about half, while even a 10-second maximal effort (eg, 100-m run, 200-m cycle) decreased PCr by 40%.[3,4] Once PCr donates its phosphate to ADP, it must return to the mitochondria to be rephosphorylated, which takes approximately 1 to 2 minutes. So, a limiting factor for performance of these very-high-intensity

Table 20.1 Events and Sports that Involve Very-High-Intensity or High-Intensity Exercise

Mode	Event (Approximate Duration)
Very-High-Intensity	
Running sprint	50-m dash (6 s), 100-m (10 s), 200-m (20 s)
Hurdles	100/110-m hurdle (12–16 s)
Jumping	High jump, long jump, triple jump, pole vault (no set duration)
Cycle sprint	200 m (10 s)
Swimming sprint	50 m (22 s)
Throwing	Shotput, javelin, discus, hammer (several seconds)
Olympic weight lifting	Snatch, clean, and jerk (≤1 sec)
Power lifting	Bench press, squat, dead lift (several seconds)
Gymnastics	Multiple events (no set duration)
Team sports with sprints	Multiple, including football, baseball (no set duration)
High-Intensity	
Running	400 m (50 s); 600 m (1 min 30 s); 800 m (2 min)
Swimming	100 m (1 min); 200 m (2 min)
Skating	1,000 m (1 min 15 s); 1,500 m (2 min)

efforts could be initial muscle PCr stores. It is logical to begin the event, game, or match with high muscle PCr. Sprint training can increase PCr stores. Another way to boost muscle creatine stores is through a supplementation strategy with oral creatine (discussed later in this chapter and in Chapter 7). Although PCr is resynthesized rapidly, replenishment may not be complete if a second very-high-intensity bout occurs close to the first. The rate of recovery for muscular PCr depends on many factors, including the magnitude of reduction, oxygen availability, pH, and substrate levels, but it can take up to a minute to regain the initial levels.

Although these reductions are meaningful, glycogen is not reduced to a level shown to be detrimental to performance of aerobic events. In addition to PCr, the other fuel that provides ATP anaerobically for high- and very-high-intensity efforts is glucose through glycolysis. The use of glycolysis for ATP generation rather than PCr increases with the duration of a sprint. A 10-second sprint depends on glycolysis for approximately 44% of the ATP used, whereas a 30-second sprint will likely get more than 50% of the ATP from this system.[3] Even so, because muscles have much more glycogen than PCr, these brief, very-high-intensity efforts do not substantially reduce muscle glycogen. The magnitude of reduction in muscle glycogen depends on the intensity and duration of an exercise bout as well as the type of activity (see Figure 20.1).[5-7] The magnitude of glycogen depletion during resistance exercise will be related to the intensity of the lift and the amount of work performed. Most of the studies used a high-volume resistance exercise workout; little research has been done on glycogen use with low-volume, high-intensity workouts.

Although unlikely that modestly reduced glycogen stores will influence performance of a single very-high-intensity effort, it could impair high-intensity efforts interspersed within a game that involves substantial aerobic exercise (eg, basketball or soccer) if it is concurrent with a low-carbohydrate diet (eg, less than 3 to 4 g/kg body weight).

Acidosis that occurs secondary to lactate production during anaerobic glycolysis is a limiting factor for performance during brief, high-intensity events. Some research suggests that acidosis directly impairs muscle force development, whereas others suggest it may have an indirect effect via impairment of enzyme activity critical for ATP generation. Other metabolic factors, such as the accumulation of intracellular phosphate with the subsequent disruption of calcium release from the sarcoplasmic reticulum, could play a role in fatigue for middle-distance events.[8]

In summary, very-high-intensity brief efforts rely primarily on PCr stores, with increasing reliance on glycogen stores occurring with longer sprints or middle-distance events, such as the 800-m sprint. This results in substantial use of the PCr stores, but typically less than one-third of the muscle glycogen stores. Accumulation of such metabolites as hydrogen ion and inorganic phosphate can contribute to fatigue for several minutes during high-intensity events.

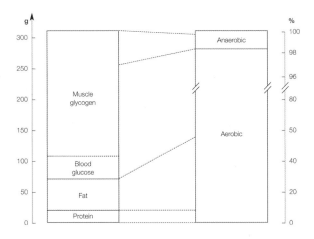

FIGURE 20.1 Percentage Muscle Glycogen Reduction for Sprints and Resistance Exercise Workout.[4-6] Left-hand scale represents the grams of substrate being utilized. Right-hand scale represents the percentage of adenosine triphosphate produced from aerobic vs anaerobic energy pathways.

NUTRITIONAL INTAKE

There are no unified studies to describe a typical diet for athletes participating in short-duration, very-high-intensity and high-intensity sports. A few studies have described the diet of very-high-intensity athletes, but the manner in which athletes are often grouped in these reports (eg, using the category swimmers, for instance, without differentiating long-distance from sprint swimmers) can make it difficult to differentiate those involved with short-duration events from those participating in long-duration events.[9] In addition, some of these data are collected on athletes from different countries, adding variation due to cultures and levels of competition.[9-14] Some studies that evaluated the diet of high-intensity or very-high-intensity athletes using dietary records are shown in Tables 20.2 (below) and 20.3 (page 454).[8-16]

Data on micronutrient intake of power athletes are even sparser than macronutrient intake data. Only two studies have reported on the micronutrient intake of international power athletes; none has reported on American athletes. Heaney and colleagues evaluated the nutrient intake of various athletes, including track and field athletes, but their analysis was an aggregate of all athletes.[17] Mineral intake (eg, calcium and iron), as well as intake of some of the fat-soluble vitamins (ie, vitamins E and A), was less than the Belgian Recommended Dietary Intake for most of the athletes.[14] Similar results were found for Greek elite high jumpers, with the male athletes consuming less than the DRI for 4 of 12 vitamins and 4 of 6 minerals. The female athletes consumed less than the US dietary reference intakes (DRI) for 7 of 12 vitamins and 5 of 6 minerals. Both sexes consumed less than the recommended level of the micronutrients vitamin D, pantothenic acid, biotin, folate, calcium, magnesium, zinc, and selenium. Interestingly, the male athletes (but not the female athletes) had inadequate vitamin C intake. The female athletes had inadequate intake of several B vitamins and iron compared with the men.[16] Maughan and colleagues reported results of an unpublished survey distributed by the anti-doping commission of the International Association of Athletics Federation that found that 88% of 310 elite track-and-field athletes reported using dietary supplements, with vitamins and antioxidant supplementation accounting for 84% of supplements used.[18] Interestingly, the percentage of short sprinters who reported using dietary supplements was the lowest of all types of athletes (77%).

Table 20.2 Reported Diet Quality and Quantity for Female Athletes Involved in Brief, High-Intensity Exercise

Type of Athlete	Energy, kcal/d (kcal/kg)	Energy from Carbohydrate, %	Carbohydrate, g/kg	Energy from Protein, %	Energy from Fat, %
Gymnasts[7]	2,298 (51.0)	42	5.4	16	42
Gymnasts[13]	1,838 (42.5)	49	5.1	15	36
Gymnasts[12]	1,678 (34.4)	66	5.8	17	18
Gymnasts[15]	1,935 (N/A[a])	49	N/A	15	36
Field athletes[11]	2,215 (26.2)	46	3.0	17	38
Throwers[9]	4,446 (53.0)	35	4.6	19	47
Throwers[10]	2,617 (40.0)	54	5.1	14	32
Sprinters[10]	2,393 (45.7)	53	5.8	15	33
Sprinters[14]	2,007 (54.7)	55	5.1	16	30
Jumpers[10]	1,982 (36.5)	51	4.5	16	33
Jumpers[16]	1,984 (34.0)	41	3.5	16	42
Swimmers[9]	4,595 (71.0)	35	6.2	26	49

[a] N/A = Not available

Type of Athlete	Energy, kcal/d (kcal/kg)	Energy from Carbohydrate, %	Carbohydrate, g/kg	Energy from Protein, %	Energy from Fat, %
Gymnasts[9]	3,310 (56.0)	43	6.1	18	38
Throwers[9]	5,353 (49.0)	34	4.1	20	47
Throwers[10]	3,591 (34.6)	55	4.1	15	30
Field athletes[11]	3,485 (36.0)	41	3.7	19	40
Sprinters[8]	2,653 (40.0)	54	5.1	15	30
Sprinters[14]	3,117 (50.9)	56	6.0	14	30
Jumpers[8]	2,863 (41.6)	54	5.2	15	31
Jumpers[16]	2,673 (35.0)	40	3.6	20	40
Swimming[9]	5,938 (80.0)	33	6.5	22	48
Swimming[15]	4,018 (N/A[a])	51	NA	14	35
Weight lifters[9]	4,597 (57.0)	38	5.4	22	40
Weight lifters[15]	3,643 (N/A)	43	NA	18	39

[a] N/A = Not available

MACRONUTRIENT AND MICRONUTRIENT DEMANDS

The effect of nutritional quality or quantity on performance of high-intensity or very-high-intensity efforts is not as well researched as performance for endurance events. The nutrition recommendations that follow are based on the theoretical limitations to performance discussed earlier, as well as the limited research that has been done.

Carbohydrate

Dietary carbohydrate can ensure that glycogen stores are adequate and that blood glucose is maintained. As discussed earlier, very-high-intensity exercise drains some muscle glycogen but not to the extent that it causes impaired performance as may occur in longer events or events involving repeated sprints. Therefore, the value of high initial muscle glycogen on a single, short, maximal effort is debatable. However, many of these athletes perform multiple events in competition, which could lead to depleted glycogen stores over the course of the day. Additionally, these athletes often participate in high-volume training, including weightlifting sessions, in which glycogen depletion may become a concern. This is why maintaining adequate glycogen stores is crucial for these athletes.

MUSCLE STRENGTH AND POWER

Glycogen levels can be depleted by 24% to 45% in a single resistance-training session, depending on the intensity and duration.[19-23] Despite this, the evidence on glycogen and muscular strength and power remains equivocal, perhaps because muscle glycogen levels are not the sole limiting factor. Some studies suggest that a low initial muscle glycogen concentration will adversely affect muscle strength and power, but a careful subsequent study suggested that some of this impairment was due to the exhaustive exercise performed, rather than the glycogen reduction itself.[24,25] It was discerned that a reduction of more than half of the muscle glycogen through diet and exercise resulted in a decrease in muscle strength and endurance, but repletion of muscle glycogen through diet did not allow recovery of muscle force. Thus, there is no good evidence that muscle glycogen has any effect on maximal, single-effort muscle strength or power.

The effect of muscle glycogen on muscle endurance is not supported in a study of 11 resistance-trained athletes who completed a resistance training workout in a carbohydrate-loaded or carbohydrate-depleted condition.[26] There was no difference in total volume lifted between the two dietary conditions, suggesting that muscle glycogen was not a limiting factor for the resistance exercises.

The effect of acute consumption of carbohydrate on muscle endurance is controversial. Several studies support the value of consuming carbohydrate just before and during a resistance exercise bout on total work performed during a workout. Resistance-trained men who consumed a glucose polymer solution before and during a repeated-set leg-extension bout tended to have better muscle endurance, as reflected by number of repetitions (149 vs 129 for carbohydrate vs placebo) and sets (17.1 vs 14.4 for carbohydrate vs placebo), but the differences were not significant.[27] Haff and colleagues reported that resistance-trained men could do approximately 8% more total work during an exercise test of 16 sets of 10 repetitions.[28] However, another study from the same laboratory using a similar design found no positive results from acute carbohydrate ingestion before and between sets of a 39-minute isotonic exercise bout.[29] This was despite the fact that the carbohydrate ingestion lessened the amount of total muscle glycogen reduction during the exercise workout.

Another study did not support the value of a single high-carbohydrate feeding (1 g/kg) on the performance of multiple-set resistance exercise when 14 participants were losing weight on a low-energy diet for 3 days.[30] The number of repetitions performed until exhaustion in the last set of leg extensions and the weight supported in the bench press portion of a four-exercise resistance workout were not different between athletes who consumed a high-carbohydrate beverage and those who drank a placebo beverage.

Most studies do not support the value of high muscle glycogen or acute carbohydrate ingestion on acute bouts of muscle strength or endurance. The majority of the studies done in a weight-room setting with multiple sets and exercise workouts have not demonstrated a benefit of a continuously high-carbohydrate diet or acute carbohydrate ingestion on performance. Some of the variation among studies may relate to the performance tests used (eg, large-muscle vs small-muscle exercises, number of repetitions, and intensity) as well as the participants (athletes trained in that event compared with those less familiar and thus less reliable in their performance of the test).

SPRINT PERFORMANCE

Few studies have examined the effect of muscle glycogen on single sprint performance. However, one study reported that a low-carbohydrate diet had a detrimental effect on high-intensity exercise over 3 days. Eight athletes produced a higher mean power output (but the same peak power) in a 30-second maximal cycling test when they consumed a 50% carbohydrate diet with approximately 3.9 g/kg compared with an isocaloric diet of only 5% carbohydrate (~0.4 g/kg) for 3 days (see Figure 20.2, page 456).[31] Few athletes are likely consuming such a low-carbohydrate diet, so the practical value of this study is limited.

Even if sprint performance is impaired by a very low-carbohydrate diet, most studies do not observe a benefit of moving from a moderate-carbohydrate diet to a high-carbohydrate diet for sprint performance. Lamb and colleagues found no benefit of a high-carbohydrate diet (80% of energy; 12.1 g/kg) compared with a moderate-carbohydrate diet (43% of energy; 6.5 g/kg) consumed for 9 days on 50-meter swim sprint performance in collegiate male swimmers.[32] Vandenberghe and colleagues found no difference in cycling time to exhaustion at supramaximal intensity (~125% VO_2 max) for a moderate-carbohydrate diet compared with a high-carbohydrate diet (70% of energy and ~7.7 g/kg vs 50% of energy and ~4.6 g/kg).[33]

Limited research suggests that sprint performance may be reduced with very low-carbohydrate diets (< 10% of energy; < 1.5 g/kg), but few athletes are likely to actually consume extremely low-carbohydrate

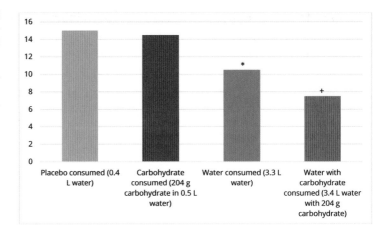

FIGURE 20.2 Decrease in Power Output for a 4-Second Maximal Power Test During a 2-Hour Endurance Exercise Bout for Treatments Varying in Hydration and Carbohydrate.[31]

*Indicates significantly different from placebo or carbohydrate consumed.
+ Indicates significantly different from all other groups.

diets. The exception could be athletes attempting to lose weight on a diet that recommends severe limits on carbohydrate intake, a practice that should be discouraged. Conversely, there is little evidence for the value of increasing dietary carbohydrate to higher than moderate levels (5 to 7 g/kg).

RECOVERY

Some athletes perform repeated events or games during a single day, so they need to recover as quickly as possible. Consumption of carbohydrate after exercise will accelerate glycogen replenishment. For example, Pascoe and colleagues showed that muscle glycogen decreased to approximately 70% of resting values after a multiset resistance exercise bout, but consumption of a carbohydrate beverage (1.5 g/kg) after exercise increased muscle glycogen to 75% of baseline after 2 hours and to 91% of baseline after 6 hours.[22] On the other hand, there was no restoration of muscle glycogen after 6 hours when a water placebo was ingested after exercise.

The evidence is not conclusive that a high-carbohydrate diet between two high-intensity exercise bouts enhances subsequent performance. Two studies using similar methodology but different participant populations yielded completely different conclusions regarding the importance of high carbohydrate intake between bouts. Haub and colleagues reported that six moderately trained men were able to maintain their maximal exercise performance of a 100-kJ cycle ergometer test to that of an initial test when they had consumed carbohydrate (0.7 g/kg) during the 60 minutes between the two tests; time to complete the 100-KJ test was longer if participants consumed a placebo during the recovery period.[34] Although this suggests a benefit of high-carbohydrate ingestion on recovery from high-intensity performance, a subsequent study with the same protocol using seven competitive cyclists found no benefit on performance after high-carbohydrate consumption between bouts.[35] Because training, especially sport-specific training, is such an important variable, it is difficult to compare the two studies. The differences between these studies emphasize the importance of using athletes specific to the event in these dietary intervention studies.

CARBOHYDRATE SUMMARY

To summarize, the information from research on dietary carbohydrate for sprinting or muscle strength translates into more flexibility for the diet of athletes involved in very-high-intensity events than for those participating in prolonged endurance exercise. Several studies show superior performance of single sprints when athletes have consumed high-carbohydrate diets (>65% of energy from carbohydrate; >7 g/kg) compared with low-carbohydrate diets (<10% of energy; <1.5 g/kg), but this is not consistent among studies. There is no consensus that a high-carbohydrate diet is superior to a moderate-carbohydrate diet for the performance of single sprints or maximum muscle power. Therefore, although glycogen stores can be supercompensated using glycogen loading, there is no evidence that this would help performance, and, in fact, it may be counterproductive, owing to weight gain that coincides with the additional carbohydrate stores. The carbohydrate content of the diet may come into play for athletes competing in multiple events over a day or for those doing substantial aerobic activity in addition to the sprints (eg, basketball). In addition, athletes who do high-volume aerobic training but compete in very-high-intensity, brief events (eg, swimmers) will need to consume substantial amounts of carbohydrate to replenish the glycogen used during training. In most cases, it is recommended that athletes involved in very-high-intensity sports or events consume approximately 5 to 7 g carbohydrate per kilogram body weight, with the lower end of the range recommended for athletes with lower energy needs and little aerobic training, and the higher end recommended for those participating in modest amounts of aerobic training in addition to the high-intensity work. The consumption of carbohydrate foods shortly after an event will enhance the rate of glycogen replacement.

Protein

Because most athletes performing brief, maximal efforts depend on high muscularity and function, nutritional strategies that enhance lean body mass are often employed throughout the year. Current data suggest that dietary protein intake necessary to support metabolic adaptation, repair, remodeling, and protein turnover generally ranges from 1.2 to 2.0 g/kg/d.[36-38] However, exceeding the recommended protein intake appears to provide no additional benefit for athletes desiring to increase their lean body mass, if consuming adequate total calories[39] Although there exists limited research, there is support for the recommendation by Phillips and Van Loon that strength athletes consume 1.8 to 2.7 g/kg of protein during a calorically restricted state.[36] However, higher intakes of protein (1.8 to 2.0 g/kg/d) are typically recommended for short periods during intensified training or when reducing energy intake.[36,40] For a more individualized recommendation, using a calculation based on kilograms of fat-free mass may be more accurate. The range of 2.3 to 3.1 g/kg of fat-free mass has been recommended to minimize loss of lean tissue, with athletes having a lower percentage of body fat tending toward the higher end of this range.[41]

Ideal muscle protein synthesis depends on the provision of substrate (amino acids) as well as the appropriate hormonal environment (eg, insulin) to enhance protein synthesis. Most studies are consistent in concluding that the consumption of protein before or after a resistance exercise bout is beneficial for protein retention and superior to the same energy as carbohydrate alone.[20,36,42,43] Research on protein intake in the immediate postexercise period, or the so-called "window of anabolic opportunity," has been confirmed by several researchers, although recent research has elucidated that the tight postexercise time (< 1 hours) may be extended when discussing anabolic gains.[44]

In fact, the postexercise window can last up to 24 hours, but most researchers agree that early feeding is more advantageous because this is when muscle protein synthesis is greatest.[45,46] Recently, the focus of research has clearly shifted from the total amount of protein consumed in a day to evaluating the timing and type of protein consumed to maximize metabolic adaptations initiated by training stimulus.[36,47] The recommendation is 0.3 g protein per kilogram body weight after key exercise sessions and every 3 to 5 hours over multiple meals.[39,48] Longitudinal training studies verify that increases in strength and muscle mass are greatest with immediate postexercise provision of protein.[49] The International Olympic Committee Consensus Statement on Sports Nutrition encourages protein consumption in the postexercise period to aid in long-term maintenance of muscle and bone and to repair tissues damaged by acute exercise.[50]

The type of protein that is best for muscle protein gains is controversial; studies have reported either no difference in muscle protein synthesis response to ingestion of different protein types or that one is superior to the others.[51-54] Muscles need to be fed essential amino acids (EAAs) in the postexercise period to reduce muscle protein breakdown.[45] High-quality dietary proteins, such as whey, casein, and soy, are effective for the maintenance, repair, and synthesis of skeletal muscle proteins.[55] The amount of EAA used in studies ranges from 8 to 10 grams. Phillips and colleagues examined the amino acid composition of high-quality protein foods (milk, meat, and eggs) and determined that 10 g of EAA translates to about 25 g of each of these proteins.[56] Most complete proteins are about 40% EAA–hence the recommendation to consume 20 to 25 g of intact, high-quality protein after exercise. Current recommendations that seem appropriate for strength athletes are 10 g of EAA (0.25 to 0.3 g/kg body weight) or 15 to 25 g protein, with more than 40 g showing no additional benefit.[38,43,47,57] See Chapter 3 for a complete review of protein.

Fat

Dietary fat intake and its direct effect on performance are of little concern for power athletes. Dietary fat intake is probably most relevant for power athletes as a means to achieve adequate energy intake and to support cardiometabolic health. Many of these athletes would find it difficult to achieve their high energy requirements if they followed a very-low-fat diet because dietary fat is two times more energy dense than carbohydrate or protein. Obviously, dietary fat and overall calories need to be limited for athletes who are trying to decrease weight. The quality of dietary fat has minimal effect on performance but should be taken into consideration as part of the athlete's overall diet and long-term health.

Since low-carbohydrate diets are typically also high-fat, implications of a high fat diet and performance are similar to those discussed earlier in this chapter regarding low-carbohydrate diets. However, research into ketogenic diets and fat adaptation has increased over the past 10 years, mostly in the context of endurance exercise. There is scant literature discussing ketogenic diets and power athletes. Havemann and colleagues found that ingestion of a high-fat diet for 6 days followed by 1 day of carbohydrate loading increased fat oxidation but reduced high-intensity sprint power performance.[58] They believe the decreased sprint performance was associated with increased muscle recruitment, elevated perceived exertion, and heart rate. Researchers have observed that following a high-fat diet decreases glycogenolysis.[59] More information is provided on this topic in Chapter 4.

Micronutrients

The micronutrient demands of athletes performing very-high-intensity and high-intensity, short-duration sports correlate to energy intake. Most athletes will meet the DRI for micronutrients as long as they are meeting their energy needs and consuming a wide variety of foods.[60] The restricted energy diets and limited intake of certain food groups (eg, dairy, meat) often consumed by these athletes may put them at risk for certain micronutrient deficiencies. Two specific considerations for power athletes are oxidative stress and joint health. Over 150 articles have been published about the association between antioxidants and exercise-induced skeletal muscle damage and impaired muscle function. Although these mostly small-scale, low-quality studies have shown that antioxidant supplementation attenuates exercise-induced oxidative stress, most have not shown an effect on muscle damage and performance.[61] It is widely known that nutrition can play an important role in joint health, but the necessity of dietary supplementation is not supported. Micronutrients that support joint health are calcium, phosphorus, zinc, and vitamins C, D, and E.[62] Refer to Chapter 5 for a detailed discussion of dietary supplements.

HYDRATION

Strenuous activity in a hot, humid environment makes it challenging to maintain hydration. American college football players, for example, come to practice dehydrated, as indicated by reduced body weight and increased urine specific gravity.[63] Similar results were found in football players whose hydration status was measured on multiple days. Fluid deficits were still present before the next practice session, indicating that additional fluid replacement may be needed between practices to avoid chronic dehydration.[64] Judelson and colleagues reviewed the research evidence for an effect of dehydration on performance of muscle strength, power, and high-intensity endurance.[65] They determined that dehydration of 3% to 4% causes a reduction in muscle strength of approximately 2%, muscle power of approximately 3%, and muscle high-intensity endurance of approximately 10%.

The value of hydration on maximal power output during prolonged endurance exercise was illustrated in a study by Fritzsche and colleagues. Eight endurance-trained cyclists exercised 122 minutes at 62% VO_2 max in a hot, humid environment on four occasions. Volume of fluid ingested was either low (~0.4 L) or high (~3.3 L) and with either 204 g or no carbohydrate. Maximal power production over 4 seconds was measured four times during each 2-hour cycling bout. Although there was no difference in maximum power production sprints during the treatments at the first power test, the decrease in power near the end of the bout was the least for the treatment with the highest fluid volume with carbohydrate (Figure 20.3).[66] The athletes could produce more power with this treatment than when they had the same volume of water alone. Both of these treatments were superior to both treatments with the small volume of water (whether containing carbohydrate or not). The researchers concluded that maximal power is best maintained by consuming high volumes of fluid with carbohydrate. This illustrates the importance of hydration to athletes involved in games that include substantial aerobic activity with sporadic sprints or high muscle-power generation.

In summary, acute dehydration is modestly harmful to sport performance involving maximal muscle strength and power. Dehydration becomes more detrimental if the high-intensity effort in a sport or exercise is longer or if sprints are interspersed within prolonged aerobic exercise, as in the case of runners. Although each athlete can respond differently to dehydration, a strong body of evidence demonstrates that even low levels of dehydration (eg, -1% body weight) can negatively affect anaerobic power and capacity, as well as strength, with the magnitude of dehydration resulting in a proportionate negative effect on performance.[66] Clearly, the effect of hypohydration on power and strength athletes requires further research.

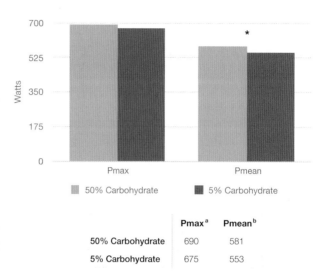

	Pmax[a]	Pmean[b]
50% Carbohydrate	690	581
5% Carbohydrate	675	553

FIGURE 20.3 Effect of 3 days of low-carbohydrate diet on 30-second cycle sprint maximum and mean power.[30]

Pmax= maximum power
Pmean = mean power.
* Indicates significant difference between dietary treatment groups.

BODY WEIGHT AND BODY COMPOSITION

Track-and-field coaches encourage athletes to increase lean mass while minimizing body fat for most events (except throwing events). Increased muscle mass has the advantage of enhanced force generation, but any extra body fat can be a disadvantage for performance. Wilmore evaluated body fat for a cross-section of athletes and reported that male sprinters and discus throwers had approximately 16% body fat, whereas shot-putters ranged from 16% to 20% body fat.[68] The female athletes in these events had more body fat than the men did, with female sprinters and jumpers at approximately 19% to 20% fat and the female throwers from 25% to 28% body fat. More recently, Mullins and colleagues found body-fat ranges of elite track athletes to be 8.4% to 16.7% for male athletes and 11.0% to 29.2% for female athletes.[69] Although these values are helpful to provide some context, there are too many other important factors that determine performance and, as discussed later in this chapter, potential unintended consequences of weight loss to encourage rigid minimum body-fat standards. Gymnasts have average ranges lower than that of most power athletes, with men ranging from 5% to 12% and women ranging from 10% to 16% body fat.[70]

There is evidence that weight loss is common in high-power athletes. Folgelholm and Hiilloskorpi reported that approximately 50% of men and women in speed sports were trying to lose weight.[71] Almost half of the elite gymnasts studied by Jonnalagadda and colleagues were on a self-prescribed diet.[12] Weight loss and negative energy balance may impair physical performance. Some researchers report no effect of short-term weight loss on performance of high-intensity exercise, whereas others report decrements. In general, rapid or substantial weight loss is more likely to impair performance than gradual or modest loss.[72] A study from Virginia Tech showed that short-term weight loss through energy restriction reduced dynamic muscle strength approximately 8% in athletes who lost 3.3 kg in 10 days.[73] Energy restrictions, especially carbohydrate restriction, will lead to weight loss due to depleted glycogen stores and subsequent water loss, as well as the loss of lean body mass. So, a substantial weight loss that is done quickly (eg, 5% within several days) is more likely to be detrimental to high-intensity performance than a more gradual weight loss.

The macronutrient mix, especially the amount of carbohydrate in a weight-loss diet, may influence performance. For example, resistance trainers who consumed a low-energy diet with 50% of energy from carbohydrate had decreased muscle endurance after 7 days of the diet, whereas those who consumed the same amount of energy but with 70% of the energy derived from carbohydrate maintained their rates of isometric fatigue at baseline levels.[74] The evidence for higher protein intakes during weight loss among strength athletes is supported for maintaining lean body mass; however, its effect on athletic performance is lacking.[40] Because energy restriction could negatively affect sports performance, body composition recommendations should be flexible and individualized for athletes with different body types and weight histories. There is no guarantee that any individual athlete will improve performance as a result of weight loss. In fact, as discussed, performance may be impaired during the weight loss. Other potential consequences of rapid weight loss include decreases in muscle mass and possible effects on linear growth, hormonal changes, and nutrient deficiencies.[20]

Female athletes dieting for weight loss are particularly susceptible to the female athlete triad: disruption of reproductive hormones, reduced bone strength concurrent with disordered eating, and poor diet (see Chapter 18). Athletes who need to lose weight should be encouraged to lose weight gradually and during the off-season to minimize any detrimental effect on performance, specifically to minimize lean body mass loss. It is standard practice to monitor weight loss through the accurate assessment and reassessment of body composition. Athletes interested in muscle mass gain need to ensure that they consume adequate energy to support their resting metabolic rate, ingest adequate protein based on lean body mass, and participate in strenuous resistance training.[20] Protein for lean mass gain is discussed in Chapter 3.

NUTRITIONAL STRATEGIES

Providing nutritional support to short-duration, very-high- and high-intensity athletes encompasses two distinct situations: training and competition. As mentioned, the training protocols of these athletes can be very different from competition. Additionally, most athletes practice some level of training periodization throughout the year, which correspondingly changes their nutritional requirements. Thus, nutritional support needs to be adjusted accordingly. In addition to performance concerns, the diet of these athletes needs to remain healthy, which means consuming a balanced, varied diet with approximately 55% of energy from carbohydrate and at least 1.2 g protein per kilogram body weight, with an abundant intake of whole grains, fruits, and vegetables.

High-Priority Considerations for Training

High-priority considerations for training include:
- maintaining energy and glycogen levels,
- maintaining adequate hydration,
- promoting maximal recovery,
- supporting training adaptations, and
- achieving an ideal power-to-weight ratio.

High-Priority Considerations for Competition

High-priority considerations for competition include:
- maintaining focus and concentration,
- maximizing reaction time, and
- managing fueling around events.

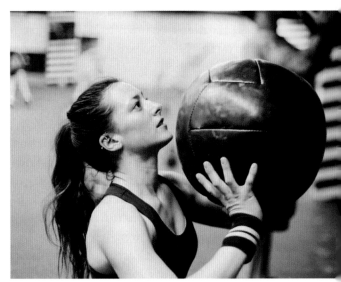

It would be prudent for the athlete to plan what to eat before, during, and after training or competition. To avoid gastrointestinal distress during the event, a balanced pre-event meal should be consumed at least 1½ hours prior, with only liquids closer to the event. A low-fiber, low-fat meal is recommended because it will leave the stomach and intestine more quickly. Inclusion of protein with carbohydrate in the meal will make it more likely that blood glucose will be at a normal concentration before the event. It is recommended that the athlete consume 1 to 4 g/kg of body weight of carbohydrate 1 to 4 hours before exercise and a small to moderate amount of protein (7 to 21 g).[38]

If a training session or competition lasts less than 60 minutes, consuming water is recommended. However, if an intense training session lasts longer than 60 minutes, the athlete may benefit from consuming high-glycemic carbohydrate found in sports drinks. Athletes competing in several events or matches during one day have a special challenge in deciding what they can tolerate that will also help their performance.

Immediately after a high-volume training session, the athlete can maximize muscle glycogen replacement and protein synthesis by consuming 0.75 to 1.5 g of carbohydrate per kilogram body weight, as well as 20 to 30 g of high-quality protein within the first 2 hours.[38] If the athlete will not be training or competing for 24 hours, the urgency of nutritional intake immediately after exercise decreases, as long as the athlete consumes adequate calories and macronutrients over the course of the next 24 hours.

Fluids should be consumed at each meal, between meals, and during workouts to maintain hydration. Measurement of body weight before and after a workout or monitoring the color of urine can be used as an index of dehydration, and effort should be made to rehydrate before the next workout or competition.

A light snack, such as yogurt with fruit, a small sandwich (without high-fat sauces or cheeses), cereal with milk, regular or dried fruit, a commercial liquid meal, granola bars, fruit bars (eg, fig), or muffins, along with sport drinks or water, are appropriate between events. Because the food provided at the concession stands at most sporting events does not fit this profile, it is best if athletes or their trainers pack snacks for the day.

All athletes, including those who compete in very-high-intensity sports, should be discouraged from consuming a very low-carbohydrate diet. This diet may impair performance and is often less healthful due to low vitamin, mineral, and fiber content.

Some athletes may know that there is less evidence for an effect of diet on performance in very-high-intensity events and therefore believe they can eat whatever they want. Practitioners making dietary recommendations for these athletes must consider the same health issues as for any other individual. Therefore, it is important that the sports dietitian assess the overall diet and provide education about making changes to improve the quality and healthfulness of the diet, as well to improve performance.

SUPPLEMENTS AND ERGOGENIC AIDS

Many athletes are tempted by various claims from supplement companies, so the sports dietitian should find out what supplements the athletes may be taking. Supplements that have no evidence of benefit, have evidence that they could be harmful, or are banned by sports governing bodies should be strongly discouraged. Additionally, the athletes need to understand that there is very little regulation over the dietary supplement industry, and the risk of contamination or banned substances is very real.

Dietary supplements that are attractive to athletes involved in very-high-intensity events or sports are those that may increase the availability of PCr, increase lean body mass, or improve reaction time or focus. Enhancement of buffering capacity may be helpful for high-intensity events lasting up to several minutes. The dietary supplement that is primarily used to maximize the PCr system is creatine. Dietary supplements that are commonly used to enhance lactic acid buffering capacity are sodium bicarbonate and β-alanine. Creatine, branched-chain amino acids, leucine, protein powders, caffeine, and β-hydroxy β-methylbuterate are dietary supplements commonly used for increasing lean body mass, although arginine and nitrate have been considered more recently. Dietary supplements that have been commonly used to improve reaction time and focus include caffeine, phosphatidylserine, taurine, tyrosine, and β-alanine. The efficacy and safety of these dietary supplements are discussed in Chapter 7.

SUMMARY

For most short-duration, very-high-intensity events, specific nutritional strategies will have less of an impact on performance than genetics, training, and motivational factors. Only very-low-carbohydrate diets or moderately low-carbohydrate diets paired with low energy intake had a detrimental effect on performance of single, maximal efforts. The benefits of nutrition for high-intensity exercise performance are most often observed when high-intensity efforts are interspersed with substantial amounts of other aerobic exercise. The training practices of these athletes are often different from those of their actual competition, and this should be taken into consideration when discussing nutritional strategies. Dehydration in the range of 1% to 2% can reduce muscle strength and power slightly and can substantially reduce muscle high-intensity endurance. Consuming more total energy, as well as protein, before or after each resistance exercise bout can improve muscle protein balance and long-term gain. Although not without controversy, most evidence suggests that supplements such as creatine, caffeine, and bicarbonate may benefit those athletes performing high-intensity exercise. Cost, efficacy, and safety should always be considered before using supplements.

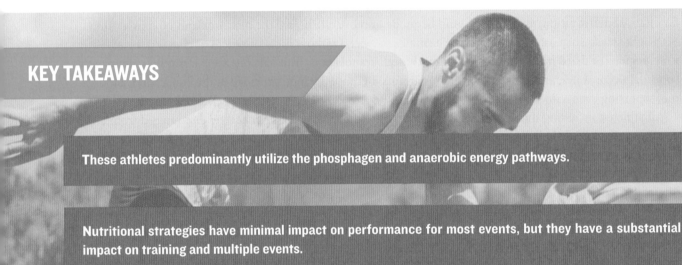

KEY TAKEAWAYS

These athletes predominantly utilize the phosphagen and anaerobic energy pathways.

Nutritional strategies have minimal impact on performance for most events, but they have a substantial impact on training and multiple events.

The athlete should utilize fueling strategies for before, during, and after exercise.

These athletes should consume a balanced diet with approximately 55% of energy from carbohydrate and at least 1.2 g protein per kilogram body weight, with an abundance of whole grains, fruits, and vegetables.

The athlete should ingest 0.3 g protein per kilogram of body weight, or approximately 20 g, after key exercise sessions and every 3 to 5 hours over multiple meals.

Dietary supplements worth consideration are creatine, sodium bicarbonate, β-alanine, β-hydroxy β-methylbuterate, branched-chain amino acids, leucine, caffeine, and protein powders.

REFERENCES

1. Lambert CP, Flynn MG. Fatigue during high-intensity intermittent exercise: application to bodybuilding. *Sports Med.* 2002;32(8):511-522.

2. Stellingwerff T, Boit MK, Res PT; International Association of Athletics Federations. Nutritional strategies to optimize training and racing in middle-distance athletes. *J Sports Sci.* 2007;25(suppl 1):17S-28S.

3. Spriet LL, Perry CGR, Talanian JL. Legal pre-event nutritional supplements to assist energy metabolism. *Essays Biochem.* 2008;44:27-43.

4. Lamb DR. *Physiology of Exercise.* 2nd ed. New York, NY: Macmillan; 1984.

5. Gaitanos GC, Williams C, Boobis LH, Brooks S. Human muscle metabolism during intermittent maximal exercise. *J Appl Physiol.* 1993;75(2):712-719.

6. Esbjörnsson-Liljedahl M, Bodin K, Jansson E. Smaller muscle ATP reduction in women than in men by repeated bouts of sprint exercise. *J Appl Physiol.* 2002;93(3):1075-1083.

7. Haff GG, Lehmkuhl MJ, McCoy LB, Stone MH. Carbohydrate supplementation and resistance training. *J Strength Cond Res.* 2003;17(1):187.

8. Ament W, Verkerke GJ. Exercise and fatigue. *Sports Med.* 2009;39(5):389-422.

9. Chen JD, Wang JF, Li KJ, et al. Nutritional problems and measures in elite and amateur athletes. *Amer J Clin Nutr.* 1989;49(suppl 5):1084-1089.

10. Sugiura K, Suzuki I, Kobayashi K. Nutritional requirements of elite Japanese marathon runners during altitude training. *Med Sci Sports Exerc.* 1999;9(2):202-212.

11. Faber M, Spinnler Benadé AJ. Mineral and vitamin intake in field athletes (discus-, hammer-, javelin-throwers and shotputters). *Int J Sports Med.* 1991;12(3):324-327.

12. Jonnalagadda SS, Bernadot D, Nelson M. Energy and nutrient intakes of the United States National Women's Artistic Gymnastics Team. *Int J Sport Nutr.* 1998;8(4):331–344.

13. Loosli AR, Gillien DM, Benson J, Bourdet K. Inadequate nutrition and chronic caloric restriction among ballet dancers. *Med Sci Sports Exerc.* 1985;17(2):201.

14. Aerenhouts D, Deriemaeker P, Hebbelinck M, Clarys P. Dietary acid-base balance in adolescent sprint athletes: a follow-up study. *Nutrients.* 2011;3(2):200-211.

15. Grandjean AC. Macronutrient intake of US athletes compared with the general population and recommendations made for athletes. *Am J Clinl Nutr.* 1989;49(suppl 5):1070-1076.

16. Bogdanis GC, Stavrinou P, Fatouros IG, et al. Short-term high-intensity interval exercise training attenuates oxidative stress responses and improves antioxidant status in healthy humans. *Food Chem Toxicol.* 2013;61:171-177.

17. Heaney S, O'Connor H, Michael S, Gifford J, Naughton G. Nutrition knowledge in athletes: a systematic review. *Int J Sport Nutr Exerc Metab.* 2011;21(3):248-261.

18. Maughan RJ, Depiesse F, Geyer H; International Association of Athletics Federations. The use of dietary supplements by athletes. *J Sports Sci.* 2007;25(suppl 1):103S-113S.

19. Slater G, Phillips SM. Nutrition guidelines for strength sports: sprinting, weightlifting, throwing events, and bodybuilding. *J Sports Sci.* 2011;29(suppl 1):67S-77S.

20. Koopman R, Saris WH, Wagenmakers AJ, van Loon LJ. Nutritional interventions to promote post-exercise muscle protein synthesis. *Sports Med.* 2007;37(10):895-906.

21. MacDougall JD, Ray S, Sale DG, McCartney N, Lee P, Garner S. Muscle substrate utilization and lactate production. *Can J Appl Physiol.* 1999;24(3):209-215.

22. Pascoe DD, Costill DL, Fink WJ, Robergs RA, Zachwieja JJ. Glycogen resynthesis in skeletal muscle following resistive exercise. *Med Sci Sports Exerc.* 1993;25(3):349-354.

23. Tesch PA, Colliander EB, Kaiser P. Muscle metabolism during intense, heavy-resistance exercise. *Eur J Appl Physiol Occup Physiol.* 1986;55(4):362-366.

24. Jacobs I, Kaiser P, Tesch P. Muscle strength and fatigue after selective glycogen depletion in human skeletal muscle fibers. *Eur J Appl Physiol Occup Physiol.* 1981;46(1):47-53.

25. Grisdale RK, Jacobs I, Cafarelli E. Relative effects of glycogen depletion and previous exercise on muscle force and endurance capacity. *J Appl Physiol.* (1985). 1990;69(4):1276-1282.

26. Mitchell JB, DiLauro PC, Pizza FX, Cavender DL. The effect of preexercise carbohydrate status on resistance exercise performance. *Int J Sport Nutr.* 1997;7(3):185-196.

27. Lambert CP, Flynn MG, Boone JB Jr, Michaud TJ, Rodriguez-Zayas J. Effects of carbohydrate feeding on multiple-bout resistance exercise. *J Appl Sport Sci Res.* 1991;5(4):192-197.

28. Haff GG, Schroeder CA, Koch AJ, Kuphal KE, Comeau MJ, Potteiger JA. The effects of supplemental carbohydrate ingestion on intermittent isokinetic leg exercise. *J Sports Med Phys Fitness.* 2001;41(2):216-222.

29. Haff GG, Koch AJ, Potteiger JA, et al. Carbohydrate supplementation attenuates muscle glycogen loss during acute bouts of resistance exercise. *Int J Sport Nutr Exerc Metab.* 2000;10(3):326-339.

30. Dalton RA, Rankin JW, Sebolt D, Gwazdauskas F. Acute carbohydrate consumption does not influence resistance exercise performance during energy restriction. *Int J Sport Nutr.* 1999;9(4):319-332.

31. Langfort J, Zarzeczny R, Pilis W, Nazar K, Kaciuba-Uscitko H. The effect of a low-carbohydrate diet on performance, hormonal and metabolic responses to a 30-s bout of supramaximal exercise. *Eur J Appl Physiol Occup Physiol.* 1997;76(2):128-133.

32. Lamb DR, Rinehardt KF, Bartels RL, Sherman WM, Snook JT. Dietary carbohydrate and intensity of interval swim training. *Am J Clin Nutr.* 1990;52(6):1058-1063.

33. Vandenberghe K, Hespel P, Vanden Eynde B, Lysens R, Richter EA. No effect of glycogen level on glycogen metabolism during high intensity exercise. *Med Sci Sports Exerc.* 1995;27(9):1278-1283.

34. Haub MD, Potteiger JA, Jacobsen DJ, Nau KL, Magee LA, Comeau MJ. Glycogen replenishment and repeated maximal effort exercise: effect of liquid carbohydrate. *Int J Sport Nutr.* 1999;9(4):406–415.

35. Haub MD, Haff GG, Potteiger JA. The effect of liquid carbohydrate ingestion on repeated maximal effort exercise in competitive cyclists. *J Strength Cond Res.* 2003;17(1):20–25.

36. Phillips SM, Van Loon LJ. Dietary protein for athletes: from requirements to optimum adaptation. *J Sports Sci.* 2011;29(suppl 1):29S-38S.

37. Houtkooper L, Abbot JM, Nimmo M; International Association of Athletics Federations. Nutrition for throwers, jumpers, and combined events athletes. *J Sports Sci.* 2007;25(suppl 1):39S-47S.

38. Thomas DT, Erdman KA, Burke LM. Position of the Academy of Nutrition and Dietetics, Dietitians of Canada, and the American College of Sports Medicine: Nutrition and Athletic Performance. *J Acad Nutr Diet.* 2016;116(3):501-528.

39. Moore DR, Robinson MJ, Fry JL, et al. Ingested protein dose response of muscle and albumin protein synthesis after resistance exercise in young men. *Am J Clin Nutr.* 2009;89(1):161-168.

40. Mettler S, Mitchell N, Tipton KD. Increased protein intake reduces lean body mass loss during weight loss in athletes. *Med Sci Sports Exerc.* 2010;42(2):326-337.

41. Helms ER, Zinn C, Rowlands DS, Brown SR. A systematic review of dietary protein during caloric restriction in resistance trained lean athletes: a case for higher intakes. *Int J Sport Nutr Exerc Metab.* 2014;24(2):127-138.

42. Tipton KD, Jeukendrup AE, Hespel P; International Association of Athletics Federations. Nutrition for the sprinter. *J Sports Sci.* 2007;25(suppl 1):5S-15S.

43. Areta JL, Burke LM, Ross ML, et al. Timing and distribution of protein ingestion during prolonged recovery from resistance exercise alters myofibrillar protein synthesis. *J Physiol.* 2013;591(9):2319-2331.

44. Cermak NM, Res PT, de Groot LC, Saris WH, van Loon LJ. Protein supplementation augments the adaptive response of skeletal muscle to resistance-type exercise training: a meta-analysis. *Am J Clin Nutr.* 2012;96(6):1454-1464.

45. Burd NA, Tang JE, Moore DR, Phillips SM. Exercise training and protein metabolism: influences of contraction, protein intake, and sex-based differences. *J Appl Physiol (1985).* 2009;106(5):1692-1701.

46. Schoenfeld BJ, Aragon AA, Krieger JW. The effect of protein timing on muscle strength and hypertrophy: a meta-analysis. *J Int Soc Sports Nutr.* 2013;10(1):53.

47. Phillips SM. Dietary protein requirements and adaptive advantages in athletes. *Br J Nutr.* 2012;108(suppl 2):158S-167S.

48. Phillips SM. A brief review of higher dietary protein diets in weight loss: a focus on athletes. *Sports Med.* 2014;44(suppl 2):149S-153S.

49. Josse AR, Atkinson SA, Tarnopolsky MA, Phillips SM. Diets higher in dairy foods and dietary protein support bone health during diet- and exercise-induced weight loss in overweight and obese premenopausal women. *J Clin Endocrinol Metab.* 2012;97(1):251-260.

50. IOC consensus statement on sports nutrition 2010. *J Sports Sci.* 2011;29(suppl 1):3S-4S.

51. Tipton KD, Elliott TA, Cree MG, Wolf SE, Sanford AP, Wolfe RR. Ingestion of casein and whey proteins result in muscle anabolism after resistance exercise. *Med Sci Sports Exerc.* 2004;36(12):2073-2081.

52. Anthony TG, McDaniel BJ, Knoll P, Bunpo P, Paul GL, McNurlan MA. Feeding meals containing soy or whey protein after exercise stimulates protein synthesis and translation initiation in the skeletal muscle of male rats. *J Nutr.* 2007;137(2):357-362.

53. Tang JE, Moore DR, Kujbida GW, Tarnopolsky MA, Phillips SM. Ingestion of whey hydrolysate, casein, or soy protein isolate: effects on mixed muscle protein synthesis at rest and following resistance exercise in young men. *J Appl Physiol. 1985.* 2009;107(3):987-992.

54. Wilkinson SB, Tarnopolsky MA, Macdonald MJ, Macdonald JR, Armstrong D, Phillips SM. Consumption of fluid skim milk promotes greater muscle protein accretion after resistance exercise than does consumption of an isonitrogenous and isoenergetic soy-protein beverage. *Am J Clin Nutr.* 2007;85(4):1031-1040.

55. Tipton KD, Elliott TA, Cree MG, Aarsland AA, Sanford AP, Wolfe RR. Stimulation of net muscle protein synthesis by whey protein ingestion before and after exercise. *Am J Physiol Endocrinol Metab.* 2007;292(1):E71-76.

56. Phillips SM, Moore DR, Tang JE. A critical examination of dietary protein requirements, benefits, and excesses in athletes. *Int J Sport Nutr Exerc Metab*. 2007;17(suppl):58S-76S.

57. Beelen M, Burke LM, Gibala MJ, van Loon JC. Nutritional strategies to promote postexercise recovery. *Int J Sport Nutr Exerc Metab*. 2010;20(6):515-532.

58. Havemann L, West SJ, Goedecke JH, et al. Fat adaptation followed by carbohydrate loading compromises high-intensity sprint performance. *J Appl Physiol*. 1985. 2006;100(1):194-202.

59. Stellingwerff T, Spriet LL, Watt MJ, et al. Decreased PDH activation and glycogenolysis during exercise following fat adaptation with carbohydrate restoration. *Am J Physiol Endocrinol Metab*. 2006;290(2):E380-E388.

60. Volpe SL. Micronutrient requirements for athletes. *Clin Sports Med*. 2007;26(1):119-130.

61. Peternelj TT, Coombes JS. Antioxidant supplementation during exercise training: beneficial or detrimental? *Sports Med*. 2011;41(12):1043-1069.

62. Clark KL. Nutritional considerations in joint health. *Clin Sports Med*. 2007;26(1):101-118.

63. Godek SF, Godek JJ, Bartolozzi AR. Hydration status in college football players during consecutive days of twice-a-day preseason practices. *Am J Sports Med*. 2005;33(6):843-851.

64. Godek SF, Bartolozzi AR, Godek JJ. Sweat rate and fluid turnover in American football players compared with runners in a hot and humid environment. *Br J Sports Med*. 2005;39(4):205-211; discussion 205-211.

65. Judelson DA, Maresh CM, Anderson JM, et al. Hydration and muscular performance: does fluid balance affect strength, power and high-intensity endurance? *Sports Med*. 2007;37(10):907-921.

66. Fritzsche RG, Switzer TW, Hodgkinson BJ, Lee S-H, Martin JC, Coyle EF. Water and carbohydrate ingestion during prolonged exercise increase maximal neuromuscular power. *J Appl Physiol*. 2000;88(2):730-737.

67. Murray B. Hydration and physical performance. *J Am Coll Nutr*. 2007;26(suppl 5):542S-548S.

68. Wilmore JH. Body composition in sport and exercise: directions for future research. *Med Sci Sports Exerc*. 1983;15(1):21-31.

69. Mullins VA, Houtkooper LB, Howell WH, Going SB, Brown CH. Nutritional status of U.S. elite female heptathletes during training. *Int J Sport Nutr Exerc Metab*. 2001;11(3):299-314.

70. Ackland TR, Lohman TG, Sundgot-Borgen J, et al. Current status of body composition assessment in sport: review and position statement on behalf of the ad hoc research working group on body composition health and performance, under the auspices of the I.O.C. Medical Commission. *Sports Med*. 2012;42(3):227-249.

71. Fogelholm M, Hiilloskorpi H. Weight and diet concerns in Finnish female and male athletes. *Med Sci Sports Exerc*. 1999;31(2):229-235.

72. Rankin JW. Weight loss and gain in athletes. *Curr Sports Med Rep*. 2002;1(4):208-213.

73. Walberg-Rankin J, Hawkins CE, Fild DS, Sebolt DR. The effect of oral arginine during energy restriction in male weight trainers. *J Strength Cond Res*. 1994;8(3):170-177.

74. Walberg JL, Leidy MK, Sturgill DJ, Hinkle DE, Ritchey SJ, Sebolt DR. Macronutrient content of a hypoenergy diet affects nitrogen retention and muscle function in weight lifters. *Int J Sports Med*. 1988;9(4):261-266.

CHAPTER 21

NUTRITION FOR HIGH-INTENSITY, INTERMITTENT SPORTS

Michele Macedonio, MS, RDN, CSSD

INTRODUCTION

The term *high-intensity, intermittent exercise* (HIIE) refers to activities that require short periods of all-out effort (eg, sprints of up to 2 to 7 seconds), punctuated with periods of less-intense effort (eg, jogging sustained over 5 to 10 minutes) and low-intensity effort (eg, walking and standing still). Team sports, such as soccer, football, basketball, lacrosse, field hockey, ice hockey, rugby, and volleyball, as well as individual sports, such as racquet sports (eg, tennis, squash), are classified as HIIE sports.[1] The common feature among team sports is the intermittent, high-intensity pattern of play. All intermittent sports require bursts of intense effort, such as jumping for a rebound in basketball, accelerating in ice hockey, or sprinting to the ball in soccer. HIIE sports vary per sport-specific game characteristics, including rules of play (eg, regarding rest periods, player substitutions); tasks such as the serve in tennis, the spike in volleyball, or the split roll dodge in lacrosse; player positions; and style of play. They also vary from match to match. Distinguishing features of each sport create various physiological challenges and nutritional needs for team-sport athletes.

Most team sports can be described as moderate to long-duration exercise punctuated with periods of high-intensity activity and periods of low to moderate active recovery or rest. Team sport players cover moderate to long distances during match play (eg, 8 to13 km in soccer).[2] Soccer is mainly aerobic in nature because of the large distances covered during competition [3-5] In comparison, a professional hockey game has 60 minutes of regulation play but usually lasts about 2.5 hours with intermissions and timeouts. The game is characterized by intense bouts of play lasting 45 to 60 seconds, seldom exceeding 90 seconds. The average ice time is less than 16 minutes for most ice hockey players, although some players may receive as much as 35 minutes of playing time. A majority of the game play is well below the lactate threshold.[6]

Intermittent sports have been classified into endurance based (eg, soccer, field hockey, lacrosse), court (eg, basketball, volleyball, tennis), batting (eg, baseball, softball, cricket), and strength and power-based (eg, American football, rugby). Success in HIIE sports is largely dependent on the ability to sustain skill execution. Aspects of cognitive function, such as attention, decision making, and response time, can affect performance. The stop-and-go nature of these sports often results in impaired performance after periods of intense effort and near the end of the competition.[5] Taken as a whole, HIIE sports require a range of exercise intensity from low to very high in varying durations during which all of the major energy systems are tapped. See Table 21.1 for example of intermitent high-intensity team sports.

Soccer has been studied extensively and provides a good base for understanding the physiological demands and nutritional implications of HIIE.[7-17] Other HIIE sports have also been studied, but not as extensively as soccer.[18-36]

Nutrient needs of athletes performing HIIE can be high but can generally be met with a diet that provides sufficient energy to meet the demands of training and competition. Careful food and fluid selection and strategic nutrient timing are key to meeting the additional nutrient demands. However, observations of the dietary practices of athletes engaged in HIIE suggest that many athletes have an inadequate diet.[37-48]

Table 21.1 Categories of Intermittent High-Intensity Team Sports [1,35]

Classification of Team Sports	Sport	Sport Distinctions	Physiological Burden
Field-Based Sports			
Endurance-based field sports	Soccer, field hockey, ice hockey, lacrosse	Large playing area; longer distances covered at high speed; change of direction; continuous activity at variable speeds	Glycogen repletion; hydration status
Strength and power field sports	American football, rugby	Cover less running distance; frequent bursts of short sprints with contact, scrimmage, and tackling bouts	Carbohydrate intake to match training goals and support performance and recovery; possibly lower carbohydrate needs for rugby union
Batting field sports	Baseball, softball, cricket	Lower overall energy demands; many hours in sun; greater rest duration between efforts; need for attention and decision making	Maintaining blood glucose during game; hydration status
Court Sports	Basketball, volleyball, tennis, badminton, team handball, racquetball, squash	Smaller playing area; shorter-duration games; frequent substitution; often several games per day or over several days; much time traveling	Training period requires high energy and fluid demands; potential for incomplete glycogen repletion due to schedule

PHYSIOLOGICAL DEMANDS OF HIGH-INTENSITY, INTERMITTENT EXERCISE

Energy Systems

Athletes engage in HIIE training to improve endurance capacity, as well as muscle strength and conditioning. Both anaerobic and aerobic energy production are important to the HIIE athlete.[2,6,21,49-51] Anaerobic energy production is essential for high-intensity exercise when the demand for adenosine triphosphate (ATP) exceeds the body's ability to produce it aerobically. At the onset of high-intensity exercise, anaerobically produced ATP provides the majority of the energy used because of the short supply of oxygen. Anaerobic production of ATP continues to play a key role in sustained high-intensity exercise (see Table 21.2, page 468).[6-14]

Both the intensity and duration of exercise increase energy demands during vigorous, stop-and-go exercise that lasts for 60 minutes or more.[10] The ability to perform sprints and short-duration recovery is an important element of performance in intermittent team sports.[6,14,19,21] Agility, which has been described as "the ability to produce whole-body movements with change of velocity or direction in response to a stimulus," has been identified as a key attribute of elite-level team sport players.[52-55] The decline in running performance during intermittent exercise is a result of fatigue. Due to the physiological demands of HIIE, fatigue occurs at different times during a game and may be the result of different mechanisms. Players experience temporary fatigue during the game after bouts of high-intensity effort and more permanent fatigue toward the end of the game.[56-58] Transient fatigue is associated with repeated high-intensity efforts and insufficient recovery (< 30 seconds), but the factors contributing to transient fatigue and its effect on subsequent running performance have not been clearly identified.[59-61]

Variations in the nature and circumstances of individual intermittent sports make it challenging to determine the exact game demands, but performance is often dependent on nutritional factors. Ongoing considerations include achieving and maintaining optimal body mass and composition and meeting the nutrient demands of the training program. Acute issues in training or competition include keeping players adequately hydrated and fueled throughout the exercise. Recovery between events is a major priority and needs to address rehydration, refueling, and repair.

Table 21.2 Approximate Relative Energy Contribution During Selected Periods of High-Intensity Exercise

Duration, s	Anaerobic, %	Aerobic, %
30	80	20
60–90	45	55
120–180	30	70

Adapted from: McArdle WD, Katch FI, Katch VL. *Exercise Physiology: Nutrition, Energy, and Human Performance.* 6th ed. Philadelphia, PA: Lippincott Williams & Wilkins; 2007.

Because of the game duration, endurance-type intermittent sports are mainly dependent on aerobic metabolism. During a 90-minute match, the average work intensity, measured by heart rate, is close to the anaerobic threshold, with mean and peak heart rates around 85% and 98% of maximum heart rate.[9,11,62,63] Total energy expended during a soccer match is directly related to the distance covered during the 90 minutes of the game, usually 8 to 13 km (5 to 8 miles).[7,9,14,49]

Elite soccer players perform 150 to 250 brief intense actions during a game, indicating that there are periods of high anaerobic energy turnover. Over the course of a soccer game, players are required to sprint, jog, stride, walk, and move sideways and backward while tackling, jumping, accelerating, and turning. Regardless of position, the greatest percentage of distance is covered at slower speeds.

Ice hockey is metabolically unique: it requires finely trained aerobic and anaerobic energy pathways. Bursts of intense muscular activity demand exceptional aerobic power and endurance and intense glycolytic activity. The involvement of the anaerobic system may depend on the efficiency of the aerobic system. Using sport-specific testing methods, Peterson and colleagues investigated the relationship between maximal oxygen uptake (VO_2 peak) and repeated on-ice sprint ability in 45 male college hockey players. Results of the study suggest that repeated on-ice sprint ability is associated with VO_2 peak and the final stage completed during the graded exercise test, pointing to the association of aerobic metabolism and fatigue in ice hockey players.[64]

Major differences have been observed in physical demands on players, due in part to team position, with a greater amount of high-intensity exercise in top-class players compared with those of a lower standard.[65] Although measurements of high-intensity running, mean recovery time, and maximal running speed are similar in elite domestic and international soccer players, they vary markedly among playing positions.[60]

Large sex differences exist for match performance characteristics of elite-level soccer players. Men cover more total distance, at higher speed thresholds, and during the most intense period of a match. Sex differences are more pronounced in women at higher speed thresholds than for total distance, with women covering a greater distance at a lower speed threshold of less than 12 km/h vs a standard of more than 15 km/h for men.[66]

Duration and relative exercise intensity are major factors in determining the fuel mixture during exercise. Exercise intensity is expressed as percentage of maximum oxygen consumption (VO_2 max), which is influenced by age, sex, genetic makeup, and level of aerobic training.[67,68] See Table 21.3.

Glycogen, an essential fuel during prolonged vigorous exercise, is required by athletes engaged in HIIE sports, especially when completing high-intensity efforts. The nature of the activity in stop-and-go team

Table 21.3 Muscle Energy Pathways During Activity of Varying Intensity[67,68]

	Muscle Energy Pathways	Duration of Activity	Type of Activity (% MHR[a])
Immediate	ATP[b] in muscles	1–6 s	Surges and sprints (≥80–90)
	ATP + PCr[c]	7–20 s	
	ATP + PCr + muscle glycogen	20–45 s	
Short term	Muscle glycogen	45–120 s	Moderate-intensity running (70–80)
	Muscle glycogen + lactic acid	120–180 s	
Long term	Muscle glycogen + free fatty acids	>30 min, limited by oxygen	Low- to moderate-intensity running (<69)

[a] MHR = maximum heart rate
[b] ATP = adenosine triphosphate
[c] PCr = phosphocreatine

sports requires use of both types of muscle fibers.[69,70] Type II (fast-twitch) fibers exhibit the greatest degree of glycogen depletion after sprint-type activities.[71] Costill and colleagues showed that in distance running, glycogen was selectively depleted in type I (slow-twitch) fibers but that type I fibers also bore some of the load.[72] From these studies, it seems that type I fibers are activated at lower workloads and that type II fibers are used during two conditions: when type I fibers are depleted of glycogen and during high-intensity output.[71,73,74]

Green examined glycogen utilization in the muscle fibers of ice hockey players. Muscle glycogen depletion averaged 60%, and this depletion indicated the utilization of both type I and type II fibers, with the greatest decline occurring in type I fibers. There was no apparent difference in the amount and pattern of glycogen depletion between forwards and defensemen.[75] Krustrup and colleagues found that muscle glycogen was reduced to 150 to 350 mmol/kg by the end of a soccer match, with half of the fibers of both types depleted or almost depleted.[76] The authors theorized that the pattern of glycogen depletion in some fibers may limit maximal sprint effort.[76]

Effects of High-Intensity, Intermittent Exercise on Substrate Utilization

The relative contribution of fat and carbohydrate depends on the intensity and duration of exercise, with an increasingly greater total and relative contribution from carbohydrate as exercise intensity increases above approximately 60% VO_2 max.[74,77] Endurance exercise training triggers metabolic adaptations that lead to a marked sparing of carbohydrate as a result of a slower utilization of glucose and muscle and liver glycogen during sustained exercise of the same intensity.[78,79] Consequently, endurance training leads to a relatively smaller reliance on carbohydrates than on fatty acids during prolonged steady-state exercise. The reduced reliance on blood glucose and muscle glycogen during exercise in a trained state is one of the mechanisms by which exercise enhances endurance.

In addition to a relative shift in substrate, the absolute amount of fat used decreases as work rate increases.[67,80] Plasma glucose and muscle glycogen utilization both increase in response to an increase in exercise intensity. Plasma glucose contributes approximately 10% to 15% of total energy at all work rates, whereas muscle glycogen supplies approximately 60% of the energy requirement in strenuous exercise at approximately 80% of VO_2 max.[67,68]

Fat as a Substrate During High-Intensity Intermittent Exercise

Studies have shown that blood free fatty acid (FFA) concentration increases during a soccer match, with greater increase in the second half than the first and after the game.[76] Blood FFA concentration during a soccer match is the net result of the uptake of FFA in various tissues and the release from adipose tissue. Hormonal responses during HIIE also exert significant influence on metabolism.[11] Bracken and colleagues studied the catecholamine response in 12 nonspecifically trained men who completed ten 6-second cycle ergometer sprints with a 30-second recovery between each sprint. Plasma epinephrine increased 6.3-fold from baseline, whereas norepinephrine increased 14.5-fold at the end of sprinting.[81] Trapp and colleagues examined the metabolic response to two forms of HIIE—short sprint and long sprint—in 16 trained and untrained women.[82] The observed increase in glycerol concentration suggests an increased reliance on fats as fuel despite increased lactate concentrations and was attributed to periods of rest and a slower pace during the second half, allowing more blood flow to adipose tissue and possibly promoting higher FFA release. This process, when coupled with hormonal changes, specifically decreased insulin, increased catecholamines, and stimulated lipolysis and release of FFA into the blood. These changes cause greater uptake of FFA and utilization of triglycerides by contracting muscles. Such adaptations favor high blood glucose concentrations and may be compensatory mechanisms for progressively decreasing muscle glycogen levels. A high uptake of glycerol in various tissues, primarily the liver, is presumed, indicating that glycerol might be an important gluconeogenic precursor. Ketone bodies may also function as a minor fat source during exercise.

Carbohydrate as a Substrate During High-Intensity, Intermittent Exercise

With increasing energy intensity, the percentage of carbohydrate used as an energy substrate increases to meet most of the energy demands of muscle contraction at an intensity near an individual's VO_2 max. The relative contribution of fat decreases with a concomitant increase in carbohydrate oxidation from 40% to 85% VO_2 max. At moderate- and high-intensity exercise (50% to 85% VO_2 max), plasma fatty acids and muscle triglycerides supply the fats that are oxidized.[67,80,83,84]

In trained athletes, during vigorous exercise there is an initial burst of glycogenolysis and a resulting production of lactic acid, followed by a slowing of the rate of glycogenolysis and a reduction in muscle and blood lactate levels.

Glycogen, an essential fuel during prolonged vigorous exercise, is required by athletes engaged in HIIE sports, especially when completing high-intensity efforts. Skeletal muscle contraction and the central nervous system depend on carbohydrate as a fuel substrate, but the body's stores of carbohydrate are limited, and often the fuel requirements of training and competition for HIIE team sports substantially exceed carbohydrate availability.

In a simulated soccer match, rate of muscle glycogen use decreased from the first to the second half, with the highest (4.0 ± 1.2 mmol/kg/min) during the warm-up and first 15 minutes of play, and becoming progressively lower during intervals from 15 to 60 minutes (1.8 ± 0.5 mmol/kg/min) and 60 to 90 minutes (0.9 ± 1.2 mmol/kg/min).[85] When muscle glycogen stores are depleted, fatigue—both physical and mental—sets in and performance is compromised.[86-88]

A study involving 20 male and female college students experienced in playing team sports performed experimental trials of varying intensities to examine the effect of 6% carbohydrate on performance and central nervous system function. Compared with a placebo, carbohydrate feedings resulted in fourth-quarter improvements, including faster sprint times, higher average jump height, enhanced motor skills, and improved mood, suggesting that carbohydrate feedings during intermittent high-intensity exercise benefit peripheral and central nervous system function.[89]

Aerobic Energy System

Researchers have attempted to determine the aerobic energy contribution during HIIE performance by measuring oxygen uptake (VO_2); however, the procedure interferes with normal play, and results are most likely imprecise. Heart rate is used to estimate oxygen uptake, but it does not always reflect the actual oxygen uptake. Factors such as dehydration, hyperthermia, and mental stress elevate heart rate without affecting oxygen uptake. Aside from its use in predicting oxygen uptake, heart rate provides a useful index of the overall physiological demands of soccer.[10]

During a match, soccer players spend a considerable amount of time working at heart rates estimated to be more than 160 beats per minute, with mean and peak heart rates around 85% and 98% of maximal values and heart rates rarely below 65% of maximum values.[9,14,90] Heart rates of ice hockey players have been reported between 79.0% and 89.5% of maximum heart rate and as much as 82.5% of maximal oxygen uptake.[6,25,91] Physiological profiles of players in other HIIE team sports, such as basketball, hockey, ice hockey, and tennis, have shown similar patterns, pointing to the importance of the aerobic energy pathway in HIIE sports. [21,34,50,92]

Intermittent exercise has an effect on oxygen consumption similar to that of submaximal continuous running.[11] Although anaerobic activity is an important component of soccer, greater demand is on aerobic metabolism. Considering total distance covered, the ratio of low-intensity to high-intensity activity is 2:1, and the relative time ratio is 7:1.[11] Sprinting occurs no more than 1.5% of total playing time.[3,16] Considering all factors, relative work rates during soccer have been estimated between 70% and 80% of VO_2 max.[9-11,14] Estimates of VO_2 max based on many studies of soccer players over the years suggest an average of 60 mL/kg/min.[70] As shown in Table 21.4, similar heart rate patterns have been found among athletes in various intermittent, high-intensity sports.[9,10,14,19,21,22,24,28,33,93,94]

Table 21.4 Heart Rate Patterns of Athletes in High-Intensity, Intermittent Sports

Sport	Maximum Heart Rate, %
Basketball[19,24]	>85
Ice hockey[28]	85–90
Racquet sports including squash, badminton[94]	80–85
Rugby[21,22]	>85
Soccer[9,10,14]	80–100
Tennis[33,93]	80–85

Anaerobic Energy System

ADENOSINE TRIPHOSPHATE AND PHOSPHOCREATINE

Considerable energy fluctuations occur when performing HIIE sports. Although the majority of work is done at submaximal intensities, high-intensity exercise plays a crucial role, and the athlete's ability to successfully carry out these high-intensity activities affects the result of the game. Creatine phosphate (PCr) concentration fluctuates throughout a match because of the intermittent nature of the game and may decrease below resting values if a number of intense bouts of exercise are accompanied by short recovery time.[76] Despite a small net utilization, PCr plays an important role as an energy buffer, providing phosphate for the resynthesis of ATP during the rapid increases in exercise intensity.[11,49] Aerobic fitness enhances recovery from HIIE through increased aerobic response, improved lactate removal, and enhanced PCr regeneration.[95]

BLOOD LACTATE

Glycolysis is activated and lactate is formed almost immediately once exercise starts.[11] Since lactate is produced at a high rate during intense activity, blood lactate concentrations have been used as indicators of anaerobic energy production in soccer.[9,11] The concentration of blood lactate fluctuates throughout a soccer match. Lactate is metabolized within the active muscle after high-intensity exercise. When high-intensity exercise is coupled with low-intensity exercise, lactate metabolism increases. Furthermore, lactate released into the blood is taken up by the heart, liver, kidney, and other tissues. Evidence suggests that lactate is an important metabolic intermediate as a substrate for oxidative metabolism in cardiac and skeletal muscle and a precursor for gluconeogenesis.[96] Thus, measurements of blood lactate concentration represent the balance of lactate released by muscle and taken up by blood and will not fully reflect lactate production during a soccer match. During HIIE, blood lactate may be high whereas muscle lactate may be relatively low.[14] Lactate production may be very high at points throughout a soccer game with mean blood lactate concentrations ranging from 2 mmol/L to10 mmol/L during a match.[9,11,76] During a tennis match, blood lactate levels were shown to have increased 50% to near, but not beyond, the anabolic threshold.[33] The authors attribute this finding to several factors, including a highly trained aerobic system and variations in play that allow blood lactate levels to clear. McInnes and colleagues reported blood lactate levels averaging 6.8 mmol/L during basketball, indicating that glycolysis is involved in energy production.[24] Blood lactate concentrations are used to estimate the contribution of anaerobic glycolysis to metabolism during team sports, with mean values reported from 3.0 to 9.0 mmol/L in soccer, 6.5 to 8.5 mmol/L in rugby, 4.94 to 6.05 mmol/L in male basketball players and 3.7 to 5.2 mmol/L in female basketball players.[14,21,50,97,98] It is important to note that blood lactate represents the balance of production, release, and removal of lactate. Lactate is metabolized by active muscles after high-intensity activity and will vary according to the intensity of play. However, not all of the lactate produced is reflected in the blood. Lactate released from active muscles into the blood is taken up by different tissues, such as the heart, liver, kidney, and inactive muscles.

ENERGY AND MACRONUTRIENT NEEDS

Energy

Energy demands are high due to the intermittent nature of stop-and-go sports, and energy intake must be adequate to support training and competition.[99] Several early reports suggested that some players may not be meeting optimal nutrient intakes.[99-104] Clark reported that professional male soccer players consumed between 2,033 and 3,923 kcal/d.[100] Data from a Major Indoor Soccer League team revealed that daily energy intakes of male players averaged 2,662 kcal and ranged from 1,618 to 4,394 kcal/d.[101] More recent data

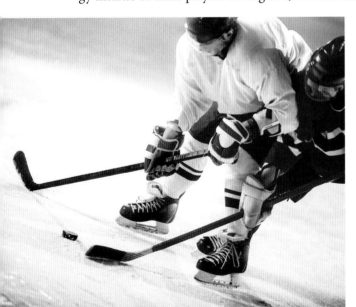

examining the diets of intermittent sports athletes support these findings and indicate that nutritional intakes of both male and female athletes participating in various HIIE sports may be inadequate.[38,40,42-44,47,102-111]

Attempts have been made to determine the energy expended during HIIE sports, but, to date, no one has provided accurate and valid data when measuring oxygen uptake. Values that have been measured are likely underestimate, and equipment probably interferes with performance. Establishing a relationship between heart rate and oxygen uptake allows for accurate indirect assessment of oxygen uptake during HIIE. A line relationship between heart rate and oxygen uptake, deemed valid for intermittent exercise, was used to estimate the work rate during a soccer match as approximately 70% VO_2 max, corresponding to an energy production of approximately 1,360 kcal for a 75 kg player with a maximum oxygen uptake of 60 mL/kg/min.[49] Stolen estimates an average exercise intensity of 85% of maximum heart rate during a soccer match, corresponding to about 75% of VO_2 max. This corresponds to an average oxygen uptake of 45.0 mL/kg/min, 48.8 mL/kg/min, and 52.5 mL/kg/min for a player performing at 60%,

65%, and 70% of VO$_2$ max, respectively. For a player who weighs 75 kg this corresponds to an energy expenditure of 1,519 kcal, 1,645 kcal, and 1,772 kcal during a match (5 kcal/L oxygen per min), assuming 60 mL/kg/min, 65 mL/kg/min, and 70 mL/kg/min, respectively.[112] Bangsbo and colleagues estimated that soccer players expended 1,608 kcal on average during each training session in the 2 weeks leading up to the men's World Cup.[14] Female soccer players experience similar exercise intensity during a match, but they expend less energy than men because women have smaller body mass.

Information regarding nutritional habits of female team sport players is limited. There are reports of insufficient energy intake among female and adolescent soccer players.[38,39,104-107,113] An examination of the dietary intake of 24 female college athletes (field hockey, cross-country, tennis, and golf) reveals less than the recommended intakes of carbohydrate and energy (1,513 ± 406 kcal/d), with iron and calcium intakes 30% below the Recommended Dietary Allowance (RDA). Fourteen of the 24 athletes were attempting to lose weight.[113] Nutter concluded that nutrition counseling is necessary to advise female players on ways to balance energy and nutrient intake with attempts to achieve a more appropriate performance weight.

Data reported in 2003 about female collegiate soccer players indicated that they met the Dietary Reference Intakes (DRIs) for total energy (37 kcal/kg of body weight), protein, and fat during the preseason and their intake was substantially higher than DRI during the playing season.[104] Although protein and fat intakes during the preseason were more than the minimum recommendations, carbohydrate intakes were not sufficient to promote glycogen repletion. In this study, protein and fat displaced carbohydrate-rich, nutrient-dense foods and helped supply the energy requirements during preseason training, but the diet failed to meet carbohydrate and micronutrient recommendations. It is important to note that total energy, carbohydrate, and micronutrient intakes during the season may not have been sufficient to support energy demands and recommended intakes and may have compromised performance.

Papadopoulous and colleagues assessed the macro- and micronutrient intakes of two Greek teams of adolescent female volleyball players, the Junior National Team and the Junior National Championship Team, and found that protein intake was satisfactory (approximately 16% of total kcal), but fat intake was generally higher than desired (approximately 37.5% of total kcal) at the expense of carbohydrate consumption (45.9% of total kcal), with mean energy intakes at less than optimal levels (2,013 kcal and 1,529 kcal, respectively).[114] As a whole, the volleyball players fell short of meeting the RDA values for calcium (935 ± 497 mg, RDA 1,200 mg), iron (7.9 ± 4.0 mg, RDA 15.0 mg), folic acid (163 ± 98 mcg, RDA 180 mcg), magnesium (207 ± 130 mg, RDA 300 mg), zinc (7 ± 5 mg, RDA 12 mg), and vitamins A (554 ± 495 retinol equivalents, RDA 800 retinol equivalents), B-1 (0.9 ± 0.5 mg, RDA 1.1 mg), B-2 (1.2 ± 0.6 mg, RDA 1.2 mg) , and B-6 (0.8 ± 0.7 mg, RDA 1.5 mg). Mean daily intake energy intake (1,648 kcal/d) was lower than the RDA (by 44 kcal/d) for very active women.[114]

Holway and Spriet summarized 30 years of published reports of the energy and macronutrient intakes of team sport athletes. The mean carbohydrate, protein, and fat intakes were 49%, 17%, and 34%, respectively, for male athletes and 50%, 15%, and 35%, respectively, for female athletes, with male athletes eating an average of 5.6 ± 1.3 g/kg/d carbohydrates and female athletes eating 4.0 l ± 0.7 g/kg/d. Generally, preseason intakes are greater than in-season intakes; larger athletes consume more energy; and carbohydrate intake, at 49%, is lower than some past recommendations of 55% to 65%.[1]

Gravina and colleagues studied the effect of macronutrient and micronutrient intake on markers of oxidative stress, muscle damage, and inflammatory and immune response in 28 female soccer players, age 21 ± 6 years old. All players engaged in training plus one match per weekend. An 8-day diet record and blood samples collected immediately after and 18 hours after four official soccer matches were analyzed. The mean reported energy intake was 2,271 ± 578 kcal/d with a macronutrient distribution that was higher in protein (15% ± 2%); lower in carbohydrate (44.3% ± 6%); and higher in fat (37% ± 7%), saturated fat (12.4 ±3%), and cholesterol (340 mg/d) than recommendations (protein 10% to 12%, carbohydrate 50% to 60%, fat 35%, cholesterol < 300 mg). Fiber intake was lower (20 ± 7 g/d) than the recommended 25 to 26 g/d. Intakes of folic acid (230 ± 100 mcg/d), vitamin D (3.3 ± 2 mcg/d,) magnesium (315 ± 97mg/d), and potassium (2973 ± 971 mg/d) were also suboptimal and lower than the DRI. Players who followed guidelines for the recommended intakes had higher levels of total antioxidant status and lower levels of creatine kinase and lactate dehydrogenase, markers of oxidative stress. The authors concluded that their data reveal an association between nutritional intake and muscle damage, oxidative stress, immunity, and inflammation markers and that adequate intakes of specific nutrients may help prevent undesirable physiological effects related to HIIE.[39]

Briggs and colleagues investigated energy intake and expenditure (triaxial accelerometer) of adolescent male academy-level soccer players age 15.4 ± 0.3 years during a competitive 7-day period. Mean energy intake (2,245 ± 321 kcal) was significantly lower than mean energy expenditure (2,552 ± 321 kcal), resulting in a daily deficit of 311 ± 397 kcal. A significant difference was observed between energy intake and energy expenditure on heavy training days (−505 ± 539 kcal) and match days (−544 ± 551 kcal). Only on rest days was a mean positive energy balance (153 ± 286 kcal) observed. Carbohydrate intake (5.6 ± 0.4 g/kg/d), mainly from starchy foods, was suboptimal, especially during training and on match days. Protein intake (1.5 ± 0.2 g/kg/d), mainly from poultry and dairy foods, was within an optimal range to support growth and development. The mean fat intake (29% ± 2%) was at the

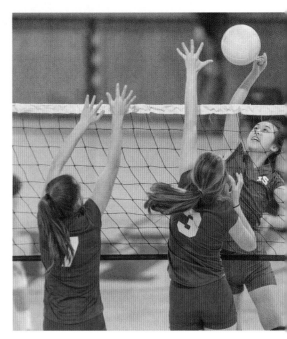

upper limit, with saturated fat values of 26 ± 3 g/d (12% total kcal). This suggests that having athletes reduce intake of saturated fat rather than total fat may be advisable. Energy deficits among young athletes have been observed in similar populations and indicate a need for nutrition education and intervention to support optimal growth, development, and performance of adolescent athletes.[115]

Carbohydrate

The large aerobic energy production in HIIE sports and the substantial anaerobic energy turnover are associated with a large consumption of substrates, predominantely carbohydrate and fat. The body's carbohydrate stores are in liver (~100 g) and skeletal muscle glycogen (~300–700 g). These endogenous carbohydrate stores are relatively small, supplying less than 5% of the body's total energy storage. When carbohydrate requirements of training or competition exceed endogenous carbohydrate stores, carbohydrate availability is compromised. In a review of studies of cyclists, Maughan and colleagues compared the effects of low-carbohydrate diets vs high-carbohydrate diets on high-intensity exercise. A low-carbohydrate diet (< 10% of total energy from carbohydrate) resulted in reduced endurance time. Conversely, diets that provided 65% to 84% carbohydrate were associated with increased performance, more consistently so with carbohydrate intakes at the higher end. Also noted was that a high-protein diet, particularly in conjunction with a low-carbohydrate diet, resulted in metabolic acidosis, which is associated with fatigue. Although many questions about the causal mechanisms remain unanswered, the authors concluded the review with two distinct messages. The first is that it is possible to improve performance of short-duration, high-intensity exercise with a high-carbohydrate, low-protein diet for a few days before competition. Second, performance of this type may be impaired by a high-protein diet with insufficient carbohydrate or an energy-restricted diet in the precompetition period.[116]

Based on the effects of nutrition interventions on molecular and cellular processes during exercise and recovery, Hawley and colleagues recommend that the diet of athletes performing HIIE approach 7 g carbohydrate per kilogram of body mass during intense training to maintain adequate muscle glycogen stores to meet the periods of strenuous demands during competition.[117]

MUSCLE GLYCOGEN

The demands on muscle glycogen are great, and early researchers almost unanimously agreed that performance improves when carbohydrate is supplied before and during HIIE. Carbohydrate used during HIIE is primarily supplied by the glycogen stored within exercising muscle, although muscles may also utilize glucose circulating in blood. Most of the early studies supported the use of a carbohydrate-electrolyte solution during HIIE but were subject to methodologic limitations. Of particular concern was the use of exercise protocols that employed the same exercise intensity, the lack of maximal- or high-intensity work, and long periods of seated recovery, which failed to replicate the pattern and physiological demands of exercise during team games, thus limiting their applicability to actual team games.[118]

Bangsbo and colleagues reported that by increasing the carbohydrate content of the diet from 39% to 65% before a soccer match, muscle glycogen levels increased and resulted in a higher work rate and improved intermittent endurance.[119] In a study of Swedish elite ice hockey players, Akermark and colleagues compared the performance of ice hockey players given a carbohydrate-enriched diet vs a mixed diet. During a 3-day period between two games, players were fed a mixed diet of approximately 40% carbohydrate or a diet of approximately 60% carbohydrate. Distance skated, number of shifts skated, amount of time skated within shifts, and skating speed improved with the higher carbohydrate intake.[28] Glycogen depletion may seriously limit players' ability to maintain high-intensity work output, distance covered, and sprinting frequency, particularly during the later stages of the game. The glycogen utilization in leg muscle is markedly increased during bouts of intense exercise. During periods of rest and low-intensity play, glycogen is resynthesized.[120]

In two studies, researchers found low levels of muscle glycogen at the end of a soccer match and reported higher glycogen use in the first half compared with the second half.[69,121] Muscle glycogen concentration was only 50% of the prematch values 2 days after the match.[69] The difference in muscle glycogen measured before and after a match represents the net glycogen utilization and does not fully reflect total glycogen turnover during play.[11,49] Toward the end of a match, players experienced fatigue and a decrease in performance. Although an exact mechanism for this phenomenon has not been identified, low levels of muscle glycogen may be a factor. Saltin observed that players with low levels of glycogen covered 24% less distance, 50% of which was covered by walking.[121] Without sufficient muscle glycogen, exercise is fueled by fat, and the intensity of that exercise is typically less than 50% of capacity.[67,122] Krustrup and colleagues measured a 150 to 350 mmol/kg dry weight drop in muscle glycogen (42% ± 6%) as a result of repeated sprinting: Postgame measures were 225 ± 22 mmol/kg dry weight compared with 449 mmol/kg dry weight) at rest. Sprint performance was reduced both temporarily after intense exercise and at the end of the match. Half of the glycogen in individual muscle fibers of both types were either depleted or almost depleted, possibly preventing maximal sprint effort.[76] The effect of low muscle glycogen is more likely to have greater consequence in intermittent sports where endogenous stores of glycogen are insufficient to meet energy demands for the full duration of play, during overtime, or during tournament competition. It is, therefore, important that athletes begin exercise with full glycogen stores and replenish glycogen stores as soon as possible after glycogen-depleting exercise. In the absence of severe muscle damage, an adequate carbohydrate intake can restore muscle glycogen stores within 24 hours of reduced exercise.[123]

BLOOD GLUCOSE

The role of liver glycogen is to regulate blood glucose to meet the needs of the whole organism, including the central nervous system. The stored glycogen in skeletal muscle provides a major portion of carbohydrate used during a soccer match, but blood glucose may also be utilized by exercising muscles and may, in fact, spare muscle glycogen.[11,124] Muscle contraction causes an increase in the uptake of glucose from the blood. As exercise duration increases, the carbohydrate from muscle glycogen decreases while that from blood glucose increases.[67] Blood glucose concentrations increase during HIIE, as long as there are sufficient liver glycogen and glucose precursors.[9,11,124]

Hypoglycemia and depletion of glycogen are associated with fatigue and reduced performance. Ferrauti and colleagues assessed the incidence of hypoglycemia in tennis players during repeated tournament and practice matches by examining the change in glucose concentrations over the test period.[125] The results indicate that glucose homeostasis is disrupted several times during tennis tournaments, leading to a decrease in glucose concentration and an increased risk of hypoglycemia, especially after a long match with only short breaks. In the absence of carbohydrate supplementation during extended play, blood glucose can decrease. To reduce the risk of hypoglycemia, a continuous intake of carbohydrate with a low glycemic index is recommended beginning with the third set through the end of the match and during changeovers.

CARBOHYDRATE RECOMMENDATIONS

A 1994 review by Hargreaves presents an overview of the early research on the role of carbohydrate in the performance of soccer players before, during, and after games and intensive training. Hargreaves concluded that a prematch diet of at least 55% of total energy as carbohydrate, accompanied by additional carbohydrate consumed during and after a match, maximizes liver and muscle glycogen stores and enhances the performance of athletes.[126]

The effects of consuming carbohydrate during HIIE have been researched.[127-133] Davison and colleagues demonstrated that 8 mL/kg of a 6% carbohydrate-electrolyte solution consumed 15 minutes prior to HIIE helped maintain higher blood glucose compared with a placebo or no fluid, resulting in delayed fatigue and improved performance.[134] More recently Phillips and colleagues demonstrated that ingesting a 6% carbohydrate-electrolyte solution significantly improves intermittent, high-intensity endurance capacity but not sprint performance of adolescents during intermittent exercise.[131] Sporting skills have been shown to decline during or following exercise.[86,135] Phillips and colleagues performed a literature review on the effects of carbohydrate intake on team sport performance. From studies mimicking the demands of team sport and using appropriate methodology, the authors concluded that a carbohydrate supplementation resulted in an increase in blood glucose concentration, significantly higher carbohydrate oxidation rates, and attenuated fat oxidation rates and FFA levels in soccer, rugby, and field hockey players.[118]

Russell and colleagues reported that a 6% sucrose-electrolyte beverage administered during a soccer match simulation attenuated declining shooting performance with improved shot speed and overall shooting performance at the end of the simulation but did not improve precision, success, ball speed, or performance in passing and dribbling. The carbohydrate beverage did not prevent an exercise-induced glycemic response when exercise was resumed after halftime.[132] Another study by Russell and colleagues documented a transient reduction in blood glucose while players consumed a carbohydrate-electrolyte beverage during team play.[136] Despite evidence that blood glucose concentrations can be maintained beyond 90 minutes and during 30-plus minutes of extra time, it is recommended that team sport athletes ingest carbohydrate during exercise to preserve endogenous glycogen and maintain running performance late in exercise.[137]

Jeukendrup noted that carbohydrates may be oxidized at different rates during exercise due to differences in absorption rates and the need to convert specific carbohydrates into substrates that can be used by skeletal muscle. Glucose, fructose, galactose, sucrose, and maltose polymers were studied originally with fructose being oxidized at slightly slower rates than glucose and galactose having a 50% slower rate of oxidation than that of glucose. Consequently, it was recommended that carbohydrates be consumed at a rate no higher than 1 g/min (30 to 60 g/h). Recent research, however, has demonstrated that ingesting multiple transportable carbohydrates that use different intestinal transporters increased carbohydrate delivery and that this carbohydrate can be oxidized at rates in excess of 1 g/min.[138]

Results were mixed in a 2015 literature review on the effects of ingesting 30 to 60 g carbohydrate per hour on intermittent sports performance for sprinting, sport-specific skills, and change of speed direction. Carbohydrate ingestion was minimally effective for jumping and cognitive function; however, carbohydrate ingestion seemed to have the greatest impact on the development of permanent fatigue and hypoglycemia, such as toward the end of a long match.[52] The available research suggests that 30 to 60 g/h of carbohydrate intake consistently enhances high-intensity intermittent performance with longer time to exhaustion and greater distance covered, and it may be more important to performance when carbohydrate is consumed before/during a high-intensity event vs a lower-intensity session.[131,139] Solid (bar) or semisolid (gel or chew) carbohydrate are oxidized at the same rate as carbohydrate solution as long as sufficient water was consumed. Carbohydrate gels can improve endurance capacity in high intensity intermittent exercise.[139] The exact amount and timing of the carbohydrate intake should be determined according to the individual's needs and a number of factors specific to the sport. For a detailed discussion and recommended guidelines for determining individual recommendations, refer to the review by Baker and colleagues.[52]

Carbohydrate recommendations are more precisely expressed on a gram per kilogram basis.[127,140,141] The current recommendations for athletes engaged in HIIE are summarized in Table 21.4.[123,141-143] Specific recommendations should be tailored to the needs of the individual athlete. Burke and colleagues[123] recommendations for carbohydrate intake by athletes according to total energy needs, specific training needs, and feedback from training performance and provide guidelines for achieving high carbohydrate availability to promote optimal performance in competition or key training sessions forms the basis of carbohydrate recommendations in the 2016 joint position statement on Nutrition and Athletic Performance.[123,143]

Before adopting any eating and drinking strategies for immediately before or during a match, players should be cautioned to experiment on training days to establish a comfortable routine to avoid any untoward consequences.

Table 21.5 Carbohydrate Guidelines for High-Intensity, Intermittent Exercise[123,141,142]

Training or Competition	Carbohydrate Intake to Promote High Carbohydrate Availability	Comments
Fueling for moderate exercise of 30–90 min	5–7 g/kg per 24 h spread over the day to promote energy availability before, during, and after training or performance	Adequate energy
Fueling for events involving < 90 min exercise	7–12 g/kg per 24 h for daily fuel needs	Adequate energy
Fueling for events involving > 90 minutes of sustained intermittent exercise	36–48 h of 10–12 g/kg per 24 h	Adequate energy
Pre-event fueling for events >60 min	1–4 g/kg; >200 g	1–4 h before competition; solid carbohydrate with a low–glycemic index may be beneficial
During exercise 1.0–2.5 h	30–60 g/h	6%–8% carbohydrate beverage or carbohydrate gel
Speedy refueling: < 8 h recovery between two fuel-demanding sessions	1.0–1.2 g/kg/h for first 4 h, then resume daily fuel needs; 0.8 g carbohydrate per kilogram per hour plus 0.2–0.4 g protein per kilogram per hour	Athletes with lower gastrointestinal threshold for carbohydrate ingestion immediately postexercise

GLYCOGEN REPLETION

In spite of measures to minimize glycogen losses, match play drastically reduces glycogen stores. Glycogen depletion is associated with fatigue and a decrease in exercise intensity. Resynthesis of depleted glycogen stores is both an important consideration and a challenge in postexercise recovery. When enough carbohydrate is supplemented immediately after exercise with sufficient recovery time, the rate of glycogen synthesis and the amount stored is optimal, increasing muscle glycogen up to sevenfold.[144-146] Several studies have suggested that the consumption of foods with a moderate to high glycemic index after exercise may be beneficial.[146-149] A large body of research supports the need for dietary carbohydrate before, during, and after exercise to fuel muscle glycogen stores and replenish liver glycogen content to help delay fatigue and maximize performance (see Chapter 2).

Protein

Studies have shown that amino acids can be oxidized for energy during endurance exercise and that amino acid oxidation is inversely related to muscle glycogen availability.[150,151] During team sports of intermittent exercise, muscle glycogen can be depleted, depending on the intensity and duration of exercise and pregame glycogen stores. The higher the intensity of exercise, the greater is the glycogen utilization and amino acid oxidation is. If the amino acids are not replaced via diet, a net loss in amino acids can occur over time, with losses in muscle strength and possibly performance.

Protein recommendations for soccer players are based on research that shows the strength component of soccer and the use of protein as an energy source. Lemon concluded that soccer players need more dietary protein than sedentary individuals and suggested a protein intake of 1.4 to 1.7 g/kg/d for competitive

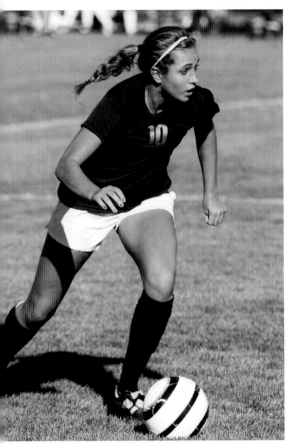

soccer players.[152] In a study of eleven 15-year-old soccer players by Boisseau and colleagues in which the mean daily energy intake of the athletes (2,345 kcal and 38.9 kcal/kg) was less than the RDA for nonactive 15-year-olds, a protein intake of 1.57 g/kg was necessary to achieve nitrogen balance.[105] A later study of 14-year-old male soccer players demonstrated that both protein intakes and energy balance were important determinants of nitrogen balance and recommended a protein intake of 1.4 g/kg/d for adolescent boys.[106] Lemon cautions against extremely high protein intakes (>2 g/kg/d) because of the lack of evidence of performance advantage.[152] A review by Wolfe addressed the use of protein supplements in exercise training and issued the same cautionary note that excessive protein intake may increase the potential for dehydration because of high urea excretion.[153] Current data suggest that the range of dietary protein intake necessary for metabolic adaptations, repair, and remodeling, as well as for protein turnover, is from 1.2 g/kg body weight and that higher intakes may be necessary for short periods of intense training or when reducing energy intake.[143]

Researchers have given attention to the possible benefits of combining protein with carbohydrate during exercise to delay fatigue and immediately after exercise to maximize muscle glycogen synthesis.[154-158] The results have been mixed, with inconclusive evidence to support the addition of protein in the presence of adequate carbohydrate intake. However, for glycogen repletion when energy intake does not provide sufficient carbohydrate, adding protein to carbohydrate during recovery may enhance overall glycogen recovery, as well as assist with muscle repair.

Fat

Of the three macronutrients, dietary fat plays the smallest role in energy distribution. Fat is certainly an important component of a balanced diet, but the absolute quantity and the percentage of energy distribution contributed by fat should be limited. It is generally recommended that fat should contribute no more than 35% of total energy. However, no performance benefits for any sports have been associated with diets providing less than 20% of total energy from fat.[143]

To achieve energy intake levels that support weight and weight-training goals, athletes often consume diets high in fat. In a review of the role of dietary macronutrients in optimizing performance, Stellingwerff observed reduced glycogenolysis during sprint exercise after 5 days of a high-fat diet followed by 1 day of carbohydrate restoration and postulated that muscle glycogen sparing observed in studies of high-fat diets followed by carbohydrate restoration might be an impairment of glycogenolysis.[159] In a review of the training adaptations via nutritional interventions, Hawley and colleagues caution against high-fat, low-carbohydrate diets as a strategy for HIIE.[117]

Among the factors that contribute to less than optimal dietary intakes of athletes are travel, all-you-can-eat buffet meals, limited time and ability to cook, and insufficient nutrition knowledge. Athletes benefit from instruction about choosing foods that support both their training and performance goals and their goals for fitness and long-term health.

Registered dietitian nutritionists (RDNs) working with athletes who participate in HIIE should observe the following guidelines on fat intake:

- Determine carbohydrate and protein intakes and then aim for 20% to 35% of energy from fat.
- Limit saturated fat to less than 10% of energy.
- Emphasize heart-healthy fats, including rich sources of essential fatty acids, especially n-3 fatty acids.
- Give practical guidelines for food selections that will control the contribution from fat, especially sources of hidden fats, such as full-fat dairy products, meats, processed foods, and foods prepared with fat, including restaurant and fast foods.
- Focus on selecting lean protein sources.
- Include tips for choosing foods away from home.

MICRONUTRIENT NEEDS

The energy demand of HIIE training and competition is considerable and requires adequate intake of all nutrients involved in energy production. There are no known micronutrient needs specific to athletes engaged in HIIE. The DRIs are appropriate goals for micronutrient intakes.[160-164] Fogelholm presents data on micronutrient status and the effects of micronutrient supplementation on exercise performance related to soccer and other team sports.[165] In an effort to understand micronutrient needs and intakes of athletes and whether there is any performance benefit to micronutrient supplementation, data were reported from nine studies examining dietary intakes of athletes involved in soccer, football, basketball, hockey, volleyball, and handball, as well as three studies assessing the effect of micronutrient supplementation. The data from these studies suggest that, overall, micronutrient intakes correlate with energy intake. Micronutrient intakes of male athletes were mostly in line with DRIs. Female athletes with energy intakes less than 2,400 kcal/d were more likely to have lower intakes than the DRIs for minerals and trace elements, such as calcium, magnesium, iron, and zinc. The data also suggest that vitamin B-6 intake was less than the DRIs for all groups studied, but this may be due to incomplete data from vitamin B-6 nutrient databases.[166]

With regard to supplementation, there was no clear evidence that micronutrient supplementation improved performance of athletes, but the number of subjects studied was small.[165] There are two exceptions to this conclusion. First, female athletes with infrequent or irregular menstruation may benefit from calcium and vitamin D supplementation to help stem the loss of bone density. In the presence of estrogen deficiency, calcium and vitamin D supplementation alone will not improve bone density. Second, iron-depleted female athletes (serum ferritin < 12 mcg/L) may benefit from daily supplementation with 100 mg elemental iron for 3 months or longer. The iron status of female athletes should be assessed annually. Those who are symptomatic (serum ferritin < 35 mcg/L) or at high risk for iron deficiency should be rescreened 3 to 4 months after the initial assessment.[167]

In general, the micronutrient status of an athlete is directly related to the quality of the dietary intake, especially energy intake. Nutter's study showed that for athletes, iron and calcium intakes were 30% less than the RDAs.[113] Similarly, data collected from male and female team athletes identify some nutrients of concern.[168] Low intakes of thiamin were observed in the diets of male athletes. Among female athletes whose daily energy intakes were less than 2,390 kcal, mineral and trace elements, such as calcium, magnesium, iron, and zinc, were suboptimal. More recently, practitioners have raised concerns about the vitamin D status of athletes, especially athletes who train and compete indoors and those whose exposure to ultraviolet light and intakes of foods rich in vitamin D are limited.[169,170]

In a 2003 investigation of collegiate female soccer players, Clark and colleagues showed that, along with insufficient carbohydrate intake, several micronutrient intakes were less than 75% of the DRI pre- and postseason.[104] Among these athletes, a greater consumption of protein- and fat-rich foods displaced more nutrient-dense complex carbohydrates. This diet becomes particularly troublesome when athletes focus on weight reduction or the maintenance of a low body weight.

The aforementioned study of female soccer players by Gravina and colleagues is the first report of the effect of macro- and micronutrient intake on markers of oxidative stress, muscle damage, and inflammatory and immune response after a soccer match. Based on nutrient analyses, players were classified into two groups, those who followed nutrition recommendations and those who did not. Among those who did not follow recommendations, fiber, folic acid, vitamin D, magnesium, and potassium intakes were below recommendations. Results of blood analyses were compared with nutrient intakes, and those authors concluded that specific nutrients, especially those associated with a carbohydrate-rich diet, may influence antioxidant capacity, as well as cell damage, immunity, and inflammation response induced by playing a soccer match.[39]

In an effort to understand the impact of magnesium on strength, Santos and colleagues analyzed 7 days of 24-hour diet records from 26 male team athletes (basketball, handball, and volleyball) age 21.1 ± 4.9 years old and compared the results with a series of strength tests. Magnesium intakes were significantly lower than recommendations, and the calcium to magnesium ratio was higher than recommendations. A regression analysis showed a direct association between magnesium intake and trunk flexion, trunk rotation, and handgrip maximal strength, as well as jumping performance tests. Magnesium's effect on muscle strength seems to be independent of total dietary intake, illustrating the importance of magnesium in muscle performance and suggesting that performance could be improved with adequate magnesium intakes.[171]

Fogelholm recommends that nutrition education for soccer players start at an early age and focus on foods and macronutrients. Additionally, periodic dietary evaluation from an RDN can detect early trouble signs, help prevent serious nutritional deficiencies, and screen for possible disordered eating.[165]

FLUID REQUIREMENTS

The major causes of fatigue in endurance sports are depletion of muscle glycogen and problems associated with thermoregulation and fluid loss. HIIE requires that players exercise at high intensities for a prolonged period, often at elevated ambient temperatures and high humidity. The added factor of clothing and equipment make heat dissipation, and thus thermoregulation, more difficult, as exemplified in the sports of American football and ice hockey.[168] Palmer and Spriet studied the hydration status and habits of elite ice hockey players and found that more than 50% of players arrived at practice in various degrees of hypohydration. In general, among players who drank sports drinks before practice and replaced 60% of lost fluid with water during practice, 30% still had a greater than 1% body mass loss. All players had high sweat rates during practice, with substantial loss of sodium in sweat that was not replaced by either the sports drink consumed before practice or the water during practice.[172]

In a study by Arnaoutis, the hydration status of 107 young soccer players was evaluated on the first day of soccer camp. Seventy-two of them agreed to undergo testing on 2 more days. Hydration assessment showed that 88.7% (95 of 107) of the youth were hypohydrated based on their first morning urine sample. Evaluation based on a urine color chart classified 93.7% (100 of 107) as hypohydrated. Measures taken before training on the third and fifth days of camp showed that 8.4% and 12.5% were euhydrated, respectively. After training, 95.8% and 97.2% were dehydrated. A majority of young players were hypohydrated and remained hypohydrated throughout camp.[173]

The energy demands of stop-and-go sports greatly reduce muscle glycogen stores and fluid reserves, which must be replenished before the next competition. Repletion of muscle glycogen depends not only on carbohydrate intake but also on fluid intake because each gram of muscle glycogen is stored with 2.7 g water.

Studies examining the effects of carbohydrate-electrolyte solutions on performance during HIIE found that muscle glycogen utilization was reduced, endurance running capacity was improved, time to fatigue was delayed, and mental function was improved when a carbohydrate-electrolyte solution was consumed.[86,89,113,174,175] Under moderate temperatures (10°C or 50°F), the sweat losses of soccer players during a match may be as much as 2 L, and in high temperatures, a mean loss of 3 L or more.[10,149] When the ambient temperature is more than skin temperature, the body builds up additional heat, and this reduces the capacity to perform prolonged exercise. Players who sweat profusely are likely to become dehydrated and fatigued toward the end of an exercise session. Players working in the heat should focus on fluid ingestion along with maintenance of hydration status. Tennis players have been shown to sweat more than 2.5 L/h and replace fluids at a slower rate during competition than during practice. In warm and hot environments, tennis players are recommended to consume a carbohydrate-electrolyte beverage at greater than 200 mL per changeover and ideally closer to 400 mL per changeover to maintain physiological homeostasis and performance.[176]

Full rehydration after exercise requires replacement of fluid and electrolytes, primarily sodium, lost in sweat. A study by Shirreffs and colleagues suggests that full rehydration after intense exercise is best achieved when the replacement fluid contains sufficient sodium and is consumed as 150% of the fluid lost through exercise.[177] An investigation examined how intermittent exercise at varying intensities, designed to simulate a soccer match, affected gastric emptying. The results revealed that a greater volume of carbohydrate-electrolyte solution emptied during the lower-intensity walking trial than during the high-intensity soccer trial, demonstrating that the intensity of activity during this type of stop-and-go team sports is sufficient to slow gastric emptying.[178] More information on hydration and fluids can be found in Chapter 6. See also Box 21.1.[177,179-184]

Box 21.1 Hydration Goals in High-Intensity, Intermittent Exercise[177,179-184]

Before Exercise
- Maximize fluid intake during the 24 h preceding training or competition.
- Drink extra fluid during the last 10 to 15 min before the game begins.
- A carbohydrate-electrolyte solution consumed 15 minutes before exercise improves endurance.

During Exercise
- Consume fluid early and at regular intervals during exercise.
- Choose cool, flavored beverages that are more palatable and contain 4% to 8% carbohydrate (30–60 g carbohydrate per hour) and electrolytes (0.5–0.7 g sodium per liter of water).

After Exercise
- Achieve rapid and complete repletion of fluid, electrolytes, and carbohydrates lost during training and exercise. Each pound lost is about 480 mL (about 16 oz) of fluid.
- Drink at least 150% or 2.5 cups of fluid for every pound lost through exercise to cover obligatory urine loss.

General precaution: Alcohol is dehydrating. Avoid alcohol within 72 hours before or after training.

Special consideration and care should be given to the fluid needs of young athletes, particularly prepubescent youth.[185] During exercise, children produce a smaller amount of heat than adults yet have a greater ration of surface area to body mass ratio (~20% higher than adults). When skin temperature is hotter than the environment, the direction of heat flux is from the body outward. However, when ambient temperatures are greater than skin temperature, children's greater surface area becomes a liability. There is an influx of heat resulting in greater heat absorption from the environment. In addition, they have less capacity for sweating, relying on dry means to dissipate heat, and they take longer to acclimatize to warm weather.[185-187] The difference in sweating rate widens with increasing exercise intensity or heat stress. These factors increase young athletes' risk for dehydration and heat illness. When children become dehydrated, their core temperatures increase faster than they do in dehydrated adults, underscoring the need for strict enforcement of hydration practices. Given the heightened risk of hyperthermia in children, the following precautions and practical measures should be taken:
- At 2 to 4 hours before exercise, consume a fluid volume of 5 to 10 mL/kg body weight to achieve urine that is pale yellow. Allow sufficient time for voiding.[143]
- For most athletes, an intake of 0.4 to 0.8 L/h will supply sufficient fluids to replace sweat losses to limit total body fluid losses to less than 2% body weight. Approximately 3.5 to 6.75 oz of fluid should be consumed at least every 15 to 20 minutes during training and exercise in the heat, with fluid needs customized to the athlete's tolerance and experience.[143]

- Fluids should be cool and palatable to encourage drinking. In one study, grape was the preferred flavor and the one that encouraged the greatest rehydration following mild dehydration.[188]
- Over drinking fluids in excess of sweat and urinary losses is the prime cause of hyponatremia (blood sodium < 135 mmol/L), also known as water intoxication.
- When large sweat losses occur (> 1.2 L/h), sodium should be ingested.
- In warm weather, avoid unnecessary layers of clothing. For example, soccer goalkeepers should remove the team jersey when wearing the goalkeeper shirt.
- Clothing should be made of wicking material. Sweat-drenched clothing should be replaced with dry clothing when possible.
- Reduce the intensity of exercise when the relative humidity and ambient temperature are high.
- Allow frequent breaks.
- Provide shelter from direct sunlight during hot weather when players are on the sidelines.
- After exercise, effective rehydration requires a fluid intake 125% to 150% for every kilogram of body weight lost.[143]
- Excessive intake of alcohol in the recovery period is discouraged due to alcohol's diuretic effect.[143]

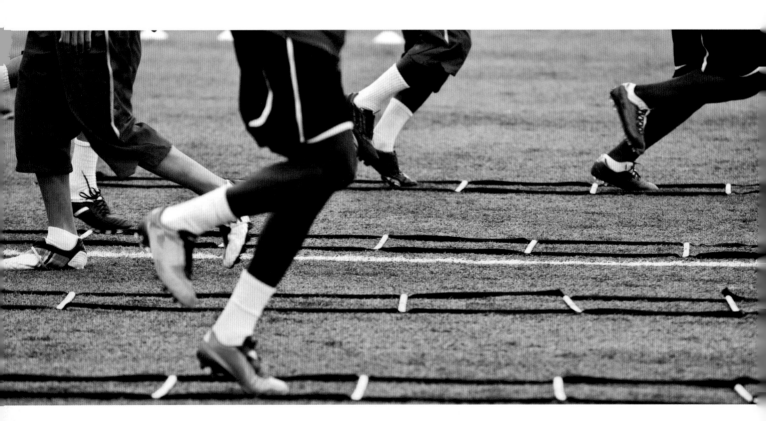

KEY TAKEAWAYS

The stop-and-go nature of HIIE places a great physiological and metabolic demand on the body and involves all three energy systems. These sports require bursts of all-out effort interspersed with periods of moderate- and low-intensity effort.

The primary goal of nutrition in such sports is to support peak performance by ensuring adequate amounts of energy and nutrients, the right blend of fuel for a given effort, adequate hydration, and a plan for the rapid replacement of fluids and muscle glycogen. Coaches and trainers must take precautions to avoid or minimize the pitfalls of HIIE, such as fatigue, hypoglycemia, impaired performance, and dehydration and its consequences.

Nutrient timing is the delivery of fuel and nutrients when the body is primed to use them most effectively. The three phases of nutrient timing are the energy phase, the anabolic phase, and the adaptation phase. Refer to Ivy for an in-depth discussion of nutrient timing and guidelines for incorporating it into a nutrition plan.[189]

Carbohydrate is the preferred fuel for much of the work in stop-and-go sports. It is crucial to supply sufficient intakes of carbohydrate before, during, and after exercise to ensure adequate energy availability to support training, performance, and recovery. The general carbohydrate recommendation is 7 g/kg/d with 7 to 12 g/kg/d during training and competition.[123] The timing of ingestion, as well as the amount of carbohydrate, helps fuel the athlete and enhances endurance and power.

Recommended daily protein intake is 1.2 to 2.0 g/kg/d. Higher intakes may be indicated during periods of intense training or reduced energy intake.[143] Excessive protein intake, generally above 2 g/kg/d, has not been shown to provide additional benefits and may limit carbohydrate intake.

The percentage of total energy as fat is best set within the guideline of 20% to 35% and should be determined after carbohydrate and protein needs are established. Heart-healthy fats should be stressed to limit saturated fats to less than 10% of total energy.

It is important to carefully choose nutrient-rich foods that also provide ample vitamins and minerals essential for health and fuel production and to support training adaptations and recovery.

Fluid intake is critical, especially because many intermittent, high-intensity sports are played in hot and humid conditions. Hydration strategies should be planned to replaced fluid and sodium lost in sweat as soon after exercise as possible.

1. Holway FE, Spriet LL. Sport-specific nutrition: practical strategies for team sports. *J Sports Sci.* 2011;29(suppl 1):115S-125S.

2. Mujika I, Burke LM. Nutrition in team sports. *Ann Nutr Metab.* 2010;57(suppl 2):26S-35S.

3. Bangsbo J, Norregaard L, Thorsoe F. Activity profile of competition soccer. *Can J Sport Sci.* 1991;16(2):110-116.

4. Carling C, Dupont G. Are declines in physical performance associated with a reduction in skill-related performance during professional soccer match-play? *J Sports Sci.* 2011;29(1):63-71.

5. Rampinini E, Impellizzeri FM, Castagna C, Coutts AJ, Wisløff U. Technical performance during soccer matches of the Italian Serie A league: effect of fatigue and competitive level. *J Sci Med Sport.* 2009;12(1):227-233.

6. Cox MH, Miles DS, Verde TJ, Rhodes EC. Applied physiology of ice hockey. *Sports Med.* 1995;19(3):184-201.

7. Reilly T, Thomas V. A motion analysis of work rate in different positional roles in professional football match play. *J Hum Mov Stud.* 1976;2(2):87-97.

8. Withers RT, Maricic Z, Wasilewski S, Kelly L. Match analysis of Australian professional soccer players. *J Hum Mov Stud.* 1982;8:159-176.

9. Ekblom B. Applied physiology of soccer. *Sports Med.* 1986;3(1):50-60.

10. Reilly T. Energetics of high-intensity exercise (soccer) with particular reference to fatigue. *J Sports Sci.* 1997;15(3):257-263.

11. Bangsbo J. The physiology of soccer—with special reference to intense intermittent exercise. *Acta Physiol Scand Suppl.* 1994;619:1-155.

12. Drust B, Reilly T, Rienzi E. Analysis of work rate in soccer. *Sports Exerc Injury.* 1988;4:151-155.

13. Shephard RJ. Biology and medicine of soccer: an update. *J Sport Sci.* 1999;17(10):757-786.

14. Bangsbo J, Mohr M, Krustrup P. Physical and metabolic demands of training and match-play in the elite football player. *J Sports Sci.* 2006;24(7):665-674.

15. Kalapotharakos VI, Strimpakos N, Vithoulka I, Karyounidis C, Diamantopoulos K, Kapreli E. Physiological characteristics of elite professional soccer teams of different ranking. *J Sports Med Phys Fit.* 2006;46(4):515-519.

16. Orendurff MS, Walker JD, Jovanovic M, Tulchin KL, Levy M, Hoffmann DK. Intensity and duration of intermittent exercise and recovery during a soccer match. *J Strength Cond Res.* 2010;24(10):2683-2692.

17. Carling C, Orhant E. Variation in body composition in professional soccer players: interseasonal and intraseasonal changes and the effects of exposure time and player position. *J Strength Cond Res.* 2010;24(5):1332-1339.

18. Pincivero DM, Bompa TO. A physiological review of American football. *Sports Med.* 1997;23(4):247-260.

19. Ben Abdelkrim N, Chaouachi A, Chamari K, Chtara M, Castagna C. Positional role and competitive-level differences in elite-level men's basketball players. *J Strength Cond Res.* 2010;24(5):1346-1355.

20. Ostojic SM, Mazic S, Dikic N. Profiling in basketball: physical and physiological characteristics of elite players. *J Strength Cond.* 2006;20(4):740-744.

21. Gabbett T, King T, Jenkins D. Applied physiology of rugby league. *Sports Med.* 2008;38(2):119-138.

22. Sirotic AC, Coutts AJ, Knowles H, Catterick C. A comparison of match demands between elite and semi-elite rugby league competition. *J Sports Sci.* 2009;27(3):203-211.

23. Gray AJ, Jenkins DG. Match analysis and the physiological demands of Australian football. *Sports Med.* 2010;40(4):347-360.

24. McInnes SE, Carlson JS, Jones CJ, McKenna MJ. The physiological load imposed on basketball players during competition. *J Sports Sci.* 1995;13(5):387-397.

25. Montgomery DL. Physiology of ice hockey. *Sports Med.* 1988;5(2):99-126.

26. Montgomery DL. Physiological profile of professional hockey players—a longitudinal comparison. *Appl Physiol Nutr Metab.* 2006;31(3):181-185.

27. Durocher JJ, Leetun DT, Carter JR. Sport-specific assessment of lactate threshold and aerobic capacity throughout a collegiate hockey season. *Appl Physiol Nutr Metab.* 2008;33(6):1165-1171.

28. Akermark C, Jacobs I, Rasmusson M, Karlsson J. Diet and muscle glycogen concentration in relation to physical performance in Swedish elite ice hockey players. *Int J Sport Nutr.* 1996;6(3):272-284.

29. Houston ME. Nutrition and ice hockey performance. *Can J Appl Sport Sci.* 1979;4(1):98-99.

30. Green HJ, Daub BD, Painter DC, Thomson JA. Glycogen depletion patterns during ice hockey performance. *Med Sci Sports.* 1978;10(4):289-293.

31. Green HJ. Metabolic aspects of intermittent work with specific regard to ice hockey. *Can J Appl Sport Sci.* 1979;4(1):29-34.

32. Konig D, Huonker M, Schmid A, Halle M, Berg A, Keul J. Cardiovascular, metabolic, and hormonal parameters in professional tennis players. *Med Sci Sports Exerc.* 2001;33(4):654-658.

33. Bergeron MF, Maresh CM, Kraemer WJ, Abraham A, Conroy B, Gabaree C. Tennis: a physiological profile during match play. *Int J Sports Med*. 1991;12(5):474-479.

34. Smekal G, von Duvillard SP, Rihacek C, et al. A physiological profile of tennis match play. *Med Sci Sports Exerc*. 2001;33(6):999-1005.

35. Bradley WJ, Cavanagh B, Douglas W, et al. Energy intake and expenditure assessed 'in-season' in an elite European rugby union squad. *Eur J Sport Sci*. 2015;15(6):469-479.

36. Johnston RD, Gabbett TJ, Jenkins DG. Applied sport science of rugby league. *Sports Med*. 2014;44(8):1087-1100.

37. Garcia-Roves PM, Garcia-Zapico P, Patterson AM, Iglesias-Gutierrez E. Nutrient intake and food habits of soccer players: analyzing the correlates of eating practice. *Nutrients*. 2014;6(7):2697-2717.

38. Gibson JC, Stuart-Hill L, Martin S, Gaul C. Nutrition status of junior elite Canadian female soccer athletes. *Int J Sport Nutr Exerc Metab*. 2011;21(6):507-514.

39. Gravina L, Ruiz F, Diaz E, et al. Influence of nutrient intake on antioxidant capacity, muscle damage and white blood cell count in female soccer players. *J Int Soc Sports Nutr*. 2012;9(1):32.

40. Iglesias-Gutierrez E, Garcia A, Garcia-Zapico P, et al. Is there a relationship between the playing position of soccer players and their food and macronutrient intake? *Appl Physiol Nutr Metab*. 2012;37(2):225-232.

41. Maroon JC, Mathyssek CM, Bost JW, et al. Vitamin D profile in National Football League players. *Am J Sports Med*. 2015;43(5):1241-1245.

42. Martinez Renon C, Sanchez Collado P. Nutritional study of a third division soccer team. *Nutr Hosp*. 2013;28(2):319-324.

43. Ono M, Kennedy E, Reeves S, Cronin L. Nutrition and culture in professional football. A mixed method approach. *Appetite*. 2012;58(1):98-104.

44. Russell M, Pennock A. Dietary analysis of young professional soccer players for 1 week during the competitive season. *J Strength Cond Res*. 2011;25(7):1816-1823.

45. Santos DA, Matias CN, Monteiro CP, et al. Magnesium intake is associated with strength performance in elite basketball, handball and volleyball players. *Magnes Res*. 2011;24(4):215-219.

46. Shriver LH, Betts NM, Wollenberg G. Dietary intakes and eating habits of college athletes: are female college athletes following the current sports nutrition standards? *J Am Coll Health*. 2013;61(1):10-16.

47. Valliant MW, Emplaincourt HP, Wenzel RK, Garner BH. Nutrition education by a registered dietitian improves dietary intake and nutrition knowledge of a NCAA female volleyball team. *Nutrients*. 2012;4(6):506-516.

48. Zapolska J, Witczak K, Manczuk A, Ostrowska L. Assessment of nutrition, supplementation and body composition parameters on the example of professional volleyball players. *Rocz Panstw Zakl Hig*. 2014;65(3):235-242.

49. Bangsbo J. Energy demands in competitive soccer. *J Sports Sci*. 1994;12(spec no):5S-12S.

50. Ben Abdelkrim N, El Fazaa S, El Ati J. Time-motion analysis and physiological data of elite under-19-year-old basketball players during competition. *Br J Sports Med*. 2007;41(2):69-75; discussion 75.

51. Sheppard JM, Gabbett TJ, Stanganelli LC. An analysis of playing positions in elite men's volleyball: considerations for competition demands and physiologic characteristics. *J Strength Cond Res*. 2009;23(6):1858-1866.

52. Baker LB, Rollo I, Stein KW, Jeukendrup AE. Acute effects of carbohydrate supplementation on intermittent sports performance. *Nutrients*. 2015;7(7):5733-5763.

53. Roczniok R, Stanula A, Maszczyk A, et al. Physiological, physical and on-ice performance criteria for selection of elite ice hockey teams. *Biol Sport*. 2016;33(1):43-48.

54. Unnithan V, White J, Georgiou A, Iga J, Drust B. Talent identification in youth soccer. *J Sports Sci*. 2012;30(15):1719-1726.

55. Mann JB, Ivey PA, Mayhew JL, Schumacher RM, Brechue WF. Relationship between agility tests and short sprints: reliability and smallest worthwhile difference in National Collegiate Athletic Association division-I football players. *J Strength Cond Res*. 2016;30(4):893-900.

56. Mohr M, Krustrup P, Bangsbo J. Fatigue in soccer: a brief review. *J Sports Sci*. 2005;23(6):593-599.

57. Mohr M, Krustrup P, Andersson H, Kirkendal D, Bangsbo J. Match activities of elite women soccer players at different performance levels. *J Strength Cond Res*. 2008;22(2):341-349.

58. Krustrup P, Zebis M, Jensen JM, Mohr M. Game-induced fatigue patterns in elite female soccer. *J Strength Cond Res*. 2010;24(2):437-441.

59. Bangsbo J, Iaia FM, Krustrup P. Metabolic response and fatigue in soccer. *Int J Sports Physiol Perform*. 2007;2(2):111-127.

60. Bradley PS, Di Mascio M, Peart D, Olsen P, Sheldon B. High-intensity activity profiles of elite soccer players at different performance levels. *J Strength Cond Res*. 2010;24(9):2343-2351.

61. Abt G, Siegler JC, Akubat I, Castagna C. The effects of a constant sprint-to-rest ratio and recovery mode on repeated sprint performance. *J Strength Cond Res.* 2011;25(6):1695-1702.

62. Krustrup P, Mohr M, Ellingsgaard H, Bangsbo J. Physical demands during an elite female soccer game: importance of training status. *Med Sci Sports Exerc.* 2005;37(7):1242-1248.

63. Reilly T, Thomas V. Estimated daily energy expenditures of professional association footballers. *Ergonomics.* 1979;22(5):541-548.

64. Peterson BJ, Fitzgerald JS, Dietz CC, et al. Aerobic capacity is associated with improved repeated shift performance in hockey. *J Strength Cond Res.* 2015;29(6):1465-1472.

65. Mohr M, Krustrup P, Bangsbo J. Match performance of high-standard soccer players with special reference to development of fatigue. *J Sports Sci.* 2003;21(7):519-528.

66. Bradley PS, Dellal A, Mohr M, Castellano J, Wilkie A. Gender differences in match performance characteristics of soccer players competing in the UEFA Champions League. *Hum Mov Sci.* 2014;33:159-171.

67. Romijn JA, Coyle EF, Sidossis LS, et al. Regulation of endogenous fat and carbohydrate metabolism in relation to exercise intensity and duration. *Am J Physiol.* 1993;265(3 pt 1):E380-E391.

68. Roberts TJ, Weber JM, Hoppeler H, Weibel ER, Taylor CR. Design of the oxygen and substrate pathways. II. Defining the upper limits of carbohydrate and fat oxidation. *J Exp Biol.* 1996;199(pt 8):1651-1658.

69. Jacobs I, Westin N, Karlsson J, Rasmusson M, Houghton B. Muscle glycogen and diet in elite soccer players. *Eur J Appl Physiol.* 1982;48(3):297-302.

70. Tumilty D. Physiological characteristics of elite soccer players. *Sports Med.* 1993;16(2):80-96.

71. Gollnick PD, Armstrong RB, Sembrowich WL, Shepherd RE, Saltin B. Glycogen depletion patterns in human skeletal muscle fibers after heavy exercise. *J Appl Physiol.* 1973;34(5):615-618.

72. Costill D, Gollnick PD, Jansson ED, Saltin B, Stein EM. Glycogen depletion pattern in human muscle fibers during distance running. *Acta Physiol Scand.* 1973;89(3):374-384.

73. Gollnick PD, Piehl K, Saubert CW IV, Armstrong RB, Saltin B. Diet, exercise, and glycogen changes in human muscle fibers. *J Appl Physiol.* 1972;33(4):421-425.

74. Brooks G, Mercier J. Balance of carbohydrate and lipid utilization during exercise: the "crossover" concept. *J Appl Physiol.* 1994;76(6):2253-2261.

75. Green HJ. Glycogen depletion patterns during continuous and intermittent ice skating. *Med Sci Sports.* 1978;10(3):183-187.

76. Krustrup P, Mohr M, Steensberg A, Bencke J, Kjaer M, Bangsbo J. Muscle and blood metabolites during a soccer game: implications for sprint performance. *Med Sci Sports Exerc.* 2006;38(6):1165-1174.

77. Brooks GA. Importance of the "crossover" concept in exercise metabolism. *Clin Exp Pharmacol Physiol.* 1997;24(11):889-895.

78. Coggan AR, Kohrt WM, Spina RJ, Bier DM, Holloszy JO. Endurance training decreases plasma glucose turnover and oxidation during moderate-intensity exercise in men. *J Appl Physiol (1985).* 1990;68(3):990-996.

79. Hurley BF, Nemeth PM, Martin WH III, Hagberg JM, Dalsky GP, Holloszy JO. Muscle triglyceride utilization during exercise: effect of training. *J Appl Physiol (1985).* 1986;60(2):562-567.

80. Sidossis LS, Gastaldelli A, Klein S, Wolfe RR. Regulation of plasma fatty acid oxidation during low- and high-intensity exercise. *Am J Physiol.* 1997;272(6 pt 1):E1065-E1070.

81. Bracken RM, Linnane DM, Brooks S. Plasma catecholamine and nephrine responses to brief intermittent maximal intensity exercise. *Amino Acids.* 2009;36(2):209-217.

82. Trapp EG, Chisholm DJ, Boutcher SH. Metabolic response of trained and untrained women during high-intensity intermittent cycle exercise. *Am J Physiol Regul Integr Comp Physiol.* 2007;293(6):R2370-R2375.

83. Martin WH III, Dalsky GP, Hurley BF, et al. Effect of endurance training on plasma free fatty acid turnover and oxidation during exercise. *Am J Physiol.* 1993;265(5 pt 1):E708-E714.

84. Weber J, Brichon G, Zwingelstein G, et al. Design of the oxygen and substrate pathways. IV. Partitioning energy provision from fatty acids. *J Exp Biol.* 1996;199(pt 8):1667-1674.

85. Bendiksen M, Bischoff R, Randers MB, et al. The Copenhagen Soccer Test: physiological response and fatigue development. *Med Sci Sports Exerc.* 2012;44(8):1595-1603.

86. Welsh RS, Davis JM, Burke JR, Williams HG. Carbohydrates and physical/mental performance during intermittent exercise to fatigue. *Med Sci Sports Exerc.* 2002;34(4):723-731.

87. Newsholme EA, Blomstrand E, Ekblom B. Physical and mental fatigue: metabolic mechanisms and importance of plasma amino acids. *Br Med Bull.* 1992;48(3):477-495.

88. Bergström J, Hermansen L, Hultman E, Saltin B. Diet, muscle glycogen and physical performance. *Acta Physiol Scand.* 1967;71(2):140-150.

89. Winnick JJ, Davis JM, Welsh RS, Carmichael MD, Murphy EA, Blackmon JA. Carbohydrate feedings during team sport exercise preserve physical and CNS function. *Med Sci Sports Exerc.* 2005;37(2):306-315.

90. Smodlaka VN. Cardiovascular aspect of soccer. *Phys Sportsmed.* 1978;6:66-70.

91. Stanula AJ, Gabryś TT, Roczniok RK, Szmatlan-Gabryś UB, Ozimek MJ, Mostowik AJ. Quantification of the demands during an ice-hockey game based on intensity zones determined from the incremental test outcomes. *J Strength Cond Res.* 2016;30(1):176-183.

92. Yagüe PL, Del Valle ME, Egocheaga J, Linnamo V, Fernandez A. The competitive demands of elite male rink hockey. *Biol Sport.* 2013;30(3):195-199.

93. Therminarias A, Dansou P, Chirpaz-Oddou MF, Gharib C, Quirion A. Hormonal and metabolic changes during a strenuous match: effect of ageing. *Int J Sports Med.* 1991;12(1):10-16.

94. Docherty D. A comparison of heart rate responses in racquet games. *Br J Sports Med.* 1982;16(2):96-100.

95. Tomlin DL, Wenger HA. The relationship between aerobic fitness and recovery from high-intensity intermittent exercise. *Sports Med.* 2001;31(1):1-11.

96. Brooks GA. Current concepts in lactate exchange. *Med Sci Sports Exerc.* 1991;2(8):895-906.

97. Matthew D, Delextrat A. Heart rate, blood lactate concentration, and time-motion analysis of female basketball players during competition. *J Sports Sci.* 2009;27(8):813-821.

98. Scanlan AT, Dascombe BJ, Reaburn P, Dalbo VJ. The physiological and activity demands experienced by Australian female basketball players during competition. *J Sci Med Sport.* 2012;15(4):341-347.

99. Williams C, Nicholas CW. Nutrition needs for team sport. *Sport Sci Exch.* 1998;11(3):70.

100. Clark K. Nutritional guidance to soccer players for training and competition. *J Sports Sci.* 1994;12(spec no):43S-50S.

101. Macedonio M. Nutrition management of the Cleveland Force soccer team. Summary report. Unpublished data. 1987.

102. Brewer J. Aspects of women's soccer. *J Sports Sci.* 1994;12(spec no):35S-38S.

103. Economos CD, Bortz SS, Nelson ME. Nutrition practices of elite athletes. *Sports Med.* 1993;16(6):381-399.

104. Clark M, Reed DB, Crouse SF, Armstrong RB. Pre- and post-season dietary intake, body composition, and performance indices of NCAA division I female soccer players. *Int J Sport Nutr Exerc Metab.* 2003;13(3):303-319.

105. Boisseau N, Le Creff C, Loyens M, Poortmans JR. Protein intake and nitrogen balance in male non-active adolescents and soccer players. *Eur J Appl Physiol.* 2002;88(3):288-293.

106. Boisseau N, Vermorel M, Rance M, Duché P, Patureau-Mirand P. Protein requirements in male adolescent soccer players. *Eur J Appl Physiol.* 2007;100(1):27-33.

107. Iglesias-Gutiérrez E, García-Rovés P, García A, Patterson AM. Food preferences do not influence adolescent high-level athletes' dietary intake. *Appetite.* 2008;50(2-3):536-543.

108. Noda Y, Iide K, Masuda R, et al. Nutrient intake and blood iron status of male collegiate soccer players. *Asia Pac J Clin Nutr.* 2009;18(3):344-350.

109. Mielgo-Ayuso J, Zourdos MC, Calleja-Gonzalez J, Urdampilleta A, Ostojic SM. Dietary intake habits and controlled training on body composition and strength in elite female volleyball players during the season. *Appl Physiol Nutr Metab.* 2015;40(8):827-834.

110. Papadopoulou SK, Papadopoulou SD. Nutritional status of top team-sport athletes according to body fat. *Nutr Food Sci.* 2010;40(1):64-73.

111. Nikic M, Pedisic Z, Satalic Z, Jakovljevic S, Venus D. Adequacy of nutrient intakes in elite junior basketball players. *Int J Sport Nutr Exerc Metab.* 2014;24(5):516-523.

112. Stolen T, Chamari K, Castagna C, Wisloff U. Physiology of soccer: an update. *Sports Med.* 2005;35(6):501-536.

113. Nutter J. Seasonal changes in female athletes' diets. *Int J Sport Nutr.* 1991;1(4):395-407.

114. Papadopoulou SK, Papadopoulou SD, Gallos GK. Macro- and micro-nutrient intake of adolescent Greek female volleyball players. *Int J Sport Nutr Exerc Metab.* 2002;12(1):73-80.

115. Briggs MA, Cockburn E, Rumbold PL, Rae G, Stevenson EJ, Russell M. Assessment of energy intake and energy expenditure of male adolescent academy-level soccer players during a competitive week. *Nutrients.* 2015;7(10):8392-8401.

116. Maughan RJ, Greenhaff PL, Leiper JB, Ball D, Lambert CP, Gleeson M. Diet composition and the performance of high-intensity exercise. *J Sports Sci.* 1997;15(3):265-275.

117. Hawley JA, Tipton KD, Millard-Stafford ML. Promoting training adaptations through nutritional interventions. *J Sports Sci.* 2006;24(7):709-721.

118. Phillips SM, Sproule J, Turner AP. Carbohydrate ingestion during team games exercise: current knowledge and areas for future investigation. *Sports Med.* 2011;41(7):559-585.

119. Bangsbo J, Norregaard L, Thorsoe F. The effect of carbohydrate diet on intermittent exercise performance. *Int J Sports Med.* 1992;13(2):152-157.

120. Nordheim K, Vollestad NK. Glycogen and lactate metabolism during low-intensity exercise in man. *Acta Physiol Scand.* 1990;139(3):475-484.

121. Saltin B. Metabolic fundamentals in exercise. *Med Sci Sports Exerc.* 1973;5(3):137-146.

122. Kirkendall DT. Effects of nutrition on performance in soccer. *Med Sci Sports Exerc.* 1993;25(12):1370-1374.

123. Burke LM, Hawley JA, Wong SH, Jeukendrup AE. Carbohydrate for training and competition. *J Sports Sci.* 2011;29(suppl 1):17S-27S.

124. Coyle EF. Substrate utilization during exercise in active people. *Am J Clin Nutr.* 1995;61(suppl 4):968S-979S.

125. Ferrauti A, Pluim BM, Busch T, Weber K. Blood glucose responses and incidence of hypoglycaemia in elite tennis under practice and tournament conditions. *J Sci Med Sport.* 2003;6(1):28-39.

126. Hargreaves M. Carbohydrate and lipid requirements of soccer. *J Sports Sci.* 1994;12(spec no):13S-16S.

127. Ali A, Williams C, Nicholas C, Foskett A. The influence of carbohydrate-electrolyte ingestion on soccer skill performance. *Med Sci Sports Exerc.* 2007;39(11):1969-1976.

128. Backhouse SH, Ali A, Biddle SJ, Williams C. Carbohydrate ingestion during prolonged high-intensity intermittent exercise: impact on affect and perceived exertion. *Scand J Med Sci Sports.* 2007;17(5):605-610.

129. Carter J, Jeukendrup AE, Mundel T, Jones DA. Carbohydrate supplementation improves moderate and high-intensity exercise in the heat. *Eur J Physiol.* 2003; 446(2):211-219.

130. de Sousa MV, Simões HG, Oshiiwa M, Rogero MM, Tirapegui J. Effects of acute carbohydrate supplementation during sessions of high-intensity intermittent exercise. *Eur J Appl Physiol.* 2007;99(1):57-63.

131. Phillips SM, Turner AP, Gray S, Sanderson MF, Sproule J. Ingesting a 6% carbohydrate-electrolyte solution improves endurance capacity, but not sprint performance, during intermittent, high-intensity shuttle running in adolescent team games players aged 12-14 years. *Eur J Appl Physiol.* 2010;109(5):811-821.

132. Russell M, Benton D, Kingsley M. Influence of carbohydrate supplementation on skill performance during a soccer match simulation. *J Sci Med Sport.* 2012;15(4):348-354.

133. Kingsley M, Penas-Ruiz C, Terry C, Russell M. Effects of carbohydrate-hydration strategies on glucose metabolism, sprint performance and hydration during a soccer match simulation in recreational players. *J Sci Med Sport.* 2014;17(2):239-243.

134. Davison GW, McClean C, Brown J, et al. The effects of ingesting a carbohydrate-electrolyte beverage 15 minutes prior to high-intensity exercise performance. *Res Sports Med.* 2008;16(3):155-166.

135. Russell M, Benton D, Kingsley M. The effects of fatigue on soccer skills performed during a soccer match simulation. *Int J Sports Physiol Perform.* 2011;6(2):221-233.

136. Russell M, Benton D, Kingsley M. Carbohydrate ingestion before and during soccer match play and blood glucose and lactate concentrations. *J Athlet Train.* 2014;49(4):447-453.

137. Harper LD, Briggs MA, McNamee G, et al. Physiological and performance effects of carbohydrate gels consumed prior to the extra time period of prolonged simulated soccer match-play. *J Sci Med Sport.* 2015;19(6):509-514.

138. Jeukendrup AE. Carbohydrate and exercise performance: the role of multiple transportable carbohydrates. *Curr Opin Clin Nutr Metab Care.* 2010;13(4):452-457.

139. Phillips SM. Carbohydrate supplementation and prolonged intermittent high-intensity exercise in adolescents: research findings, ethical issues and suggestions for the future. *Sports Med.* 2012;42(10):817-828.

140. Burke LM, Cox GR, Cummings NK, Desbrow B. Guidelines for daily carbohydrate intake: do athletes achieve them? *Sports Med.* 2001;31(4):267-299.

141. Burke LM. Fueling strategies to optimize performance: training high or training low? *Scand J Med Sci Sports.* 2010;20(suppl 2):48-58.

142. Cermak NM, van Loon LJ. The use of carbohydrates during exercise as an ergogenic aid. *Sports Med.* 2013;43(11):1139-1155.

143. Thomas DT, Erdman KA, Burke LM. Position of the Academy of Nutrition and Dietetics, Dietitians of Canada, and the American College of Sports Medicine: nutrition and athletic performance. *J Acad Nutr Diet.* 2016;116(3):501-528.

144. Ivy J. Optimization of glycogen stores. In: Maughan RJ, ed. *Nutrition in Sport.* Malden, MA: Blackwell Science; 2000:97-111.

145. Mondazzi L, Arcelli E. Glycemic index in sport nutrition. *J Am Coll Nutr.* 2009;28(suppl):455S-463S.

146. Burke LM, Collier GR, Davis PG, Fricker PA, Sanigorski AJ, Hargreaves M. Muscle glycogen storage after prolonged exercise: effect of the frequency of carbohydrate feedings. *Am J Clin Nutr.* 1996;64(1):115-119.

147. Rankin J. Glycemic index and exercise metabolism. *Sports Sci Exch.* 1997;10(1)64.

148. Burke LM, Hargreaves M, Collier GR. Muscle glycogen storage after prolonged exercise: effect of the glycemic index of carbohydrate feedings. *J Appl Physiol (1985).* 1993;75(2):1019-1023.

149. Coyle EE. Timing and method of increased carbohydrate intake to cope with heavy training, competition and recovery. *J Sports Sci.* 1991;9(spec no):29-51.

150. Evans WJ, Fisher EC, Hoerr RA, Young VR. Protein metabolism and endurance exercise. *Phys Sportsmed.* 1983;11(7):63-72.

151. Lemon PW, Mullin JP. Effect of initial muscle glycogen levels on protein catabolism during exercise. *J Appl Physiol Respir Environ Exerc Physiol.* 1980;48(4):624-629.

152. Lemon PW. Protein requirements of soccer. *J Sports Sci.* 1994;12(spec no):17S-22S.

153. Wolfe RR. Protein supplements and exercise. *Am J Clin Nutr.* 2000;72(suppl 2):551S-557S.

154. Lambert E, Goedecke J. The role of dietary macronutrients in optimizing endurance performance. *Curr Sports Med Rep.* 2003;2(4):194-201.

155. Ivy JL, Goforth HW Jr, Damon BM, McCauley TR, Parsons EC, Price TB. Early postexercise muscle glycogen recovery is enhanced with a carbohydrate-protein supplement. *J Appl Physiol.* 2002;93(4):1337-1344.

156. Davis JM, Welsh RS, De Volve KA, Alderson NL. Effects of branched-chain amino acids and carbohydrate on fatigue during intermittent, high-intensity running. *Int J Sports Med.* 1999;20(5):309-314.

157. Lemon PW. Beyond the zone: protein needs of active individuals. *J Am Coll Nutr.* 2000;19(5):513S-521S.

158. Gunnarsson TP, Bendiksen M, Bischoff R, et al. Effect of whey protein- and carbohydrate-enriched diet on glycogen resynthesis during the first 48 h after a soccer game. *Scand J Med Sci Sports.* 2013;23(4):508-515.

159. Stellingwerff T, Spriet LL, Watt MJ, et al. Decreased PDH activation and glycogenolysis during exercise following fat adaptation with carbohydrate restoration. *Am J Physiol Endocrinol Metab.* 2006;290(2):E380-388.

160. Institute of Medicine. *Dietary Reference Intakes for Vitamin A, Vitamin K, Arsenic, Boron, Chromium, Copper, Iodine, Iron, Molybdenum, Nickel, Silicon, Vanadium, and Zinc.* Washington, DC: National Academies Press; 2001.

161. Institute of Medicine. *Dietary Reference Intakes for Calcium, Phosphorus, Magnesium, Vitamin D, and Fluoride.* Washington, DC: National Academies Press; 1997.

162. Institute of Medicine. *Dietary Reference Intakes for Calcium, Phosphorous, Magnesium, Vitamin D, and Fluoride.* Washington, DC: National Academies Press; 2010

163. Institute of Medicine. *Dietary Reference Intakes for Thiamin, Riboflavin, Niacin, Vitamin B6, Folate, Vitamin B12, Pantothenic Acid, Biotin, and Choline.* Washington, DC: National Academies Press; 1998.

164. Institute of Medicine. *Dietary Reference Intakes for Vitamin C, Vitamin E, Selenium, and Carotenoids.* Washington, DC: National Academies Press; 2000.

165. Fogelholm M. Vitamins, minerals and supplementation in soccer. *J Sports Sci.* 1994;12(spec no):23S-27S.

166. Reynolds RD. Determination of dietary vitamin B-6 intake: is it accurate? *J Am Diet Assoc.* 1990;90(6):799-801.

167. Nielsen P, Nachtigall D. Iron supplementation in athletes. Current recommendations. *Sports Med.* 1998;26(4):207-216.

168. Kulka T, Kenney L. Heat balance limits in football uniforms: how different uniform ensembles alter the equation. *Phys Sportsmed.* 2002;30(7):29-39.

169. Willis K, Peterson N, Larson-Meyer D. Should we be concerned about the vitamin D status of athletes? *Int J Sport Nutr Exerc Metab.* 2008;18(2):204-224.

170. Cannell J, Hollis B, Sorenson M, Taft T, Anderson J. Athletic performance and vitamin D. *Med Sci Sports Exerc.* 2009;41(5):1102-1110.

171. Santos DA, Dawson JA, Matias CN, et al. Reference values for body composition and anthropometric measurements in athletes. *PLoS One.* 2014;9(5):e97846.

172. Palmer MS, Spriet LL. Sweat rate, salt loss, and fluid intake during an intense on-ice practice in elite Canadian male junior hockey players. *Appl Physiol Nutr Metab.* 2008;33(2):263-271.

173. Arnaoutis G, Kavouras SA, Kotsis YP, Tsekouras YE, Makrillos M, Bardis CN. Ad libitum fluid intake does not prevent dehydration in suboptimally hydrated young soccer players during a training session of a summer camp. *Int J Sport Nutr Exerc Metab.* 2013;23(3):245-251.

174. Nicholas CW, Tsintzas K, Boobis L, Williams C. Carbohydrate-electrolyte ingestion during intermittent high-intensity running. *Med Sci Sports Exerc.* 1999;31(9):1280-1286.

175. Nicholas CW, Williams C, Lakomy H, Phillips G, Nowitz A. Influence of ingesting a carbohydrate-electrolyte solution on endurance capacity during intermittent, high-intensity shuttle running. *J Sports Sci.* 1995;13(4):283-290.

176. Kovacs M. A review of fluid and hydration in competitive tennis. *Int J Sports Physiol Perform*. 2008;3(4):413-423.

177. Shirreffs SM, Taylor AJ, Leiper JB, Maughan RJ. Post-exercise rehydration in man: effects of volume consumed and drink sodium content. *Med Sci Sports Exerc*. 1996;28(10):1260-1271.

178. Leiper JB, Prentice AS, Wrightson C, Maughan RJ. Gastric emptying of a carbohydrate-electrolyte drink during a soccer match. *Med Sci Sports Exerc*. 2000;33(11):1932-1938.

179. Convertino VA, Armstrong LE, Coyle EF, American College of Sports Medicine. Position stand. Exercise and fluid replacement. *Med Sci Sports Exerc*. 1996;28(1):i-vii.

180. Greenleaf JE, Castle BL. Exercise temperature regulation in man during hypohydration and hyperthermia. *J Appl Physiol*. 1971;30(6):847-853.

181. Maughan R, Leiper J. Fluid replacement requirements in soccer. *J Sports Sci*. 1994;12(spec no):29S-34S.

182. Shi X, Gisolfi CV. Fluid and carbohydrate replacement during intermittent exercise. *Sports Med*. 1998;25(3):157-172.

183. Horswill CA. Effective fluid replacement. *Int J Sport Nutr Exerc Metab*. 1998;8(2):175-195.

184. Burke LM, Hawley JA. Fluid balance in team sports. Guidelines for optimal practices. *Sports Med*. 1997;24(1):38-54.

185. Petrie HJ, Stover EA, Horswill CA. Nutritional concerns for the child and adolescent competitor. *Nutrition*. 2004;20(7-8):620-631.

186. American Academy of Pediatrics. Committee on Sports Medicine and Fitness. Climatic heat stress and the exercising child and adolescent. *Pediatrics*. 2000;106(1 pt 1):158-159.

187. Falk B, Dotan R. Children's thermoregulation during exercise in the heat: a revisit. *Appl Physiol Nutr Metab*. 2008;33(2):420-427.

188. Meyer F, Bar-Or O, Salsberg A, Passe D. Hypohydration during exercise in children: effect of thirst, drink preferences, and rehydration. *Int J Sport Nutr Exerc Metab*. 1994;4(1):22-35.

189. Ivy JL, Ferguson-Stegall LM. Nutrient timing: the means to improved exercise performance, recovery, and training adaptation. *Am J Lifestyle Med*. 2014;8(4):246-259.

CHAPTER 22

NUTRITION FOR ENDURANCE AND ULTRAENDURANCE SPORTS

Eve Pearson, MBA, RDN, CSSD

INTRODUCTION

Endurance events encompass a wide range of competitions, including half marathon and marathon runs, Olympic distance triathlons, cross-country ski races, adventure races, obstacle course races, and road and mountain cycling events. Ultraendurance events involve races that last from 4 to 24 hours and include marathon rowing, running 31 to 100 miles, cycling 100-plus miles, the longest obstacle course races (eg, Toughest Mudder and Spartan Beast), and triathlons ranging from Half Ironman events to the Ultraman distance. Multistage or multiday ultraendurance events entail competing over consecutive days, such as the Tour de France bicycle race (~2,500 miles over 22 days), the Race Across America (RAAM) cycling event (3,000 miles), the US Barkley Marathons (one of the toughest 100-mile run courses with a 60-hour time cutoff), the self-supported mountain bike race Tour Divide (2,745 miles), and some adventure races.

Endurance racing has become very popular, even among nonelite athletes, many of whom participate in these races for fun and to finish rather than to compete. These recreational athletes also need an individualized nutrition and hydration plan. Keep in mind that although the majority of the research discussed in this chapter involves elite athletes; the results of these studies provide a starting point from which adjustments can be made for the individual needs of recreational athletes as well.

ENERGY SYSTEMS AND FUEL USAGE

Endurance athletes have unique nutrient demands because of their high energy expenditures, and they must cope with a variety of challenges to achieve their fuel and fluid replacement goals. The predominant energy system for endurance athletes is the aerobic energy system with brief, intermittent involvement of the anaerobic energy systems. During prolonged exercise, the oxidative metabolism of carbohydrate (muscle glycogen and plasma glucose) and fat (intramuscular triglycerides and plasma fatty acids) provide the vast majority of adenosine triphosphate for muscle contraction. Although amino acid oxidation occurs to a limited extent during endurance exercise, carbohydrate and fat are the most important oxidative substrates.[1,2]

During high-intensity endurance events, the exercise intensity is often 85% of VO_2 max or more, and carbohydrate (primarily muscle glycogen) is the primary fuel source. An endurance athlete can sustain exercise at 85% of VO_2 max for approximately 90 minutes without exogenous fuel. During ultraendurance events, the exercise intensity averages 65% of VO_2 max, where fat oxidation reaches its peak for male athletes. An ultraendurance athlete can sustain exercise at 65% of VO_2 max for approximately 8 hours with exogenous fuel.[2] The length of time at % VO_2 max will vary with modality, training, sex, and environmental conditions; it varies widely among athletes.[3] See Chapter 4 for more on fat utilization during exercise at different intensities and duration.

Energy needs among endurance athletes vary based on a variety of factors, making it important to fully assess the athlete and create an individual plan. Fueling strategies should be fine-tuned based on exercise intensity, duration, mode, and environmental conditions.

Energy Needs

Endurance athletes should consume adequate daily energy, especially carbohydrate, during various phases of training to maintain a desirable training intensity and thus maximize training adaptations. As shown in Table 22.1, these athletes have high energy requirements.[4-9] In addition, a review by Burke and colleagues showed that male elite cyclists consume approximately 51 to 63 kcal/kg/d, and female elite cyclists consume approximately 39 to 50 kcal/kg/d.[10]

Table 22.1 Daily Energy Intakes of Endurance and Ultraendurance Athletes

Type of Athlete	Energy Intake for Training
Male elite ultraendurance triathletes[a,4]	4,079 kcal/d
Male marathon runners[b,4]	3,570 kcal/d
Male elite Kenyan distance runners[5]	3,478 kcal/d
Male Japanese distance runners[8]	3,784 kcal/d
Male elite road cyclists [c,6]	5,333 kcal/d
Female elite road cyclists[7]	3,261 kcal/d
Male adventure racer[9]	44.6 ± 8.0 kcal/kg/d
Female adventure racer[9]	48.1 ± 19.8 kcal/kg/d

[a] 8.1 miles swimming, 202 miles cycling, 47 miles running per week.
[b] 91.6 miles per week.
[c] 405 miles per month.

To meet energy demands, endurance athletes often need to eat meals and snacks continuously throughout the day, especially surrounding their training sessions. Testing specific foods and fluids before, during, and after training sessions allows the athlete to determine effective fueling strategies for competition.[11-13]

If needed, the athlete should lose excess body fat in the off-season or early in the training cycle for ideal timing.[14] Failure to match energy intake to energy expenditure during training impairs endurance performance, most likely as a result of muscle and liver glycogen depletion. Compared with male endurance athletes, female endurance athletes are more likely to consume insufficient energy.[10] However, Martin and colleagues[8] reported that most elite female cyclists modulated energy intake based on energy expenditure.

Because recreational athletes typically train around their professional job and personal responsibilities, finding time for eating adds a layer of difficulty in their schedule. Often, their meal and snack times are dictated by work and personal demands, meetings, or other commitments. All of this makes it increasingly important to educate them on the importance of pre- and posttraining fuel to meet daily energy demands.

Daily Macronutrients

The endurance athlete's carbohydrate, protein, and fat needs also vary, similar to energy needs, based on exercise intensity, duration, mode, and environmental conditions. Calculate the athlete's protein and carbohydrate needs based on kilograms per body weight, and adjust fat accordingly using the guidelines that follow.

CARBOHYDRATE

Adequate carbohydrate stores (muscle, liver glycogen, and blood glucose) are critical for optimum endurance performance. Fatigue during endurance exercise is often associated with muscle glycogen depletion or hypoglycemia. Thus, nutritional strategies that optimize carbohydrate availability before, during, and after exercise are recommended to improve endurance performance.[1] Nutrient-rich carbohydrate foods and fluids should be emphasized because they contain other nutrients, such as vitamins and minerals, that are important for the overall diet as well as exercise recovery.[13]

The athlete's carbohydrate and energy intake should be adjusted or periodized to meet the requirements of the particular training cycle or phase for his or her sport, possibly on a daily basis. Excessive energy intake, including carbohydrate, during light training can cause an increase in body fat, which may have a negative effect on performance. Conversely, inadequate carbohydrate and energy intake during heavy training can cause loss of lean tissue, depleted carbohydrate stores, and impaired performance. The recommended daily carbohydrate intake for endurance athletes is found in Box 22.1.

Box 22.1 Daily Carbohydrate Intake Recommendations for Endurance and Ultraendurance Athletes

Daily carbohydrate intake should be in the range of 5 to 12 g/kg body weight. Adjust intake goals taking into consideration the athlete's total energy needs, specific training needs, and feedback from training performance.

Carbohydrate intake should be spread over the day (before, during, and after exercise) to promote fuel availability for key training sessions.

The amount of carbohydrate per day can vary daily if the athlete's training varies in length and intensity (eg, in one week, an athlete may have two 4- to 5-h/d training sessions, two 1-h/d training sessions, and three 1- to 3-h/d training sessions, making the athlete's carbohydrate requirements vary daily).

The following are examples of daily guidelines for various activity levels:

- 5 to 7 g/kg: moderate-intensity training programs for 1 h/d
- 6 to 10 g/kg: moderate- to high-intensity endurance exercise for 1 to 3 h/d
- 8 to 12 g/kg: moderate- to high-intensity exercise for 4 to 5 h/d

---

Results of dietary surveys of male endurance athletes published between 1990 and 1999 suggest that they consume an appropriate amount of carbohydrate (7.6 g/kg/d). Results of dietary surveys of female endurance athletes published between 1990 and 1999 suggest that they are less likely to consume adequate carbohydrate because of lower energy intakes (5.7 g/kg/d).[13] Table 22.2 (page 494) provides average daily macronutrient intake in endurance athletes. [4,5,7-9,15-20]

Results of a few studies after 2000 suggest that male runners and male and female cyclists also consume adequate carbohydrate (9 g/kg, 11 g/kg, and 9 g/kg, respectively) during training. However, one study suggested that both male and female adventure racers are likely consuming inadequate amounts of carbohydrates (5.7 g/kg and 6.9 g/kg, respectively). [5,7-9,20]

Training for endurance events involves hours of prolonged exercise that may include multiple daily training sessions. The stress of such rigorous training can decrease appetite, resulting in reduced consumption of energy and carbohydrate.[13,21] As discussed in Chapter 2, athletes who train heavily and have difficulty eating enough can consume a high-carbohydrate liquid supplement.

To demonstrate this, Brouns and colleagues evaluated the effect of a simulated Tour de France on food and fluid intake, energy balance, and substrate oxidation. Although the cyclists consumed 630 g of carbohydrate (8.6 g/kg/d), they oxidized 850 g carbohydrate per day (11.6 g/kg/d). In spite of ad libitum intake of conventional foods, the cyclists were unable to ingest sufficient carbohydrate and calories to compensate for their increased energy expenditure. When the diet was supplemented with a 20% carbohydrate beverage, carbohydrate intake increased to 16 g/kg/d and carbohydrate oxidation rose to 13 g/kg/d.[21]

In addition, Lindeman reported that a male cyclist who competed in the RAAM obtained most of his total energy intake from a high-carbohydrate liquid supplement (23% carbohydrate).[19] Saris and colleagues reported that approximately 30% of the total carbohydrate consumed by Tour de France cyclists came from high-carbohydrate beverages (eg, sports drinks, soft drinks, and liquid meals).[15]

Athletes who have extremely high carbohydrate requirements and suppressed appetites due to heavy endurance training or competition should include compact, low-fiber forms of carbohydrate, such as pasta, white rice, sports nutrition bars and gels, baked goods (cake, tarts, biscuits), cereal, granola bars, and sugar-rich foods (eg, candy in their diet). Carbohydrate-rich fluids, such as sports drinks, juices, low-fat chocolate milk, high-carbohydrate liquid supplements, soft drinks, commercial liquid meals, milk shakes, yogurt drinks, and fruit smoothies, may also be appealing to athletes who are very tired and dehydrated.[13,22]

Table 22.2 Average Daily Macronutrient Intake in Endurance and Ultraendurance Athletes

Type of Athlete	Carbohydrate, g/kg body weight	Protein, g/kg body weight	Fat, g/kg body weight (Percentage of Energy Intake)
Male elite ultraendurance triathletes, training[4]	9.0	2.0	1.8 (27%)
Male marathon runners[4]	8.0	2.0	2.0 (32%)
Male elite Kenyan distance runners[5]	9.0	2.1	1.0 (17%)
Male elite road cyclists[7]	Training: 11.0 Racing: 12.0	Training: 2.9 Racing: 2.6	Training: 2.8 (30%) Racing: 2.2 (25%)
Female elite road cyclists[8]	Training: 9.0 Racing: 9.9	Training: 2.6 Racing: 2.2	Training and racing: 1.0 (17%)
Male Tour de France cyclists[15]	12.0	3.1	2.1 (23%)
Male Pony Express Trail cyclists,[a] racing[16]	18.0	2.7	3.5 (27%)
Male Tour de Spain cyclists, racing[17]	12.6	3.0	2.3 (26)
Male Sydney to Melbourne runner,[b] racing[18]	17.0	2.9	3.2 (27%)
Male Race Across America cyclist,[c] racing[19]	22.6	3.6	1.0 (9%)
Male Race Across America cyclist (4th-place finish),[d] racing[20]	24.8	2.8	2.3 (16%)
Male Adventure Racer[e,9]	5.7	1.9	1.5 (30%)
Female Adventure Racer[e,9]	6.9	2.0	1.5 (28%)

[a] 2,050 miles in 10 days.
[b] 628 miles in 8.5 days.
[c] 10 days, 7 hours, and 53 minutes.
[d] 9 days, 16 hours, and 45 minutes.
[e] 149 hours, 33 minutes.

A large range of foods can be recommended provided that they are easy to consume, portable, and easy to store, ensuring athlete compliance. Additional carbohydrate foods used by Tour de France cyclists and one ultraendurance runner include sweet cakes, bread, muesli, yogurt, pancakes, toast, porridge, sandwiches with protein fillings, instant noodle meals, muffins, fruit, sweets, and pastries. Daily carbohydrate intake can be in liquid, semisolid, or solid form and will depend on each athlete's preference and tolerance.[14]

PROTEIN

Although acute endurance exercise results in the oxidation of several amino acids, the total amount of amino acid oxidation amounts to only 1% to 6% of the total energy cost of exercise. A low-energy and low-carbohydrate intake will increase amino acid oxidation and total protein requirements.[23,24]

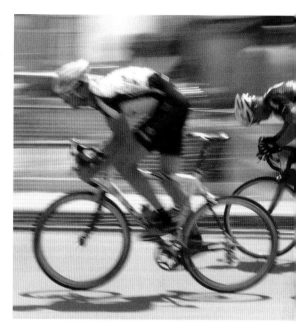

During low- to moderate-intensity endurance activity, protein intake of 1.2 g/kg/d is sufficient when energy and carbohydrate intake are adequate.[24] Elite male endurance athletes may require 1.5 to 1.8 g/kg/d to maintain nitrogen balance.[24-27] Several studies suggest higher levels, up to 2.0 g/kg/d may be necessary when energy is restricted[28-30] or when male endurance athletes are in heavy training blocks.[21]

Studies of male endurance athletes suggest that they are consuming an appropriate amount of protein. The data on female endurance athletes are extremely limited, as shown in Table 22.2.

The athlete's sex affects protein metabolism. During endurance exercise, women oxidize more lipids and less carbohydrate and protein compared with equally trained and nourished men. Due to sex-based hormonal responses that promote fat metabolism in women and carbohydrate-protein metabolism in men, female endurance athletes may have a 10% to 20% lower protein requirement compared with their male counterparts.[23] Furthermore, during the follicular phase of the menstrual cycle, protein needs may increase to 1.6 g/kg/d to maintain nitrogen balance or when energy or carbohydrate intake is low.[31]

Research suggests that, due to its high oxidation rate, the amino acid leucine has been found to be of great importance to endurance athletes, more so in male athletes than their female counterparts.[32] Foods containing the highest amounts of leucine are eggs, soy protein, seaweed, elk, tuna, chicken and turkey breast meat, cod, buffalo, and haddock.

Although most endurance athletes get sufficient protein (including leucine), those with low-energy or reduced-carbohydrate intakes and vegetarians or vegans could benefit from nutrition counseling to optimize and increase dietary protein intake.[23]

FAT

The Food and Nutrition Board of the Institute of Medicine established an Acceptable Macronutrient Distribution Range for fat at 20% to 35% of total energy intake.[30] Research indicates that this range is also acceptable for endurance athletes. Studies of male endurance athletes suggest that they are consuming an appropriate amount of fat. The data on female endurance athletes are extremely limited, as shown in Table 22.2.

A big question among endurance athletes and their coaches is relevance of fat adaptation. While more research needs to be done in this area, in a review article, Yeo and colleagues found that some well-trained athletes have responded positively when attempting to increase fat metabolism during training and races, while others have not.[31] Most studies fail to find performance advantages or disadvantages, even when fat adaptation occurs. There are reports of gastrointestinal distress when using medium-chain triglyceride oils for improved fat metabolism.[32] This concept of fat adaptation is practiced among coaches and athletes alike, thereby making it important to assess each athlete individually and determine the best approach. This topic is discussed in more detail in Chapter 4.

Water

The Institute of Medicine has declared Adequate Intake levels of fluids (from a combination of water, other beverages, and food) to be 13 cups for men and 9 cups for women each day, while the 2004 Dietary Reference Intake (DRI) recommends 16 cups for men and 12 cups for women.[33] Note that these recommendations refer to sedentary individuals. As demonstrated in Chapter 6, there is no one fluid recommendation that will suffice for everyone, especially endurance athletes. When working with endurance athletes, begin with this initial recommendation, and add more daily fluids based on sweat rate, which is discussed later in this chapter. Each athlete needs a specific daily hydration plan based on his or her training plan.

Athletes can easily monitor their daily hydration status by checking the color of their urine, daily changes in body weight, and pre- and posttraining weights. Another subjective, inexpensive measurement of hydration status in the recent literature is urine specific gravity (USG). Darkly colored urine is an indication of dehydration, while light colored urine generally represents a euhydrated state, making this a simple discussion with athletes. When considering daily weight changes, especially before and after training sessions, having multiple days of data is helpful. When athletes participate in multiple sports within an event (eg, triathlon), collect weight-change data for each event (eg, swim, bike, run).

While USG has not been recognized as a valid measure of hydration status on its own, collecting and monitoring the data regularly can be an additional tool if athletes are not severely dehydrated. A USG less than 1.020 indicates that an athlete is hydrated and a measurement greater than 1.030 indicates dehydration.[34,35]

Using data from three simple field tests in a Venn diagram decision tool may be the best approach.[36] It combines body mass (weight), urine, and thirst. A combination of any two markers means dehydration is likely, and the presence of three markers means dehydration is very likely. Additional information on hydration can be found in Chapter 6.

Micronutrients

While there are limited data on the micronutrient intake of endurance athletes, those who consume adequate total energy usually meet or exceed population reference values, such as the DRIs for vitamins and minerals.[6,10,17,20,22,37] According to a few studies, intake of thiamin and riboflavin might be inadequate[15,16,18]; however, the researchers conceded that any questions and concerns about food quality and nutrient density became immaterial considering micronutrients from supplements, whether from pills or injections.[15]

Endurance athletes who regularly restrict energy or eat a limited variety of foods may be at risk for suboptimal micronutrient intakes. Some endurance and ultraendurance athletes may have increased requirements due to excessive losses in sweat or urine. Consuming a nutrient-dense diet containing fruits, vegetables, whole grains, legumes, lean meats, and dairy foods during training helps to ensure adequate micronutrient intake.[40]

Supplementation with single micronutrients is not recommended unless there is a medical necessity (eg, iron to treat iron-deficiency anemia).[38] When supplementing, athletes should not exceed the Tolerable Upper Intake Level for any nutrient to prevent possible adverse effects on health and performance.

SODIUM

Due to the nature of endurance training, endurance athletes may have greater sodium needs. Like water, daily sodium intake can be addressed by starting with typical recommendations of no more than 2,300 mg/d.[33] Sodium requirements vary significantly based on intensity and time of training sessions, sodium concentrations in sweat, and sweat rate. When devising a plan, sweat rate should be considered, and sweat sodium losses have been shown to average 800 mg/L of sweat lost, with a range of sodium losses ranging from 10 to 70 mEq/L.[39] Heat acclimatization improves the ability to reabsorb sodium and chloride, thus people who are heat acclimatized usually have lower sweat sodium concentrations for any given sweating rate. Considering these multiple factors, daily sodium requirements for endurance athletes may exceed normal sodium dietary guidelines, especially during multihour training days. The athlete's current eating habits should be considered when discussing sodium because most people far exceed the recommended 2,300 mg/d, making it likely there will be no need to increase daily sodium on low to moderate training days.

IRON

Endurance training can increase iron requirements (due to increases in hemoglobin, myoglobin, and iron-containing proteins involved in aerobic metabolism), iron losses (through sweating, gastrointestinal bleeding, mechanical trauma such as foot strike hemolysis), and upregulated hepcidin postexercise.[40-42] The debilitating effects of iron-deficiency anemia on endurance performance are well-established. Anemia impairs erythropoiesis (red blood cell formation), thereby limiting oxygen delivery to the muscles and decreasing VO_2 max and endurance performance.[43-45]

The effects of iron depletion (stage 1 iron deficiency) on endurance performance are less clear. At the very least, iron depletion can progress to iron-deficiency anemia if untreated. Endurance and ultraendurance athletes, especially female athletes and runners of both sexes, are at risk for depleting their iron stores.[44] Although depleted iron stores should not affect VO_2 max because hemoglobin levels are not compromised, inadequate tissue iron stores may reduce oxidative metabolism in the muscle and impair endurance performance.[46,47]

One indicator for tissue iron deficiency, known as serum transferrin receptor, suggests that even stage 1 iron deficiency (depleted iron stores) may compromise aerobic and endurance capacity. Hinton and colleagues found that iron supplementation in iron-depleted, nonanemic women significantly improved endurance capacity, serum ferritin, and serum transferrin receptor concentrations, but the supplementation did not affect hemoglobin concentrations.[46] Further analysis of these data showed that tissue iron deficiency impaired adaptations to endurance training.[47] Subjects with the most tissue iron depletion also showed the greatest improvement in endurance capacity after supplementation.[48] An increase in plasma and storage iron increases the synthesis of hepcidin, therefore a decrease in hepcidin may be an early marker of iron deficiency.[52]

Athletes at risk for iron deficiency should have routine checks of their iron status. A low plasma ferritin level (< 20 mcg/dL) or serum hepcidin levels less than 20 ng/mL indicate tissue iron deficiency, which can impair endurance.[50] The athlete's iron stores can be increased through diet and iron supplementation to prevent the negative consequences of iron deficiency.[43]

CALCIUM AND VITAMIN D

Inadequate dietary calcium and vitamin D increase the risk of low bone mineral density and stress fractures. Female endurance and ultraendurance athletes who have low energy intakes, eliminate dairy products, or have menstrual dysfunction are at high risk for low bone mineral density. Vitamin D status can be easily checked via a routine blood draw by the athlete's physician or sports medicine team. Supplementation with calcium and vitamin D should be determined after nutrition assessment.[45]

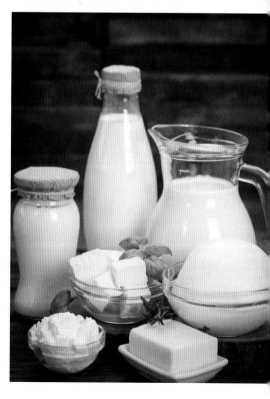

MAGNESIUM

While the direct correlation between performance and magnesium status is still unclear, a deficient magnesium status in endurance sports may result in cellular damage.[51] It is clear that losses via sweat and urine in prolonged endurance exercise could lead to a deficit, weakening muscles and affecting neuromuscular function.[52] This has led some researchers to report that a magnesium intake 10% to 20% higher may be necessary for endurance athletes.[51]

ANTIOXIDANTS

The dietary antioxidant vitamins C and E play an important role in protecting cell membranes from oxidative damage. Although endurance exercise is associated with increased oxidative stress, it also increases the body's enzymatic and nonenzymatic antioxidant defenses as an adaptation to training.[53] In fact, there may be negative effects from the routine consumption of antioxidant supplements during endurance training. Several studies found that suppression of free radical generation during exercise can attenuate some of the signals for endogenous adaptation to endurance training.[54,55] Until research suggests otherwise, it is prudent to recommend that endurance and ultraendurance athletes consume an antioxidant-rich diet, rather than supplements, to protect against oxidative damage.[53-55]

TRAINING AND RACE-DAY NUTRITION RECOMMENDATIONS

While training and racing are combined in this section, there are several important differences to note. First, energy requirements for competition days are often higher than during training, especially for ultraendurance events (eg, Ironman triathlon, 100-mile runs) and multiday events, as shown in Table 22.3.[15-20,56-60] It is neither necessary nor practical to replace 100% of calories during ultraendurance events. However, during multiday events (eg, Tour de France, RAAM), energy intake should match energy expenditure as much as possible to promote glycogen restoration, preservation of lean tissue, an adequate intake of macro- and micronutrients, and best continued performance.[6] Second, during training, endurance athletes should try different products to see what works best for them. The athlete should never try anything new on race day. Therefore, in training, the race-day plan comes together, and the athlete can practice the plan to implement on race day. Typically, a weekly endurance training schedule will include one or two long training sessions of 3 or more hours. These are the perfect days to replicate race-day nutrition.

While endurance athletes are reported to have a calorie deficit during events and training less than 24 hours, it is important to note, in training, energy will be replaced before or after the training session. The athlete should develop and refine a fueling and hydration plan months ahead of the priority race by experimenting during training and in lower-priority races. The fueling plan should be tested while training at race pace and in environmental conditions that simulate the race conditions for best results.[12] Athletes should not consume untested foods or fluids during the race because the results may be severe gastrointestinal distress and poor performance. Endurance athletes should consume liquid, semisolid, or solid fuel before feeling hungry or tired, usually within the first hour of training, depending on the timing of the meal before the training session. Consuming small amounts at frequent intervals (every 15 to 20 minutes) helps prevent gastrointestinal upset, maintains blood glucose levels, and promotes hydration.[12,18] The athlete's foods and fluids should be easily digestible, familiar (tested in training), and enjoyable (to encourage eating and drinking).[12,16,18,22]

Kimber and colleagues determined that the average energy expenditure of triathletes in the New Zealand Ironman triathlon was much greater than their average energy intake, creating a substantial energy deficit for both men (5,973 kcal) and women (5,213 kcal). This finding indicates that the triathletes obtained a large amount (59%) of their energy during the Ironman from endogenous fuel stores. The authors noted that total energy expenditure was similar between sexes when adjusted for fat-free mass.[56] A more recent study of male triathletes showed a race-day energy deficit ranging from 6,070 to 8,651 kcal.[61]

Glace and colleagues found that male ultrarunners incurred an energy deficit of 7,513 kcal in 24.3 hours during a 100-mile run.[57] In another study, Glace and colleagues found that male and female ultrarunners incurred an energy deficit of 2,516 kcal in 26.2 hours during a 100-mile run.[58]

For multiday events, Saris and colleagues found that mean daily energy intake (5,785 kcal) closely matched energy expenditure (6,069 kcal) and maintained body weight and composition for five male cyclists competing in the Tour de France.[15] Two case studies, one involving a runner and the other involving two cyclists, found that the athletes maintained their body weight and composition over 9 to 10 days of ultraendurance exercise, suggesting that energy intake was adequate to meet energy demands.[16,18]

Remarkably, an athlete who ran around Australia only lost about 5 kg after averaging approximately 47 miles/d for 191 days. O'Connor noted that a typical day's intake provided about 100 g of protein, more than 1,000 g of carbohydrate, and 120 g of fat.[22]

An additional point to consider when devising a race nutrition strategy is that male and female athletes differ with respect to carbohydrate-loading before racing. Female athletes oxidize more fat and less carbohydrate during endurance training, compared with their male counterparts.[62] According to a review by Burke and colleagues, carbohydrate-loading appears to be most effective in men running over 30 km.[63] The research available regarding woman and carbohydrate loading is scarce and inconclusive, likely due to small sample sizes; however, a few studies demonstrated improvements in performance. In addition, carbohydrate loading in women is only effective if consuming adequate energy and carbohydrate leading into the race. The regimen can be viewed as an extended period of fueling up to prepare for competition. Carbohydrate-loading guidelines are provided in Chapter 2.

Table 22.3 Energy Intake and Energy Expenditure of Endurance and Ultraendurance Athletes

Type of Athlete	Energy Intake and Expenditure During Competition, kcal/d
Male New Zealand Ironman triathletes[12]	Intake: 3,940 Expenditure: 10,036
Female New Zealand Ironman triathletes[54]	Intake: 3,115 Expenditure: 8,570
Male ultrarunners[a,55]	Intake: 6,047 Expenditure: 13,560
Male and female ultrarunners[b,56]	Intake: 7,022 Expenditure: 9,538
Male Tour de France cyclists[15]	Intake: 5,785 Expenditure: 6,069
Male Pony Express Trail cyclists[c,16]	Intake: 7,125 Expenditure: Not reported
Male Tour de Spain cyclists[17]	Intake: 5,595 Expenditure: Not reported
Male Race Around Australia runner[d,54,57]	Intake: ~6,000[54] Expenditure: 6,321[57]
Male Sydney to Melbourne runner[e,18]	Intake: 5,952 Expenditure: Not reported
Male Race Across America cyclist[f,19]	Intake: 8,429 Expenditure: Not reported
Male Race Across America cyclist (4th-place finish)[g,20]	Intake: 9,612 Expenditure: Not reported
Female Race Across America cyclist (1st-place finish)[h,58]	Intake: 7,950 Expenditure: Not reported

[a] 100-mile run; 24.3 hours.
[b] 100-mile run; 26.2 hours.
[c] 2,050 miles in 10 days.
[d] 9,053 miles in 191 days.
[e] 628 miles in 8.5 days.
[f] 10 days, 7 hours, and 53 minutes.
[g] 9 days, 16 hours, and 45 minutes.
[h] 12 days, 6 hours, and 21 minutes.

Before Training and Racing

Consuming carbohydrate before an endurance event helps to maintain blood glucose levels during prolonged exercise. The athlete should consume 1 to 4 g carbohydrate per kilogram of body weight 1 to 4 hours before exercise. García-Rovés and colleagues noted that the Tour de Spain cyclists consumed 4.5 g/kg approximately 3 hours before competition.[17]

Foods typically consumed prior to endurance and ultraendurance events include liquid meals, muesli, porridge, milk, yogurt, fruit and fruit juice, toast, jam, pancakes, waffles, bagels and biscuits, and jam or honey.[15,17,18,22]

During Training and Racing

Consuming carbohydrate is neither practical nor necessary during endurance exercise lasting less than 45 minutes. Small amounts of carbohydrate from sports drinks or foods or a carbohydrate mouth rinse may enhance performance during sustained high-intensity endurance exercise lasting 45 to 75 minutes. Athletes should consume 30 to 60 g carbohydrate pe hour from carbohydrate-rich fluids or foods during endurance sports and exercise lasting 1 to 2.5 hours. As the duration of the event increases, so does the amount of carbohydrate required to enhance performance. During endurance and ultraendurance exercise lasting 2.5 to 3 hours and longer, athletes should consume up to 80 to 90 g carbohydrate per hour from products that provide multiple transportable carbohydrates.[64] Based on Jeukendrup's 2010 review, it appears that a glucose/fructose or maltodextrin/fructose mix provides the most benefit, allowing for 1.75 g/min carbohydrate oxidation.[65]

Consuming carbohydrate during training enables the athlete to maintain a desirable training pace (and therefore maximize training adaptations), as well as practice fueling strategies for competition. Athletes should individually determine a fueling plan that meets their nutritional goals (including hydration) and minimizes gastrointestinal distress by consuming food or fluids in 10- to 20-minute intervals, as previously stated. Table 22.4 shows the carbohydrate intake during various ultraendurance events.[15-18,22,59-61]

Table 22.4 Carbohydrate Intake During Ultraendurance Events	
Type of Athlete	**Carbohydrate Intake, g/h**
Male and female New Zealand Ironman triathletes[54]	Men: 82 Women: 62
Male ultrarunners[c,55]	44
Male and female ultrarunners[d,15]	54
Male Tour de France cyclists[15]	94
Male Pony Express Trail cyclists[a,16]	60–75
Male Tour de Spain cyclists[17]	25
Male Sydney to Melbourne runner[b,18]	39
Male 24-hour mountain bike racer[22]	75

[a] 2,050 miles in 10 days.
[b] 628 miles in 8.5 days.
[c] 100-mile run, 24.3 hours.
[d] 100-mile run, 26.2 hours.

Kimber and colleagues found that New Zealand Ironman triathletes consumed substantially more energy during the bike segment (2,233 kcal for women; 2,896 kcal for men) than during the run segment of the race (883 kcal for women; 1,049 kcal for men. Energy intake during cycling provided 73% of the total energy intake. This is not surprising because foods and fluid are easier to consume and digest while on the bike, and the cycling portion is approximately 54% of the total race time. The bike portion of an Ironman also provides the opportunity to obtain energy and fluid in preparation for the marathon run.[56]

Saris and colleagues found that Tour de France male cyclists consumed nearly half of their daily energy during the race, and (as noted previously in this chapter) about 30% of the total carbohydrate consumed came from high-carbohydrate beverages.[15] Gabel and colleagues found that two male cyclists consumed about 24% of their total energy intake from high-carbohydrate beverages (eg, sports drinks, fruit juices) during a 10-day, 2,050-mile ride.[16] Eden and Abernathy reported that the male ultradistance runner in the Sydney to Melbourne race utilized a combination of high-carbohydrate solid foods and a sports drink during running to meet his energy requirements.[18]

Although high-carbohydrate beverages help increase carbohydrate and energy intake during endurance and ultraendurance events, they may also cause gastrointestinal distress when consumed in large volumes. Lindeman noted that a male RAAM cyclist's reliance on a 23% carbohydrate solution to meet the majority of his energy needs contributed to gastrointestinal distress during the race despite consistent dilution.[19]

Gastrointestinal distress during training or racing is attributable to the types of carbohydrate being consumed in addition to the osmotic pressure exerted in the small intestine when consuming particular drinks and products.[66-69] The perfect sports drink or product for every athlete in every condition does not exist. This is why it's so important to help formulate the best plan for each individual athlete and his or her preferences, avoiding gastrointestinal distress and maximizing performance.

It is essential to have a variety of carbohydrate-rich foods and fluids available during ultraendurance and multiday events to prevent flavor fatigue and an associated decrease in energy intake. Alternating between sweet choices (eg, gels, sodas, candy) and savory/salty choices (eg, vegetable soup or broth, pretzels, baked chips) helps to maintain the athlete's desire to eat. Consuming solid food with small amounts of protein and fat (eg, a turkey, cheese, or peanut butter sandwich) also helps provide satiety and variety.[22]

Consuming a small amount of protein during prolonged exercise improves protein balance. Koopman and colleagues found that the combined ingestion of protein (0.25 g/kg/h) and carbohydrate (0.7 g/kg/h) before, during, and after prolonged moderate-intensity exercise (6 hours at 50% of VO_2 max) improved net protein balance at rest, during exercise, and during subsequent recovery in endurance athletes; however, this did not necessarily equate to better performance.[70]

Gabel and colleagues reported that the two men who cycled 2,050 miles in 10 days achieved an optimal intake because of the variety and palatability of foods that were available during the event.[16] The cyclists consumed sports drinks, fruit juices, sodas, potato chips, crackers, fruit, cookies, sandwiches, and candy. Eden and Abernathy noted that the foods eaten during the Sydney to Melbourne race were based on what the male runner had enjoyed eating during training and what he could tolerate while competing. The runner consumed a sports drink, pasta with meat sauce, rice, bread, biscuits, cheese, vegetable soup, muffin with egg and cheese, fruit, and fruit juice.[18] O'Connor noted that the athlete who completed the run around Australia consumed sports drinks, fruit juice, soft drinks, high-carbohydrate supplements, milk shakes, and liquid meals during the run.[22]

High-fiber foods should be limited during competition to avoid gut distress such as abdominal bloating, cramping, and diarrhea.[12] Lindeman noted that a male RAAM cyclist's high fiber intake (57 g/d) from consuming fiber-rich sports bars and fruit may have contributed to his gastrointestinal distress during the race.[19]

When the athlete's gut blood flow is low (eg, during intense cycling or running), the athlete should emphasize carbohydrate-rich fluids (sports drinks, liquid meals, high-carbohydrate liquid supplements, fruit juices, and carbohydrate gels) to promote rapid gastric emptying and intestinal absorption. When the athlete's gut blood flow is moderate (eg, during moderate-paced cycling or slow running), the athlete may be able to consume easily digested carbohydrate-rich foods such as sports bars, fruit, and grain products (fig bars, bagels, graham crackers) in addition to liquid foods and fluids.[71] Recreational athletes often travel away from their home training base for races, which can create uncertainly in their results. They may train in a hot, humid environment and travel to race in a cooler, drier part of the country or world. They may train at low elevation in an area with little elevation change but race in the mountains. This makes it extremely important to gather data (eg, average heart rates, sweat tests) year-round, not only during the time of year the race will occur. This might also dictate the type of fueling and hydration plan the athlete should practice at home. For example, if there will be a large amount of elevation change, liquid nutrition might be easier to consume while climbing vs eating solid food. If the athlete will race at altitude, he or she may require a higher energy intake compared with what they would consume where they normally train. These are just a few of the reasons it is important to know about the environmental conditions where the race will occur, the time of year, and some details about the race course.

After Training

Restoring muscle and liver glycogen stores, replacing fluid and electrolyte losses, and promoting muscle repair are important for recovery after strenuous endurance training and multiday events.

When there is less than 8 hours between workouts or competitions that deplete muscle glycogen stores, the athlete should start consuming carbohydrate immediately after the first exercise session to maximize the effective recovery time between sessions. The athlete should consume carbohydrate at a rate of 1 to 1.2 g/kg/h for the first 4 hours after glycogen-depleting exercise. Consuming small amounts of carbohydrate frequently (every 15 to 30 minutes) further enhances muscle glycogen synthesis. During longer periods of recovery (24 hours), it does not matter how carbohydrate intake is spaced throughout the day as long as the athlete consumes adequate carbohydrate and energy.[64] Liquid forms of carbohydrate may be desirable when athletes have decreased appetites due to fatigue or dehydration.

In addition to carbohydrate, the athlete's initial recovery snack or meal should include 15 to 25 g high-quality protein.[64] The protein can be consumed through liquids, such as a recovery drink, or through solid food, such as a meal or snack. Consuming protein with recovery snacks and meals helps to increase net muscle protein balance, promote muscle tissue repair, and enhance adaptations involving synthesis of new proteins.[72] Adding a small amount of protein (~0.3 g/kg/h) to a suboptimal carbohydrate intake (<1 g/kg/h) also accelerates muscle glycogen restoration.[73] Recovery meals and snacks contribute toward the athlete's daily protein and carbohydrate requirements.[13] In consideration of multiday events, García-Rovés and colleagues noted that the Tour of Spain cyclists consumed carbohydrate at a rate of 1.1 g/kg/h and protein at a rate of 0.35 g/kg/h for the first 6 hours after the race.[17] This combined dose of carbohydrate and protein helped promote muscle glycogen restoration and muscle tissue repair.

The foods consumed during recovery meals and snacks should contribute to the athlete's overall nutrient intake. Nutritious carbohydrate-rich foods and lean sources of protein and dairy also contain vitamins and minerals that are essential for health and performance. These micronutrients are important for post-exercise recovery processes. Athletes should avoid consuming large amounts of foods high in fat or protein when total energy requirements or gastrointestinal distress limits food intake during recovery. These foods can displace carbohydrate-rich foods and reduce muscle glycogen storage.[13]

It is common for endurance athletes not to feel hungry after long training sessions, especially in hot weather. Working with them to try a liquid recovery option could be important to improve compliance and ensure that the athlete consumes an adequate amount of recovery calories and macronutrients.

FLUID AND SODIUM NEEDS DURING TRAINING AND RACING

There are limited data on fluid and sodium intakes and body-weight changes during endurance events, although new research is being conducted. As illustrated in the daily nutrition section of this chapter, fluid and sodium requirements for endurance athletes have large degrees of variability. The same holds true for during training and racing, thereby making it necessary to consider each athlete's needs individually. Additionally, sweat rates in training may not closely reflect sweat rates on race day of an endurance event due to many factors.[74] It is not possible to develop a one-size-fits-all fluid and electrolyte replacement schedule because of the multiple factors that influence sweating rate and sweat electrolyte concentration.[39] Endurance and ultraendurance athletes who have high sweat rates and a high sweat-sodium concentration ("salty sweat") can sustain substantial losses of sodium.[75] However, the high sodium sweat losses could be due to a high daily sodium intake, and it remains unclear if this affects all athletes the same.[76]

Symptomatic exercise-associated hyponatremia (plasma sodium concentration < 135 mmol/L) can occur in prolonged endurance exercise lasting more than 4 hours. Contributing factors to exercise-associated hyponatremia include drinking an amount of fluid that exceeds sweat and urinary water losses and excessive loss of total body sodium.[52] According to the 2015 Third International Exercise-Associated Hyponatremia Consensus Statement, those at higher risk are smaller persons and possibly those who regularly using nonsteroidal antiinflammatory drugs (NSAIDs), though more research is needed on NSAID use.[77] In

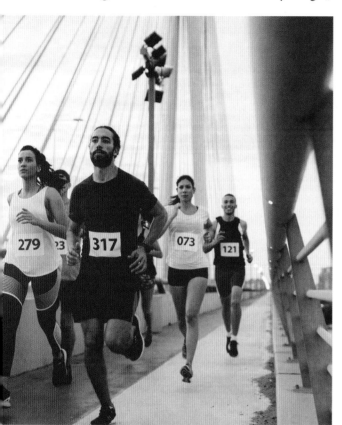

addition, several studies indicate that female athletes are at higher risk for exercise-induced hyponatremia than their male counterparts.[78,79]

In events that last less than 4 hours, hyponatremia is primarily caused by overdrinking before, during, and after the event.[75,80] During a marathon, symptomatic hyponatremia is more likely to occur in smaller and less lean participants who run slowly, sweat less, and drink excessively before, during, and after the race, as well as female athletes.[76,78-80]

Endurance athletes can experience health problems from either dehydration or overdrinking. Dehydration is more common and can impair exercise performance and contribute to serious heat illness. However, symptomatic hyponatremia is more dangerous and can cause grave illness or death. Because of the considerable variability among individuals in sweat rates and sweat electrolyte content, athletes should customize their fluid replacement plans.[39]

Before Training

Endurance athletes should also begin exercise with normal hydration and plasma electrolyte levels. Prior to exercise, an athlete should drink approximately 5 to 7 mL of fluid per hour per kilogram of body weight about 4 hours before exercise; 7 mL/kg is equivalent to approximately 1 oz for every 10 lb of body weight. Drinking several hours before exercise allows adequate time for the urine output to return toward normal.[47]

Athletes should experiment with different preexercise foods and fluids during training. Before competition, the athlete should choose familiar, well-tolerated, and palatable foods and fluids.[11]

During Training

During prolonged ultraendurance exercise (eg, Ironman triathlon), total sodium losses can induce symptomatic hyponatremia if the athlete is drinking either not enough or too much fluid.[39] High sweat rates and a high sweat-sodium concentration confer a greater risk of developing hyponatremia because less fluid intake is required to produce dangerously low blood sodium levels.[75]

Hydration during endurance exercise is necessary to prevent the detrimental effects of excessive dehydration (> 2% body weight loss) and electrolyte loss on exercise performance and health. A loss of 1% to

2% of body weight is likely to occur from factors unrelated to sweat losses (substrate oxidation) and is acceptable.[12] Dehydration increases physiological stress as measured by core temperature, heart rate, and perceived exertion, and these effects are accentuated during exercise in warm to hot and humid weather. The greater the body-water shortage, the greater the physiological strain and greater the impairment of endurance performance.[39] However, in a 2013 meta-analysis of field research, Goulet and colleagues demonstrated that body mass losses of ≤ 4% body weight in outdoor, real-world, time-trial exercise is unlikely to impair performance.[81] In addition, a weight loss of up to 3% may be tolerable and may not impair performance in cool weather.[39] Glace and colleagues estimated that body fat loss (according to skinfold measurements) accounted for about 1.13 kg of the 1.6 kg lost (2% of body weight) during a 100-mile run. In a second study, Glace and colleagues found that high fluid intakes during a 100-mile run were associated with decreased serum sodium levels and increased risk of mental status change, suggesting possible fluid overload.[57]

To prevent hyponatremia, endurance athletes should avoid overconsumption of fluids and associated weight gain.[39] Consuming a sodium-containing sports drink helps to maintain plasma sodium levels and may reduce the risk of hyponatremia during prolonged exercise.[82,83] It is recommended that the drink contain 20 to 50 mmol/L of sodium.[84] This is equivalent to 460 mg/L to 1,150 mg/L. This practice is especially important for heavy or salty sweaters, as well as for training sessions exceeding 2 hours.

Athletes participating in endurance exercise lasting longer than 3 hours should be particularly meticulous about establishing their fluid replacement schedule. As the exercise duration increases, the cumulative effects of slight disparities between fluid intake and loss can cause extreme dehydration or hyponatremia.[39] Athletes training for an hour or less may not need hydration during training, depending on the environment and the pre- and posthydration plan.

During training, athletes should experiment with different fluid replacement drinks and adjust their drinking strategies based on the workout intensity, duration, and environmental conditions. Drinking appropriately during workouts enables the athlete to maintain a desirable training pace (and maximize training adaptations), protects against heat illness, and allows the athlete to practice proper drinking strategies for competition.[5] The athlete may also choose water as the hydration source, with gels, gummies, or other sports nutrition products for the electrolytes and carbohydrates.

After Training

Ideally, the athlete should fully restore fluid and electrolyte losses between exercise sessions.[39] Consuming sodium during recovery promotes fluid retention and stimulates thirst.[85] Precise sodium losses are harder to determine than water losses because each athlete has vastly different rates of sweat electrolyte losses. Although drinks containing sodium (eg, sports drinks) may be beneficial, many foods can supply the needed electrolytes. Extra salt can be added, only when necessary, to meals and recovery fluids when sweat sodium losses are high; ½ tsp (2.5 g) salt supplies 1,000 mg sodium.[39] Keep in mind that this may not be an issue that needs to be addressed for many recreational athletes. Be sure to consider the athlete's individual needs for the best nutrition and hydration plan.

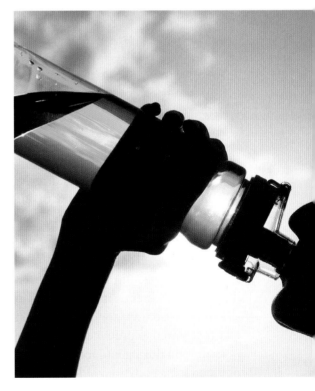

Athletes should drink 24 oz of fluid for each pound lost to achieve rapid and total recovery from dehydration.[86] The additional volume (150% of sweat losses) is required to compensate for the increased urine production that goes along with the rapid intake of large volumes of fluid.[39,86] Additional information on fluid and sodium needs is provided in Chapter 6.

There are a few overarching similarities between all endurance events that sports dietitians should consider when working with endurance athletes. An elite athlete's time to finish an event can differ tremendously from a recreational athlete's. For many recreational athletes, finish times are double that of their elite counterparts.

More often than not, an elite athlete has the opportunity to acclimatize in the race environment before event day. This is rarely the case for a recreational athlete. It is important to know the details of the race location and weather for the race; some races have extreme temperature shifts throughout race day(s), making it necessary to make adjustments throughout the race.

For most endurance races, professional athletes or those competing at the elite level have a special feed zone and their exact nutrition bottle or food is handed to them by volunteers or teammates, depending on the sport. This makes it easy to plan for this level of athlete. Recreational athletes have to bring their own nutrition, rely on products provided on the course, or have a club teammate who is not racing hand them nutrition in designated feed zones. In many races, disqualification occurs if aid is not received in the designated feed zones.

Each type of athlete and group of athletes has their own rituals, desires, and beliefs, making it important for athlete education to become a priority. Sports dietitians should encourage practice and application during long training sessions. Get to know the sport culture to be able to build a rapport with each athlete individually.

One unique consideration in regards to sports nutrition products for each type of event is the weather. If it is very cold, gummies and gels will solidify, making them difficult to chew or swallow. Solid food will also feel dry and tough to consume in the cold weather. Body heat can keep the product warm if it is near the athlete's body, as opposed to being stored in their equipment (eg, bike or pack).

At endurance and ultraendurance events, it is not uncommon for athletes to unknowingly drop their nutrition on the ground or not be able to find it easily for various reasons. Having extra fuel or salt tabs at fed stations or in a pocket or pack is always a good idea.

Lastly, for endurance events, it is crucial that the athlete practices his or her race nutrition and hydration plan many times before race day. If the athlete is wearing a heart rate monitor, a timer can be set to remind the athlete to eat and drink the same way that was practiced.

For practical application of nutrition, the following sections present specific details that are unique to different sports. Each sport is divided into endurance and ultraendurance, and if there is a multiday event for that sport, it is addressed as well.

Adventure Racing

Adventure racing, also called expedition racing, is typically a team sport involving different distances, times, and disciplines (eg, trekking, mountain biking, paddling, and climbing).

ENDURANCE

Shorter sprint adventure races can last 3 to 6 hours, making this an endurance sport. Athletes are responsible for nutrition and hydration because there are no aid stations on the course. A lightweight pack is necessary to carry hydration, and the shorter distance lends itself to a faster pace and higher heart rate. What the athlete chooses to consume depends on athlete preference and what he or she practiced in training. One easy nutrition plan is to combine energy with hydration in the pack because the course is short enough for this possibility. If this method is not possible because of athlete preference, quick, low-fiber carbohydrates are easy and light to carry.

ULTRAENDURANCE

The next level of endurance adventure race lasts 12 or 24 hours. These races typically have a gear checklist that all athletes must have in their pack, making it heavy at times. At this level, there are teams of two to four racers. There is a transition area between sections of the course where the athlete can leave nutrition and hydration of choice to keep their pack as light as possible. This allows them to add additional fuel and hydration between each section of the race.

Obstacle Course Racing

Obstacle course racing involves foot racing with various physical challenges in the form of obstacles. The most popular obstacle course races in the United States to date are Tough Mudder, Spartan Race, and BattleFrog.

ENDURANCE

The Spartan Super (8 to 10 miles, 25 or more obstacles) and the Spartan Beast (13 to 17 miles, 30 or more obstacles), Tough Mudder (10 to 12 miles) and BattleFrog 8K race fall into the endurance category.

Spartan race finish times are dependent on the location and terrain of the race. Some Spartan Beast races are won in approximately 2 hours and others take up to 3:45 to win. Due to the wide variety of Spartan race terrain (eg, some flat and some mountainous), availability of aid stations at each race are not consistent, which makes it difficult to depend on course nutrition and hydration support. There is no time limit on Spartan Super or Beast races.

The Tough Mudder races are typically more consistent; all courses are roughly 8 to 12 miles long and have 20 to 25 obstacles. Racers can often carry sports drinks and water throughout the course. Winners typically finish in less than 2 hours, but any competitors who have not reached a specific time limit at the designated halfway point are given a modified course route that allows them to cross the finish line. Tough Mudder is more conducive to athletes using course nutrition and hydration support.

The BattleFrog 8K course has at least 22 obstacles, and the BattleFrog Elite (16K) is two loops of the 8K course. There are aid stations on the course. Some athletes prefer to wear a hydration pack during obstacle course racing, while others rely on the course-provided nutrition. Either way, devising an exact plan for the athlete using the this chapter's recommendations is crucial.

One last consideration in nutrition planning for this type of race is the wave starts. Groups of athletes are released at 15- to 30-minute time increments to put space between participants. Additionally, start times run in waves between 8 AM and 3 PM.

ULTRAENDURANCE

Spartan's World Championship race, called the Ultra Beast, takes place over 26 miles and 50 or more obstacles, and the fastest finish time is approximately 7 hours. The race starts between 6 AM and 6:30 AM, and the course closes at 9 PM. This is a two-loop course; at the halway point, athletes are allowed to access a drop bin, a box of goods created prior to the race in which athletes can store extra clothing, food, drinks, etc. If they choose to carry their own nutrition and hydration while racing, athletes can also refuel during the loops as they need to. There are some aid stations on the course. To date, the race has been held in Killington, Vermont; Olympic Valley, California; and Maui, Hawaii.

The World's Toughest Mudder consists of a 5-mile course; the winner is the athlete who finishes the most laps in 24 hours. The most recent winner completed over 100 miles. Because of this course is a loop, it is easy for athletes to control their nutrition and hydration schedule. The race location changes every year and could be international.

The BattleFrog consists of 8K loops. At every race there is an Xtreme category, and the winner is the athlete who completes the most loops between 8:30 AM and 3:30 PM. Again, due to the loop format, athletes are more likely to be able to follow their nutrition and hydration schedule more closely.

Cross-Country Skiing

Although cross-country skiing is widely practiced as a recreational activity, cross-country ski competition involves a variety of formats for races over courses of varying lengths, including marathons.

ENDURANCE

The sheer nature of the uniform and the need for gloves during a race make it difficult for the athlete to open certain types of nutrition packages. It is possible to carry a waist pack with a water bottle and access this regularly. The bottle could contain most of the calories the athlete needs, as well as their hydration. In this case, liquid nutrition may be the most viable option.

Endurance Cycling

Road bicycle racing involves both team and individual competitions and, by nature, is significantly longer than running events.

ENDURANCE

Endurance cycling events are fast and furious in the elite field, making it very difficult for the athlete to consume nutrition, especially when a volunteer is responsible for handing out the nutrition products.

These events are typically 75 to 125 miles, and teams usually work together in a draft legal race structure (cyclists rotate through a line, taking turns riding up front "pulling" before peeling off and latching onto the back). A team member or a volunteer at designated feed zones can hand nutrition and hydration to the cyclist, or there may be a caravan where teammates can hand the athlete nutrition and hydration. For the nonelite cyclists, endurance cycling events range from 100K to 100 miles for cyclists. Athletes typically carry their nutrition and hydration or take only water or sports drinks at aid stations, choosing to finish the race faster rather than they would if they stopped at aid stations for nutrition. For the athlete's safety, if the nutrition plan includes solid food choices, it is important to have packages open and accessible.

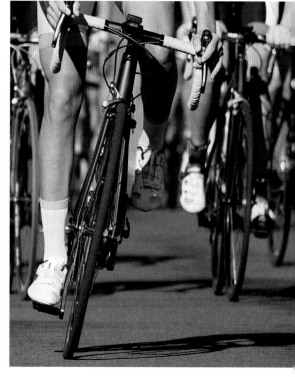

ULTRAENDURANCE

There are many types of ultraendurance cycling events. Some consist of a specific number of hours of a time trial, such as 6, 12, or 24 hours. These races consist of a loop, and the winner is the person who completes the most loops in the set amount of time. Some races are draft legal and some are not, which sometimes affects the athlete's ability to reach for and implement their nutrition on the bike. Elite athletes do not participate in these types of races, but they are very popular among recreational athletes.

Some races have a set number of miles, totaling 100, 200, 400, or 500 miles or other increments, with a maximum of 250 miles for a single-day event. While an elite racer can finish 100 miles in approximately 3 hours 30 minutes, it may take a recreational athlete as many as 8 hours to finish. This ultimately dictates the type of nutrition plan each athlete would adhere to. Most courses will have aid stations containing some or all of the following: sports drinks, salt tablets, pickle juice, baked goods, salty snacks, soda, candy, peanut butter sandwiches, and boiled potatoes. The elite field receives their planned nutrition handed to them at designated feed zones as they are riding through, while the recreational athletes occasionally stop at aid stations to rest, refuel, and rehydrate for a long day.

A hydration pack may be necessary, depending on the spacing of aid stations and individual sweat losses. Riders can fit two to four bottles on their bikes and can carry one or two bottles in their race jerseys. However, for every bottle of fluid, the athlete is adding weight to the bike, which can make carrying too many bottles a hard sell. Asking the right questions helps the sports dietitian better make a better plan for the athlete. As a reminder, the recreational athletes are at most risk for fluid and electrolyte imbalances and hyponatremia.

Endurance Running

Endurance running, also called long-distance running, can include track running, road running, and cross-country running. It is primarily an individual sport.

ENDURANCE

Endurance running consists of road and trail races around a half marathon (13.1 miles) to full marathon (26.2 miles) distance. There is wide variability in finish times for these distances depending on each athlete's experience and goal. The largest attended road races now have corrals with wave starts.

For road races, there are typically aid stations on the course at designated spaces throughout the race. Some aid stations are sponsored, especially with large races. This helps the sports dietitian plan ahead for how the athlete should use nutrition and hydration from the course. The information is available on the race website. Otherwise, there are many different fuel belts and bottles for carrying nutrition and hydration to ensure that the athletes have what they need and what they trained with.

The availability of water is typically reliable on a race course, and only toccasionally does the event run out when temperatures reach unusual highs. The availability of sports drinks may not be as reliable because of the way they are mixed (concentrations are diluted or strong), and races tend to run out of sports drinks before water. One other issue with on-course nutrition is that the flavors of the sports drink, gummies, or gels the race distributes may not be the same flavor the athlete trained with, which may make it difficult to consume.

Most trail runs have a mass start. For trail races, the aid stations are spaced farther apart due to trail access points. There are many more options for athletes to choose from, including solid, liquid, sugary, and salty snacks. The limited number of stations, however, makes it easier for the athlete to potentially eat too much at one time and not properly space out nutrition as discussed previously. This is especially true for slower runners. To improve the athlete's trail running plan for those using on-course nutrition, educate them to take small amounts of aid from each aid station, allowing them to spread out energy intake over time. For trail running, encourage the athlete to carry a handheld bottle or race hydration pack for the best hydration plan.

ULTRAENDURANCE

This distance is typically no more than 135 miles of running for a single-day event. Examples are the road race (eg, Badwater ultramarathon) or the trail race (eg, Western States Endurance Run). There are a large number of these races in the United States and the world, although the elite field is small, making many of the entrants recreational. Even though these distances involve constant running, many participants will not finish in a 24-hour time frame. The fastest times at Badwater are just shy of 24 hours for men. While a 100-mile trail run, such as Western States, is won in 15 hours, the slowest runner will finish in double that time.

For some trail ultraendurance races, the course is set up in a loop structure making, it easy for the athlete to access his or her own nutrition and hydration products of choice and not rely on the course support. This is important for athletes with certain constraints (eg, celiac disease, past gastrointestinal distress). During a 100K trail race, it is not uncommon for a runner to have a pacer, usually a friend or multiple friends who can help remind the runner to eat and drink in the event his or her motor skills are declining.

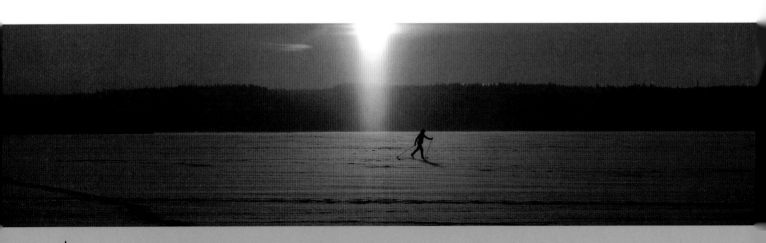

Many ultraendurance runners carry two handheld race bottles or wear a hydration pack. Even with a hydration pack, it is difficult for athletes to know how much they are drinking because the pack is not clear. Discussing their hydration plan in terms of swallows or sips per 10 minutes, or similar, is helpful.

Marathon Rowing

Rowing, also referred to as crew in the United States, involves propelling a boat (racing shell) on water using oars. Athletes compete in a number of boat classes, ranging from an individual shell to an eight-person shell.

ENDURANCE

Finishing times can range from just over 3 hours up to 6 hours. It is somewhat easy for a rower to put nutrition and hydration in the boat. If the nutrition plan includes solid food choices, it is important to have packages open and easy to get to. This is another sport where the athlete's hands are being used, so the quicker the athlete can consume nutrition the better, especially when racing as a single. One final consideration is wind. Some races can be extremely windy, making consuming nutrition and hydration even more difficult, in addition to increasing the athlete's workload and energy output.

Triathlon

A triathlon is a multiple-stage competition that includes the completion of three endurance disciplines in immediate succession over various distances. Although several combinations exist, the most popular combination is swimming, cycling, and running.

ENDURANCE

Olympic distance triathlons fall in this category. Average age group times range from about 2 hours 30 minutes to 3 hours 10 minutes depending on the course, with the last athletes coming in around 4 hours. The course has aid stations on the bike and run portion, and some races are sponsored, so specific products are available at aid stations. This information is typically available on the race website. Volunteers are responsible for handing out hydration and nutrition, but they are not always experienced. Getting hydration on the bike can be difficult as is, especially when the athlete is also inexperienced.

Unlike ultraendurance triathlons, each split is longer than 1 hour, making it difficult to follow an hourly plan. It is much easier to discuss nutrition in terms of "on the bike," "in transition," or "on the run," instead of following a plan based on an hourly clock. This still allows for nutrition and hydration every 10 to 20 minutes, but the athlete will not have to think about time as much during the race. For example, advice could be, "Consume X calories of X product at the beginning, middle, and end of the bike portion of the race."

ULTRAENDURANCE

These events take over 4 hours to finish and could be a Half Ironman (1.2-mile swim, 56-mile bike, 13.1-mile run) or Ironman distance (2.4-mile swim, 112-mile bike, 26.22-mile run). In these races, it is important to consider the differences in nutrition tolerance during the bike and run phases of the race. Athletes can generally consume more calories per hour cycling than running.[13] Ironman triathlon competitors often decrease their calorie intake toward the end of the bike segment so they can start the run with a fairly empty gut. During the run segment of a triathlon, the athletes usually consume only sports drinks, gels, gummies, broth, and water to reduce the risk of gut distress.

Many races have implemented a wave start. Find out in which wave the athlete begins because it could be an hour after the official race start, and this dictates the prerace meal. Additionally, there are course cutoff times where athletes are removed from the course if they don't make it to a point by a certain time.

The aid stations are similar to those in Olympic distance courses. On an Ironman course, the bike and run portions have special needs station at the halfway point, and athletes are allowed to to put any nutrition or hydration product of choice in their numbered bag. The numbering makes it easy for the volunteer to quickly identify the bag when the athletes enter the special needs area. Athletes are not required to stop to get their bag, but it sometimes helps to have extra nutrition and hydration available in case something unexpected occurs.

Most ultraendurance nutrition plans should be discussed with the athlete in terms of "per hour on the bike" and "per hour on the run" for best compliance.

The sports dietitian should be aware of the athlete's hydration system on his or her bike. Some athletes have hydration systems between the handlebars that make it very easy to drink. Others have cages for water bottles on the bike frame and others store hydration behind the seat. Knowing this information will help with planning.

It is not uncommon for some athletes to wear fuel belts or carry a handheld water bottle on the run portion of the course, which enables them to use their product of choice vs relying on the on-course nutrition. It also improves fluid consumption because they do not have to wait until aid stations to drink.

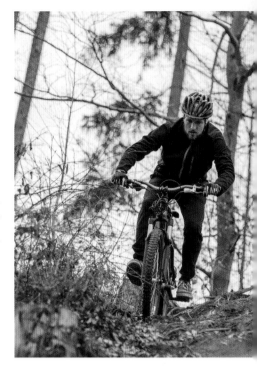

Endurance Mountain Biking

Mountain biking events are off-road and categorized into two main categories: cross-country and downhill. Cross-country is considered an endurance sport.

ENDURANCE AND ULTRAENDURANCE

In mountain biking, a marathon can range from 37 to 99 miles, as defined by Union Cycliste Internationale. However, there are many single-day mountain bike races over 99 miles. Mountain bike races can also be 6-, 12-, or 24-hour events; the winner is the rider who completes the most loops of a course in that time frame. Times can vary wildly for distance races due to different terrain; for example the most recent Leadville Trail 100 (a 100-mile race) was won in just under 6 hours while the Wilderness 101 (just one mile longer) was most recently won in just under 7 hours. Marathon races are usually cross-country races; they have a mass start. There are typically course cutoff times: If cyclists do not make it to certain points by certain times, they are removed from the course. There are aid stations throughout the course to refuel and rehydrate. These aid stations are similar to trail-running aid stations and have many different options to choose from.

It is typical for the recreational athlete to carry a hydration pack. Even with a hydration pack; however, it is difficult for the athlete to know how much they are drinking because the pack is not clear. Therefore, sports dietitians will find it helpful to discuss the hydration plan with athletes in terms of swallows or sips per 10 minutes,or something similar.

It is crucial to know the course to help the athlete be compliant with a nutrition plan. For example, if there will be long periods of climbing in the mountains, it is unrealistic for the athlete to eat solid food during that time. In this case compliance can be improved if the sports dietitian recommends that the athlete to consume liquids during that portion of the race. In some longer mountain bike races, the athlete dismounts the bike at aid stations to refuel and rehydrate before continuing.

Multiday Events

Cycling is the most common multiday sport, with professional stage races like the Tour de France and recreational races such as the Register's Annual Great Bicycle Ride Across Iowa or RAAM. For mountain biking, a race such as Tour Divide falls in this category. Adventure races take place over multiple days, and occasionally there are endurance run events over multiple days.

The importance of proper fueling and hydration during ultraendurance and multiday events cannot be overemphasized. The athlete's fueling and fluid replacement strategies can be the difference between completing the event and dropping out of the race.[22]

During the event, the athlete's primary nutritional requirements are water, carbohydrate, and sodium.[13,22] Athletes should limit foods that are high in fat, protein, and fiber during the race to decrease the risk of gastrointestinal distress.[13] The following pointers are also helpful:

- The food plan should be built around the athlete's food preferences and should include a variety of foods (savory, salty, and sweet) rather than a restricted assortment.[16,18,22,63]
- Food and fluid intake should be closely monitored during multiday events.[16,18,22,63] The crew should be prepared to enforce an eating and drinking schedule. If necessary, separate timers can be set for both liquid and solid feedings.[63]
- Food records and body weight should be assessed daily during multiday events. By tracking the athlete's food and fluid intake and body weight, the crew can take immediate corrective action, without overfeeding or causing gastrointestinal distress, if the athlete starts to fall behind on fluid or energy intake.[16,63]
- Solid food should be easy to handle, chew, and digest.[22] Beverages should promote rapid absorption of fluids and nutrients.[42] Concentrated nutrition, such as high-carbohydrate supplements or liquid meals, may be offered immediately before scheduled rest.[19,63,77]

The advice of a sports dietitian is recommended to determine the multiday athlete's nutritional requirements and develop an individualized dietary plan. The sports dietitian can also help monitor the athlete's nutrition during multiday events and help enforce food and fluid intake when necessary.[16,18,19,22]

SUMMARY

Endurance athletes should consume adequate energy and carbohydrate (5 to 12 g/kg/d) during training to maintain a desirable training intensity and thus maximize training adaptations. They have increased protein requirements (~1.2 to 1.6 g/kg/d) and should consume 20% to 35% of calories from fat.

Endurance athletes who consume adequate total energy usually meet or exceed population reference values, such as the DRI for vitamins and minerals. Consuming a nutrient-dense diet containing fruits, vegetables, whole grains, legumes, lean meat, and dairy foods during training and competition also helps to ensure adequate micronutrient intake. Endurance training can increase the need for certain micronutrients, such as iron and magnesium.

Drinking during endurance exercise is necessary to prevent the detrimental effects of excessive dehydration (>2% body weight loss) and electrolyte loss on exercise performance and health. Athletes should have customized fluid replacement plans because of the considerable variability in sweating rates and sweat electrolyte content among individuals.

Carbohydrate loading can improve performance in endurance events exceeding 90 minutes. For most athletes, a carbohydrate-loading regimen will involve 2 to 3 days of a high-carbohydrate intake (10 to 12 g carbohydrate per kilogram) and tapered training. Consuming carbohydrate before exercise can help performance by topping off muscle and liver glycogen stores. The preexercise meal should contain approximately 1 to 4 g carbohydrate per kilogram, consumed 1 to 4 hours before exercise. The athlete should also slowly drink about 5 to 7 mL/kg at least 4 hours before activity.

Consuming carbohydrate during exercise can improve performance by maintaining blood glucose levels and carbohydrate oxidation. Small amounts of carbohydrate from sports drinks, foods, or a carbohydrate mouth rinse may enhance performance during sustained high-intensity endurance exercise lasting 45 to 75 minutes. Athletes should consume 30 to 60 g carbohydrate per hour during endurance sports and exercise lasting 1 to 2.5 hours. During endurance and ultraendurance exercise lasting 2.5 to 3 hours and longer, athletes should consume up to 80 to 90 g carbohydrate per hour from multiple transportable carbohydrates.

Consuming carbohydrate following exercise facilitates rapid refilling of carbohydrate stores. During the early period of recovery (0 to 4 hours), the endurance athlete should consume 1 to 1.2 g/kg/h. The athlete's initial recovery snack or meal should also include 15 to 25 g high-quality protein to promote muscle tissue repair. Endurance athletes should drink 24 oz of fluid for each pound lost and should consume adequate sodium to achieve rapid and total recovery from dehydration.

Endurance athletes should practice adjusting their fueling strategies based on workout intensity, duration, and environmental conditions. Testing specific foods and fluids before, during, and after training sessions also allows the athlete to determine effective fueling strategies for competition.

Endurance athletes should consume adequate energy and carbohydrate (5 to 12 g/kg/d) during training to maintain a desirable training intensity and thus maximize training adaptations.

Endurance athletes who consume adequate total energy usually meet or exceed population reference values, such as the **DRI** for vitamins and minerals.

Drinking during endurance exercise is necessary to prevent the detrimental effects of excessive dehydration and electrolyte loss on exercise performance and health. The best start is to minimize body weight loss to < 2% and adjust from there.

Carbohydrate loading can improve performance in endurance events exceeding 90 minutes.

Consuming carbohydrate during exercise can improve performance by maintaining blood glucose levels and carbohydrate oxidation.

Endurance athletes should practice adjusting their fueling strategies based on workout intensity, duration, and environmental conditions.

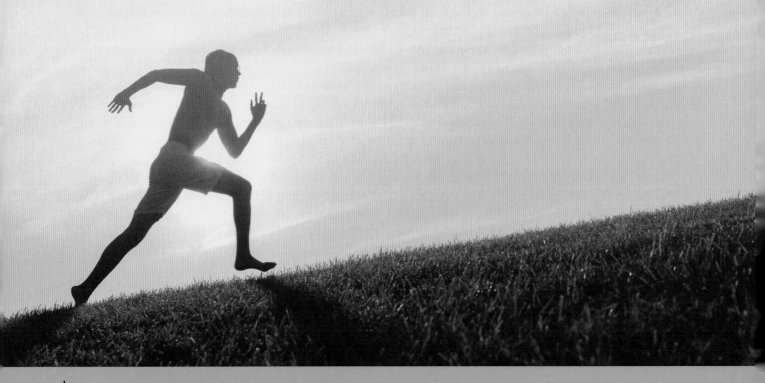

REFERENCES

1. Hargreaves M. Exercise physiology and metabolism. In: Burke L, Deakin V, eds. *Clinical Sports Nutrition*. 3rd ed. Sydney, Australia: McGraw-Hill; 2006:1-20.

2. Coyle EF. Substrate utilization during exercise in active people. *Am J Clin Nutr*. 1995;61(suppl 4):968S-979S.

3. Jeukendrup AE, Achten J. Maximal fat oxidation during exercise in trained men. *Int J Sports Med*. 2003;24(8):603-608.

4. Burke LM, Gollan RA, Read RSD. Dietary intakes and food use of groups of elite Australian male athletes. *Int J Sport Nutr*. 1992;1:378-394.

5. Fudge BW, Westerterp KR, Kiplamai FK, et al. Evidence of negative energy balance using doubly labelled water in elite Kenyan endurance runners prior to competition. *Br J Nutr*. 2006;95(1):59-66.

6. Motonaga K, Yoshida S, Yamagami F, Kawano T, Takeda E. Estimation of total daily energy expenditure and its components by monitoring the heart rate of Japanese endurance athletes. *J Nutr Sci Vitaminol (Tokyo)*. 2006;52(5):360-367.

7. Garcia-Roves PM, Terrados N, Fernandez S, Patterson AM. Comparison of dietary intake and eating behavior of professional road cyclists during training and competition. *Int J Sport Nutr*. 2000;10(1):82-98.

8. Martin MK, Martin DT, Collier GR, Burke LM. Voluntary food intake by elite female cyclists during training and racing: Influence of daily energy expenditure and body composition. *Int J Sport Nutr Exerc Metab*. 2002;12(3):249-267.

9. Zalcman I, Guarita HV, Juzwiak CR, et al. Nutritional status of adventure racers. *Nutrition*. 2007;23(5):404-411.

10. Burke LM. Nutritional practices of male and female endurance cyclists. *Sports Med*. 2001;31(7):521-532.

11. Burke L. Preparation for competition. In: Burke L, Deakin V, eds. *Clinical Sports Nutrition*. 3rd ed. Sydney, Australia: McGraw-Hill; 2006:355-384.

12. Maughan RJ. Fluid and carbohydrate intake during exercise. In: Burke L, Deakin V, eds. *Clinical Sports Nutrition*. 3rd ed. Sydney, Australia: McGraw-Hill; 2006:385-414.

13. Burke L. Nutrition for recovery after training and competition. In: Burke L, Deakin V, eds. *Clinical Sports Nutrition*. 3rd ed. Sydney, Australia: McGraw-Hill; 2006:415-453.

14. O'Connor H, Caterson I. Weight loss and the athlete. In: Burke L, Deakin V, eds. *Clinical Sports Nutrition*. 3rd ed. Sydney, Australia: McGraw-Hill; 2006:135-173.

15. Saris WH, van Erp-Baart MA, Brouns F, Westerterp KR, ten Hoor F. Study on food intake and energy expenditure during extreme sustained exercise: the Tour de France. *Int J Sports Med*. 1989;10(suppl 1):26S-31S.

16. Gabel KA, Aldous A, Edgington C. Dietary intake of two elite male cyclists during a 10- day, 2,050-mile ride. *Int J Sport Nutr*. 1995;5(1):56-61.

17. Garcia-Roves PM, Terrados N, Fernández SF, Patterson AM. Macronutrients intake of top level cyclists during continuous competition—change in the feeding pattern. *Int J Sports Med*. 1998;19(1):61-67.

18. Eden BD, Abernethy PJ. Nutritional intake during an ultraendurance running race. *Int J Sport Nutr*. 1994;4(2):166-174.

19. Lindeman AK. Nutrient intake of an ultraendurance cyclist. *Int J Sport Nutr*. 1991;1(1):79-85.

20. Knechtle B, Enggist A, Jehle T. Energy turnover at the Race Across America (RAAM)–a case report. *Int J Sports Med*. 2005;26(6):499-503.

21. Brouns F, Saris WH, Stroecken J, et al. Eating, drinking, and cycling. A controlled Tour de France simulation study, Part II. Effect of diet manipulation. *Int J Sports Med*. 1989;10(suppl 1):41S-48S.

22. Burke LM. Feeding ultraendurance athletes: an interview with Dr. Helen O'Connor and Gregory Cox. (Interview.) *Int J Sport Nutr Exerc Metab*. 2002;12:490-494.

23. Tarnopolsky M. Protein and amino acid needs for bulking up. In: Burke L, Deakin V, eds. *Clinical Sports Nutrition*. 3rd ed. Sydney, Australia: McGraw-Hill; 2006:73–111.

24. Tarnopolsky M. Protein requirements for endurance athletes. *Nutrition*. 2004;20(7-8):662-668.

25. Brouns F, Saris WH, Stroecken J, et al. Eating, drinking, and cycling. A controlled Tour de France simulation study, Part I. *Int J Sports Med*. 1989;10(suppl 1):32S-40S.

26. Tarnopolsky MA, Macdougall JD, Atkinson SA. Influence of protein intake and training status on nitrogen balance and lean body mass. *J Appl Physiol (1985)*. 1988;64(1):187-193.

27. Friedman JE, Lemon PW. Effect of chronic endurance exercise on retention of dietary protein. *Int J Sports Med*. 1989;10(2):118-123.

28. Houltham SD, Rowlands DS. A snapshot of nitrogen balance in endurance-trained women. *Appl Physiol Nutr Metab*. 2014;39(2):219-225.

29. Phillips SM. Dietary protein requirements and adaptive advantages in athletes. *Br J Nutr*. 2012;108(suppl 2):158S-167S.

30. Panel on Macronutrients, Panel on the Definition of Dietary Fiber, Subcommittee on Upper Reference Levels of Nutrients, Subcommittee on Interpretation and Uses of Dietary Reference Intakes, and the Standing Committee on the Scientific Evaluation of Dietary Reference Intakes, Food and Nutrition Board, Institute of Medicine of the National Academies. *Dietary Reference Intakes for Energy, Carbohydrate, Fiber, Fat, Fatty Acids, Cholesterol, Protein, and Amino Acids*. Washington, DC: National Academies Press; 2005.

31. Yeo WK, Carey AL, Burke L, Spriet LL, Hawley JA. Fat adaptation in well-trained athletes: effects on cell metabolism. *Appl Physiol Nutr Metab*. 2011;36(1):12-22.

32. Burke LM, Hawley JA. Fat and carbohydrate for exercise. *Curr Opin Clin Nutr Metab Care.* 2006;9(4):476-481.

33. Panel on Dietary Reference Intakes for Electrolytes and Water, Standing Committee on the Scientific Evaluation of Dietary Reference Intakes, Food and Nutrition Board, Institute of Medicine of the National Academies. *Dietary Reference Intakes for Water, Potassium, Sodium, Chloride, and Sulfate.* Washington, DC: National Academies Press; 2004.

34. Armstrong LE. Assessing hydration status: the elusive gold standard. *J Am Coll Nutr.* 2007;26(suppl 5):575S-584S.

35. Fernandez-Elias VE, Martinez-Abellán A, López-Gullón JM, et al. Validity of hydration non-invasive indices during the weightcutting and official weigh-in for Olympic combat sports. *PloS One.* 2014;9(4):e95336.

36. Cheuvront SN, Sawka MN. Hydration assessment of athletes. *Sports Sci Exch.* 2005;18(2):1-10.

37. Singh A, Evans P, Gallagher KL, Deuster PA. Dietary intakes and biochemical profiles of nutritional status of ultramarathoners. *Med Sci Sports Exer.* 1993;25(3):328-334.

38. Fogelholm M. Vitamin, mineral, and antioxidant needs of athletes. In: Burke L, Deakin V, eds. *Clinical Sports Nutrition.* 3rd ed. Sydney, Australia: McGraw-Hill; 2006:313-342.

39. Sawka MN, Burke LM, Eichner ER, Maughan RJ, Montain SJ, Stachenfeld NS. Exercise and fluid replacement. *Med Sci Sports Exerc.* 2007;39(2):377-390.

40. Peeling P. Exercise as a mediator of hepcidin activity in athletes. *Eur J Appl Physiol.* 2010;110(5):877-883.

41. Peeling P, Dawson B, Goodman C, et al. Cumulative effects of consecutive running sessions on hemolysis, inflammation and hepcidin activity. *Eur J Appl Physiol.* 2009;106(1):51-59.

42. Peeling P, Sim M, Badenhorst CE, et al. Iron status and the acute post-exercise hepcidin response in athletes. *PloS One.* 2014;9(3):e93002.

43. Deakin V. Iron depletion in athletes. In: Burke L, Deakin V, eds. *Clinical Sports Nutrition.* 3rd ed. Sydney, Australia: McGraw-Hill; 2006:263-312.

44. Schumacher YO, Schmid A, Grathwohl D, Bultermann D, Berg A. Hematological indices and iron status in athletes of various sports and performances. *Med Sci Sports Exerc.* 2002;34(5):869-875.

45. Rodriguez NR, DiMarco NM, Langley S, et al. Nutrition and athletic performance. *Med Sci Sports Exerc.* 2009;41(3):709-731.

46. Hinton PS, Giordano C, Brownlie T, Haas JD. Iron supplementation improves endurance after training in iron-depleted, nonanemic women. *J Appl Physiol (1985).* 2000;88(3):1103-1111.

47. Brownlie T, Utermohlen V, Hinton PS, Giordano C, Haas JD. Marginal iron deficiency without anemia impairs aerobic adaptation among previously untrained women. *Am J Clin Nutr.* 2002;75(4):734-742.

48. Brownlie T, Utermohlen V, Hinton PS, Haas JD. Tissue iron deficiency without anemia impairs adaptation in endurance capacity after aerobic training in previously untrained women. *Am J Clin Nutr.* 2004;79(3):437-443.

49. D'Angelo G. Role of hepcidin in the pathophysiology and diagnosis of anemia. *Blood Res.* 2013;48(1):10-15.

50. Ziemann E, Kasprowicz K, Kasperska A, Zembroń-Lacny A, Antosiewicz J, Laskowski R. Do high blood hepcidin concentrations contribute to low ferritin levels in young tennis players at the end of tournament season? *J Sports Sci Med.* 2013;12(2):249-258.

51. Laires MJ, Monteiro CP, Matias CN, Santos DA, Silva AM, Bicho M. Magnesium status and exercise performance in athletes. *J Trace Elem Electrolytes.* 2014;31(1):13-20.

52. Resina A, Gatteschi L, Castellani W, Galvan P, Panise G, Rubenni MG. Effects of aerobic training and exercise on plasma and erythrocyte magnesium concentration. In: Kies CV, Driskell JA, eds. *Sports Nutrition: Minerals and Electrolytes.* London: CRC Press; 1995:189-203.

53. Watson T. The science of anti-oxidants and exercise performance. In: Burke L, Deakin V, eds. *Clinical Sports Nutrition.* 3rd ed. Sydney, Australia: McGraw-Hill; 2006:343-353.

54. Gomez-Cabrera MC, Domenech E, Romagnoli M, et al. Oral administration of vitamin C decreases muscle mitochondrial biogenesis and hampers training-induced adaptations in endurance performance. *Am J Clin Nutr.* 2008;87(1):142-149.

55. Ristow M, Zarse K, Oberbach A, et al. Antioxidants prevent health-promoting effects of physical exercise in humans. *Proc Natl Acad Sci U.S.A.* 2009;106(21):8665-8670.

56. Kimber NE, Ross JJ, Mason SL, Speedy DB. Energy balance during an Ironman triathlon in male and female triathletes. *Int J Sport Nutr Exerc Metab.* 2002;12(1):47-62.

57. Glace B, Murphy C, McHugh M. Food and fluid intake and disturbances in gastrointestinal and mental function during an ultramarathon. *Int J Sport Nutr Exerc Metab.* 2002;12(4):414-427.

58. Glace BW, Murphy CA, McHugh MP. Food intake and electrolyte status of ultramarathoners competing in extreme heat. *J Am Coll Nutr.* 2002;21(6):553-559.

59. Hill RJ, Davies PS. Energy expenditure during 2 wk of an ultraendurance run around Australia. *Med Sci Sports Exerc.* 2001;33(1):148-151.

60. Clark N, Tobin J Jr, Ellis C. Feeding the ultraendurance athlete: practical tips and a case study. *J Am Diet Assoc.* 1992;92(10):1258-1262.

61. Barrero A, Erola P, Bescos R. Energy balance of triathletes during an ultraendurance event. *Nutrients.* 2015;7(1):209-222.

62. Tarnopolsky MA. Gender differences in substrate metabolism during endurance exercise. *Can J Appl Physiol.* 2000;25(4):312-327.

63. Burke LM, Millet GE, Tarnopolsky MA. Nutrition for distance events. *J Sports Sci.* 2007;25(suppl 1):29S-38S.

64. Burke LM, Hawley JA, Wong SH, Jeukendrup AE. Carbohydrates for training and competition. *J Sports Sci.* 2011;29(suppl 1):17S-27S.

65. Jeukendrup AE. Carbohydrate and exercise performance: the role of multiple transportable carbohydrates. *Curr Opin Clin Nutr Metab Care.* 2010;13(4):452-457.

66. Gisolfi CV, Lambert GP, Summers RW. Intestinal fluid absorption during exercise: role of sport drink osmolality and [Na+]. *Med Sci Sports Exerc.* 2001;33(6):907-915.

67. Gisolfi CV, Summers RW, Lambert GP, Xia T. Effect of beverage osmolality on intestinal fluid absorption during exercise. *J Appl Physiol (1985).* 1998;85:1941-1948.

68. Hunt JB, Elliott EJ, Fairclough PD, Clark ML, Farthing MJ. Water and solute absorption from hypotonic glucose-electrolyte solutions in human jejunum. *Gut.* 1992;33(4):479-483.

69. Shi X, Summers RW, Schedl HP, Chang RT, Lambert GP, Gisolfi CV. Effects of solution osmolality on absorption of select fluid replacement solutions in human duodenojejunum. *J Appl Physiol (1985).* 1994;77(3):1178-1184.

70. Koopman R, Pannemans DL, Jeukendrup AE, et al. Combined ingestion of protein and carbohydrate improves protein balance during ultraendurance exercise. *Am J Physiol Endocrinol Metab.* 2004;287(4):E712-E720.

71. Laursen PB, Rhodes EC, Buchanan JM. Physiological analysis of a high intensity ultraendurance event. *Strength Cond J.* 1999;21(1):26-38.

72. Phillips SM, Moore DR, Tang JE. A critical examination of dietary protein requirements, benefits, and excesses in athletes. *Int J Sport Nutr Exerc Metab.* 2007;17(suppl):58S-76S.

73. Betts JA, Williams C. Short-term recovery from prolonged exercise exploring the potential for protein ingestion to accentuate the benefits of carbohydrate supplements. *Sports Med.* 2010;40(11):941-959.

74. Maughan RJ, Shirreffs SM, Leiper JB. Errors in the estimation of hydration status from changes in body mass. *J Sports Sci.* 2007;25(7):797-804.

75. Montain SJ, Cheuvront SN, Sawka MN. Exercise associated hyponatremia: quantitative analysis for understanding the aetiology. *Br J Sports Med.* 2006;40(2):98-106.

76. Allsopp AJ, Sutherland R, Wood P, Wootton SA. The effect of sodium balance on sweat sodium secretion and plasma aldosterone concentration. *Eur J Appl Physiol Occup Physiol.* 1998;78(6):516-521.

77. Hew-Butler T, Rosner MH, Fowkes-Godek S, et al. Statement of the Third International Exercise-Associated Hyponatremia Consensus Development Conference, Carlsbad, California, 2015. *Clin J Sport Med.* 2015;25(4):303-320.

78. Eijsvogels TMH, Scholten RR, van Duijnhoven NTL, Thijssen DHJ, Hopman MTE. Sex difference in fluid balance responses during prolonged exercise. *Scand J Med Sci Spor.* 2013;23(2):198-206.

79. Wagner S, Knechtle B, Knechtle P, Rüst CA, Rosemann T. Higher prevalence of exercise-associated hyponatremia in female than in male open-water ultraendurance swimmers: the "Marathon-Swim" in Lake Zurich. *Eur J Appl Physiol.* 2012;112(3):1095-1106.

80. Hew TD, Chorley JN, Cianca JC, Divine JG. The incidence, risk factors, and clinical manifestations of hyponatremia in marathon runners. *Clin J Sport Med.* 2003;13(1):41-47.

81. Goulet ED. Effect of exercise-induced dehydration on endurance performance: evaluating the impact of exercise protocols on outcomes using a meta-analytic procedure. *Br J Sports Med.* 2013;47(11):679-686.

82. Vrijens DM, Rehrer NJ. Sodium-free fluid ingestion decreases plasma sodium during exercise in the heat. *J Appl Physiol (1985).* 1999;86(6):1847-1851.

83. Twerenbold R, Knechtle B, Kakebeeke T, et al. Effects of different sodium concentrations in replacement fluids during prolonged exercise in women. *Br J Sports Med.* 2003;37(4):300-303.

84. Sharp RL. Role of sodium in fluid homeostasis with exercise. *J Am Coll Nutr.* 2006;25(suppl 3):231S-239S.

85. Nose H, Mack GW, Shi XR, Nadel ER. Involvement of sodium retention hormones during rehydration in humans. *J Appl Physiol (1985).* 1988;65(1):332-336.

86. Shirreffs SM, Maughan RJ. Volume repletion after exercise-induced volume depletion in humans: replacement of water and sodium losses. *Am J Physiol.* 1998;274(5 pt 2):F868-F875.

CHAPTER 23

EMERGING OPPORTUNITIES IN SPORTS NUTRITION

Elizabeth Abbey, PhD, RDN

INTRODUCTION

When he was a swimmer in college, James first became interested in nutrition after working with his university's sports dietitian, who helped him to manage a new diagnosis of celiac disease. After completing a dietetics internship and passing the board exam, James is a newly minted registered dietitian nutritionist (RDN) with the goal of earning the certified specialist in sports dietetics (CSSD) credential and pursuing a career in sports nutrition. However, he lives in an area where there are few opportunities to work with high-level athletes and is not in a situation where he can move to a larger market. James has found work as a relief RDN at the local hospital but would like a position that would connect him with a more active population so he can start logging CSSD hours. Outside of working with college or professional athletes, James is not sure what opportunities exist for sports dietitians and how to break into the field.

Does James's situation sound familiar? While the prevalence of RDNs in collegiate and professional athletics continues to grow, in reality, most sports dietitians work with individuals of all skill and activity levels.

When sports dietitians look beyond our traditional athlete populations, there are limitless, untapped opportunities. Several active populations—some new and some that have been around for some time—are increasingly seeking out RDNs for their expertise. These include people involved in CrossFit, obstacle races, motorsports, dance, and marching bands as well as first responders. Clearly, there is overlap between some of these groups and other sports (eg, CrossFit and very-high- and high-intensity, short-duration sports), and you are encouraged to refer to those chapters for more background on the physiological underpinnings of those activities. The purpose of this chapter is not to provide exhaustive detail on each of these sports or populations but to give a general overview of the unique considerations for each of these groups, practical tips from RDNs who currently work with them, and suggestions for how to make inroads into these fields. Hopefully, you will be encouraged to explore these and other emerging opportunities in sports nutrition.

CROSSFIT

Description

Since the first CrossFit gym opened in the late 1990s, similar programs have flooded the market.[1] For simplicity's sake, this section will focus on CrossFit, but the same basic principles can apply to other high-intensity interval training (HIIT) programs. CrossFit is a "sport of fitness" that involves "constantly varied, high-intensity, functional movement" with the goal of increasing power.[2] This is achieved by collectively increasing load, distance, and speed. While HIIT is not new, the recent explosion of CrossFit may be attributed to the variety of workouts, camaraderie, and competition among participants. To fully engage in the CrossFit community, participants are encouraged to join an affiliate gym, called a "box," which is staffed by accredited CrossFit trainers. Individuals can also participate without a membership by accessing the "workout of the day" (WOD) online. Top-level CrossFitters can vie for the crown of the Fittest Man and Woman on Earth at the annual CrossFit Games, where they compete in mystery challenges. Qualifying is a three-stage process that begins at the local box, followed by regional events, and finally the national finals.[3] While the chiseled, Special Forces commando is the CrossFit image that typically comes to mind, CrossFit has attracted individuals from all backgrounds and skill levels. Andrea Chapin, an RDN based in California, has seen many ex-collegiate athletes, military personnel, and first responders among the CrossFitters she has counseled (email communication, July 20, 2015). Opportunities to work with Crossfit athletes are not limited to the top-level Crossfitters, as thousands of people participate in Crossfit as a way to improve their fitness level. There is even a CrossFit Kids program with scaled workouts for youth from ages 3 to 18.[4] Box 23.1 explains common CrossFit terms.

Box 23.1: A Selection of Common CrossFit Terms and Abbreviations[5]	
Beast	An athlete with exceptionally good work capacity and/or work ethic
Box	The name for a CrossFit gym, so-named because they are often in industrial-type warehouses
CF Games	CrossFit Games: annual competition to find the fittest man and woman on Earth
Firebreather	An elite-level CrossFit athlete
GPP	General physical preparedness: fitness
Girls	Several CrossFit benchmark workouts that are given female names but are not named after actual people
Heroes	Several CrossFit benchmark workouts that are named after actual military figures, law enforcement officers, and firefighters who have died in the line of duty—typically very difficult
Metcon	Metabolic conditioning: training with the intent to enhance performance of the three metabolic pathways
Paleo	A theory of nutrition that humans are suited to eat only foods that have been available in nature and eaten by hominoids for millions of years
Paleolithic lifestyle	A theory that we should try to replicate the lifestyle of our Paleolithic ancestors including: following the Paleo Diet, sleeping longer and more often with no or minimal electric light, minimizing stress, minimizing repetitive work, walking a lot, moving heavy things often, exercising near maximum intensity every once in a while, and maintaining social connections
WOD	Workout of the day: combination of exercises that changes from day-to-day

Basic Physiological Demands

CrossFit is unique in that every WOD is different, as they range in time from as little as 10 minutes to over an hour (Jennifer Vattimo, RDN, LDN, CrossFit coach, email communication, July 16, 2015).[3] CrossFit is appealing to many because people can get a good workout relatively quickly. Participants usually take two rest days every week. The types of activities vary widely from Olympic lifting, powerlifting, and body weight training to sports such as gymnastics, swimming, and running. While all WODs are performed at a high to very high intensity and therefore rely heavily on anaerobic energy production, aerobic energy production is also important during longer workouts. Refer to Chapters 20 and 21 on sport-specific nutrition guidelines for a more thorough overview of the physiological considerations for these types of activities.

Typical Diets

Nutrition is a key component of the CrossFit training program. CrossFitters are encouraged to avoid processed foods and focus on a higher-protein diet with low glycemic index carbohydrates.[3] While the Zone Diet, developed by Barry Sears, PhD, was commonly promoted during the early years of CrossFit and is still mentioned on its website, the diet most frequently associated with CrossFit today is the Paleolithic-style (Paleo) diet. The recommended macronutrient distribution for the Zone Diet is 30% protein, 30% fat, and 40% carbohydrates. In terms of a dinner plate, this translates into roughly ⅓ lean protein, ⅔ non-starchy fruits and vegetables, and a dash of monounsaturated fat.[6,7] One of the primary claims of this diet is that it is anti-inflammatory. While there are some similarities between the Zone and Paleo diets (ie, higher protein intake and an emphasis on fruits, vegetables, and monounsaturated fats), there are distinct differences. See Box 23.2 for an overview of the Paleo Diet.[8-19]

Nutrition Issues

ENERGY AVAILABILITY AND HYDRATION

Chapin found that while many of the CrossFitters she has encountered claim to follow the Paleo Diet, interpretation of the diet guidelines differ widely. In particular, she notes that many participants think carbohydrates should be avoided (Andrea Chapin, RDN, email communication, July 20, 2015). Vattimo says

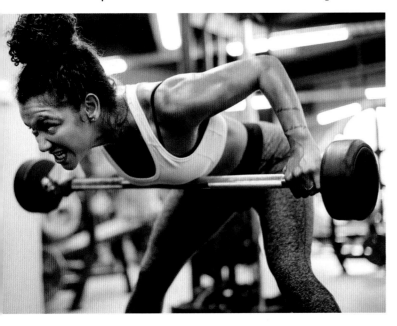

many of the athletes she has worked with have complained of tiredness and lack of energy while on the Paleo Diet (Jennifer Vattimo, RDN, LDN, email communication, July 16, 2015). Restriction of certain types of carbohydrates and food groups may prevent an athlete from meeting his or her nutritional needs. Besides recommending a specific type of diet, the CrossFit prescription advocates reducing caloric intake as a means of chronic disease prevention and longevity.[3] While this may be helpful for those whose primary goal is weight loss, it may leave an athlete feeling fatigued, especially if she or he is not consuming adequate carbohydrates.

If a CrossFitter consumes anything during a workout, it is likely water. Even that may be difficult due to the sustained intensity of the workout. The hot environment of many gyms may also put participants at a higher risk for dehydration and heat illness. Fluid intake pre- and postworkout, in addition to appropriate recovery nutrition, should be emphasized. See Chapter 6 for fluid guidelines.

SUPPLEMENTS AND ERGOGENIC AIDS

Vattimo has observed that many of her CrossFit athletes take supplements. Whey protein, typically ingested postworkout, is the most popular supplement (Jennifer Vattimo, RDN, LDN, email communication, July 16, 2015). On top of whey, supplements marketed as preworkout energy boosters (usually with some sugars and caffeine) are also widely consumed (Andrea Chapin, RDN, email communication, July 20, 2015). No scientific studies have been published on supplement use among CrossFitters; however, many online CrossFit articles and blogs speak to supplement use. While real food is the primary objective, many CrossFitters supplement with the following: creatine monohydrate, protein powder, fish oil, branched-chain amino acids, β-alanine, zinc, and magnesium.[20-22]

Box 23.2 The Paleo Diet

Popularized by Loren Cordain, PhD, the Paleo Diet is based on eating modern foods that mimic the food groups eaten by our preagricultural, hunter-gatherer ancestors.[8] In *The Paleo Diet for Athletes: The Ancient Nutritional Formula for Peak Athletic Performance*, authors Cordain and Joe Friel, MS, describe this approach as not an actual diet but a lifelong pattern of eating that will improve athletic performance, normalize body weight, and reduce the risk for many chronic diseases and conditions, such as heart disease, cancer, osteoporosis, diabetes, and some autoimmune diseases.[9]

The primary rules of this plan are to avoid grains, sugars, dairy products, legumes and beans, salt, processed foods, and processed meats. Green-light foods include fresh fruits and vegetables, nuts and seeds (except peanuts), eggs, meats, seafood, and oils high in mono- and polyunsaturated fats. This translates into higher protein and fat (~40% each) and lower carbohydrate (~20% to 25%) intake.[9] The authors explain that this is ergogenic because (1) it is higher in branched-chain amino acids (BCAAs) to stimulate muscle synthesis and repair; (2) it prevents muscle breakdown by reversing metabolic acidosis; (3) it is high in antioxidants and phytochemicals that promote immune function; and (4) it best replenishes glycogen stores through consumption of carbohydrates only during exercise and immediately postexercise.

The Paleo Diet has a myriad of variations. Stricter adherents may choose to eat only organic produce and meat, as well as higher amounts of wild game. Cheating is not discouraged as long as at least 85% of weekly calories adhere to the Paleo guidelines. Cordain and Friel also make concessions for the consumption of high-carbohydrate sports drinks, gels, and bars during longer endurance exercise and immediately after exercise to replenish glycogen stores.[9] A carb-to-protein (especially BCAAs) ratio of approximately 4:1 during the 30-minute recovery window is recommended. These exceptions aside, a majority of daily calories are expected to come from the standard Paleo guidelines.

Despite the popularity of the Paleo Diet among athletes, the human research on the effectiveness of this diet has been almost exclusively focused on adults with comorbidities such as overweight or obesity, cardiovascular disease, and type 2 diabetes and not as an ergogenic aid for athletes.[10] While there are definitely positive aspects of going Paleo for athletes (increased focus on whole foods, fewer processed and high-sugar foods, more unsaturated fats, and potential weight loss), its restrictiveness (without making exceptions) may lead to inadequate carbohydrate intake for endurance activity and low intake of essential nutrients, such as calcium. There is overwhelming evidence that daily carbohydrate intake, particularly of 5 to 12 g/kg body weight (depending on exercise intensity and volume) maintains glycogen stores and achieves optimal carbohydrate availability.[11] It is also impossible to ignore the many documented health benefits of several foods that are off limits to Paleo adherents, such as whole grains, beans, and legumes.[12-15]

The acid-base claims of this diet are also questionable. The focus on a net acid-producing diet (measured by the potential renal acid load [PRAL] of a food) assumes that foods that impact urinary pH have the same effect on blood pH, which has not been shown to be the case.[16] As long as an individual has healthy, functioning kidneys, blood pH remains quite stable. There is also a lack of evidence supporting the theory that high levels of urinary calcium excretion are indicative of increased bone resorption.[17] Finally, if one were to consider the PRAL values of individual foods, one would see that all animal products would be classified as acidic, yet they are still included in the Paleo plan.[9] In summary, the evidence behind the acid-base assertions of this diet is weak and should continue to be critically evaluated.

The potential high cost and feasibility of the Paleo Diet may be roadblocks for some athletes. A study on the feasibility of the Paleo Diet for low-income consumers found that a 9.3% increase in income was required to meet the recommended dietary intakes for all nutrients except calcium.[18] Adherence may also be a problem. In a 2-year randomized controlled trial of 70 postmenopausal women who were obese and following either the Paleolithic-type diet or the Nordic Nutrition Recommendations, the Paleo group had short-term improvements in body composition that were not sustained at 24 months.[19] In particular, the high levels of protein intake were not sustained.

All athletes could benefit from eating fewer processed foods, as prescribed in the Paleo Diet. If an athlete has poor eating habits to begin with, following a Paleo Diet could encourage more healthful food choices. The level of activity, diet history, time commitments, and overall goals of the athlete should be considered when counseling him or her on this way of eating.

Expert Nutrition Tips

CrossFitters tend to be extremely focused, driven individuals willing to push their bodies to the limit. They usually have also received a lot of misinformation in regards to nutrition and can take that to an extreme. As with counseling any athlete, Chapin says it is important to "keep an open mind and work from the beginning to build a strong rapport." When an athlete chooses to follow a specific diet, such as Paleo, she emphasizes providing guidance on evidence-based sports nutrition and, if necessary, working with the athlete to modify the diet plan to fit his or her unique needs (Andrea Chapin, RDN, email communication, July 20, 2015).

How to Get Your Foot in the Door

RDNs interviewed for this chapter suggested that a common theme for success was to be proactive and initiate contact. Very rarely will the athletes come to you; you need to go where the athletes are. This involves contacting your local CrossFit affiliate box and offering a series of nutrition seminars or presentations. Many CrossFit affiliates host events and invite vendors to come—ask to participate and set up an interactive booth to showcase your business (Andrea Chapin, RDN, email communication, July 20, 2015). Finally, when working with any new clientele group, go and observe a workout. Signing up for at least an introductory workout series will best acquaint you with the physical demands and jargon of CrossFit. CrossFitters are a loyal, highly connected group. Fostering connections in the "sport of fitness" may open several doors for a motivated RDN.

OBSTACLE COURSE RACES

Description

Between 2009 and 2013, participation in nontraditional running events (eg, theme races and obstacle races) increased 40-fold to over 4 million participants in the United States annually.[23] In 2013, more people took part in nontraditional races than marathons and half-marathons combined. Theme races (eg, mud, color, zombie) tend to be short (5K) and attract individuals whose main goals are to finish and have a good time with friends. Obstacle races, on the other hand, are more intense and geared toward athletes who are looking for a new challenge that combines endurance with strength and skill. The two most popular obstacle course races are Tough Mudder and Spartan Race. Both are team-oriented endurance events with obstacle courses throughout. While Tough Mudder runs are typically 10 to 12 miles (there is a 24-hour option), Spartan Races can vary from a sprint (4 to 5 miles with 20 to 25 obstacles) to an Ultra Beast (26 to 30 miles with 60 to 70 obstacles) (Amy Culp, RDN, CSSD, email communication, August 3, 2015).[24] The exact obstacles are not disclosed until the day of the race, though signature challenges are usually included (eg, barbed wire crawl, mud pit, rope climbs, live wires, and fire rings). Most obstacle course races are for-profit events (participants pay for their entry), and typically some amount of the profit is donated to charity. Though they attract athletes of varied backgrounds, most participants are young adults, and there appears to be a high level of participation among CrossFitters and individuals with military experience (Carol Lapin, MS, RD, LD, email communication, July 24, 2015). In Tough Mudder races, times are not recorded. Spartan Races, however, provide an elite racing division that has an annual scoring system culminating in a world championship race with prize money available (Amy Culp, RDB, CSSD, email communication, August 3, 2015). This division attracts former Olympic athletes and elite triathletes and runners.

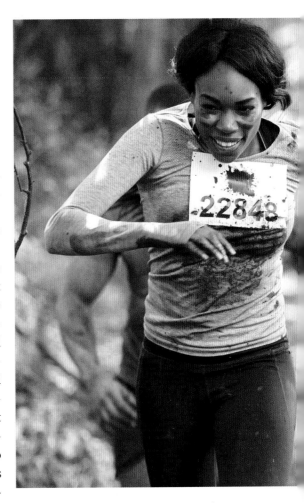

Basic Physiological Demands

Due to the varied nature of obstacle course races, racers do not fit neatly into one physiological category. Athletes are expected to quickly transition between sprinting, jumping, climbing, crawling, and lifting over the course of many miles through any number of terrain types (they usually involve some amount of mud). The physical demands of these events can be equated to that of a marathon or ultramarathon but with additional strength concerns (Carol Lapin, email communication, July 24, 2015, and Amy Culp, RDB, CSSD, August 3, 2015). These races primarily require endurance, but nutritional guidance should also consider recommendations for very high, short-duration as well as high-intensity, intermittent sports (see Chapters 20 and 21). For obstacle course races that require more time to complete than a typical marathon, refer to information on ultraendurance sports in Chapter 22. Since these events last multiple hours, the daily macronutrient guidelines for an endurance athlete, or ultraendurance athlete if competing in longer events, are recommended. One exception to this would be to consider increasing protein intake to a range of at least 1.4 to 1.7 g/kg body weight to match the guidelines for a strength athlete, particularly during difficult training.[25,26] As discussed in previous chapters, the timing of protein intake before and after exercise is an important consideration to promote training adaptations and to speed recovery.

Nutrition Issues

ENERGY AVAILABILITY AND HYDRATION

Carol Lapin is a past chair of the Sports, Cardiovascular, and Wellness Nutrition (SCAN) dietetic practice group of the Academy of Nutrition and Dietetics and a Tough Mudder finisher. In her experience, the race organizers were not able to tell her what sports drinks and food would be available on the course. Even when fluids are available, the unpredictable nature of these events can make adhering to a prescribed fueling regimen difficult. Consuming any sports foods on the course may also be impractical since participants want to avoid carrying bulky items that could get caught on obstacles or caked in mud (email communication, July 24, 2015, and October 9, 2015).[27]

Amy Culp, RDN, CSSD, is a sports dietitian at the University of Texas who consults with obstacle course racers, particularly Spartan racers (email communication, August 3, 2015). Most Spartan Races have water stations every 2 to 3 miles (most of these offer only water and no additional supplementation, such as sports drink or gels). Some races loop the same route multiple times, and participants may have access to a drop bin in which they can store supplies. However, if an athlete wants food or electrolytes on the course, they must carry them. For Ultra Beast distances, participants are required to carry a personal hydration system.

Postrace parties usually have plenty of alcohol available but may be lacking in foods optimal for recovery and rehydration (Carol Lapin, email communication, July 24, 2015).[27] Obstacle course racers need to expect the unexpected even more than when participating in traditional races. Fueling for these events is another part of the overall challenge and may give well-prepared athletes a distinct advantage.

BODY COMPOSITION

Since obstacle races are a unique blend of endurance and strength, athletes are constantly trying to achieve the ideal strength-to-weight ratio (Amy Culp, RDN, CSSD, email communication, August 3, 2015). Some climbing obstacles may require participants to carry an additional 18 to 23 kg for women and 35 to 45 kg for men. Culp has seen some participants struggle with disordered eating and eating disorders (EDs). Many obstacle racers are high-achieving perfectionists, which is a common phenotype of individuals with EDs.[28] RDNs working with this population should see that the energy needs of their clients are being met and be cognizant of symptoms of disordered eating patterns and body dysmorphia. For more detail, see Chapter 18.

Expert Nutrition Tips

- Participants need to do their homework and see if they will have access to a drop bin during the race and plan accordingly. They should always come to the race having eaten beforehand and prepared with their own postrace snacks—they should not assume that there will be anything available.[27]
- Depending on the race distance, participants may consider training with only water as a fluid replacement if it is known that no sports drinks or foods will be offered on the course. Lapin's race was during a hot and humid summer in Houston, Texas, and she credits her acclimatization to the

conditions as a significant contributor to her completing the race without experiencing heat illness (Carol Lapin, MS, RD, LD, email communication, July 24, 2015, and October 9, 2015).

- With the exception of the sprint distance, Culp emphasizes calorie replacement every 45 minutes, as well as frequent hydration and electrolyte replacement (Amy Culp, RDN, CSSD, email communication, August 3, 2015). The easiest foods to carry and consume while racing are gels. If drop bins are available along the course, easily digestible carbohydrates, such as bananas, sports drinks, gels, and lower-fiber energy bars, are good choices. Electrolyte tablets may also be recommended, depending on the sweat rate of the athlete, the climate, and other race foods and beverages. For longer Spartan Race distances such as Ultra Beasts, more substantial, energy-dense food options containing electrolytes are recommended, such as peanut butter and jelly sandwiches, trail mix, chicken noodle soup, or egg and cheese biscuit sandwiches. Before any competition, participants should practice with the foods they plan on consuming during the race. For specific guidelines, see Chapter 22.

How to Get Your Foot in the Door

Obstacle races are currently an untapped area for sports RDNs (Amy Culp, RDN, CSSD, email communication, August 3, 2015). Attending an obstacle race as a participant or observer is the best way to learn about the event and potentially make some client contacts. Since many participants also tend to be involved in CrossFit, have a military background, or were former collegiate athletes, tapping into those networks through a gym or social media is a good idea as well. Lapin highly recommends having the CSSD credential and experience working with both endurance and strength athletes (Carol Lapin, MS, RD, LD, email communication, July 24, 2015). Culp points out that there has never been a sport quite like obstacle course racing, so simply applying the same principles one would with a marathon runner is not enough (Culp, RDN, CSSD, email communication, August 3, 2015). Being well-versed in the types of obstacles, race lingo, and even the best types of clothes, shoes, and equipment are important for counseling and gaining credibility with clients.

MOTORSPORTS

Description

Box 23.3 provides an overview of the main motorsport categories.[29,30]

Basic Physiological Demands

The physiological demands of race care driving, based on oxygen consumption (VO_2) and heart rate, have been found to be similar to that of other sports, such as basketball and soccer.[31] In a study with seven professional, open-wheel drivers on both a roadway and an oval course, the average VO_2 and heart rate responses were approximately 79% and 82% of maximum, respectively. It is believed, in part, that the elevated heart rate observed in this population is due to emotional stress in addition to physical effort. Drivers can reach speeds of 322 km/h for roughly 3 to 4 hours at potentially high temperatures (~50°C).[32] It is important to note, however, that different styles of racing require different physical demands. Open-wheel racing on a non–oval-shaped course is particularly difficult because the drivers are constantly reacting to turns of varying degrees and high g-forces, whereas oval racing is more consistent.

Nutrition Issues

HYDRATION AND THERMOREGULATION

While all athletes should be concerned about proper hydration, this is especially true when operating a machine traveling at extremely high speeds—mental acuity is crucial. Motorsport athletes may compete for

Box 23.3 Basic Motorsport Categories and Racing Circuits[29,30]

Open wheel	A vehicle in this class has wheels that are outside of the car's main body, and it typically has a single-seat cockpit that encloses the driver's body leaving the head exposed to the air (includes Formula One and Indy).
Formula One	This class of open-wheel, closed-road course racing is the most glamorous and expensive class of motor racing and the most popular motorsport outside of the United States. Races are usually around 300 km and last less than 2 hours.
Indy Racing	This class of open-wheel, oval-track racing in the United States is organized by IndyCar. The Indianapolis 500 is the signature race.
Enclosed wheel	A vehicle in this class has wheels that are inside the car's main body (includes stock, touring cars, and sports cars).
NASCAR (National Association for Stock Car Auto Racing)	Vehicles are raced over an oval speedway track. The Sprint Cup series is the sport's highest level of competition and involves 36 points races that count in the overall season standings; races stretch over 10 months, February through November. The longest races are 500 miles and can last several hours.
Touring car	These vehicles are modified street cars that race over closed-road courses or street circuits. The cars are usually based on family cars (eg, hatchbacks) but are very similar to sports cars.
Stock car	In the traditional sense, this is a car that has not been modified from its original factory configuration, though the vehicles are now based on a shared custom design, for example NASCAR.
Sports car	This modified street car is raced over closed-road courses or street circuits. The cars are usually based on more powerful and expensive sports cars rather than touring cars.
Rally car racing	This form of racing takes place on roads (usually unpaved) with modified-production or specialty-built road-legal cars. Events can last several days and cover hundreds of miles. It is one of the most popular motorsports among amateurs. Unlike most other motorsports, there is a codriver.
Motocross	This is a form of off-road motorcycle racing that is held on enclosed, off-road loops.

several hours without a break, which makes it difficult to consume foods and fluids during competition. Depending on the type of car and race, some drivers may be able to drink water and sports drinks through hydration systems installed in the cars. Small amounts of solid foods may be consumed during a pit stop, which averages about 15 seconds, or if there is a red flag (eg, a race delay for a crash).[29,33] Such situations, however, are few and far between, so making sure that the driver is adequately fueled and hydrated before racing is crucial.

Not only is it very difficult for drivers to safely ingest fluids and food during the race but the fire-protective clothing they must wear can also significantly impede heat loss.[32] This cloth is capable of resisting temperatures up to 700°C, but it blocks ventilation to the surface of the skin. As the driver sweats, the clothing becomes soaked, and the transference of environmental heat to the driver's skin is increased, which exacerbates the problem.[34] Other environmental exposures are also of concern. In a study of eight elite motorsport athletes driving a simulator, the combined effect of carbon monoxide and heat exposure resulted in greater sweat loss and increased core temperature compared with exposure to heat alone.[35] The specific mechanism for this effect is unknown.

ENERGY AVAILABILITY AND BODY COMPOSITION

In a sport focused on speed, any extra weight is dead weight. This is especially true with the ultra-light sports cars used in Formula One racing.[36] Motorsport drivers want to optimize their strength, especially the upper body, while minimizing their overall weight. Achieving a low percent body fat is a common goal among this population (Laura Kruskall, PhD, RDN, CSSD, LD, FACSM, email communication, August 21, 2015). While some drivers may see the role that optimal fitness can play in improving their finishes, many have the eating habits and overall fitness of the general population. Danielle LaFata, MA, RDN, CSSD, is the director of performance nutrition for the Pro/Elite Division of EXOS, an athletic performance consulting company. She has worked with a wide range of elite athletes, including sports car, NASCAR, and rally car drivers. In her experience, most drivers do not understand how to put together a proper training regimen, including nutrition, to support their efforts on the track (email communication, October 5, 2015). Even if the motivation is there, the long season (10 months for NASCAR) and constant travel can make it difficult to develop a healthy and consistent diet. It is important to not only work with the individual driver to develop a realistic eating plan but also the crew managers who may coordinate the food choices available.

PIT CREWS

While motorsports are often considered individual events, they are, in many ways, team sports. A race car driver will not be successful without a strong pit crew. In recent years, there has been increased attention to the physical training of pit crews.[37] During a pit stop, the crew must refuel the vehicle, change tires, and make adjustments, all within approximately 15 seconds. In a sport where every second counts, the physical fitness of the pit crew is crucial to the team's success. In some cases, elite teams recruit former professional and collegiate athletes to be pit crew members. They train as high-intensity power athletes who must optimize strength and speed. There are no known studies published on the nutritional habits of this population, though descriptive data indicate that they tend to lose lean body mass in the off-season.[37] Pairing a strength program with nutritional strategies to optimize the development and maintenance of lean body tissue could have a significant impact on the success of the team.

Expert Nutrition Tips

- LaFata notes that what separates a good driver from a great driver is his or her ability to focus for a full race. Racing involves significant physical and mental stress. LaFata frames her nutrition recommendations in the context that optimal fuel will help decrease the negative effects experienced before and after racing: fatigue, decreased stamina and focus, impaired reaction time, and poor recovery. Drivers often feel fatigued for days after a race, so nutrition strategies that aid in recovery should be a primary focus for them (Danielle LaFata, MA, RDN, CSSD, email communication, October 5, 2015).
- Weighing the driver before and after racing is a good way to develop a pre- and postrace hydration plan. The drivers that LaFata has worked with may lose 1.4 to 2.7 kg in only a few hours. Dehydration is a sure and quick way to fatigue their muscles and brains. A hydrated driver is a more mentally aware driver (Danielle LaFata, MA, RDN, CSSD, email communication, October 5, 2015).
- A race car driver needs to have the mind-set of an elite athlete and work toward the fitness level of a professional. Even if race car drivers understand the need for peak physical conditioning, they may not eat like professional athletes. Drivers understand the importance of optimal fuel in their cars but also need reminding that the bodies run better on premium fuel (Danielle LaFata, MA, RDN, CSSD, email communication, October 5, 2015).

How to Get Your Foot in the Door

Among motorsport athletes, RDNs are a relatively untapped resource. Racing teams that work with an RDN often do so under the umbrella of other exercise professionals, such as certified strength and conditioning specialists, athletic trainers, and personal trainers. Having a background in these areas or building a network of professionals in exercise training is a definite plus. RDNs who want to break into this profession have to do their homework on the specific motorsport and be able to sell their services to a potentially skeptical audience. Partnering with other exercise professionals is an easier way to gain buy-in. Motorsport RDNs should be self-starters who are confident in their abilities and are authoritative and firm in their recommendations. Working with motorsport athletes is not for the timid.

DANCE

Basic Physiological Demands

Ballet, jazz, modern, tap, hip-hop, ballroom, folk—the types of dance are as varied as the individuals who participate. Similar to other figure sports (eg, gymnastics and figure skating), dance involves intermittent bursts of moderate-to-intense activity and predominantly utilizes the anaerobic system.[38] Among female professional dancers, dance intensity can reach greater than 11 metabolic equivalents (METs), though most of a dancer's day is spent around 3 METs.[39] Dancers are unusual among athletes in that even with a full day of rehearsal, they may only burn a few hundred calories per hour due to the stop-and-go nature of the activity. Their nutritional needs exceed that of the less-active, general population; however, their body type expectations and potential societal pressures may create barriers to meeting these needs (Rachel Fine, MS, RDN, CSSD, email communication, September 30, 2015). Refer to Chapter 21 for specific recommendations on nutrition for intermittent, high-intensity sports.

Nutrition Issues

ENERGY AVAILABILITY AND BODY COMPOSITION

A majority of the research literature on dance has focused on female ballet dancers, particularly because of concerns over low energy intake and body composition. Among the types of dance, ballet dancers tend to be the leanest and may have very low body fat percentages resulting in higher rates of amenorrhea among female dancers.[38,40] Contributing to this is that dancers tend to have low energy intake (70% to 80% of recommended) and high rates of EDs. Energy intake among dancers has been reported to be lower than matched controls, particularly among professional dancers.[40] In a study comparing 15 professional ballet dancers to nondancing control subjects matched by age, body mass index (BMI), and fat-free mass (FFM), the energy intake of the dancers was significantly less (1,577 ± 89 kcal/d vs 2,075 ± 163 kcal/d). In addition, they had significantly lower resting metabolic rates (RMRs) and bone mineral densities (BMDs). This supports work by Kaufman and colleagues, who observed a significant positive correlation between RMR/FFM and BMD in the arms and spines of dancers compared with those of control subjects. The lower RMRs/FFMs were predicted by dancers ever having amenorrhea.[41]

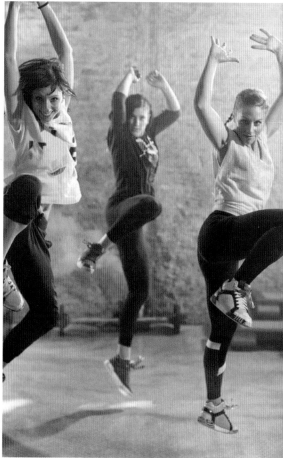

Several studies have been published over the past 50 years on the prevalence of EDs in this population. In a meta-analysis of 33 international studies published since 1966, the prevalence of EDs among dancers in general was 12% (range = 13.1% to 20.5%) and 16.4% (range = 1.9% to 26.6%) for ballet dancers.[42] Compared with nondancer control subjects, dancers had a three times higher risk of having an ED, particularly anorexia nervosa and eating disorders not otherwise specified. All included studies were of female dancers, and a majority of them were dance students rather than professionals. Though it was not statistically assessed in this analysis, a higher number of cases of EDs occured among students not attending elite ballet schools. Whether students in preprofessional programs are less likely to develop EDs or those with EDs are less likely to make it to the elite levels is unknown.

Wyon and colleagues assessed BMI and nutrition knowledge in student and professional ballet dancers and found that those dancers with disordered eating behaviors had lower levels of nutrition knowledge.[43] In addition, the student dancers had lower BMIs (possibly due to less muscle mass) and higher scores (high = concern) on a common ED screening tool (Eating Attitude Test-26 [EAT-26]). These results raise red flags, particularly among dance students, preprofessional and professional dancers should continue to be monitored closely. In studies of professional American ballet dancers, participants still had significantly higher EAT-26 scores than matched controls.[40,41] In one systematic review of disordered eating behaviors in dancers, the lifetime prevalence of EDs in professional dancers was 50%.[44] In a small (n = 15) group of professional ballet dancers, 40% met the criteria for the female athlete triad.[40] Among 31 collegiate modern dancers, the incidence of EDs was 12.9%.[45] Even if we use the more conservative estimates by Arcelus, Witcomb, and Mitchell, the rates of EDs in this population warrant vigilance among those who work with these athletes.[42] Fortunately, there has been increased awareness of this issue among professional dance companies and efforts to address EDs and healthy eating. In 2011, the Dance/USA Taskforce on Dancer Health issued a report to: (1) educate both dancers and staff on healthy nutrition; (2) prevent nutritional problems before they arise; and (3) recognize and manage nutritional disorders.[46]

Shannon Sterne, MS, MA, RDN, is a dancer, choreographer, and teacher at Case Western Reserve University who has counseled dancers at all levels, from recreational to professional. She has seen many types of disordered eating in this population, from fad diets to restrictive eating behaviors resulting in relative energy deficiency in sport. Among students in particular, Sterne has observed frequent meal skipping when they have back-to-back classes and rehearsals. Dancers usually do not like to have a full stomach before practices and performances due to tight clothing and demanding choreographies (email communication, July 29, 2015).[38] In addition, preperformance anxiety may have a negative impact on appetite, and performance days can be incredibly busy with the venues often lacking ideal options. It is therefore common for dancers to not eat within a couple of hours of a performance. While performances themselves are relatively short, the demanding schedule could make maintaining adequate energy levels difficult.

Like other athletes, dancers may follow a variety of diet trends. Deanna Busteed, MS, RD, CSSD, has had experience working with both high school and collegiate dancers and cheer teams. Due to concerns over weight gain and maintaining a lean physique, she has noticed that many of these athletes choose to follow vegetarian, high-protein/low-carb, or Paleo diets (email communication, July 15, 2015). Sterne also sees weight-loss supplement use among dancers who follow fad diets, as well as weight-gain supplements among mostly male dancers desiring to improve muscle mass (email communication, July 29, 2015).

Rachel Fine, MS, RDN, CSSD, is a dancer herself and works with dancers of all levels. She sees a great deal of variation in what dancers may eat, but one commonality among many of them is an obsession with healthy eating (email communication, September 30, 2015). See Chapter 18 for more on disordered eating and eating disorders.

INJURIES AND BONE HEALTH

Injuries have been studied more among ballet dancers than other types of dancers. In a study of 266 male and female preprofessional, full-time dance students, the risk of injury was 76% over a 1-year period.[47] The vast majority of the injuries (72%) was due to overuse and involved the joints and ligaments (46%), followed by muscle, tendon, and myofascia (30%), and then bone (19%). Bone injuries resulted in the greatest amount of time lost from full participation—an average of 177 days for tibial stress fractures. Along with low energy availability and menstrual disturbances among female dancers, dancers experienced a prevalence of low BMD and osteopenia ranging from 10% to 46.5%.[44] Some researchers, however, have observed higher or no different BMDs in dancers compared to non-dancer controls.[48-50] There is evidence, though, that dancers' BMDs are less than those of athletes involved in other weight-bearing sports and that the non-weight-bearing sites are particularly at risk.[49,51]

MICRONUTRIENT INTAKE

If dancers are not consuming adequate calories, they are at risk for various micronutrient deficiencies, with calcium, vitamin D, and iron being of particular concern. Adequate calcium intake is crucial for optimal bone health. In a study of 37 professional dance students, those who had the highest intakes of dietary calcium also had the highest BMD values.[48] Adolescents may be particularly at risk for low dietary calcium. Khan and colleagues found that retired professional dancers self-reported inadequate calcium intake during their adolescence.[49] Besides poor dietary intake, the lack of sun exposure among dancers also puts them at risk for vitamin D deficiency.[52] Wolman and colleagues studied 19 professional ballet dancers in the winter and found that all were either insufficient or deficient in serum 25(OH)D.[53] While Doyle-Lucas and colleagues did not observe differences in macro- or micronutrient intakes between elite female dancers and lean controls (only energy intake was lower), the mean reported intakes for calcium (851 mg), vitamin D (5 mcg), and iron (13 mg) were still lower than recommended, even for nonathletes.[40]

Expert Nutrition Tips

- While both Sterne (email communication, July 29, 2015) and Fine (email, communication September 30, 2015) take a "food first" approach, they frequently advise their clients to take a vitamin D or vitamin D plus calcium supplement due to the high risk of deficiency.[53] For those with restrictive diets, an iron-containing multivitamin/mineral may also be warranted.

- Among high-level dancers who tour, finding appropriate foods is another major concern. Sterne encourages her clients to pack meal-replacement bars for emergencies and scout out dining options in advance (email communications, July 29, 2015).

- It's important for an RDN to understand not only the physical demands of the sport but the psychological aspects as well. This can vary significantly depending on the level of the dancer and the genre. Sterne explains, "This art form is often very deeply intertwined with the dancer's ego and a drive for perfection. Sometimes dancing is more important than their health". She encourages clients to view their bodies as instruments that need enough fuel to function at their peak (email communication, July 29, 2015).

- Fine notes that RDNs who work with this population need to be both compassionate and realistic. The RDNs need compassion to understand the psychology behind aesthetic sports—it is very difficult to get dancers away from the ideal body image goal. And the RDNs need to be realistic and frank about the importance of maintaining a *healthy* weight to prevent malnutrition and injury. Her goal for clients is that they achieve a happy, nonrestrictive, and realistic lifestyle where dessert is an acceptable indulgence (email communication, September 30, 2015).

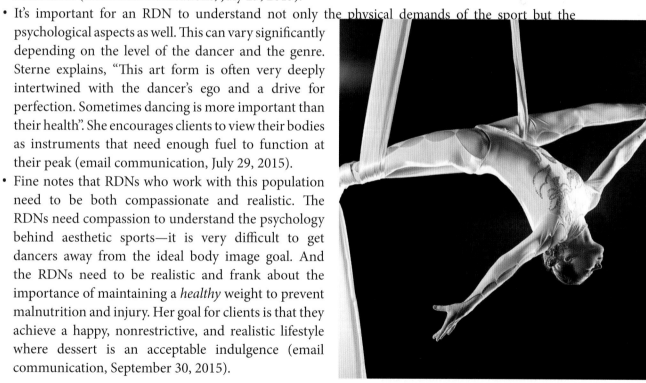

How to Get Your Foot in the Door

In Sterne's experience, most professional companies either cannot afford to have an RDN on staff or do not prioritize it (email communication, July 29, 2015). However, that does not mean that companies are not open to working with an RDN. In their 2011 report, Dance/USA recommended that professional dance companies have a nutrition specialist as part of the in-house team.[46] This person is encouraged to provide educational sessions to dancers and staff at least at the beginning of the season with periodic check-ins. Recommended seminar topics include: self-awareness and body image, eating disorders, cooking demonstrations and healthy food preparation, smoking cessation, stress management, and special interests to women (eg, amenorrhea). An RDN with a broad range of experience in health-related topics would have a definite advantage. Contacting a dance company and seeing how they are addressing these recommendations is a good place to start. Also, many dance schools will offer a 1-hour nutrition class during their summer intensive program (Shannon Sterne, email communication, July 29, 2015; Deanna Busteed, email communication, July 15, 2015). Sterne suggests that RDNs who want to work with dancers individually should contact dance schools and offer to teach a special weekend workshop for a given age group or topic (email communication, July 29, 2015). This is one way to generate interest in nutrition and establish rapport with the dancers and hopefully make them more willing to reach out for private counseling. Finally, networking with other health care professionals such as orthopedists, physical therapists, and ED therapists is a great way to attract future referrals and ensure a balanced treatment program for the client (Deanna Busteed, email communication, July 15, 2015).

MARCHING BAND

Description

Marching band includes any group of instrumentalists who perform for entertainment or competition.[54] Historically, the first organized marching bands were military bands. This style is characterized by marching in straight formations and can include specific field units such as drum and bugle corps and pipe bands. It is commonly seen in parades. Corps style bands differ from military bands in that the step sizes and formations are constantly changing and the music style can vary from marches to contemporary rock music. Corps style is probably the most intense and competitive category of marching band. Finally, show bands are focused on crowd entertainment, such as half-time shows at football games.[55] While the corps band season runs from May to August, high school and collegiate military and show bands perform at least through the fall football season and usually march in spring parades. In addition to the instrumentalists, corps and show bands typically have a color guard and dancers. A college marching band may have upward of 300 participants of all shapes, sizes, and levels of fitness.

Basic Physiological Demands

Classifying marching band in terms of its physiological demands can be tricky. When considering 12-hour rehearsal days as well as parade marching, it is an endurance activity. Erdmann and colleagues estimated the exercise intensity of adolescent marching band members in a lab setting as 4.5 to 6 METs. This is similar to recreational activities such as tennis, easy swimming, golfing, and mowing the lawn. Elite level drum corps members, however, are likely on par with intermittent, high-intensity sports.[55] Drum corps programs are 10 to 12 minutes, and a summer tour usually consists of 25 to 40 competitions.[56] It is worth noting the energy cost will vary widely depending on the instrument (eg, bass drum vs flute) and role (instrumentalist vs flag bearer) played. Performance anxiety has also been shown to contribute to elevated heart rates before and during a performance.[57] Finally, as with other outdoor sports, performers will be exposed to all types of weather from sweltering heat and humidity to wind, rain, and snow (Melissa Church, MS, RDN, email communication, September 3, 2015). Refer to Chapters 21 and 22 for more information on the energy demands for intermittent and endurance sports.

Nutrition Issues

BODY COMPOSITION AND CHRONIC DISEASE RISK

Marching band members vary considerably in their fitness levels and overall health. In a study on the association between diet and cardiovascular disease (CVD) risk factors among 232 university marching band, dance team, and cheer squad members (n = 225 for band members), 45% were classified as overweight or obese (BMI ≥ 25 kg/m²) and 30% of women and 4.3% of men had high waist-to-hip ratios.[58] In a more recent national survey of college students, the prevalence of overweight and obesity was estimated to be approximately 40%, indicating that university marching band members are not necessarily in any better physical condition than the average college student.[59] Risk for CVD and other chronic conditions among this population is also a concern because 7.8% of participants had high blood glucose (>110 mg/dL), 10.3% had high total blood cholesterol (>200 mg/dL), and 14.7% had high systolic blood pressure (>140 mm Hg).[58] These values are lower than those reported in another study on the general college population using the National Heart, Lung, and Blood Institute (NHLBI) guidelines for metabolic syndrome diagnosis, though the NHLBI guidelines are more stringent.[60,61] Depending on the criteria used, this could mean that the risk for cardiovascular or metabolic diseases among university marching band members may be underestimated.[58]

It is important to note that drum and bugle corps members appear to have lower BMIs compared to members of other forms of marching band, which is likely due to the higher intensity of the sport. In a longitudinal study of Drum Corps International world-class performers (n = 501), 37% had BMIs that would classify them as overweight or obese.[56] By the end of the competitive season (3 months later), only 23% were classified as overweight or obese. After a 1-year follow-up, however, participants' BMIs had returned to their initial levels.

DIETARY PATTERNS AND HYDRATION

To date, there has been one study published on the dietary habits of marching band members.[58] From a self-administered survey based on the 2000 Dietary Guidelines for Americans, 85% of participants consumed fewer than five fruits and vegetables per day. Both higher grain (includes non–whole grains) and alcohol intake were positively associated with higher BMI. No data has been collected on the total energy

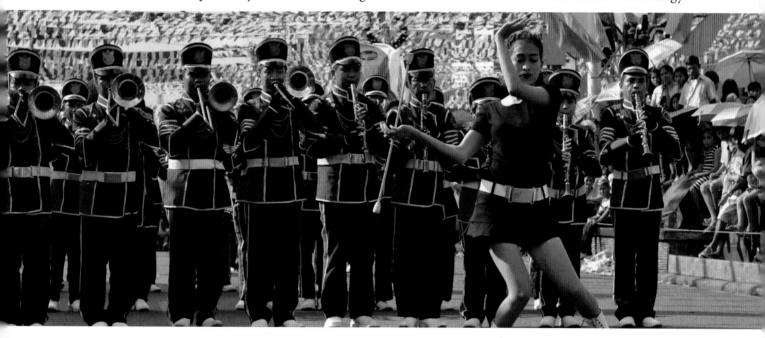

intake of this population and how it aligns with total energy expenditure. Among high school band programs, parents and booster clubs often provide meals during long competition days or band members tend to eat from stadium concession stands (Melissa Church, email communication, September 3, 2015). When meals are provided, choices may be limited and difficult for participants who have specialized dietary needs or requests (eg, gluten-free or vegetarian).

Marching band members are at a particular risk for fluid imbalance, especially during early season training camps where they may spend all day outside.[55,58,62] Sharma and colleagues found that less than 30% of marching band members consumed eight glasses of water per day.[58] In a noncontrolled assessment of hydration management among high school marching band students, barriers to adequate fluid intake included the logistical difficulties of taking the time to break formation, participants not wanting to call attention to themselves if they are having a problem, and the lack of training in health-related issues of most music directors.[62]

Expert Nutrition Tips

- Melissa Church, MS, RDN, has worked with high school marching band members and cites consuming adequate energy and fluids as primary concerns among this group. Besides getting band directors on board, she sees parents and booster club members as potential allies. As with any large group, there will be a wide range of food preferences and special dietary needs. Some parents and boosters are less nutrition savvy than others, so there is a role for the RDN in educating and giving guidance to these supporters. RDNs can provide suggestions on ideal prerehearsal snacks, meal options for special diets, and eating on the road (email communication, September 3, 2015).

- Most bands require participants to bring water bottles during rehearsals, though it is important that time is set aside for water breaks (Melissa Church, email communication, September 3, 2015). In her work with high school marching band members, Vepraskas found that providing them with fuel belts to hold their water bottles was an easy way to provide fluids without interrupting rehearsals.[62] Subjective feedback from these students included improved mental acuity, more productive rehearsals, feeling better overall, and fewer episodes of heat-related stress.

How to Get Your Foot in the Door

The literature on the health of marching band members is sparse, but there is an increasing awareness on the importance of their overall health. The National Association of Schools of Music, which is the national accrediting agency for music and music-related disciplines, requires that music program policies, protocols, and operations reflect attention to health and injury prevention among musicians.[63] RDNs can use this accreditation requirement as a way to market their skill set. For most marching band directors outside of the collegiate realm, proper fueling likely is not even on their radars. While they are often receptive to nutritional guidance and resources, they usually need to have its importance explained to them. This takes time and effort on the part of the RDN to work with band directors, parents, and boosters. Church was fortunate to have an inside connection because her husband is a band director. However, it was not until she attended a session on *Athletes in the Arts* at the Food and Nutrition Conference and Expo that she was motivated to become more involved with this population. Church sees networking with other SCAN RDNs and band directors as a key to successfully getting one's name out there. Introduce yourself to area directors and offer to do a short presentation at band camp or at a parent/booster meeting. To work with marching bands, RDNs have to go where the action is (email communication, September 3, 2015).

OTHER PERFORMING ARTISTS

Actors and vocalists are another relatively untapped group in the field of sports nutrition. Andrea Chernus, MS, RDN, CSSD, has worked with many Broadway actors, dancers, and vocalists in her private practice in New York City. She notes that "appearance is a big issue, so looking healthy—glowing skin, shiny hair, a fit and trim body—these are all concerns for this group." In addition, singers and stage actors have to pay particular attention to remaining well hydrated and protecting their vocal cords by avoiding foods and beverages that can aggravate reflux. Some clients may be incredibly fit or need to achieve a particular body type in a relatively short time, while others may be quite sedentary. They also tend to be on tight budgets and have chaotic schedules that can make meal planning difficult. Chernus recommends that RDNs interested in working with this population be open-minded, good listeners, and ideally have some training in EDs. Contacting the people who provide the training for these artists (eg, theater schools and companies, vocal coaches, and dance studios) is a great place to start. In particular, consulting with youth programs is a good way to educate future artists before poor eating habits become ingrained (email communication, July 15, 2015).

Description

First responders (firefighters, police officers, and paramedics) are in professions that, for the most part, can be quite sedentary. However, they need to be able to perform vigorous activity and lift heavy loads at a moment's notice. Of this category, firefighters typically undergo the highest levels of physical stress due to their heavy equipment (at least 20 additional kgs), heat exposure, and potentially long hours on a call.[64] Wildland firefighters in particular must not only be strong but also have a solid endurance base to handle multiple days on duty. Contrast this with a police officer or paramedic who may spend almost the entire day in a vehicle; the nutritional needs of these individuals are extremely different.

Basic Physiological Demands

Except for special cases like wildland firefighting and extended fire calls, the physiological demands for most first responders would be classified has very high-intensity and high-intensity, short-duration activities. Donovan and colleagues estimates that firefighting may require up to 12 METs, making it a very intense activity.[65] Refer to Chapters 20 and 21 for a more thorough overview of the physiological considerations for these types of activities.

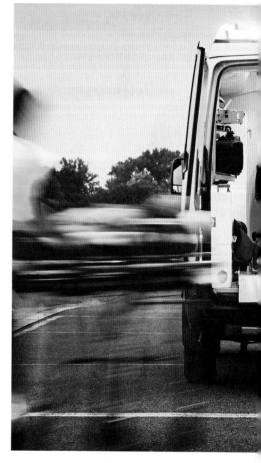

Nutrition Issues

ENERGY AVAILABILITY AND WEIGHT MANAGEMENT

The leading cause of on-duty death among firefighters is sudden cardiac death.[66,67] While some of this may be attributed to congenital abnormalities, poor physical health—especially overweight and obesity—is a major risk factor. Poston and colleagues found higher rates of obesity (average BMI > 28 kg/m²) in a group of 677 career and volunteer firefighters compared to the general population, even when controlling for percent body fat.[68] This indicates that their high BMIs were not likely due to greater amounts of lean tissue. Hartley and colleagues found that 40.5% of police officers in Buffalo, New York, were obese, and 26.7% had metabolic syndrome.[69] Conversely, some first responders are high-level athletes who frequently participate in marathons and obstacle races. The nutrition needs of this population can therefore vary widely and should be handled case by case.

The few published studies on the dietary practices of first responders have involved weight loss and healthy-living interventions.[70-72] Elliot and colleagues found baseline levels of daily fruit and vegetable consumption among 599 male firefighters in the Portland, Oregon, metro area was actually quite high at approximately 5.5 servings.[71] Anecdotal evidence, however, suggests that this may not be representative of most first responders and likely varies based on geography and the culture of the department.

Derek Hughes, MS, RDN, wellness coordinator for the Broward Sheriff's Office in Ft Lauderdale, Florida, works with over 5,400 employees in law enforcement, detention, and fire and rescue services. He identifies the main nutritional issues as poor daily feeding habits for general health and weight management. In his experience, many first responders consume diets high in starches, added sugars, processed foods, and sugar-sweetened beverages. Some emerging diet trends that Hughes has seen, particularly among firefighters and police officers, are Paleo-style diets, fruit and vegetable smoothies, and use of supplements such as protein powders, vitamin D, and fish oil. Access to healthy options may be limited (email communication, July 30, 2015). Firefighters are at the mercy of what is prepared at the firehouse, and police and corrections officers may only have access to vending machines and possibly a microwave during their 8-hour-plus shifts. Paramedics literally eat on the road and often have no kitchen equipment available (Jennifer O'Donnell-Giles, MS, RDN, CSSD, email communication, July 24, 2015). This unpredictability creates many barriers to healthy eating.

Another nutritional concern is how to effectively fuel firefighters during large structural fires and tactical units during long call-outs. Meals may be interrupted, and the first responder may go long periods without food or fluids. When they finally do have a break, they may be more prone to make poor food choices and binge eat. The nature of their jobs can make calorie distribution throughout the day very imbalanced (Derek Hughes, email communication, July 30, 2015). In a randomized, prospective 12-week diet study of 38 overweight police officers, Demling and DeSanti observed that 70% of officers consumed over 50% of total daily calories just before bed and only 10% as the first meal of the day.[70] Jennifer O'Donnell-Giles, MS, RDN, CSSD, who has worked with firefighters through her private practice has noticed similar trends (email communication, July 24, 2015). Her clients frequently skip breakfast, grab something quick like a sandwich for lunch, and then have a very large, often carb-heavy dinner.

HYDRATION

Hydration is obviously a major concern for firefighters, though other first responders are frequently exposed to extreme temperatures and elevated heat indexes as well. Research is limited on the hydra-

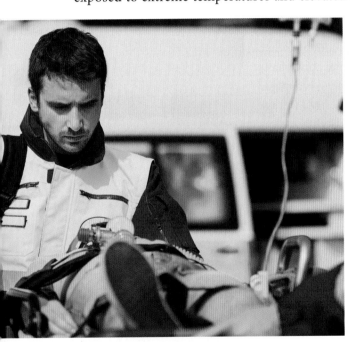

tion statuses of individuals in these professions, with most studies focused on firefighters. The protective clothing they wear restricts evaporative heat loss, and this, along with increased skin perfusion in response to thermal strain, significantly taxes the cardiovascular system.[73] Among wildland firefighters, Raines and colleagues observed that most individuals reported to work hypohydrated though they were able to reach euhydration by ad lib fluid consumption during their shifts.[74-76] This does not mean that firefighters can just rely on their thirst mechanisms alone. There are cases of firefighters experiencing heat exhaustion despite aggressive fluid intake.[77]

UNIQUE CONCERNS

Overall, alcohol consumption seems to be quite high in this population, potentially due to the stress of the job. Intake of caffeine-containing products, particularly with shift-work, also appears high (Derek Hughes, email communication, July 30, 2015). It has been widely documented that shift work may have many negative impacts on overall health, such as increased risk of overweight and obesity, CVD, and type 2 diabetes to name a few.[78-81] Shift work has been associated with poor eating habits and higher rates of inflammation.[82-84] The high stress nature of these jobs may also negatively affect mental and emotional health. The rate of depression in one cohort of police officers was double that of the general population (12%), and 33% of officers reported sleeping fewer than 6 hours per night on average.[69] The prevalence of posttraumatic stress disorder in emergency workers is estimated to be 20% compared to 5% of the general population.[85] The chronic stress, shift work, and exposure to environmental toxins may contribute to the numerous chronic health conditions that have been observed in this population.[78]

- Encourage first responders to have an assortment of healthy, satiating snacks such as trail mix with nuts and dried fruit readily available to eat during their inconsistent shifts. The more convenient and easy to grab-and-go, the better.
- To cut back on the amount of starches and refined grains consumed, Hughes encourages simple swaps such as spaghetti squash, quinoa, and bean-based dishes (email communication, July 30, 2015). He also emphasizes the appropriate portions for body size and energy output.
- Because the nature of the job is not likely to change, Jennifer O'Donnell-Giles, MS, RDN, CSSD, says it is important to work with clients to design plans that fit their lifestyles and value systems (email communication, July 24, 2015). If they eat out a lot, help them make good choices at the restaurants and delis they frequent.
- Hughes notes that first responders frequently deal with gruesome and intense situations, and many may use humor to cope. Important personality traits for an RDN would be a good sense of humor and a flexible, but determined nature. First responders appreciate straight-forwardness rather than dancing around the truth. This does not mean, however, that they want to be all business all the time (email communication, July 30, 2015). O'Donnell-Giles recommends making your sessions fun by coming up with easy and attainable challenges for them (email communication, July 24, 2015). They are hard-working people who often have a competitive streak, which can work to your advantage if you tap into it.

How to Get Your Foot in the Door

Because most emergency service organizations have limited budgets for wellness, having a versatile skill set that includes a range of services that overlap with health and fitness is a big plus. Hughes got his start with his current employer as a fitness specialist, which then grew to include nutrition while he was in graduate school. His positions originated with federal grants that morphed into permanent positions when strong outcomes and employee satisfaction justified the work (email communication, July 30, 2015). O'Donnell-Giles had a similar experience. She worked with firefighters as part of a state grant that included nutrition counseling and personal training (email communication, July 24, 2015). Working with police and fire departments to apply for grant funding is one way to potentially secure a long-term position. RDNs can penetrate this arena by offering to provide educational presentations for staff, speaking at roll-call meetings, or getting involved with wellness fairs at various government agencies (Derek Hughes, email communication, July 30, 2015). Finally, several gyms and online fitness and training programs now cater to first responders. Find out what is available in your area and online, and don't be afraid to pitch your expertise to these companies.

See Box 23.4 for a list of helpful resources covering a range of topics and emerging opportunities in sports nutrition.

CrossFit

- CrossFit: www.crossfit.com
- CrossFit Journal: http://journal.crossfit.com
- The Paleo Diet: http://thepaleodiet.com

Obstacle Course Races

- Mud Run Guide: www.mudrunguide.com
- Obstacle Racing Media: http://obstacleracingmedia.com
- Spartan Race: www.spartan.com/en
- Tough Mudder: https://toughmudder.com

Motorsports

- Federation Internationale De L'Automobile: www.fia.com

Dance

- Stack Nutrition: www.stack.com/c/nutrition-2Dance
- American College Dance Association: www.acda.dance
- Athletes and the Arts: http://athletesandthearts.com
- Dance/USA Task Force on Dancer Health: www.danceusa.org/dancerhealth
- International Association for Dance Medicine and Science: www.iadms.org
- The Centre for Dance Nutrition: www.dancernutrition.com
- USA Dance: http://usadance.org/

Marching Band

- Athletes and the Arts: http://athletesandthearts.com/
- College Band Directors National Association: www.cbdna.org
- Drum Corps International: www.dci.org
- National Association of Music Parents: www.amparents.org/
- National Association of Schools of Music: http://nasm.arts-accredit.org
- World Association of Marching Show Bands: www.wamsb.org

First Responders

- American Heart Association Workplace Health Solutions: www.heart.org/HEARTORG/GettingHealthy/WorkplaceWellness/Workplace-Wellness_UCM_460416_SubHomePage.jsp
- FireRescue 1 Health and Wellness: www.firerescue1.com/health
- Harvard School of Public Health, SafeWell: http://centerforworkhealth.sph.harvard.edu/projects/safewell
- National Volunteer Fire Council Heart Healthy Firefighter Program: www.healthy-firefighter.org/

The traditional sports that we most often associate with sports nutrition comprise a small percentage of the opportunities available. This chapter has not covered all the opportunities that exist.

Any individual or group involved in regular, organized physical activity could benefit from the expertise of a sports dietitian.

While RDNs clearly see the impact that they can make with these groups, it will take some convincing of these athletes, coaches, and organizing bodies, as well as collaborations with other health and fitness professionals who are already established in each field. The research literature on these emerging sports, as it relates to nutrition, is sparse. To make a case, RDNs should begin to collect data and ensure that guidelines are evidence-based.

Self-motivated, curious, and entrepreneurial RDNs have much to offer and gain from working with these emerging sports.

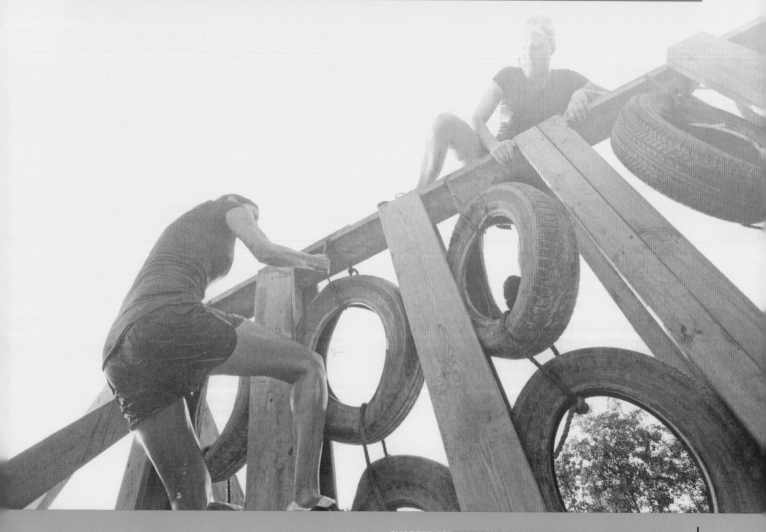

1. Origins of CrossFit. The Box website. www.theboxmag.com/article/origins-of-crossfit-9629. Published October 2012. Accessed July 16, 2015.

2. Glassman G. Understanding CrossFit. *CrossFit J.* 2007;56:1-2.

3. CrossFit, Inc website. www.crossfit.com. Accessed July 16, 2015.

4. CrossFit Kids website. https://kids.crossfit.com. Accessed July 20, 2015.

5. CrossFit reflex. http://crossfitreflex.com/getting-started/crossfit-dictionary. CrossFit Dictionary website. Accessed September 2, 2015.

6. The Zone Diet. Zone website. www.zonediet.com/the-zone-diet/. Accessed July 28, 2015.

7. Cheuvront S. The Zone Diet and athletic performance. *Sports Med.* 1999;27(4):213-228.

8. The Paleo Diet website. http://thepaleodiet.com. Accessed July 20, 2015.

9. Cordain L, Friel J. *The Paleo Diet for Athletes.* 2nd ed. New York, NY: Rodale Books; 2012.

10. Hertzler S. The Paleo Diet: Stone Age nutrition for today's athlete? *SCAN Pulse.* 2014;33(4):11-17.

11. Burke L, Hawley J, Wong S, Jeukendrup A. Carbohydrates for training and competition. *J Sports Sci.* 2011;29(suppl 1):17S-27S.

12. Widmer R, Flammer A, Lerman L, Lerman A. The Mediterranean diet, its components, and cardiovascular disease. *Am J Med.* 2015;128(3):229-238.

13. Chiva-Blanch G, Badimon L, Estruch R. Latest evidence of the effects of the Mediterranean diet in prevention of cardiovascular disease. *Curr Atheroscler Rep.* 2014;16(10):446.

14. Craig W, Mangels A. Position of the American Dietetic Association: vegetarian diets. *J Am Diet Assoc.* 2009;109(7):1266-1282.

15. Slavin J. Position of the American Dietetic Association: health implications of dietary fiber. *J Am Diet Assoc.* 2008;108(10):1716-1731.

16. Poupin N, Calvez J, Lassale C, Chesneau C, Tomé D. Impact of the diet on net endogenous acid production and acid-base balance. *Clin Nutr.* 2012;31(3):313-321.

17. Fenton T, Tough S, Lyon A, Eliasziw M, Hanley D. Causal assessment of dietary acid load and bone disease: a systematic review & meta-analysis applying Hill's epidemiologic criteria for causality. *Nutr J.* 2011;10:41.

18. Metzgar M, Rideout T, Fontes-Villalba M, Kuipers R. The feasibility of a Paleolithic diet for low-income consumers. *Nutr Res.* 2011;31(6):444-451.

19. Mellberg C, Sandberg S, Lindahl B, et al. Long-term effects of a Palaeolithic-type diet in obese postmenopausal women: a 2-year randomized trial. *Eur J Clin Nutr.* 2014;68(3):350-357.

20. Wildman R. Clean supplementation. THe Box website. www.theboxmag.com/article/clean-supplementation-9462. Published October 22, 2012. Accessed September 5, 2015.

21. Catris M. CrossFitters: the 3 letters you need to know in supplements. Breaking Muscle website. http://breakingmuscle.com/supplements/crossfitters-the-3-letters-you-need-to-know-in-supplements. Accessed September 5, 2015.

22. Ferguson A. What are the best CrossFit supplements and do you need them? Think Healthiness website. www.thinkhealthiness.com/best-crossfit-supplements. Published January 26, 2015. Accessed September 5, 2015.

23. 2014 State of the sport—part I: non-traditional running events. Running USA website. www.runningusa.org/non-traditional-running-events-special-report. Published April 27, 2014. Accessed July 28, 2015.

24. Spartan Race website. www.spartan.com. Accessed July 28, 2015.

25. Rodriguez N, DiMarco N, Langley S. Position of the American Dietetic Association, Dietitians of Canada, and the American College of Sports Medicine: nutrition and athletic performance. *J Am Diet Assoc.* 2009;109:509-527.

26. Ranchordas M. Nutrition for adventure racing. *Sports Med.* 2012;42(11):915-927.

27. Lapin C. Tough Mudder finisher … over 50 Mudders welcomed! CSL Nutritional Services website. 2013. http://cslnutritionalservices.com/2013/10/tough-mudder-finisher-over-50-mudders-welcomed/. Accessed July 24, 2015.

28. Halmi K, Sunday S, Kaye W, et al. Perfectionism in anorexia nervosa: variation by clinical subtype, obsessionality, and pathological eating behavior. *Am J Psychiatry.* 2000;157(11):1799-1805.

29. Gifford C. *Racing: The Ultimate Motorsport Encyclopedia.* Boston, MA: Kingfisher Publications; 2006.

30. What is rally? Rally America website. www.rally-america.com/what_is_rally. Accessed August 22, 2015.

31. Jacobs P, Olvey S, Johnson B, Cohn K. Physiological responses to high-speed, open-wheel racecar driving. *Med Sci Sports Exerc.* 2002;34(12):2085-2090.

32. Carlson L, Ferguson D, Kenefick R. Physiological strain of stock car drivers during competitive racing. *J Thermal Biol.* 2014;44:20-26.

33. Ganguli T. Race car drivers eating during a race gives new meaning to fast food. *Orlando Sentinel.* May, 22, 2009. http://articles.orlandosentinel.com/2009-05-22/sports/ganguli_1_race-eat-snack. Accessed August 27, 2015.

34. Rodrigues L, Magalhaes F. Car racing: in the heat of competition. *Rev Bras Med Esporte.* 2004;10(3):212-215.

35. Walker S, Ackland T, Dawson B. The combined effect of heat and carbon monoxide on the performance of motorsport athletes. *Comp Biochem Physiol A.* 2001;128(4):709-718.

36. Snape J. Built for speed. *Men's Fitness.* www.mensfitnessmagazine.com.au/2012/08/built-for-speed-2. Published 2012. Accessed August 29, 2015.

37. Ferguson D, Davis A, Lightfoot J. Optimizing the physical conditioning of the NASCAR Sprint Cup pit crew athlete. *J Strength Cond Res.* 2015;29(3):567-577.

38. Sousa M, Carvalho P, Moreira P, Teixeira V. Nutrition and nutritional issues for dancers. *Med Probl Perform Art.* 2013;28(3):119-123.

39. Twitchett E, Angioi M, Koutedakis Y, Wyon M. The demands of a working day among female professional ballet dancers. *J Dance Med Sci.* 2010;14(4):127-132.

40. Doyle-Lucas A, Akers J, Davy B. Energetic efficiency, menstrual irregularity, and bone mineral density in elite professional female ballet dancers. *J Dance Med Sci.* 2010;14(4):146-154.

41. Kaufman B, Warren M, Dominguez J, Wang J, Heymsfield S, Pierson R. Bone density and amenorrhea in ballet dancers are related to a decreased resting metabolic rate and lower leptin levels. *J Clin Endocrinal Metab.* 2002;87(6):2777-2783.

42. Arcelus J, Witcomb G, Mitchell A. Prevalence of eating disorders amongst dancers: a systemic review and meta-analysis. *Eur Eat Disorder Rev.* 2014;22(2):92-101.

43. Wyon M, Hutchings K, Wells A, Nevill A. Body mass index, nutritional knowledge, and eating behaviors in elite student and professional ballet dancers. *Clin J Sport Med.* 2014;24(5):390-396.

44. Hincapié C, Cassidy J. Disordered eating, menstrual disturbances, and low bone mineral density in dancers: a systematic review. *Arch Phys Med Rehabil.* 2010;91(11):1777-1789.

45. Friesen K, Rozenek R, Clippinger K, Gunter K, Russo A, Sklar S. Bone mineral density and body composition of collegiate modern dancers. *J Dance Med Sci.* 2011;15(1):31-36.

46. Gibbs R. Guidelines for professional dance companies on healthy nutrition. *Dance/USA Taskforce on Dancer Health.* www.danceuk.org/media/cms_page_media/204/2-2011GuidelinesforProfessionalDanceCompaniesonHealthyNutritiondocfinal1.pdf. Published 2011. Accessed September 7, 2015.

47. Ekegren C, Quested R, Brodrick A. Injuries in pre-professional ballet dancers: incidence, characteristics and consequences. *J Sci Med Sport.* 2014;17(3):271-275.

48. Yannakoulia M, Keramopoulos A, Matalas A. Bone mineral density in young active females: the case of dancers. *Int J Sport Nutr Exerc Metab.* 2004;14(3):285-297.

49. Khan K, Green R, Wark J, et al. Retired elite female ballet dancers and nonathletic controls have similar bone mineral density at weightbearing sites. *J Bone Miner Res.* 1996;11(10):1566-1574.

50. Karlsson M, Johnell O, Obrant K. Bone mineral density in professional ballet dancers. *Bone Miner.* 1993;21(3):163-169.

51. Quintas M, Ortega R, López-Sobaler A, Garrido G, Requejo A. Influence of dietetic and anthropometric factors and of the type of sport practised on bone density in different groups of women. *Eur J Clin Nutr.* 2003;57(suppl 1):58S-62S.

52. Constantini N, Arieli R, Chodick G, Dubnov-Raz G. High prevalence of vitamin D insufficiency in athletes and dancers. *Clin J Sport Med.* 2010;20(5):368-371.

53. Wolman R, Wyon M, Koutedakis Y, Nevill A, Eastell R, Allen N. Vitamin D status in professional ballet dancers: winter vs. summer. *J Sci Med Sport.* 2013;16(5):388-391.

54. Left foot is always first. Marcing Band website. http://mickaelab-marchingbandphysics.weebly.com/marching3.html. Accessed January 3, 2016.

55. Pape L. More than just marching band: musical athletes redefine 'sport.' *Austin Fit Magazine.* www.austinfitmagazine.com/October-2014/More-Than-Just-Marching-Band. Published October 7, 2014. Accessed September 3, 2015.

56. Levy J, Statham W, VanDoren L. BMI changes among marching artists: a longitudinal study. *Med Prol Perform Art.* 2013;28(4):236-241.

57. Jin Y, Obert M, Siivola C, LeBlanc A. Effect of audience on music performance anxiety. *J Res Music Ed.* 1997;45(3):480-496.

58. Sharma S, Bush J, Bertman D, et al. Diet and cardiovascular risk in university marching band, dance team and cheer squad members: a cross-sectional study. *J Int Soc Sport Nutr.* 2008;5:9.

59. American College Health Association. National College Health Assessment II: Spring 2014 Reference Group Executive Summary. www.acha-ncha.org/docs/ACHA-NCHA-II_ReferenceGroup_ExecutiveSummary_Spring2014.pdf. Published 2014. Accessed August 31, 2015.

60. Morrell J, Lofgren I, Burke J, Reilly R. Metabolic syndrome, obesity, and related risk factors among college men and women. *J Am Coll Health.* 2012;60(1):82-89.

61. National Heart, Lung, and Blood Institute, National Institute of Health. How is metabolic syndrome diagnosed? Available from: www.nhlbi.nih.gov/health/health-topics/topics/ms/diagnosis. Published November 2011. Accessed September 1, 2015.

62. Vepraskas C. Beat the heat: managing heat and hydration in marching band. *J Sch Nurs.* 2002;18(4):237-243.

63. *National Association of Schools of Music Handbook 2014-15.* Reston, VA: National Association of Schools of Music; 2014.

64. Lyon J. Adding up a firefighter's gear. *CDAPress. com.* www.cdapress.com/lifestyles/article_128f858b-792a-5ae1-b574-e5a47e3b39b7.html. Published December 26, 2010. Accessed July 30, 2015.

65. Donovan R, Nelson T, Peel J, Lipsey T, Voyles W, Israel R. Cardiorespiratory fitness and the metabolic syndrome in firefighters. *Occup Med.* 2009;59(7):487-492.

66. Kales S, Soteriades E, Christophi C, Christiani D. Emergency duties and deaths from heart disease among firefighters in the United States. *New Engl J Med.* 2007;356(12):1207-1215.

67. Yang J, Teehan D, Farioli A, Baur D, Smith D, Kales S. Sudden cardiac death among firefighters ≤45 years of age in the United States. *Am J Cardiol.* 2013;112(12):1962-1967.

68. Poston W, Haddock C, Jahnke S, Jitnarin N, Tuley B, Kales S. The prevalence of overweight, obesity, and substandard fitness in a population-based firefighter cohort. *J Occup Environ Med.* 2011;53(3):266-273.

69. Hartley T, Burchfiel C, Fekedulegn D, Andrew M, Knox S, Violanti J. Associations between police officer stress and the metabolic syndrome. *Int J Emerg Ment Health.* 2011;13(4):243-256.

70. Demling R, DeSanti L. Effect of a hypocaloric diet, increased protein intake and resistance training on lean mass gains and fat mass loss in overweight police officers. *Ann Nutr Metab.* 2000;44(1):21-29.

71. Elliot D, Goldberg L, Kuehl K, Moe E, Breger R, Pickering M. The PHLAME (Promoting Healthy Lifestyles: Alternative Models' Effects) firefighter study: outcomes of two models of behavior change. *J Occup Environ Med.* 2007;49(2):204-213.

72. Macdonald A, Rossiter M, Jensen J. Nutrition and shiftwork: evaluation of new paramedics' knowledge and attitudes. *Can J Diet Pract Res.* 2013;74(4):198-201.

73. McLellan T, Selkirk G. The management of heat stress for the firefighter: a review of work conducted on behalf of the Toronto Fire Service. *Ind Health.* 2006;44(3):414-426.

74. Raines J, Snow R, Petersen A, Harvey J, Nichols D, Aisbett B. Pre-shift fluid intake: effect on physiology, work and drinking during emergency wildfire fighting. *Appl Ergon.* 2012;43(3):532-540.

75. Raines J, Snow R, Petersen A, Harvey J, Nichols D, Aisbett B. The effect of prescribed fluid consumption on physiology and work behavior of wildfire fighters. *Appl Ergon.* 2013;44(3):404-413.

76. Raines J, Snow R, Nichols D, Aisbett B. Fluid intake, hydration, work physiology of wildfire fighters working in the heat over consecutive days. *Ann Occup Hyg.* 2015;59(5):554-565 .

77. Cuddy J, Ruby B. High work output combined with high ambient temperatures caused heat exhaustion in a wildland firefighter despite high fluid intake. *Wilderness Environ Med.* 2011;22(2):122-125.

78. Krajnak K. Potential contribution of work-related psychosocial stress to the development of cardiovascular disease and type II diabetes: a brief review. *Environ Health Insights.* 2014;8(suppl 1):41-45.

79. Fekedulegn D, Burchfiel C, Violanti J, et al. Shiftwork and sickness absence among police officers: the BCOPS study. *Chronobiol Int.* 2013;30(7):930-941.

80. Gu F, Han J, Schernhammer E, et al. Total and cause-specific mortality of U.S. nurses working rotating night shifts. *Am J Prev Med.* 2015;48(3):241-252.

81. Ramin C, Devore E, Wang W, Pierre-Paul J, Wegrzyn L, Schernhammer E. Night shift work at specific age ranges and chronic disease risk factors. *Occup Environ Med.* 2015;72(2):100-107.

82. Lowden A, Moreno C, Holmbäck U, Lennernäs M, Tucker P. Eating and shift work - effects on habits, metabolism and performance. *Scan J Work Environ Health.* 2010;36(2):150-162.

83. Hemiö K, Puttonen S, Viitasalo K, Härmä M, Peltonen M, Lindström J. Food and nutrient intake among workers with different shift systems. *Occup Environ Med.* 2015;72(7):513-520.

84. Puttonen S, Viitasalo K, Härmä M. Effect of shiftwork on systemic markers of inflammation. *Chronobiol Int.* 2011;28(6):528-535.

85. Hegg-Deloye S, Brassard P, Corbeil P, et al. Current state of knowledge of post-traumatic stress, sleeping problems, obesity and cardiovascular disease in paramedics. *Emerg Med J.* 2014;31(3):242-247.

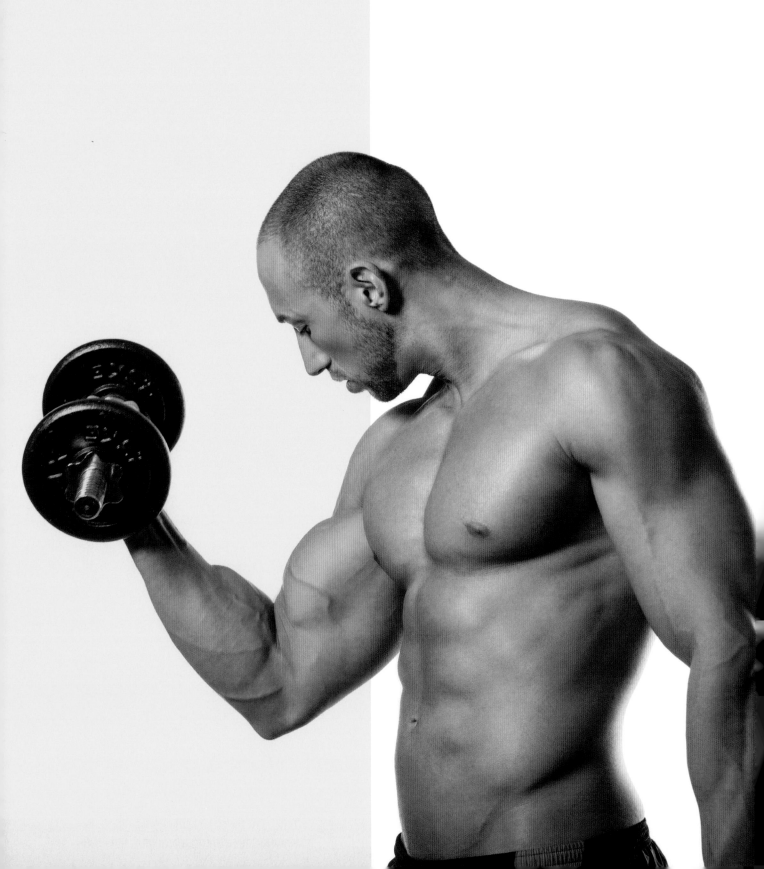

SECTION 5

AT A GLANCE

The preceding chapters help professionals understand the physiological and nutritional demands of related sports, but sports dietitians may find that they need a quick and easy reference for a specific sport. The At a Glance section features summaries for 18 sports. The summaries include brief descriptions of the sports and the URLs for websites where more information is available. General nutrition guidelines are included and can serve as a basis for an individualized plan. Common nutritional concerns are highlighted and briefly explained. These summaries may be helpful when preparing sports nutrition presentations for teams or as a topical guideline for an individual counseling session with an athlete.

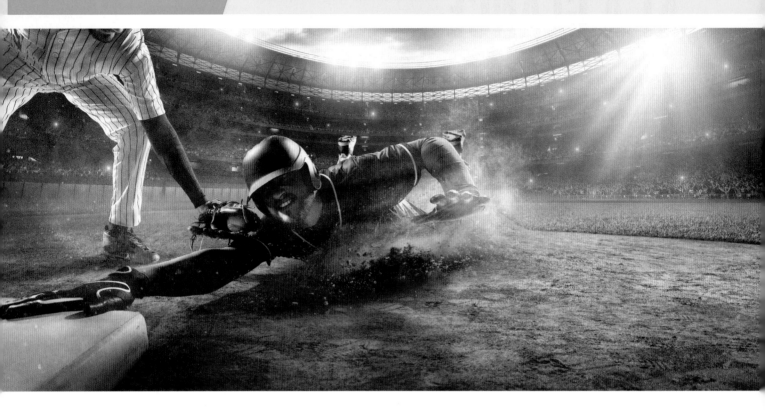

Baseball and Softball are skill sports requiring fine-motor control, superb coordination, and quick reaction time, as well as anaerobic power and general fitness conditioning. Baseball and Softball are not high energy–demand sports because they do not involve continuous activity. Professional baseball players begin spring training in February and softball begins in May. The regular season of professional baseball is April through September, followed by postseason play in October.. The professional softball season runs from late May through late August. Collegiate and youth baseball/softball are spring sports in school, and some players continue throughout the summer in recreational leagues. Learn more about baseball at the Major League Baseball website (www.mlb.com) and softball at the National Pro Fastpitch website(www.profast pitch.com).

GENERAL NUTRITION GUIDELINES

Energy:	Baseball/Softball are relatively low-energy–expenditure sport.
Carbohydrate:	Recommended intake is between 3 and 5 g/kg/d.
Protein:	Recommended intake is between 1.2 and 1.7 g/kg/d.
Fat:	Recommended intake is approximately 1.0 g/kg/d.

COMMON NUTRITIONAL CONCERNS

Weight Gain

Professional players may skip meals and then overeat, consume excess alcohol, and eat high-calorie snacks such as sunflower seeds, during the game, all habits that can contribute to weight gain. Many overeat and reduce activity during the off-season.

Fluid Intake

Baseball and softball is often played in hot, humid conditions and is one of the only sports without a time limit. Dehydration is a daily concern.

Pregame Meal

Players often arrive for games without having eaten and must eat food that is accessible, which is often high in calories, fat, sugar, and salt. Minor league players have a limited budget and seek out inexpensive food, which is often low in nutritional quality.

Postgame Meal

Late-night eating, large postgame meals, and alcohol intake often result in weight gain. Minor league and collegiate players typically eat fast food to break up long bus rides.

Frequent Travel

Frequent travel makes it difficult to maintain a routine and increases exposure to high-calorie foods low in nutritional quality.

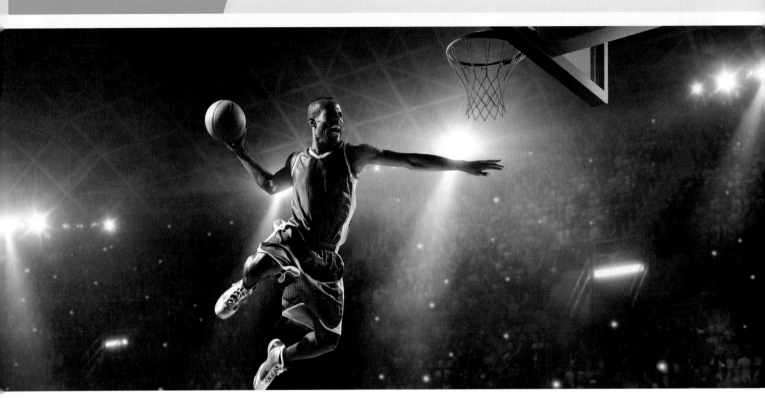

Basketball is an intermittent, high-intensity sport requiring strength, power, cardiovascular fitness, agility, and skill. It is usually played in four quarters with a break at halftime, although overtime periods are necessary if the game is tied. All of the body's energy systems are used to fuel the sport: adenosine triphosphate-creatine phosphate to jump and pass, the lactic acid system for multiple sprints, and the aerobic system to support several hours of play. The game may be played casually or with great intensity and duration and in a variety of venues, from the playground to the National Basketball Association (NBA) arena. Learn more about the sport at the NBA's website (www.nba.com).

GENERAL NUTRITION GUIDELINES

Energy:	Energy needs of basketball players differ, depending on body size, intensity of training, cross-training, and playing time, but in general basketball is a high energy–expenditure sport.
Carbohydrate:	Recommended intake is more than 5 g/kg/d. Recommendation increases to between 7 and 12 g/kg/d during heavy training or competition.
Protein:	Recommended intake is between 1.4 and 1.7 g/kg/d.
Fat:	The remainder of kcals should be consumed as fat with an emphasis on heart-healthy fats.

COMMON NUTRITIONAL CONCERNS

Energy Intake

NBA players may need 6,000 to 7,000 kcal/d whereas other players, such as high school or recreational players, need considerably less. Low energy and nutrient intakes over the long season may contribute to fatigue, especially during playoffs, and to weight loss.

Carbohydrate Intake

Basketball players need a large amount of carbohydrate daily to replenish glycogen used during demanding training sessions and games.

Fluid Intake

Training and games are often held in hot environments. Dehydration can lead to early fatigue and heat illness. Fluid intake should balance fluid losses.

Restoration of Glycogen, Fluids, and Electrolytes

Basketball seasons are long and intense. A good nutrition plan can prevent the staleness that many athletes report as the season wears on. Demanding practices, games, and training sessions deplete glycogen, fluids, and electrolytes. Glycogen stores and fluid and electrolyte losses must be replenished beginning immediately after competition or training. Some postexercise protein consumption is also encouraged. Appetite may be depressed, so liquid meal replacements may become an important option.

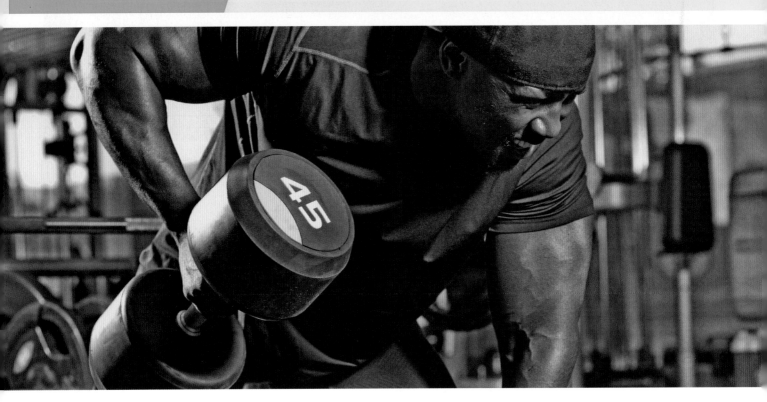

Bodybuilding is a subjectively judged sport based on muscular development and body presentation. Males and females participate in contests at the amateur and professional levels. Training and nutrition must be well-matched and will vary depending on the demands of the training period—maintaining muscle mass, building muscle mass, tapering (precontest dieting), or cutting weight immediately before competition. Learn more about the sport at the International Federation of Bodybuilding and Fitness website (www .ifbb.com).

GENERAL NUTRITION GUIDELINES

Bodybuilders are a variety of weights and sizes, and training and nutrient intakes change as they prepare for contests. Competitive bodybuilders spend about 1½ hours in the gym each day during the off-season and 2 to 3 hours per day during precompetition. Energy needs will vary with the phase and amount of training. The muscle-building phase begins after rest from the previous competitive season. The tapering phase is started approximately 12 weeks before competition with the goal of decreasing body fat and defining muscle mass, and the cutting phase is used if the tapering phase did not meet all of the goals for body composition. A maintenance phase should be used during the off-season. Sufficient carbohydrate is needed to meet the demands of training. Protein intakes generally increase during the muscle-building, tapering, and cutting periods. As energy and protein intakes change, the relative contribution of carbohydrates and fats change. These general guidelines must be highly individualized:

Energy: Energy intake and expenditure must be individually determined. Estimated energy needs are as low as 30 kcal/kg/d for females trying to lose fat weight and maintain muscle mass and as high as 60 kcal/kg/d for males trying to build muscle mass.

Carbohydrate: Recommended intake is between 5 and 7 g/kg/d.

Protein: Recommended intake is between 1.4 and 1.7 g/kg/d. (low energy intakes or individual preferences may result in higher intakes—2g/kg/d during lowest energy intake).

Fat: The remainder of kcals should be consumed as fat with an emphasis on heart-healthy fats.

COMMON NUTRITIONAL CONCERNS

Energy Intake

Baseline energy intake varies tremendously, and energy needs change as contests approach. Bodybuilders need personalized meal plans that reflect various energy (kcal) levels.

Other Macronutrients

Excessive intake of any one macronutrient may result in a low intake of another. The focus must be macronutrient balance (not just protein intake) with the understanding that the demands of training and competition change the relative balance. Emphasize the importance of carbohydrate and healthful fats for health and performance as well as an appropriate protein and energy intake.

Fluid Intake

Fluid loss must be balanced with fluid intake. Voluntary dehydration is one method that is used before competition and may be dangerous or life-threatening.

Lack of Variety

Diets tend to be repetitive and lack variety. Meal plans or suggestions for foods that contain similar energy and nutrient profiles are helpful.

Body Image and Disordered Eating

Due to the nature of the sport, there is a risk for distorted body image and disordered eating.

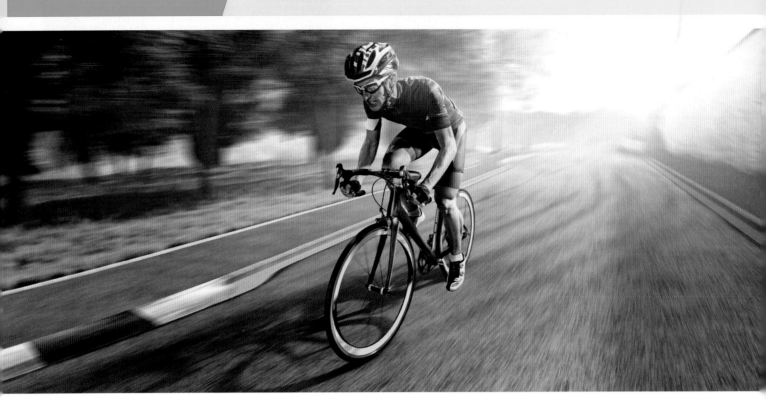

Cycling is a sport of various intensities and durations, from sprinters, whose races last only seconds, to endurance cyclists, such as Tour de France riders, who traverse more than 2,000 miles, much of it over mountainous terrain. Energy and nutrient needs vary according to the type of cycling (eg, track, road racing, mountain biking, and bicycle motocross [BMX]), the demands of training, and the intensity and duration of the race. Learn more about the sport at the USA Cycling website (www.usacycling.org).

GENERAL NUTRITION GUIDELINES

Endurance cycling guidelines can be found under Endurance and Ultraendurance Sports in this At a Glance section. Sprint cycling is a very high-intensity, short-duration sport, and the general guidelines include the following:

Energy: Individual needs should be calculated based on demands of training.

Carbohydrate: Recommended intake is between 7 and 12 g/kg/d.

Protein: Recommended intake is between 1.2 and 1.7 g/kg/d.

Fat: The remainder of kcals should be consumed as fat with an emphasis on heart-healthy fats.

Many cyclists are between the two extremes of sprinting and endurance, and energy and macronutrient requirements must be adjusted accordingly to reflect the demands of training and competition.

COMMON NUTRITIONAL CONCERNS

Energy and Carbohydrate Intake

Nutrient needs are often high, and a well-balanced diet is important. Distance cyclists need carbohydrate during the ride and must learn to consume food on the bike. Carbohydrate/electrolyte drinks, energy bars, gels, and bananas are some foods that work well, but individual preferences and tolerances must be determined by trial and error.

Fluid Intake

Meeting fluids needs is challenging—road cyclists can carry only two water bottles and can get additional fluids only at special feed zones along the course. In road cycling and mountain biking, taking one hand off the bike to drink can lead to crashes.

Dehydration is a daily concern. Sweat rates should be calculated and an individualized hydration plan should be developed. Take precautions to prevent hyponatremia, especially in hot, humid environments.

Restoration of Glycogen, Fluids, and Electrolytes

Glycogen stores and fluid and electrolyte losses must be replenished beginning immediately after competition or training. Some postexercise protein consumption is also encouraged. Appetite may be depressed, so liquid meal replacements may become an important option.

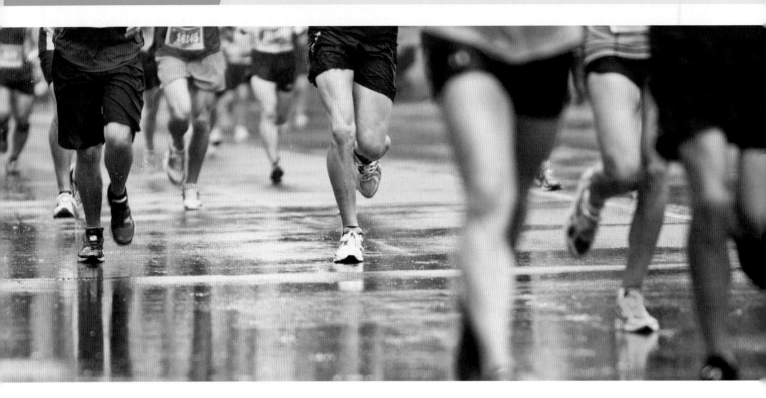

Endurance and ultraendurance sports include marathons, triathlons, and distance cycling and swimming events. All require year-round training and nutrition support. Training and nutrition must be well-matched and will vary depending on the training period—preparation, prerace, race, or active recovery. Reducing body fat or weight should be attempted during active recovery or early in the preparation period so that high-volume training or competition is not compromised. Learn more about these sports at the following websites:

- USA Track & Field (www.usatf.org/groups/roadrunning),

- USA Triathlon (www.usatriathlon.org),

- US Masters Swimming: Long-Distance Swimming (www.usms.org/longdist),

- and UltraMarathon Cycling Association (www.ultracycling.com).

GENERAL NUTRITION GUIDELINES

Energy:	This category of sports are associated with high energy-expenditure.
Carbohydrate:	Recommended intake is between 5 and 7 g/kg/d when training is reduced and as high as 10 to 12 g/kg/d during heavy training and racing season. Carbohydrate-loading (glycogen supercompensation) for competition is common.
Protein:	Recommended intake is between 1.2 and 1.7 g/kg/d, with higher levels consumed during prerace and racing seasons.
Fat:	Recommended intake is between 0.8 and 2.0 g/kg/d to match energy expenditure, with emphasis on heart-healthy fats.

COMMON NUTRITIONAL CONCERNS

Energy and Macronutrient Intake

Energy and macronutrient needs are high, and proper food intake must be an integral part of training. A structured eating plan must be developed to support training throughout the year.

Weight Gain

After the racing season is over, energy intake must be adjusted to reflect the decreased volume and intensity of training to prevent unwanted weight gain.

Body Composition

Leanness and low body weight is advantageous in sports in which the body must be moved. Excess body fat can be detrimental because, unlike muscle, it is non-force-producing mass. Rapid weight or fat loss can be detrimental to training and performance, so changes to body composition must be slow. Small reductions in daily energy intake and some increase in activities of daily living will promote slow weight loss. Weight loss is best attempted during the recovery period or early in the preparation period.

Fluid and Sodium Intake

Fluids to an endurance athlete are like water to a car's radiator—without it, both will overheat and stall. Fluid intake must be balanced to avoid dehydration and prevent hyponatremia. Sodium needs must be individually established. The inclusion of sodium in products taken during training and racing is recommended.

Lack of Variety

Variety and balance can be difficult day after day. Athletes must avoid getting in a rut. Focus on whole foods, especially on off days.

Food Intolerances

Some foods are not tolerated well during competition. Practice using various race foods and beverages during training to prevent problems during competition.

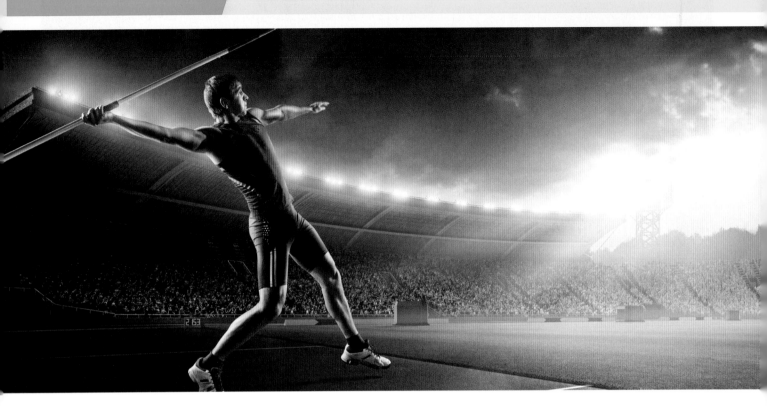

Indoor field events include high jump, pole vault, long jump, triple jump, and shot put. Outdoor field events also include discus, hammer, and javelin throws. Both males and females compete in these events. The necessary athletic skills and body composition differ between jumpers and throwers. Jumpers tend to be leaner because they must move their body through space, whereas throwers depend on their strength and body mass to propel an object through space. Jumpers consume less energy than throwers. Learn more about the sports at the USA Track & Field website (www.usatf.org).

GENERAL NUTRITION GUIDELINES

Energy:	Recommended intake varies depending on the individual and the event.
Carbohydrate:	Recommended intake is between 5 and 7 g/kg/d.
Protein:	Recommended intake is between 1.2 and 1.7 g/kg/d.
Fat:	The remainder of kcals should be consumed as fat with an emphasis on heart-healthy fats.

COMMON NUTRITIONAL CONCERNS

Body Composition and Weight Loss

Jumpers are encouraged to have a low percentage of body fat. There is a performance disadvantage to having excess body fat because fat represents non–force-producing mass. A weight-loss plan must allow for sufficient carbohydrate and protein to support training as well as weight (fat) loss.

High-Fat Diets

Throwers have a tendency to have high-fat diets. Such diets may also be high in saturated fat. All athletes should be aware of the advantages of consuming heart-healthy fats and should be encouraged to substitute such fats for saturated fats. If weight loss is desired, reducing dietary fat would be appropriate.

Fluid Intake

Several factors unique to track and field contribute to dehydration, including unsupervised workouts (which places the responsibility for hydration on the athletes), limited availability of fluids at the training facility, frequent travel from cool environments to hot climates with little time to acclimate to the change in temperature, increased fluid loss during air travel due to the low humidity in an airplane cabin, and the competitive nature of the sport, which might push an athlete to exercise even when dehydrated. Fluid loss must be balanced with fluid intake.

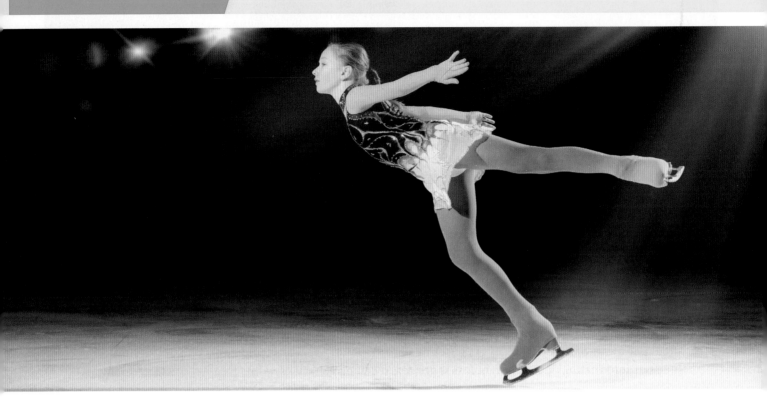

Figure skating requires strength, power, and endurance. Individual competitions are held for men and women. Couples compete in pairs and ice dancing, and there are team skating competitions. Training starts very early, sometimes at age 3 years, and many world champions are in their teens. Technique and speed are important, and the degree of skating difficulty increases as skaters reach the elite level. An elite figure skater's training includes learning new skills, like jumping and spinning, and repeated practice of those skills. High-intensity work coupled with lower-intensity skating and training 6 days a week in two sessions per day is a usual routine. Artistry plays a critical role, and there are many subjective elements considered in scoring. Competitions at the elite level include a short program that is 2 minutes and 40 seconds and a long program that is 4 minutes (females) or 4.5 minutes (males and pairs). Learn more about the sport at the US Figure Skating website (www.usfsa.org).

GENERAL NUTRITION GUIDELINES

Energy: Recommended intake should be individualized based on body composition goals.

Carbohydrate: Recommended intake is between 3 and 7 g/kg/d.

Protein: Recommended intake is between 1.2 and 1.7 g/kg/d.

Fat: The remainder of kcals should be consumed as fat with an emphasis on heart-healthy fats.

COMMON NUTRITIONAL CONCERNS

Energy Restriction

Despite the high energy demands of training, many female figure skaters limit energy intake in an effort to attain or maintain a low percentage of body fat. Weight loss must be slow, with small restrictions of energy so that muscle mass can be protected and training will not be negatively impacted.

Body Composition

A low percentage of body fat, particularly for females, is considered necessary for success because of the physical demands of the sport and appearance, which is part of the subjective scoring system. The potential for disordered eating or eating disorders is great, and early intervention is imperative.

Nutrient Intake

The consumption of nutrient-dense foods is important, especially if energy intake is restricted. Many figure skaters are children and adolescents and need adequate nutrition to support growth and development.

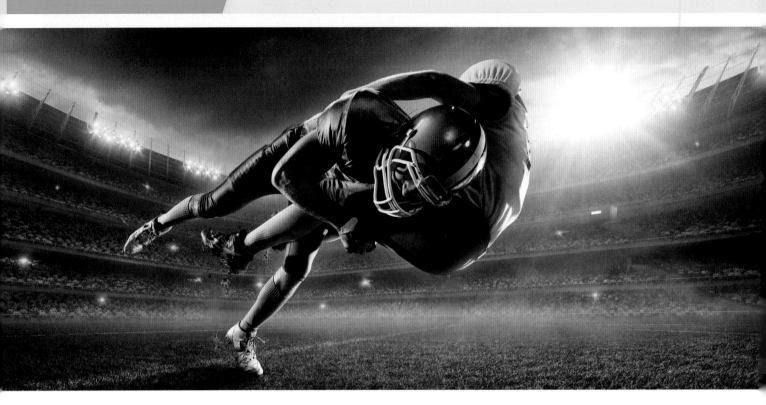

American football is played by two teams of 11 players each. Each play involves some high-intensity, short-duration activity, and there is a short rest between plays. Professional football games have four 15-minute quarters with a halftime break, but the clock is frequently stopped so the game takes about 4 hours to complete. Body composition varies by position, with receivers being lean and fast, whereas linemen depend on their strength and body mass to block. College football players usually have a smaller body mass than professional players and must increase size if they move into the professional ranks. Learn more about the sport at the National Football League website (www.nfl.com).

GENERAL NUTRITION GUIDELINES

Energy:	Energy expenditure varies depending on the level of the sport (professional, college, high school, or youth), level of training, amount of muscle mass, growth, and other factors, and must be individually determined.
Carbohydrate:	Recommended intake is more than 5 g/kg/d and 7 to 12 g/kg/d may be needed during rigorous training.
Protein:	Recommended intake is between 1.4 and 1.7 g/kg/d.
Fat:	The remainder of kcals should be consumed as fat with an emphasis on heart-healthy fats.

COMMON NUTRITIONAL CONCERNS

Energy Intake

Energy intake goals vary among athletes but can be more than 5,000 kcal/d. Many wish to change body composition by increasing muscle mass (which may require a higher energy intake) or decreasing body fat.

Off-Season Weight Gain

Players need to match their off-season energy intake with energy expenditure. Some football players arrive at training camp or spring football practice overweight and out of shape. When this is the case, they often look for quick weight-loss methods. Some of these methods may be dangerous, such as voluntary dehydration, use of drugs thought to reduce body fat, and severe restriction of food intake. A nutrition and training plan during the off-season can help athletes prevent unwanted off-season weight gain.

High Fat Intake

Some football players eat out frequently and consume a high-fat, high–saturated fat diet.

Fluid and Electrolyte Intake

Football players may play in hot, humid conditions, often early in the season before they are acclimated to the heat. Dehydration is a serious and potentially life-threatening problem. Sweating rates can be as high as 10 L/d, and a football player can lose 12 pounds in practice. Hydration can be challenging because the weight of the uniform and pads are an additional burden when exercising in the heat. If heat illness occurs, it is most likely to happen on the first day or two of preseason practice when players are not used to the heat. Fluid and electrolyte intakes must be balanced with losses. Approximately 10% of players may be cramp prone due to large losses of sodium in sweat. They may need additional sodium in addition to fluids to prevent heat cramps.

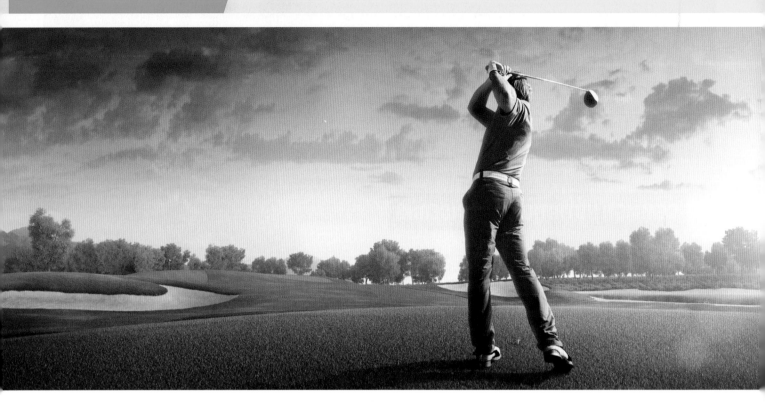

Golf is a low-endurance, precision-skill sport. It requires fine-motor control and coordination. Swinging a club requires power, and walking the course requires general fitness, especially if the golfer is carrying clubs. Golf courses vary in length, but championship courses are approximately 6,000 to 7,000 yards, and an 18-hole course takes several hours to play. Women play shorter distances because of the location of the tees. Professional tournaments include four rounds (72 holes over 4 days) with additional holes played on the last day in case of ties. Learn more about the sport at the websites for the PGA of America (www.pga .com) or the Ladies Professional Golf Association (www.lpga.com).

GENERAL NUTRITION GUIDELINES

Golfers do not have significantly increased demands for energy or nutrients; thus, general nutrient guidelines are used and adjusted on an individual basis.

Energy: Golf is considered a relatively low–energy-expenditure sport.

Carbohydrate: Recommended intake is between 3 and 5 g/kg/d.

Protein: Recommended intake is between 1.2 and 1.7 g/kg/d (often nearer the lower end of the range).

Fat: Recommended intake is approximately 1.0 g/kg/d or the remainder of kcals should be consumed as fat with an emphasis on heart-healthy fats.

COMMON NUTRITIONAL CONCERNS

Energy Intake

The focus is typically on energy balance, although some players may wish to reduce energy intake to lose body fat. Slow weight loss should not affect performance, but severe restriction could lead to inadequate total energy intake and/or low blood glucose, which could negatively affect performance.

Fluid Intake

Golf often takes place in hot, humid conditions. Dehydration is a daily concern, and golfers are encouraged to consume fluids between holes.

Precompetition Meal

Players need to eat a meal prior to play because they will be on the course for many hours. Start times vary and may be changed due to weather delays. Breakfast is vital because golfers often start early in the morning. Golfers should have a plan for a pregame meal that considers volume, macronutrient composition, and timing of intake that can be adjusted if the start time changes. Avoid the high-fat and high-sugar foods at the halfway house or in the clubhouse. Golfers usually carry snacks, such as energy bars or sports drinks, to prevent hunger while playing.

Frequent Travel

Frequent travel makes it difficult to maintain a routine and increases exposure to high-calorie, low–nutrient-dense foods.

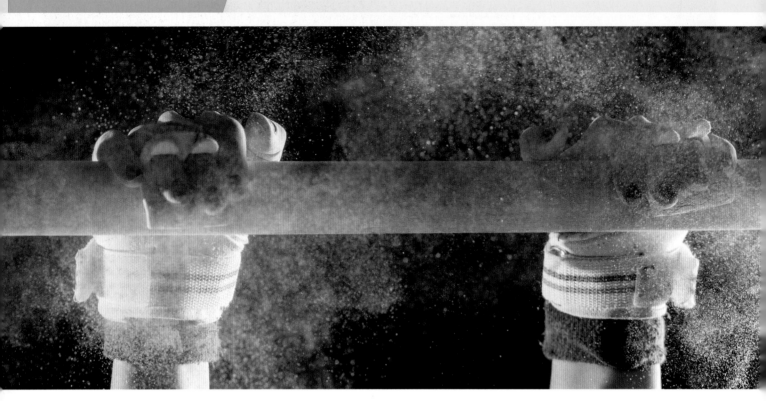

Gymnastics involves activities that are typically characterized as high-intensity to very high-intensity and short duration. In competition, athletes perform and then rest before beginning a new event. Gymnastics requires strength, power, and flexibility. Training is demanding, often involving many repetitions of individual skills or routines, but athletes can rest when it is not their turn to perform. Female gymnasts tend to be shorter and lighter than most other athletes and other females their age. A high percentage of lean body mass and a low percentage of body fat are desirable, not only to perform the skills but also because such bodies are aesthetically appealing. It is biologically easier for males to attain the currently held "ideal" body type than for females. Learn more about the sport at the USA Gymnastics website (www.usa-gym nastics.org).

GENERAL NUTRITION GUIDELINES

Energy:	Intake should be individualized based on body composition goals.
Carbohydrate:	Recommended intake is between 3 and 7 g/kg/d.
Protein:	Recommended intake is between 1.2 and 1.7 g/kg/d.
Fat:	The remainder of kcals should be consumed as fat with an emphasis on heart-healthy fats.

COMMON NUTRITIONAL CONCERNS

Energy Restriction

Despite the high energy demands of training, surveys suggest that many female gymnasts limit energy intake. If body fat loss is an appropriate goal, it must be slow, with small restrictions of energy so that muscle mass can be protected and training will not be negatively affected.

Body Composition

A low percentage of body fat, which may be difficult for females to attain or maintain, is considered necessary for success because of appearance and the physical demands of the sport. Amenorrhea may be present and is a warning sign associated with excessive energy restriction or anorexia. The potential for disordered eating and eating disorders is great, and early intervention is imperative.

Nutrient Intake

The consumption of nutrient-dense foods is important, especially if energy intake is restricted. Many gymnasts are children and adolescents and need adequate nutrition to support growth and development.

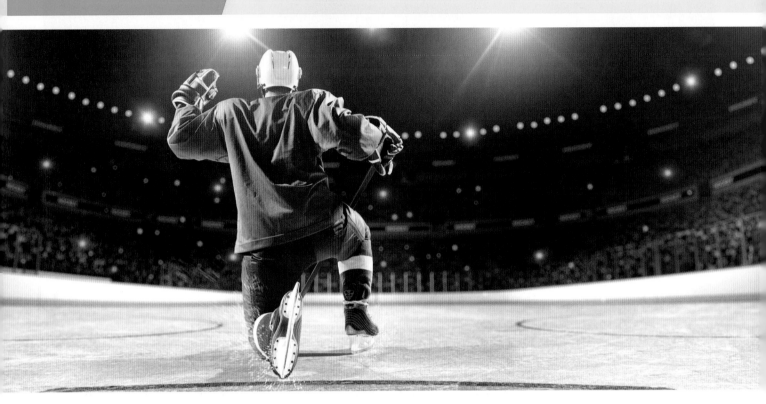

Ice hockey requires anaerobic power, aerobic conditioning, strength, agility, and speed. Similar to other intermittent, high-intensity sports, there are constant changes in speed and direction, but ice hockey differs from soccer or basketball in that there is full body contact. A game consists of three 16-minute periods, but frequent player substitutions reduce playing time to at least half of the game time. Learn more about the sport at the websites for the National Hockey League (www.nhl.com) and USA Hockey (www.usahockey .com).

GENERAL NUTRITION GUIDELINES

Energy:	Intake recommendation varies based on level of training, but ice hockey is generally considered a high–energy-expenditure sport.
Carbohydrate:	Recommended intake is more than 5 g/kg/d and 8 to 10 g/kg/d during training and competition to ensure adequate glycogen in quadriceps.
Protein:	Recommended intake is between 1.4 and 1.7 g/kg/d.
Fat:	The remainder of kcals should be consumed as fat with an emphasis on heart-healthy fats.

COMMON NUTRITIONAL CONCERNS

Carbohydrate and Protein Intake

Hockey players need a large amount of carbohydrate daily to replenish glycogen used during demanding training sessions and games. Protein is important to repair the wear and tear on muscles that occurs in hockey. Constant body-checking can take its toll on muscles, bones, tendons, and teeth.

Hydration During Exercise

Hydration during training and competition is important because players can sweat profusely under all of their gear even though they are on ice. Many hockey players spit out fluids instead of swallowing them. Sipping on fluids between shifts can help prevent dehydration and improve performance.

Restoration of Glycogen, Fluids, and Electrolytes

Demanding practices, games, and training sessions deplete glycogen, fluids, and electrolytes. Glycogen stores and fluid and electrolyte losses must be replenished beginning immediately after competition or training. Some postexercise protein consumption is also encouraged. Appetite may be depressed. Liquid meal replacements may be beneficial.

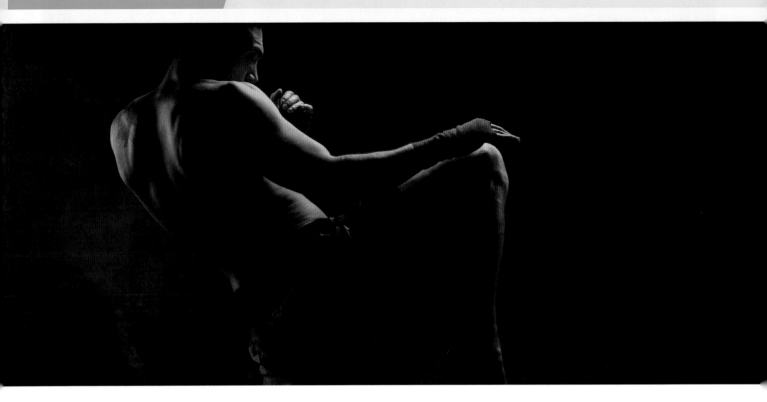

Martial arts is a broad term that describes several combat sports; boxing, fencing, judo, and tae kwon do may be the best known because they are Olympic sports, but there are hundreds of types of martial arts. Each art is different, but most involve strength, flexibility, and agility, and some also include explosive movements. Each art requires a strong level of mental and physical fitness. Many have weight classes, and some martial artists use a variety of methods to make weight. Participants in some competitions, such as judo or tae kwon do, compete several times over the course of a day. Learn more about the sports at the USA Dojo website (www.usadojo.com).

GENERAL NUTRITION GUIDELINES

Energy:	Intake should be individualized based on body composition and weight goals.
Carbohydrate:	Recommended intake is between 5 and 7 g/kg/d.
Protein:	Recommended intake is between 1.2 and 1.7 g/kg/d.
Fat:	The remainder of kcals should be consumed as fat with an emphasis on heart-healthy fats.

COMMON NUTRITIONAL CONCERNS

Making Weight

As with any sport that has weight categories, rapid reduction of body weight, including extreme methods such as fasting, fluid restriction, or semi-starvation, may be an issue. Rapid weight loss is more likely to be detrimental to performance than gradual weight loss. A weight-loss plan must allow for sufficient carbohydrate and protein to support training.

Nutrient Intake

The consumption of nutrient-dense foods is important, especially if energy intake is restricted. Meal timing and adequacy of intake during meets (multiple bouts during one day) should be addressed.

Fluid Intake

Dehydration is a daily concern. Fluid loss should be balanced with fluid intake. If an athlete uses dehydration to lose weight, restoration of fluid and electrolyte balance is critical.

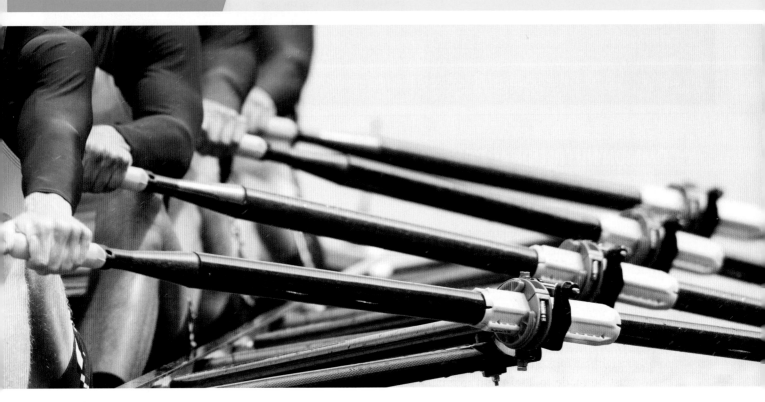

A typical crew race is 2,000 meters lasting 5½ to 8 minutes and requiring strength, power, and endurance. The crew season begins in the fall with preseason training. Winter is a time of intense training and muscle building, whereas the spring racing season is known for its long daily practices leading up to a rest day and weekend competition. Summer is the off-season. There are lightweight and open (heavy) weight categories. Learn more about the sport at the US Rowing website (www.usrowing.org).

GENERAL NUTRITION GUIDELINES

Energy:	Rowing is considered a relatively high–energy-expenditure sport.
Carbohydrate:	Recommended intake is between 5 and 7 g/kg/d.
Protein:	Recommended intake is between 1.2 and 1.7 g/kg/d.
Fat:	Recommended intake is approximately 1.0 g/kg/d. Fat, in the form of heart-healthy fats, may be increased to meet high energy needs while training and decreased during the off-season.

COMMON NUTRITIONAL CONCERNS

Energy Intake

Fatigue and lack of appetite may result in involuntary underconsumption of energy. Lightweight rowers may voluntarily restrict energy to make weight.

Making Weight

Lightweight rowers who are genetically lean and biologically small can comfortably meet the requirements for lightweight rowing. Problems with disordered eating and eating disorders occur when extraordinary efforts must be made to attain and maintain a low body weight. Voluntary dehydration may also be an issue. Learning to manage weight in the off-season is preferred to cutting weight in season. Dangerous weight-cutting practices and disordered eating are found in both male and female rowers.

Consumption of Foods with Low Nutrient Density

Rowers have high energy needs, and both male and female heavyweight rowers quickly discover that they must eat a lot of food to maintain energy balance. High-fat, high-sugar snack foods and beverages can provide the energy needed but not the nutrients.

Balancing Fluid Intake with Fluid Losses

Dehydration is a daily concern. Rowers have water bottles in the boat during training, but they do not have access to them during long training pieces (approximately 30 to 45 minutes each). It is unlikely that rowers can maintain fluid balance during training. Therefore, they should pay special attention to drinking sufficiently before and after training.

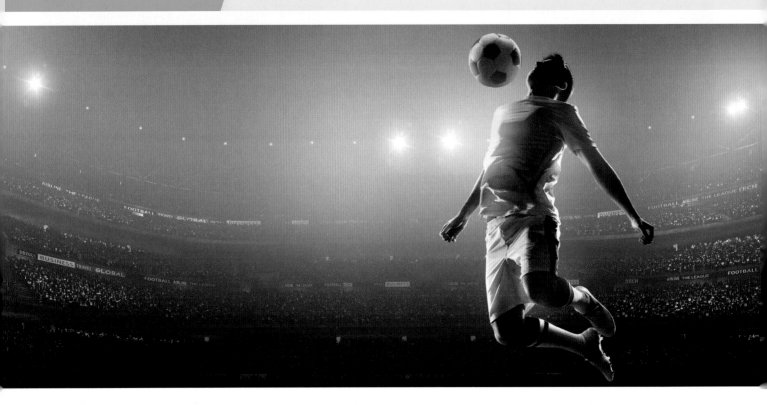

Soccer involves short, intense bursts of activity combined with moderately intense exercise and occasional rest periods. When played outdoors, the field is larger than a football field, and the average soccer player will cover between 8 and 12 km (5 to 7 miles). The game consists of two 45-minute halves with a 15-minute halftime and may go into overtime, although the game is shorter for younger players. Learn more about the sport at the websites for US Soccer (www.ussoccer.com) and international soccer (www.fifa.com).

GENERAL NUTRITION GUIDELINES

Energy:	Soccer is considered a relatively high–energy-expenditure sport.
Carbohydrate:	Recommended intake is approximately 5 g/kg/d and 7 to 12 g/kg/d during training and competition.
Protein:	Recommended intake is between 1.4 and 1.7 g/kg/d.
Fat:	The remainder of kcals should be consumed as fat with an emphasis on heart-healthy fats.

COMMON NUTRITIONAL CONCERNS

Energy Intake

Energy expenditure is high during training and games. A 75-kg male soccer player may expend more than 1,500 kcal in a game. Many players, both male and female, do not consume an adequate energy intake, which can lead to early onset of fatigue and poor nutrient intake.

Fluid Intake

Players should consume fluid early and at regular intervals during the game. Needs are especially high in hot, humid conditions. Carbohydrate/electrolyte solutions are beneficial during the game. Special attention should be paid to youth soccer players because they do not sweat as much as adults, and the risk for dehydration and heat illness is high. Youth players should consume fluid at least every 15 to 20 minutes during practice and frequently during games.

Restoration of Glycogen, Fluids, and Electrolytes

Glycogen stores and fluid and electrolyte losses must be replenished beginning immediately after competition or training. Soccer games are often scheduled close to each other with little time between games to replace muscle glycogen. Recovery nutrition helps soccer players make it through the season without fatigue. Some postexercise protein consumption is also encouraged. Appetite may be depressed, so liquid meal replacements may become an important option.

Frequent Travel

Frequent travel makes it difficult to maintain a routine and increases exposure to high-energy, low–nutrient-dense foods.

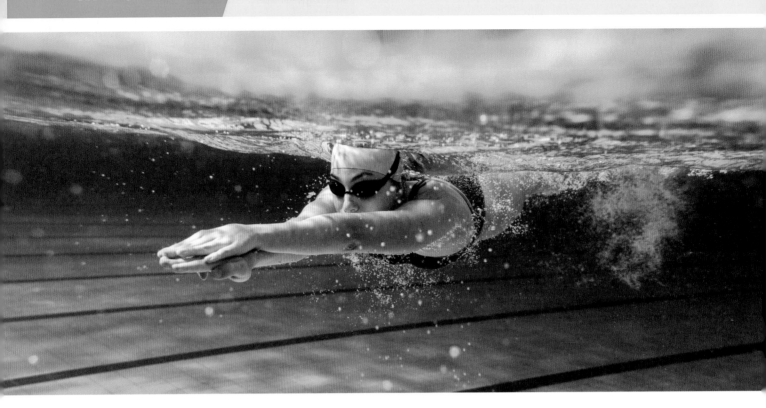

Swimming is a sport of various intensities and durations. Swimming events include 50 and 100 meters (sprints), 200 and 400 meters (middle distances), and 800 and 1,500 meters (distance). Long-distance swimming encompasses the swim portion of the full triathlon (2.4 miles) and ultraendurance events, such as swimming the English Channel (~24 miles). All swimmers have demanding training, so adequate daily energy and nutrient intake are important. Learn more about the sport at the USA Swimming website (www.usaswimming.org).

GENERAL NUTRITION GUIDELINES

Recommendations must be tailored to the individual based on the level of training and the distance. For swimming events ranging from 50 to 1,500 meters, the general guidelines include the following:

Energy: Intake should be individualized based on demands of training.

Carbohydrate: Recommended intake is between 7 and 12 g/kg/d.

Protein: Recommended intake is between 1.2 and 1.7 g/kg/d.

Fat: Recommended intake is approximately 1.0 g/kg/d or the remainder of kcals should be consumed as fat with an emphasis on heart-healthy fats.

Long-distance swimming guidelines can be found under Endurance and Ultraendurance Sports in this At a Glance section.

COMMON NUTRITIONAL CONCERNS

Energy and Carbohydrate Intake

Energy and nutrient needs are high, and a well-balanced diet is important. Chronic undereating can be a problem. Swimmers often complain of chronic fatigue; hard training coupled with poor nutrition leads to fatigue. Aim for a minimum of 500 g of carbohydrate each day during the competitive season. Frequent meals or snacks are important.

Fluid Intake

Dehydration is a daily concern and can occur within 30 minutes of swimming. Many swimmers ignore fluid intake because they are surrounded by water, but the environmental conditions of swimming (warm pool water, warm air temperatures, and high humidity) can lead to dehydration.

Restoration of Glycogen, Fluids, and Electrolytes

Glycogen stores and fluid and electrolyte losses must be replenished beginning immediately after competition or training. Some postexercise protein consumption is also encouraged. Two-a-day swim practices are often conducted, and rapid replenishment of glycogen and fluid balance is critical.

Body Composition

Appropriate percentage of body fat varies depending on the distance. Reducing body fat should be a slow process because too great a reduction in energy, carbohydrate, and protein intakes can negatively affect training and performance.

Risk for Disordered Eating and Eating Disorders

Swimmers are at risk for developing disordered eating and eating disorders. Refer to qualified health professionals when necessary.

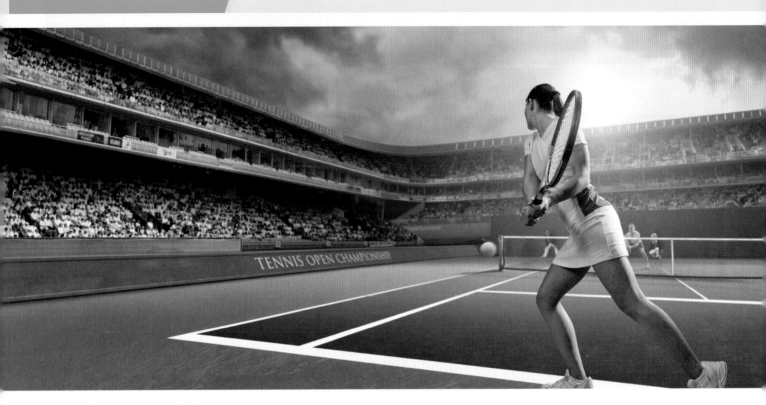

Tennis requires anaerobic power, aerobic conditioning, strength, and agility. The game may be played casually or with great intensity and duration; thus, training and nutrient requirements vary tremendously. One (singles) or two (doubles) players are on each side. Male professional singles players must win three of five sets and singles matches typically last 2 to 4 hours. Females play the best of three sets. Most singles players hit from the baseline, and long rallies require excellent fitness. Most tournaments span 1 week, but major tournaments last 2 weeks. Most points in tennis take less than 10 seconds, but there are only 25 seconds of rest between points and 90 seconds between games, so endurance is needed for long matches. Tennis requires about 300 to 500 bursts of energy over the course of a match, so maintaining energy levels and hydration are critical for success. Recreational players play at a variety of intensities, and some do not have significantly increased demands for energy or nutrients. Learn more about the sport at the US Tennis Association website (www.usta.com).

GENERAL NUTRITION GUIDELINES

Energy:	Recommendations vary depending on the level of training and the intensity and duration of play. Professional and collegiate players have high energy expenditures.
Carbohydrate:	Recommended intake is between 7 and 12 g/kg/d.
Protein:	Recommended intake is between 1.2 and 1.7 g/kg/d.
Fat:	Recommended intake is approximately 1.0 g/kg/d or the remainder of kcals should be consumed as fat with an emphasis on heart-healthy fats.

COMMON NUTRITIONAL CONCERNS

Fluid and Electrolyte Intake

Practice and play typically take place in hot and humid conditions. Dehydration is a daily concern. Some players may be cramp prone due to large losses of sodium in sweat. They may need additional sodium in addition to fluids to prevent heat cramps. Tennis players who are prone to cramps can try adding ½ teaspoon of table salt to 32 oz of sports drink or choose an endurance"formula sports drink that contains more sodium than regular sports drinks.

Restoration of Glycogen, Fluids, and Electrolytes

Demanding practices, training sessions, and match play deplete glycogen, fluids, and electrolytes. Glycogen stores and fluid and electrolyte losses must be replenished beginning immediately after competition or training. Some postexercise protein consumption is also encouraged. Near the end of the tournament, replenishment is especially important for peak performance.

Prematch Meal

Players, especially males, will be on the court for many hours, and they need to eat a meal before play. Start time may not be known (due to the length of other matches), and play may be stopped and restarted with short notice due to rain. Tennis players should have a plan for a prematch meal that considers volume, macronutrient composition, and timing of intake. The meal can be adjusted based on start time.

Multiple Matches in One Day

Tennis players may play more than one match in a day. This is especially true for younger athletes who compete in tournaments. Mini-meals or snacks may be needed because sports drinks alone may not be substantial enough.

Frequent Travel

Frequent travel makes it difficult to maintain a routine and increases exposure to high-calorie, low–nutrient-dense foods.

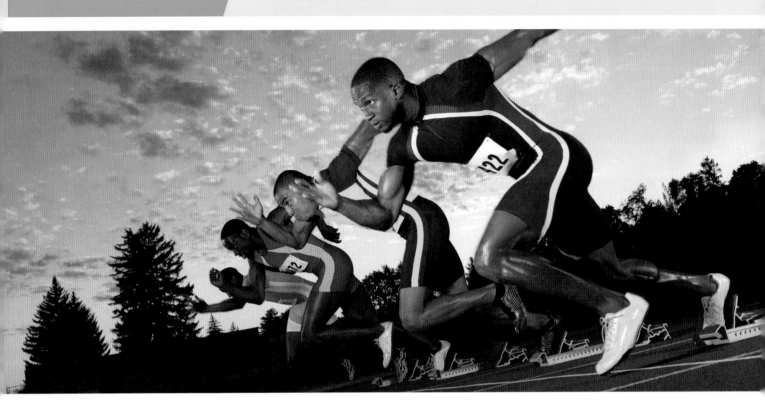

Track events range from the very fast 100-meter race to the much longer 10,000-meter run or 20,000-meter walking events. Nutrition recommendations must consider the distance involved. Daily workouts are intense. Athletes may compete several times a day. For most very high-intensity, brief events, diet has less impact than other factors such as genetics and training. Compared with distance runners, middle-distance runners have more moderate carbohydrate needs. Learn more about the various track events and the demands of training at the USA Track & Field website (www.usatf.org).

GENERAL NUTRITION GUIDELINES

Energy:	Recommendations should be individualized based on body composition goals.
Carbohydrate:	For very high-intensity, brief events (100 to 400 meters) recommended intake is between 5 and 7 g/kg/d. For high-intensity, short-duration events (800 to 10,000 meters) recommended intake is between 5 and 7 g/kg/d.
Protein:	Recommended intake is between 1.2 and 1.7 g/kg/d.
Fat:	Recommended intake is approximately 1.0 g/kg/d or the remainder of kcals should be consumed as fat with an emphasis on heart-healthy fats.

COMMON NUTRITIONAL CONCERNS

Energy Intake

In general, daily energy expenditure is high due to demanding training. Reported daily intakes are often less than estimated needs.

Weight Loss

High muscularity is valued, so many track athletes are attempting to lose body fat. Rapid weight loss is more likely to be detrimental to performance than gradual weight loss. A weight-loss plan must allow for sufficient carbohydrate and protein to support training.

Potential for Disordered Eating or Eating Disorders

Pressure to attain or maintain a low percentage of body fat or an undue focus on body appearance increases the risk for athletes, particularly female middle-distance runners, to develop disordered eating or eating disorders.

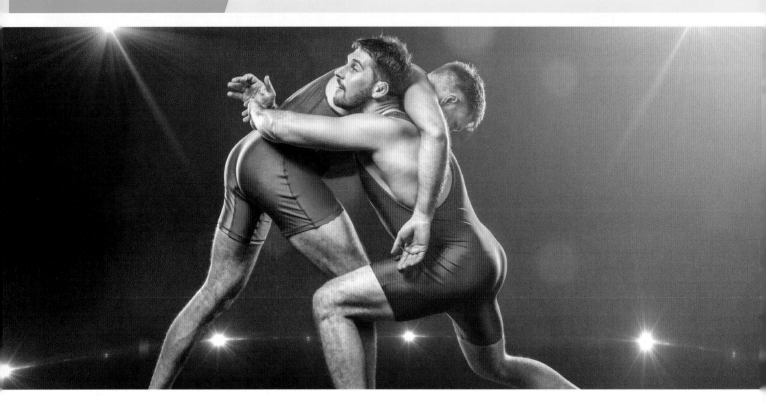

Wrestling involves hand-to-hand combat and requires strength and stamina. A high power-to-weight ratio is desirable. The sport features weight divisions, and some wrestlers "make weight" using drastic measures. Deaths have resulted through the combined use of a variety of techniques, including voluntary dehydration and starvation. Rule changes have been instituted to reduce excessive weight loss, including assessing body fat at the beginning of the season, determining a minimum competitive weight, and holding weigh-ins close to the start of competition. No longer just a men's sport, women's wrestling became an Olympic sport in 2004, and the number of high school and collegiate female wrestlers is expected to grow. Learn more about the sport at the websites for USA Wrestling (http://themat.com), National Collegiate Athletic Association (www.ncaa.com/sports/wrestling), and the National Federation of State High School Associations (www.nfhs.org).

GENERAL NUTRITION GUIDELINES

Energy:	Recommendations should be individualized based on body composition and weight goals.
Carbohydrate:	Recommended intake is between 5 and 7 g/kg/d.
Protein:	Recommended intake is between 1.2 and 1.7 g/kg/d. Protein requirements may increase to 2g/kg/d during periods of lowest energy intake to achieve weight loss.
Fat:	The remainder of kcals should be consumed as fat with an emphasis on heart-healthy fats.

COMMON NUTRITIONAL CONCERNS

Energy Intake

Appropriate energy intake must be individually determined. A focus on performance and health, not just weight, can help wrestlers view energy intake from a positive perspective.

Cutting Weight or Making Weight

Weight-cutting practices can be severe and life-threatening, although new rules have resulted in less extreme weight-cutting behaviors than in the past. Collegiate wrestlers use more extreme methods than high school wrestlers. Wrestlers in lower weight classes have relatively larger weight changes than those in heavier weight classes. Fasting, fluid restriction, and semistarvation are popular methods to make weight at all levels. Saunas, sweat suits (although banned), and diuretics may also be used. Nutrition counseling across the season is important to develop individualized plans, discuss weight loss methods, and monitor weight changes.

Nutrient Intake

The consumption of nutrient-dense foods is important, especially if energy intake is restricted. Wrestlers have demanding training programs, and sufficient macronutrient and micronutrient intakes are important to support training, performance, and health. Many wrestlers are adolescents and need adequate nutrition to support growth and development.

Fluid Intake

Dehydration is a daily concern. Fluid loss should be balanced with fluid intake. If dehydration is used as a weight-loss method, restoration of fluid and electrolyte balance is critical. Some wrestlers believe they can lose weight for the weigh-in and then rehydrate before a match. That is a false belief because it takes up to 6 hours to reach normal hydration.

Acknowledgment:
Thank you to Jen Vattimo, RD, for reviewing this section, cross-checking it with current recommendations, and assuring that the organizational information is current.

Selected Sports Nutrition–Related Position Papers, Practice Papers, and Consensus Statements

Academy of Nutrition and Dietetics Positions

The following are available at www.eatright.org/positions:

- Nutrition and Athletic Performance (joint position statement of the Academy of Nutrition and Dietetics, Dietitians of Canada, and the American College of Sports Medicine.)
- Functional Foods
- Nutrient Supplementation
- Nutrition Intervention in the Treatment of Eating Disorders
- Total Diet Approach to Healthy Eating
- Vegetarian Diets
- Interventions for the Treatment of Overweight and Obesity in Adults

American College of Sports Medicine Positions

The following are available at http://journals.lww.com/acsm-msse/pages/collectiondetails.aspx?TopicalCollectionId=1:

- Exercise and Type 2 Diabetes
- Exercise and Physical Activity for Older Adults
- The Female Athlete Triad
- Appropriate Physical Activity Intervention Strategies for Weight Loss and Prevention of Weight Regain for Adults
- Exertional Heat Illness during Training and Competition
- Exercise and Fluid Replacement
- Physical Activity and Bone Health
- Exercise and Hypertension

National Athletic Trainers' Association Positions

The following are available at www.nata.org/position-statements:

- Preventing, Detecting, and Managing Disordered Eating in Athletes
- Management of the Athlete with Type 1 Diabetes Mellitus
- Safe Weight Loss and Maintenance Practices in Sport and Exercise

International Olympic Committee Consensus Statements

The following are available at www.olympic.org/medical-and-scientific-commission:

- The IOC Consensus Statement: Beyond the Female Athlete Triad—Relative Energy Deficiency in Sport (RED-S)
- IOC Consensus Statement on Sports Nutrition 2010
- Consensus Statement on Body Composition Health and Performance in Sport

Sports Nutrition–Related Websites

Academy of Nutrition and Dietetics: www.eatright.org

Athletics and Fitness Association of America: www.afaa.com

Amateur Athletic Union: www.aausports.org

SHAPE America Society of Health and Physical Education: www.shapeamerica.org

American College of Sports Medicine: www.acsm.org

American Council on Exercise: www.acefitness.org

American Diabetes Association: www.diabetes.org

American Medical Society for Sports Medicine: www.amssm.org

American Running Association: www.americanrunning.org

Australian Sports Commission's AIS: www.ausport.gov.au/ais

Body Positive: www.bodypositive.com

Endurance Nation: www.endurancenation.us

Dietitians of Canada: www.dietitians.ca

Gatorade Sports Science Institute: www.gssiweb.com

IDEA Health & Fitness Association: www.ideafit.com

Korey Stringer Institute at University of Connecticut: www.ksi.uconn.edu

MomsTeam.com: www.MomsTeam.com

National Athletic Trainers' Association: www.nata.org

National Eating Disorders Association: www.nationaleatingdisorders.org

National Recreation and Park Association: www.nrpa.org

Nicholas Institute of Sports Medicine and Athletic Trauma: www.nismat.org

Physical Activity Guidelines for Americans: www.health.gov/paguidelines

Runner's World: www.runnersworld.com

ShapeUpUS.org: www.shapeupus.org

Special Olympics: www.specialolympics.org

Sports, Cardiovascular, and Wellness Nutrition (dietetic practice group of the Academy of Nutrition and Dietetics): www.scandpg.org

Sports Dietitians Australia: www.sportsdietitians.com.au

SportsOracle: www.sportsoracle.com

SportScience: www.sportsci.org

Sports Science Insights: www.sportsscienceinsights.com

UltraMarathon Cycling Association: www.ultracycling.com

The Vegetarian Resource Group: www.vrg.org

Note: This list includes websites that may be valuable to sports dietitians and other health professionals. The inclusion of a website does not constitute an endorsement of that site.

At the time of publication, all URLs were correct.

CONTINUING PROFESSIONAL EDUCATION

This edition of *Sports Nutrition: A Handbook for Nutrition Professionals* offers readers 4 hours of Continuing Professional Education (CPE) credit. Readers may earn credit by completing the interactive online quiz at: https://publications.webauthor.com/sports_nutrition_sixthedition.

INDEX

6-carbon glucose molecule, 07

16-carbon fatty acid, 07

24-hour recall, 159, 162–163, 250

A

abdominal fat, 221, 224, 225, 238, 300

abdominal skinfold measurement, 181

Academy of Nutrition and Dietetics

    on dietary fat, 334

    fact sheets from, 271, 404

    on fluid/electrolyte replacement, 113

    position papers, 113, 170, 249, 375

    protein recommendations, 230

    Sports, Cardiovascular and Wellness Nutrition DPG, 271

    on vegetarian and vegan lifestyles, 99–100

    on weight management, 281

Acceptable Macronutrient Distribution Range (AMDR)

    for fat, 62–64, 65

Acetyl coenzyme A, 7, 8, 66, 81, 84

acidosis, from high-intensity events, 452

ACSM, *see American College of Sports Medicine*

ACSM's Guidelines for Exercise Testing and Prescription, 154, 179

actin, 03, 11

action stage, of change, 164

active insulin, 432, 433

actors, 531

acute response, to exercise, 02–05

acyl carrier protein, 84

adenosine diphosphate (ADP), 05, 60, 192, 193

adenosine monophosphate protein kinase, 41

adenosine triphosphate (ATP), 05, 06, 07, 08, 28, 29, 66, 192, 193, 194–196, 451–452, 467, 469

adenosine triphosphate-phosphocreatine system, 06

Adequate Intakes (AI), 80, 83, 90, 111, 112, 474

adjusting insulin, 428, 433, 437

adolescence, 239–241, 243, 244, 245, 246, 247, 249, 399, 401

aerobic energy

    and free-radical production, 84

    hallmark adaptations with, 44

    in high-intensity sports, 467–469, 470, 471, 474

    protein for, 41, 44, 50-51

    in ultraendurance sports, 491

aerobic metabolic pathways, 06

aerobic metabolism, 07

aerobic training, 44

aging, and exercise, 66, 297, 298–299, 302–303

air displacement plethysmography, 160–161, 179, 182–183

AIS, *see Australian Institute of Sport*

albuminuria, 441

alcohol use, 116–117, 191, 246, 250, 251, 275–279, 360, 371, 372, 481, 532, 543

α-linolenic acid, 61, 62, 74

altitude and ambient temperature, 441

AMDR, *see Acceptable Macronutrient Distribution Range*

amenorrhea, 343, 359, 525

American Academy of Pediatrics, 113, 170, 240, 248, 253, 257

American College Health Association, 276

American College of Obstetricians and Gynecologists, 360, 366, 373, 376

American College of Sports Medicine

    energy expenditure values, 201–202

    exercise certification, 13–14, 187

    on exercise for older adults, 298

    on exercise in pregnancy, 374

    fat recommendations, 334

    on fluid/electrolyte replacement, 112–113, 114, 248

    guidelines for nutriiton assessment, 154

    on overtraining, 11–12

    protein recommendations, 230

    on weight management, 281, 420

American Council on Exercise, 14–15

American Diabetes Association, 420

amino acids, 39,–40, 41, 43, 44, 45, 46, 47, 48, 49, 50, 51–52, 122, 134, 135, 193, 280, 290, 331, 334, 367, 424, 457, 477–478, 495

amphetamines, 277

anabolic steroids, 226, 277

anaerobic energy, 452, 467, 468, 471–472, 491

anaerobic glycolysis, 06–07, 452

anaerobic metabolic pathways, 06, 67, 451, 452, 468, 469

anaerobic sprints, 09

android obesity, 160

androstenedione, 141, 144

phylloquinone, 99

physical activity energy expenditure (PAEE), 192, 195, 199, 201, 202, 203, 207, 208

Physical Activity Guidelines for Americans, 12, 15, 16

physical activity levels (PALs), 192, 203, 205, 206, 230, 241, 330

physical examination, 154, 227, 243

phytochemicals, 84, 410

plasma malondialdehyde concentrations, 86

plasma osmolality, 109, 119, 122, 126, 307

polycystic ovary syndrome (PCOS), 225, 422–423

polysaccharide, 96

polyunsaturated fatty acids (PUFAs), 42, 61–62, 63, 65, 73, 252, 335, 367

postpartum recommendations, 375–376

potassium, 90, 111, 112, 117, 125, 251, 343

power-to-weight ratio, 160, 218, 219, 221–222, 228, 576

prealbumin, 167

preconception weight status, 357–359

prediction equations for RMR, 200

pregnancy

    contraindicated foods, 371–373

    exercise during, 374

    macronutrient requirements, 366–367

    micronutrient requirements, 368–370

    nutrition considerations during 364–366

    physiological changes during, 360–364

    weight gain during, 373–374

prepubertal stage, 242

progressive overload, 9

prohormones, 136, 141, 144, 145

protein

    for children/adolescents, 251

    in endurance exercise, 40–41, 44–45

    for endurance/ultra-endurance sports, 45

    during exercise, 41, 44–45

    for high-intensity exercise

    for masters athletes, 303–304

    pre-exercise intake, 41

    for the preganant athlete, 367

    postexercise, 42

    quantity of intake, 48–51

    in resistance exercise, 40, 41–44

    timing of intake, 41–45

    for vegetarian athletes, 331–334

protein supplements, 137, 257, 340

prothrombin, 99

protons, 192, 193, 194

psychological benefits of sports, 238–242

psychosocial stigma of obesity in children/adolescents, 242

pubertal development, 243–245

pulmonary ventilation, 04, 05, 10

purging, 164, 388–389, 392, 399, 401

pyridoxal, 82

pyridoxal 5'-phosphate, 82

pyridoxamine, 82

pyridoxamine 5'-phosphate, 82

pyridoxine, 82, 305

pyruvate, 06, 08, 71, 81, 84, 145

pyruvic acid, 06, 07

Q

quercetin, 144

quinoa, 48

R

Ramadan, 320

raw fish, 371

RDAs, *see Recommended Dietary Allowances*

RDNs, *see registered dietitians nutritionists*

Recommended Dietary Allowances (RDAs)

    definition, 80

    for fat-soluble vitamins, 87

    for minerals, 88, 90

    for protein in vegetarin athletes, 331–334, 338

    for water-soluble vitamins, 83

recovery

    in adenosine triphosphate-phosphocreatine system, 06, 471

    for athletes with diabetes, 425

    carbohydrate intake during, 29, 31–32

    for elite athletes, 314, 315

    glycemic effects, 25

    for high-intensity sports, 29, 456

    for high-intensity, intermittent sports, 467–468

    protein intake effects, 43, 44, 48, 49, 50

    principles of exercise training, 08–09

    for student athletes, 267, 268, 276, 279

    variation/periodization, 10

sweating, 80, 90, 108, 109, 111, 112–114, 115, 117, 119, 120, 121, 122, 123, 124, 125, 126, 127, 180, 243, 244, 247–248, 307, 480–482, 496, 503, 504

swimming, 221, 222, 224, 278, 301, 374, 393, 451, 454, 509, 550–551, 570–571

synephrine, 139–141

T

T1D, *see type 1 diabetes*

T2D, *see type 2 diabetes*

TAC, *see Total Antioxidant Capacity*

tachycardia, 04, 398

TDEE, *See Total Daily Energy Expenditure*

technology, in nutrition assessment, 163

tennis, 466, 471, 472, 475, 481, 572–573

testosterone, supplements to increase, 144, 280

thermic effect of food, 195, 201

thermoregulation, 04, 107, 112, 114, 123, 247–248, 480, 522–523

thiamin, 81–82, 83, 100, 362

thiamine diphosphate, 81

thiazide diuretics, 307

thigh skinfold measurement, 181

third trimester, energy requirement, 365

thirst, 109, 110, 112–114, 116, 118, 119–120, 121, 122, 123, 170, 307, 435

thyroid, 87, 88, 89, 195, 199, 370, 439–440

TIBC, *see Total Iron Binding Capacity*

tobacco, 277, 278, 279

tocopherols, 86, 87

tocotrienols, 86

Tolerable Upper Intake Levels (ULs), 80, 81, 84, 87, 88, 94, 97, 99

Torres, Dara, 308

total antioxidant capacity (TAC), 86–87

total cholesterol, 167, 283, 307

total daily energy expenditure (TDEE)

    changes in energy balance,208–210

    determination of, 202–204, 228

    in energy balance scale, 199–204

    in vegetarian athletes, 329–331

    and weight gain, 208

    and weight loss, 207–208

total iron binding capacity (TIBC), 169, 338

trace minerals, needs for athletes, 88

track and field, 278, 296, 450, 453, 459, 508, 548–549, 552–553, 574–575

training at altitude, 96, 98, 117, 118, 319, 337

training blocks, *see periodization*

training days *versus* competition days, nutritional needs, 165

training load, of elite athletes, 314–315

"training low" concept, 33–34, 70

training tables, 267, 268, 270, 272, 273, 286, 287–288

trans fatty acids, 62, 63, 64, 65, 66, 335, 359

Transtheoretical Model, 155, 164

travel, challenges of, 318, 319

tricarboxylic acid cycle (TCA cycle), *see Krebbs cycle*

triceps skinfold measurement, 161

triglycerides, 06, 60, 61, 62, 66, 67, 71, 72, 75, 167, 225, 334, 470

type 1 diabetes (T1D), 283, 420, 421, 422, 425, 428–429, 430, 433, 435, 436, 437, 438, 439, 440

type 2 diabetes (T2D), 178, 225, 239, 240, 420, 421–422, 425, 426, 428–429, 430, 435, 436

U

UL, *see Tolerable Upper Intake Level*

Ultraendurance sports

    carbohydrates for performance, 30, 31

    energy needs in, 492

    energy systems in, 491

    hydration needs, 121, 496

    nutrient needs in, 341, 483–485

    nutrition recommendations, training and race day, 498–502

    protein intake, 45

    vitamin meeds in, 97, 496–498

UltraMarathon Cycling Association, 550

undercooked meat and poultry, 371

underwater weighing (UWW), 161, 178, 179, 182, 183

underweight, 160, 177, 227, 358–359, 373

United States Olympic Committee (USOC), 169

United States Olympic Committee Protocol, 168, 169

United States Olympic Committee Sports Dietetics Assessment Form, 156–158

unpasteurized foods, 371, 372

unsaturated fatty acids, 61, 63, 304, 519

upper respiratory tract infections, 83, 85, 136

urine osmolality, 121, 168, 371

urine specific gravity (USG), 114, 125, 168, 407, 458, 496

US Anti-Doping Agency, 146, 280

US Department of Agriculture, 106, 166, 338